CLINICAL INTERPRETATION OF LABORATORY TESTS

CLINICAL INTERPRETATION OF LABORATORY TESTS

FRANCES K. WIDMANN, M.D.

ASSOCIATE PROFESSOR OF PATHOLOGY
DUKE UNIVERSITY SCHOOL OF MEDICINE
DURHAM, NORTH CAROLINA

ASSISTANT CHIEF, LABORATORY SERVICE
VETERANS ADMINISTRATION HOSPITAL
DURHAM, NORTH CAROLINA

EDITION 8

F.A. DAVIS COMPANY/PHILADELPHIA

Library of Congress Cataloging in Publication Data

Widmann, Frances K   1935–
  Clinical interpretation of laboratory tests.

  Edition 7, by R. H. Goodale, published under title:
Goodale's Clinical interpretation of laboratory tests.
  Includes bibliographical references and index.
  1. Diagnosis, Laboratory.   I. Goodale, Raymond
Hamilton, 1898–   Goodale's Clinical interpretation of
laboratory tests. II. Title. [DNLM: 1.   Diagnosis,
Laboratory.   QY4.3 W641c]
RB37.G64 1979   616.07'5   78-21975
ISBN 0-8036-9322-2

PREFACE

The range of laboratory tests continues to expand. More tests are done; more money is spent; more data are generated than ever before. How can the individual clinician, caring for individual patients, hope to make optimal use of the laboratory and assimilate the information thus generated? In an era of intense specialization and maxi-experts who limit themselves to mini-subjects, the patient is the ultimate generalist. His complaints and concerns cover all areas. The clinician caring for the patient must be conversant with the diagnostic procedures that he, or others, employs to illuminate these concerns.

This book comes from the pen of an individual, rather than the pens of a group, but draws upon the work of many persons in the field. My aim is to assist primary care providers to select laboratory procedures and evaluate results as they apply to the many possible problems that individual patients embody. The emphasis is on pathophysiology of disease states, not the technical details of laboratory procedures. In this way, I hope to provide both clinician and laboratory worker with a conceptual framework that puts disease and diagnosis into perspective. The laboratory worker and the clinician approach the patient from very different starting points, but both have the same goal in mind: optimal patient care.

This eighth edition of *Clinical Interpretation of Laboratory Tests* has a format different from that of its predecessors. Rather than divide the book into two divisions, Laboratory Principles and Clinical Findings, I have organized the chapters into the sectional categories that most laboratories employ: Hematology, Immunology, Chemistry, Microbiology, etc. All of the material on hematology, immunology, blood banking, and coagulation is new for this edition, as are the chapters on liver function tests and pregnancy. More than half of the previous edition has thus been completely replaced. In other chapters, new sections extensively replace or augment material from the seventh edition, especially in considering blood lipids, serum isoenzymes, anaerobic microbiology, mechanisms of antibiotic activity, and Legionnaires' disease.

As always, I owe much to colleagues and students, especially the students in Duke University's Medical Technology, Pathologist's Assistant, and Physician's Associate programs. Their lively interest and intellectual curiosity remind me continually that all our facts, theories, and answers are only the foundation for further questions. The drawings are from the very helpful and cooperative pen of Mr. Donald Powell. I am particularly indebted to Linda Brogan, who did most of the typing, along with Diane Evans and Marjorie Penny. Their cheerful assistance was invaluable.

A book like this is never finished. Even as it goes to press, there are exciting new items I would like to work in. Judith Kim and Nancy Schmidt of the F. A. Davis Company did everything possible to help me with this eighth edition, and I thank them for their efforts.

Frances K. Widmann, M.D.

CONTENTS

SECTION 1

HEMATOLOGY

CHAPTER 1

HEMATOLOGIC METHODS

Blood constitutes 6 to 7 percent of total body weight—nearer to 7 percent in men and 6 percent in women. Plasma, the fluid portion of blood, comprises 45 to 60 percent of this total, while red blood cells occupy most of the remaining volume. White blood cells and platelets, although functionally essential, occupy a relatively small proportion of total blood mass. Hematology traditionally limits itself to the cellular elements of blood and the physiologic derangements that affect their functions. Hematologists also study blood volume, the flow properties of blood, and the physical relationships between red cells and plasma. The innumerable substances dissolved or suspended in the plasma fall into other laboratory disciplines.

The principal function of circulating blood is transportation; temperature regulation and the regulation of fluid and acid-base equilibrium are functions somewhat distinct from the purely transportive role. Red blood cells remain within the blood throughout their normal lifetime; they effectively transport oxygen without leaving the cardiovascular tree. White cells, on the other hand, perform their physiologic roles within tissue; while in the blood, they are merely in transit. Platelets exert their effects at the wall of blood vessels; circulating platelets do not, as far as we know, perform any specific function in the blood stream itself.

HEMATOPOIESIS AND BONE MARROW EXAMINATION

Except for some lymphocytes, blood cells in normal adults are manufactured in the marrow of a relatively few bones, notably the sternum, ribs, vertebral bodies, pelvic bones, and the proximal portions of humerus and femur. In the fetus, mesodermal derivatives in other locations actively produce blood cells. The liver, the spleen, and the marrow cavities of nearly all bones are active hematopoietic sites in the newborn. Adult reticuloendothelial tissues retain the potential for hematopoiesis, although in a healthy state, reserve sites are not activated. Under conditions of hematopoietic stress in later life, liver, spleen, and an expanded bone marrow may resume producing blood cells.

Evaluating Hematopoiesis

Hematopoietic activity can be evaluated by examining bone marrow tissue, by measuring systemic uptake and incorporation of known precursor materials, and by using x-ray or radioisotope techniques to identify and characterize sites of hematopoietic activity. Microscopic examination of aspirated marrow is usually the first step, and the results determine whether other procedures are indicated. Obtaining bone marrow requires introducing a needle through the outer bony layers into the semisolid marrow and withdrawing a sample for examination.

ASPIRATION AND BIOPSY

In the adult, marrow is most accessible in the sternum and the anterior and posterior iliac crests. In very young children, the proximal portion of the tibia gives good results, while in older children, the vertebral bodies often are used. Hematopoietic bone marrow contains fat and other connective tissue as well as blood-forming cells. It is fluid enough to be aspirated through a needle, but only the first few drops should be used for examination because, in the later aliquots, fluid blood dilutes the marrow material. Tiny fragments of connective tissue as well as free-floating cells will be withdrawn. The morphology of these free cells provides much useful information but does not indicate the in situ relationship of hematopoietic cells to bone, fat, connective tissue, or other elements.

Sometimes marrow cellularity and tissue relationships can be estimated from paraffin sections of the clotted, aspirated material, but often a larger sample of intact tissue is needed. Specially designed biopsy needles make it possible to remove a cylinder of intact marrow tissue and overlying bone. This usually is done from the iliac crests, but if some other site is known or suspected to be abnormal, that site can be sampled. Occasionally, open surgical biopsy is necessary.

Meticulous aseptic technique is necessary, since infectious material introduced into bone marrow rapidly reaches the entire circulation. Skin and subcutaneous tissues usually are anaesthetized by local injection, but the patient often experiences some discomfort when the needle penetrates the periosteum; many patients perceive a "pulling" sensation at the moment of aspiration. Once the needle is withdrawn, firm pressure is needed to prevent hemorrhagic complications. Applying pressure is easiest over the sternum and most difficult over the iliac crests, especially in an obese individual.

M:E RATIO

Cells normally present in hematopoietic marrow include granulocytes and erythrocytes in all stages of maturation; megakaryocytes, the large, multinucleated cells from whose cytoplasm platelets develop; moderate numbers of lymphocytes; and occasional plasma cells. Although circulating blood contains 1000 times as many red cells as white cells (5 million red cells/mm.^{3}, as compared with 5,000 to 10,000 white cells/mm.^{3}), nucleated white cells in the bone marrow outnumber nucleated erythrocytic cells by about 3 to 1. This is called the M:E (myeloid to erythroid) ratio. Many factors contribute to this disproportion.

Red cells require 5 to 6 days for bone marrow development, but the nucleus disappears after 2 to 3 days.[5] Maturing red cells enter the circulating blood very promptly, even before the last maturational events have occurred. Red cells remain in the circulation for about 120 days before senescence and destruction. Nucleated granulocytic cells are numerous in the marrow because granulocytes have conspicuous nuclei throughout the 5 to 7 days of marrow development and large numbers of mature cells remain within the marrow as a "storage pool." On an average, granulocytes spend only 1 day in the circulating blood and have a total life span of only 9 to 15 days. The combination of massive granulocyte turnover, persistence of the nucleus, and marrow retention of mature cells makes the myeloid series the predominant nucleated form when marrow is examined. The normal M:E ratio is between 2:1 and 4:1.[40,50]

MARROW DIFFERENTIAL

Different sources give somewhat different values for normal proportions of marrow cells. The reasons for this variation are numerous.

Criteria for classifying cells differ; data about truly normal bone marrows are relatively sparse; the range of variation among normals is wide; and techniques for examination are various. Terminology for granulocyte maturation is fairly standard, but erythroid cells are described in several different terminologies (see Table 1). Table 2 indicates the range of "normal values" for cells in aspirated marrow. Paraffin-embedded tissue sections are unsuitable for detailed morphologic differentiation, but the approximate M:E ratio, the number of megakaryocytes, and the existence of severe cellular disproportions can easily be observed.

Sometimes aspirated material does not contain hematopoietic cells. This condition, called a "dry tap," occurs when hematopoietic activity is so sparse that virtually no cells exist to be withdrawn or when the marrow contains so many tightly packed, sticky, highly immature cells that gentle suction cannot dislodge them. If aspiration is unsuccessful, needle biopsy or open biopsy readily reveals what is wrong with the marrow.

INDICATIONS

Bone marrow examination is virtually diagnostic in multiple myeloma and in most leukemias, both acute and chronic. Lymphomas are best diagnosed by lymph node examination, but, after the diagnosis has been made, it often is desirable to determine whether there is lymphoma in the bone marrow. Bone marrow frequently is examined to search for metastatic spread of carcinoma; dissemination of systemic infections, especially tuberculosis; or the existence of generalized diseases that affect macrophages, such as lipid or glycogen storage diseases. Evaluating the marrow for evidence of increased or decreased cellular proliferation helps to determine whether deficient production or increased destruction is causing a patient's anemia or cytopenia, although this may not reveal the reason for the difficulty. In conditions of megaloblastic erythroid maturation or disordered iron metabolism, the bone marrow morphology may be highly revealing.

If the bone marrow shows little erythropoietic activity, the patient is said to have *hypoplastic anemia*. This is a description, not a diagnosis, and the cause for depressed erythropoiesis still must be sought. Common causes include chronic infection, hypothyroidism, chronic renal failure, advanced liver disease, and a range of "idiopathic" conditions. If an anemic patient has *erythropoietic hyperplasia*, many conditions must be considered. Marrow hyperactivity is characteristic

Table 1. Maturation of Erythrocytes

	Nucleus	Cytoplasm	Size (μm.)
Pronormoblast (Rubriblast)	Dispersed or granular chromatin Nucleoli present	Scant, medium blue No hemoglobin	18–25
Basophilic normoblast (Prorubricyte, early erythroblast)	Chromatin clumped in spoke-like pattern No nucleoli	Deep blue Polyribosomes numerous No hemoglobin	14–18
Polychromatophilic normoblast (Rubricyte, late erythroblast)	Chromatin in irregular lumps Occupies less than one-half of cell	Grayish-purple or greenish-purple Modest number of ribosomes, some unaggregated Hemoglobin present	12–15
Orthochromic normoblast (metarubricyte, normoblast)	Densely pyknotic Occupies one-fourth or less of cell	Grayish-pink Few polyribosomes, some unaggregated ribosomes Substantial hemoglobin	9–13
Reticulocyte	No nucleus	Uniformly pink, faintly gray Scattered residual RNA structures	9–10
Mature erythrocyte	No nucleus	Pink with central pallor No RNA	6–8

of iron deficiency anemia; thalassemias; hemoglobinopathies; pernicious anemia and other diseases of folate and B_{12} metabolism; hypersplenism; enzyme deficiencies such as G-6-PD deficiency, hereditary spherocytosis, and other membrane abnormalities; and destructive processes like antibody-mediated, bacterial, or chemical hemolysis. In pernicious anemia and other disorders of vitamin B_{12} or folic acid metabolism, developing red cells have a peculiar appearance called *megaloblastic maturation*. Except for this readily detected morphologic abnormality, the appearance of the hyperplastic marrow usually gives few clues to the specific diagnosis.

Table 2. Differential Counts of Nucleated Bone Marrow Cells*

	Range of Mean Values[†]	Range of Ranges Given
Myeloblast	0.3–2	0–5
Promyelocyte	1.4–5	0–8
Myelocyte	4.2–8.9	0–15
Metamyelocyte	6.5–22	3–32
Band	13–24	12–34
Mature granulocyte		
Neutrophil	15–20	5–32
Eosinophil	0.5–2	0–6
Basophil	0–0.2	0–5
Lymphocyte	14–16	3–26
Monocyte	0.3–2.4	0–6
Plasma cell	0.3–1.3	0–3.9
Pronormoblast	0.2–0.6	0–1.3
Basophilic normoblast	1.4–2	0–4
Polychromatophilic normoblast	6–21	4–29
Orthochromic normoblast	1–3	0–4.6
M/E ratio	2.3–3.5 to 1	1.5–8 to 1

*Figures are for adults and are taken from several series as reported in Williams[54] and Wintrobe.[55]
†Values are expressed as percent of nucleated cells present.

Regulation of Marrow Activity

ERYTHROPOIETIN

Red-cell production is largely regulated by *erythropoietin*, a heat-stable α-globulin produced by the kidney. Reduced tissue oxygen levels stimulate secretion of erythropoietin. It is unclear where and how tissue hypoxia conveys the need for erythropoietin to the kidney; such communication may occur within the kidney itself.[5] Very slight changes in oxygenation have this effect. Tissue oxygen levels may change as a result of altered blood hemoglobin concentration, altered oxygen affinity of hemoglobin, reduction in hemoglobin oxygen saturation, or changes in pattern or spread of blood flow. When hemoglobin and tissue oxygenation are normal, small amounts of erythropoietin are excreted in urine. Anemic or hypoxic patients usually have much increased urinary erythropoietin levels.

Erythropoietin acts upon hematopoietic stem cells, inducing them to differentiate toward red cell development.[37,46] Erythropoietin causes increased numbers of cells to differentiate into red cell precursors; it enhances hemoglobin synthesis and iron incorporation; it increases the speed of cellular maturation; and it provokes release of reticulocytes into the circulating blood at an earlier stage of development than is normal. The best index of erythropoietin activity is the level of circulating reticulocytes. In an anemic patient, absence of reticulocytosis indicates inadequate response to the anemic stimulus.

OTHER ERYTHROPOIETIC STIMULANTS

Erythropoietin is not the only stimulus to red cell production. Patients without kidneys who are maintained for long periods on hemodialysis continue to produce red cells.[39] However, no specific substance or activity has been documented to influence red cell production directly. Androgens play a role in erythropoiesis, but this consists largely of enhancing the production or the physiologic activity of erythropoietin. Similarly, the presence of red cell degradation products seems to exert a "feedback" action that encourages red cell manufacture, but this, too, seems to act through erythropoietin mediation. The roles of the hypothalamus and of anterior pituitary hormones probably are intertwined with erythropoietin as well.

GRANULOCYTE PRODUCTION

The level of circulating granulocytes responds promptly to physiologic or pathologic stimulation. Mature granulocytes can be released from the storage pool within minutes, followed somewhat later by enhanced granulocyte production. No white cell-active substance comparable to erythropoietin has been found. No clear-cut pathways of granulocyte regulation have been documented even though neutrophil degradation products, microbial products, and cellular breakdown products all seem to influence granulocyte kinetics. Relative and absolute numbers of circulating granulocytes rise, and increased numbers of immature granulocytes are seen in peripheral blood after an effective granulocytic stimulus occurs. Normally, no more than 5 percent of circulating granulocytes are immature, and all of these are at the band stage. Under intense granulocytic stimulation, large numbers of bands, some metamyelocytes, and occasionally even myelocytes find their way into the circulation.

Reticulocytes

As red cells mature, several days are needed for the hemoglobin-containing cell to rid itself of residual cytoplasmic RNA after the nucleus has been expelled. Part of this process occurs in the bone marrow and part in the circulation. During this last phase of maturation, the RNA-containing cell is slightly larger than the mature cell; it contains miscellaneous fragments of mitochondria and other organelles, as well as ribosomal RNA. These cells, called *reticulocytes,* can often be distinguished on Wright-stained smears by their size and slightly gray or purple appearance (Fig. 1). The reticulofila-mentous material that gives these cells their name is seen only after supravital staining, but essentially the same material is responsible for several kinds of tinctorial abnormalities easily seen on routine smears. *Polychromatophilia,* a diffuse grayish or blue discoloration, and *basophilic stippling,* a punctate form of blue discoloration, owe their occurrence to this ribosomal material. A slightly alkaline pH, highly concentrated stains, or prolonged staining conduces to baso-philic stippling, while acidic pH and rapid staining with strong fixing agents result in polychromatophilic cells with little stippling. Supra-vital staining precipitates the reticulofilamentous material and makes it easy to distinguish immature from mature cells.

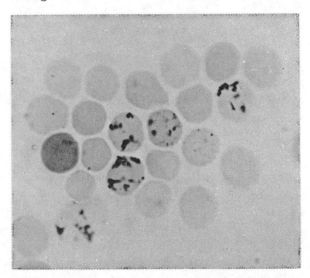

Figure 1. Reticulocytes in the peripheral blood of a patient with severe hemolysis. The brilliant cresyl blue stain makes cytoplasmic RNA remnants visible; with Wright's stain, reticulocytes have a uniform, slightly gray cast.

RETICULOCYTE COUNT

Normal cells spend 1 to 2 days circulating as a reticulocyte and 120 days circulating in mature form.[5] In normal blood, between 0.5 and 2.5 percent of circulating red cells are reticulocytes. A 0.5 to 2.5 percent reticulocyte count indicates normal marrow activity if the hemoglobin level is normal. An elevated reticulocyte count in the presence of normal hemoglobin levels indicates that red cells are being lost or destroyed but that the marrow has stepped up red cell production to compensate. With low hemoglobin levels, a "normal" reticulocyte count of 0.5 to 2.5 percent indicates that the response to anemia is inadequate. This can result from defective erythropoietin production or bone marrow hyporesponsiveness or both. Patients with chronic hemolytic diseases (especially hemoglobin S disease) and, to a much lesser extent, hereditary spherocytosis may experience "aplastic crises" in which red cell destruction continues but red cell production stops and their normally high level of reticulocytes drops abruptly.

SIGNIFICANT CHANGES

When the marrow has normal cells and adequate stores of iron and other precursors, the degree of reticulocytosis parallels the degree of blood loss or red cell destruction. Patients with defects of cellular maturation or hemoglobin production sometimes have *ineffective erythropoiesis*. In these conditions, the bone marrow is enormously hyperplastic, but the reticulocyte count is disproportionately low because many cells never mature sufficiently to enter the peripheral blood. Pernicious anemia and thalassemia are classic causes of ineffective erythropoiesis; severe iron deficiency produces a less marked degree of the same effect.

After blood loss or effective therapy for certain kinds of anemia, a rising reticulocyte count indicates that the marrow is normally responsive. A single hemorrhagic episode causes reticulocytosis beginning within 24 to 48 hours and reaching a peak at 4 to 7 days.[30] Normal levels resume when hemoglobin levels stabilize, usually by 30 days. Persistent reticulocytosis or a second rise in reticulocyte levels indicates continuing or recurrent blood loss.

In iron-deficient patients and especially in those whose insufficiency has resulted from prolonged blood loss, therapeutic iron administration produces reticulocytosis within 3 days. The count should remain elevated until normal hemoglobin values are achieved.

Similarly, vitamin B_{12} therapy for pernicious anemia causes a prompt, continuing reticulocytosis; if this fails to occur, the diagnosis and therapy should be reconsidered promptly.

CORRECTED RETICULOCYTE COUNTS

Some workers believe that expressing reticulocytes as a percentage of total red cells is misleading when the total number of red cells is abnormal. One remedy is to translate the observed percentage of reticulocytes to what it would be if normal numbers of red cells were present. Thus a patient with 6 percent reticulocytes and a hematocrit of 30 percent would have a "corrected reticulocyte count" of only 4 percent, because only two-thirds of the normal number of red cells are present. The formula for corrected reticulocyte count is:

$$\text{Percentage of observed reticulocytes} \times \frac{\text{Patient's hematocrit}}{45} = \text{Corrected reticulocyte count}$$

where 45 equals the theoretically normal hematocrit.

Another approach is to report the number of circulating reticulocytes as an absolute number rather than as a percentage of total red cells. This must be done by multiplying the total red count by the percentage of reticulocytes, since there is no generally acceptable method of identifying and counting reticulocytes independently. A range of 60,000 to 90,000/mm.^{3} is considered to be the normal absolute value.[55]

One refinement is to correct for the fact that reticulocytes enter the circulation more rapidly when erythropoietic stress is intense. With pronounced stimulation, younger non-nucleated cells enter the circulation and circulate longer as recognizable reticulocytes. The normal circulation time for reticulocytes is considered to be 1 day at the normal hematocrit of 45 percent. Circulation time increases as hematocrit drops: 1.5 days at 35 percent, 2 days at 25 percent and 2.5 days at 15 percent.[55] The formula for the *reticulocyte production index* (RPI) is:

$$\frac{\text{Observed reticulocyte percentage}}{\text{Reticulocyte maturation time (days)}} \times \frac{\text{Patient's hematocrit}}{\text{Normal hematocrit (45\%)}} = \text{RPI}$$

where the result is expressed as the proportion of normal reticulocyte production.

A person with a hematocrit of 45 percent and a reticulocyte level of 1 percent would have an RPI of 1. A patient with 8 percent reticulocytes and a hematocrit of 15 percent would have an RPI of $8/2.5 \times 15/45 = 1\frac{1}{3}$, indicating only modestly increased red cell production. Another patient with 8 percent reticulocytes, but with a 25 percent hematocrit would have an RPI of $8/2 \times 25/45 = 2.2$, while still another patient with 8 percent reticulocytes, and a hematocrit as high as 35 percent would be given an RPI of $8/1.5 \times 35/45 = 3.2$, or 3.2 times normal. The same reticulocyte percentage reflects rather different marrow response in different patients when the RPI is employed.

In everyday practice, the observed percentage of reticulocytes is the simplest and most useful piece of information on which to base diagnosis and evaluate therapy.

ERYTHROCYTE PRODUCTION

Hemoglobin Synthesis

The parts of a hemoglobin molecule have very different synthetic pathways. Each hemoglobin molecule has four identical heme moieties attached to four globin chains, of which two are α chains and the other two differ with hemoglobin type: β for hemoglobin A, δ for hemoglobin A_2, and γ for hemoglobin F. Different genes regulate peptide structure and rate of synthesis for each globin chain. Hemoglobinopathies are due to genes that code for abnormal amino acid sequence (see p. 91), while defects in manufacturing processes produce thalassemias (see p. 99).

Heme synthesis involves the stepwise synthesis of a porphyrin framework followed by the insertion of ferrous iron into each of the four heme groups. Availability of iron is a crucial factor in maintaining hemoglobin levels, and iron lack is a common cause of clinical illness. Disordered porphyrin synthesis occurs less often and may have a genetic or exogenous basis.

PORPHYRIN METABOLISM

Porphyrin consists of four symmetrical, ringed, 4-carbon structures called pyrrole rings. Synthesis requires initial construction of a straight-line chain of carbon-containing groups, which is closed into a single pyrrole ring. Four pyrroles link together, after several changes and exchanges of substituent groups, to form the final iron-free compound, protoporphyrin. Constituent carbon groups derive initially from glycine and succinyl coenzyme A, which in turn originate from the tricarboxylic acid cycle.

We shall merely list the steps and compounds involved in heme synthesis. *Succinyl coenzyme A* and *glycine* combine to form *alpha-amino, beta-keto adipic acid,* which is decarboxylated to form *delta-amino levulinic acid* (ALA). The straight-line compound ALA is the first precursor distinctively associated with heme synthesis. Two molecules of ALA combine to form *porphobilinogen,* a single-ring molecule, and four porphobilinogen rings condense to form the tetrapyrrole *uroporphyrinogen.* Subsequent steps in synthesis include conversion of uroporphyrinogen to *coproporphyrinogen,* conversion of coproporphyrinogen to *protoporphyrin,* and coupling of protoporphyrin with iron for the happy ending—the production of *heme.*

Unused coproporphyrin and uroporphyrin are excreted in urine and feces. If heme synthesis is abnormal, abnormal quantities of these and other precursors are excreted. Identification and measurement will be discussed in later chapters (see pp. 579 and 581). The clinical states associated with abnormal heme production rarely include anemia; chemical and metabolic derangements are the major findings.

Iron Metabolism

About 65 percent of the body's normal 4000 mg. of iron (somewhat less in women) resides in hemoglobin and about 3 percent is in myoglobin. A tiny but vital fraction is in the mitochondrial enzymes that mediate electron transfer, and the remainder exists in storage form as *hemosiderin* or *ferritin.* If available iron diminishes, storage sources are emptied; if the deficit continues, hemoglobin synthesis declines and anemia ensues. It is clinically unnecessary to measure total body iron. Iron deficiency is documented by observing decreased or absent stainable iron in bone marrow sections. Increased storage iron is apparent in sections of bone marrow or liver and can be documented dynamically by inducing massive excretion of iron following therapeutic doses of an iron-mobilizing chelating agent.

Except after blood transfusion, the only way iron enters the body is orally. Under normal conditions, only 10 percent of ingested iron is absorbed, but up to 20 percent of ingested iron can be absorbed in cases of iron deficiency. It is never possible to absorb all ingested iron, no matter how great the need. Iron absorption is rarely measured specifically. Usually it is sufficient to measure the amount of iron in the blood and the amount of transport protein capable of binding the iron. If abnormal dynamics are suspected, one can measure the plasma iron turnover, or the rate at which iron is incorporated into developing red cells.

SERUM IRON AND IRON-BINDING CAPACITY

Iron travels in the blood stream bound to *transferrin*, a β-globulin manufactured by the liver. Serum iron is usually measured colorimetrically in a technically demanding procedure subject to errors from artefact.

If glassware or water is contaminated with iron, values will be too high. Free serum hemoglobin elevates the iron level enormously, even quantities too slight to be seen with the naked eye. Falsely low values occur if iron is trapped during precipitation of serum proteins. Normal serum iron values are 75 to 170 μg./dl. for men and slightly lower for women.

Iron-binding capacity is expressed as the quantity of iron present in serum after transferrin is exposed to excess iron. Levels for fully saturated transferrin range between 300 and 400 μg. of iron/dl. With normal iron stores and protein metabolism, transferrin is usually 30 to 35 percent saturated. The normal range is between 20 and 45 percent saturation. Saturation levels follow a diurnal pattern; they are highest in the morning and lowest in late afternoon and early evening. Blood for serum iron and iron-binding capacity should be drawn in the morning, in the fasting state, and 24 hours or more after discontinuing iron-containing medications.

INTERPRETATION OF RESULTS

When total body iron is low, transferrin levels increase, but the relative and absolute amount of serum iron declines. Low serum iron levels, sometimes down to 10 or 15 μg./dl., characterize iron deficiency. The percentage of saturation is extremely low because more transferrin is available for less iron. Iron turnover and the percentage of serum iron utilized in red cell production both increase — a way of getting the most possible "mileage" out of the little iron available.

Serum iron levels are low in the anemias of chronic illness, and those that complicate persistent infection, malignant neoplasms, collagen-vascular diseases, and chronic renal diseases. In these conditions, however, transferrin levels also tend to be low. The percentage of saturation does not drop dramatically as it does with iron deficiency. Transferrin levels rise in late pregnancy and in women taking oral contraceptives, an increase seen with other transport proteins as well. If iron stores are adequate, the percentage of saturation remains normal or only slightly decreased. Because iron deficiency is common in pregnancy and in women during the active reproductive years, both relative and absolute iron levels should be scrutinized during pregnancy.

Both serum iron and saturation percentage are elevated in hemochromatosis, a genetic defect of iron regulation, and in iron excess induced by multiple red cell transfusions. Severe hemolytic conditions also cause elevated iron levels.

Vitamin B_{12} and Folic Acid

The metabolism of vitamin B_{12} (cyanocobalamin) and folic acid (pteroylmonoglutamic acid) is a subject too complex for complete exposition in this chapter. Both are vitally implicated in the synthesis and intermolecular exchanges of one- and two-carbon fragments. These reactions affect synthesis of purines and pyrimidines, and thus they interact with the reactions involved in DNA synthesis. Deficiency states cause abnormal nuclear and cytoplasmic development of the *megaloblastic* type. This is especially prominent in red cell precursors, although granulocytes and rapidly proliferating cells outside the marrow are also involved.

METABOLIC INTERRELATIONS

Vitamin B_{12} is synthesized solely by microorganisms. Humans acquire their supplies by eating animal products, but animals are themselves unable to synthesize it. Normal body stores are sufficient to withstand a year or more of zero intake, although states of rapid growth or cell turnover increase B_{12} requirements. Relatively few reactions in human metabolism are known unequivocally to be B_{12}-dependent. Among these are the *methylmalonyl CoA mutase* reaction, which mediates isomeric conversion between methylmalonyl CoA and succinyl CoA; and methylation of *homocysteine* to *methionine*, a conversion that not only produces methionine, but generates tetrahydrofolate. The methylmalonate-succinate conversion is essential to the interconversion pathways between lipids and carbohydrates. Defective homocysteine methylation causes a relative deficit of methionine, a substance available from other sources. A more significant defect is failure to regenerate tetrahydrofolic acid from N^5-methyltetrahydrofolic acid.

Tetrahydrofolic acid is the reduced form of *folic acid*, the catalytic, self-regenerating compound that mediates one-carbon transfers. Folic acid is present in many foods of vegetable origin, but body stores are small and mammals cannot synthesize it. The major effect of folic acid deficiency is impaired thymidine synthesis. Thymidine is part of DNA but not of RNA; thus, altered thymidine metabolism specifically affects DNA and leaves RNA production unaffected.[3] Folate deficiency also impairs histidine catabolism, an abnormality that causes no clinical disability but does cause large quantities of the metabolite *formiminoglutamic acid* (FIGlu) to accumulate.

LABORATORY DETERMINATIONS

The classic technique for measuring folic acid has been a bioassay that measures growth of specific strains of Lactobacillus. Normal values are 7 to 19 ng./ml. of serum, and 165 to 600 ng./ml. of packed red cells.[3] Microbial bioassay is less precise for vitamin B_{12}, but normal levels seem to range between 200 and 900 pg./ml. serum. Radioimmunoassay and radioisotope dilution techniques make determinations less demanding technically, but the tests are totally dependent on having reagents of high specificity. With folic acid deficiency, serum levels fall to 1 ng./ml. or even lower. However, serum folic acid levels remain normal in vitamin B_{12} deficiency. When serum B_{12} levels fall to 100 pg./ml. or below, megaloblastic marrow development can be seen; in full-blown pernicious anemia, values may go as low as 20 pg./ml. or less.[29]

Until recently, accurate B_{12} and folic acid determinations were expensive and time-consuming. Therefore the assessment of possible deficiencies relied heavily on measuring diagnostically significant metabolites. Formiminoglutamic acid is elevated in folic acid deficiency. Urinary excretion of more than 17 mg. of FIGlu per day indicates folate-dependent impaired histidine metabolism.[3] Occasionally, patients with vitamin B_{12} deficiency and normal folate levels may also have elevated FIGlu excretion. Urine levels of methylmalonate give a good indication of B_{12} deficiency; excretion of more than 9 or 10 mg./day indicates defective activity of B_{12}-dependent methylmalonyl-CoA mutase.[4]

Diagnostic information can be obtained by observing the clinical effects of selected replacement therapy. When megaloblastic anemia is due to vitamin B_{12} deficiency, 1 μg. of injected B_{12} causes megaloblastic nuclear development to revert to normal within 48 hours, beginning as early as 8 to 12 hours, and pronounced reticulocytosis occurs within 3 days. When folic acid deficiency is at fault, B_{12} does not correct the hematologic picture. Physiologic doses of folic acid (200 μg./day), on the other hand, cause prompt hematologic response. Very large doses of folic acid (5 to 15 mg./day) will correct the hematologic changes of B_{12}-deficiency anemia, but excessive folic acid may overtax other B_{12}-dependent reactions. Folic acid inappropriately administered to vitamin B_{12}-deficient patients can accentuate the neurologic symptoms that accompany B_{12} deficiency.[4]

SCHILLING TEST

Absorption of dietary vitamin B_{12} requires that it become bound to *intrinsic factor*, a glycoprotein elaborated by the gastric mucosa.[2] Pernicious anemia, the commonest and most severe form of B_{12} deficiency, involves a deficiency of intrinsic factor as well as reduced vitamin B_{12} absorption. Intestinal malabsorption syndromes also can cause clinically significant B_{12} deficiency. The Schilling test is used to establish (1) whether B_{12} absorption is defective and (2) whether absorptive mechanisms are intact but intrinsic factor is deficient. With normal absorption, the body acquires far more B_{12} than it needs, and the excess is excreted in the urine. Urinary excretion increases if B_{12} requirements have already been met. With impaired absorption, orally administered vitamin does not get into the system and therefore does not appear in the urine. ^{57}Co-labeled vitamin B_{12} is used to follow the ins and outs of orally administered B_{12}. To ensure that immediate body needs have been met, a loading dose of unlabeled vitamin is injected before the test dose is given.

PERFORMANCE OF THE TEST

The patient is given 0.5 or 1.0 μg. of ^{57}Co-labeled vitamin B_{12} by mouth after parenteral injection of 1000 μg. of unlabeled vitamin, and all the urine is collected for the next 24 hours. Complete collection and accurate measurement are important, for the test depends upon measuring the absolute amount of radioactivity excreted. The amount of radiolabeled vitamin excreted is compared with the amount given, and the result is expressed as a percentage of excretion. Normal individuals excrete from 15 to 40 percent of the smaller (0.5 μg. dose and 5 to 40 percent of the larger (1.0 μg.) dose within 24 hours.[1] Patients with impaired absorption excrete no more than 7 percent of the smaller dose and 0 to 3 percent of the larger dose.

PROBLEMS IN INTERPRETATION

This procedure, like other tests depending on urinary excretion, is difficult to interpret if there is severe renal disease. With reduced urine formation, less radioactive material is excreted in the allotted time, regardless of the amount absorbed. If there is known renal disease, the test can be prolonged to a 48- or 72-hour collection. Eventually, nearly all the absorbed material will be excreted. A more frequent problem is failure to collect all urine in the 24-hour period. This produces a small total amount of measured radioactivity and makes it appear that less has been absorbed.

ADDITION OF INTRINSIC FACTOR

When initial testing reveals reduced vitamin B_{12} absorption, the next step should be to investigate the cause. The Schilling test can be repeated with 60 μg. of intrinsic factor administered orally along with the vitamin B_{12}. If urinary ^{57}Co excretion rises to normal when intrinsic factor is added, the diagnosis of intrinsic factor deficiency is established. A second low excretion indicates some other cause of malabsorption—either intestinal disease or abnormal competition for vitamin B_{12} in the bowel lumen.

Before a Schilling test is done, other diagnostic procedures should already have been completed. The parenteral dose of 1000 μg. of vitamin B_{12} produces therapeutic effects and can induce marked bone marrow changes. Bone marrow aspiration should precede the Schilling test. The reticulocytosis induced by B_{12} administration additionally supports the diagnosis, if it occurs.[29]

PERIPHERAL BLOOD: RED CELLS

Red cells transport hemoglobin, and hemoglobin transports oxygen. The amount of oxygen that tissues receive depends on the amount and the function of available hemoglobin, on effective blood flow patterns, and on the state of the tissue and fluid through which oxygen diffuses. Only the first consideration is in the province of hematology. The three primary variables are the amount of hemoglobin present in whole blood, expressed in grams of hemoglobin per deciliter of whole blood; the proportion of whole blood that red cells contribute, expressed as the hematocrit, or percentage of red cells in whole blood volume; and the absolute number of red cells in whole blood, usually expressed as a number (in millions) per cubic millimeter of blood. In international units, this is expressed as the number of red cells per liter of blood. Thus a red count of 5,000,000/mm.^{3} is expressed in SI units as $5 \times 10^{12}/L$.

   Corpuscular indices are calculations which allow characterization of size and hemoglobin content in individual cells. The indices include *mean corpuscular volume* (MCV), calculated as the volume of packed cells divided by the red cell count and expressed as cubic microns (femtoliters [fl] in SI units); *mean corpuscular hemoglobin* (MCH), calculated as the hemoglobin concentration of whole blood divided by the number of red cells present and expressed as picograms (pg.) or micro-micrograms ($\mu\mu$g.); and the *mean corpuscular hemoglobin concentration* (MCH), calculated as the hemoglobin concentration of whole blood divided by the volume of packed red cells and expressed as a percentage of cell volume (in SI units, as grams of hemoglobin per deciliter of red cells).

Manual Methods

HEMOGLOBIN

Hemoglobin is best evaluated from the absorbance, at a 540 nm. wavelength, of the highly colored hemoglobin solution. This requires lysing the red cells to release the hemoglobin and converting all forms of the molecule (oxyhemoglobin, deoxyhemoglobin, methemoglobin, and carboxyhemoglobin) to a single, stable form. Conversion to cyanmethemoglobin is the method most widely used,[32] because reagents and instruments can be controlled most easily against stable, reliable standards. Limitations of this technique lie, as always, in accurate sample dilution and reagent preparation and in careful calibration of instruments. For adult men, normal levels are 13 to 17 gm. of hemoglobin/dl.; the normal range for women is 12 to 16 gm./dl.

   Hemoglobin is a heavy molecule and contributes substantially to the weight of blood. It is possible to estimate the hemoglobin concentration by determining the specific gravity of whole blood. This rather "rough and ready" technique is often used to determine whether or not a person can safely donate blood. For this purpose, an absolute figure is not needed; only an indication that a minimum safe level is present. These levels are 1.053 for women, corresponding to hemoglobin level of approximately 12.5 gm./dl., and 1.057 for men, corresponding to 13.5 gm./dl. The test consists of allowing a drop of whole blood to fall through a copper sulfate solution made up to a specific gravity of 1.053 or 1.057. If the drop sinks, its specific gravity equals or exceeds that of the copper sulfate solution; if it rises to the top, its specific gravity is less. Inaccuracies arise if the copper sulfate solution changes its specific gravity, either through contamination or evaporation, or if there is anything besides hemoglobin in the blood that significantly affects specific gravity. Myeloma proteins, other abnormal globulins, and x-ray contrast materials are the most likely offenders.

HEMATOCRIT

Packed red cell volume can be measured on venous or capillary blood, in macro or micro technique. In the classical Wintrobe method, anticoagulated venous blood is pipetted into a tube 100 mm. long, which is centrifuged at 2260 G. for 30 minutes.[55] The volume of packed red cells and plasma is read directly from the millimeter marks along the side of the tube. This reference method is not suitable for routine clinical use. In the micro method, either venous or capillary blood is used to fill a capillary tube approximately 7 cm. long and 1 mm. in diameter. This is centrifuged for 4 to 5 minutes at 10,000 G., and the proportions of plasma and red cells are determined by means of a calibrated reading device.

The micro method is quick and easy, but the centrifuge must be controlled for optimum centrifugal force and the tube must be carefully positioned and read against the read-out scale. Both techniques allow visual estimation of the volume of white cells and platelets that constitute the buffy coat between red cells and plasma. The supernatant plasma should be observed for jaundice or hemolysis.

RED CELL COUNT

Counting red cells in a small volume of enormously diluted blood is so time-consuming and so inaccurate that it is rarely performed. Before automated techniques were available, a few laboratories had a few meticulous workers whose results were reliable and reproducible, but the general run of manual red counts gave results of very dubious validity.

Automated Methods

Automated techniques allow cell numbers and hemoglobin content to be measured in a rapid, reproducible fashion. The hematocrit is calculated indirectly by manipulating the values for observed cell size and number, electrical conductivity, and other variables. Automation does not eliminate problems of sample dilution and of standardizing equipment, but it markedly increases speed and reproducibility as compared with manual techniques.[3] Since automated red counts are highly accurate, and electronic calculators are part of the instruments, computation of corpuscular indices has become a routine part of the complete blood count.

INTERPRETATION

Anemia generally means any condition in which a patient's oxygen-carrying capacity is below normal for the appropriate age and sex. Increase in size or number of red blood cells is also abnormal, although distinctly less common. Hemoglobin or hematocrit values are commonly used to express the degree of anemia. These two values usually are parallel, but disproportion may occur if cells have abnormal size or shape, or if hemoglobin manufacture is defective. Such disproportions become apparent through abnormalities of corpuscular indices.

The size (MCV) and hemoglobin content (MCH) of individual cells are important in evaluating anemias or other hematologic abnormalities. Cells may be described as *normochromic, hypochromic,* or (rarely) *hyperchromic,* indicating that individual cells have normal, reduced, or increased amounts of hemoglobin. Cell size is indicated by the terms *normocytic, microcytic,* and *macrocytic.* The indices reflect calculated mean values. When disease exists, there may be variation among the cells such that the average figure is misleading, but such variability should be detected when cells are examined on the stained blood film.

In prepubertal children, normal hemoglobin and red cell levels are the same for males and females. Beginning at the second decade, however, values go up for males and down for females. In males, hemoglobin and hematocrit rise with puberty, remain constant to age 40 or 50, decline slowly until age 70, and then decline somewhat more rapidly.[35] In females, the drop in hemoglobin and hematocrit that begins with puberty reverses at about age 50, but rising normal values never return to the prepubertal levels or reach the level found in males of the same age. The difference between adult males and adult females is due partly to menstrual blood loss in women, and partly to the effects of androgens in men. Castration of adult men usually causes hemoglobin and hematocrit to decline to levels near those of adult females.[55]

Morphology

Much diagnostic information can be gained by examining red cells on a well-prepared, stained blood film. The normal red cell is a biconcave disc, 6 to 8 μm. in diameter. Hemoglobin imparts a reddish-orange appearance to the stained cell. The outer portions of the cell stain more deeply than the center because there is greater depth of hemoglobin solution around the periphery than in the flattened center. The normal cell shades gradually from deep pink at the perimeter to very pale in the center. In a normal smear, all the cells are uniform in size, shape, and staining characteristics.

NUCLEATED RED CELLS

Normally maturing red cells lose their nucleus well before they leave the bone marrow. If erythropoietic stress is intense, less mature cells enter the circulation. In addition to numerous young reticulocytes, nucleated precursors occasionally enter the blood stream. The presence of *nucleated red cells* in the peripheral blood indicates either intense erythropoietic activity in the bone marrow or the existence of erythropoiesis in the spleen and other non-marrow sites, where there is less control over entry into the blood stream.[52]

INCLUSIONS AND STAINED FRAGMENTS

Residual cytoplasmic RNA can be seen on routine smears as *basophilic stippling*. In lead poisoning and thalassemia, the abnormalities of hemoglobin synthesis seem to render ribosomes more unstable than normal and thus more liable to aggregation (Fig. 2). Basophilic stippling is commonly seen in these conditions and sometimes in the anemias of complex liver disease.

Howell-Jolly bodies are fragments of residual DNA, apparently representing chromosomal fragments that detached from the dividing nucleus during cell division.[54] The spleen normally removes inclusions of this sort. Cells containing Howell-Jolly bodies are most likely to be seen after splenectomy or in patients with intense or abnormal

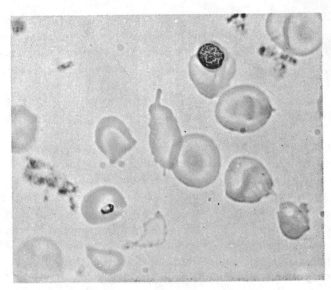

Figure 2. Severely abnormal circulating red cells of a patient with homozygous β-thalassemia. Several target cells are seen as well as a nucleated red
cell and another cell with a retained nuclear fragment. There is, in addition,
pronounced variation in cell size and shape. The indistinct clumps of particles
are platelets, which are often elevated in conditions of pronounced bone
marrow hyperactivity.

cell production due to hemolysis or inefficient erythropoiesis. *Cabot
rings*, slender curves of reddish-purple material, appear to have the
same significance, but their chemical composition is not known.

Heinz bodies are masses of denatured hemoglobin, invisible on
Wright-stained smears but easily seen with phase microscopy, Giemsa
staining, or after supravital staining. Denatured hemoglobin precipitates if there is severe oxidative stress or if excess globin chains
accumulate. Normal cells exposed to severe oxidative stress, or
enzyme-deficient cells exposed to modest oxidative stress, produce
Heinz bodies which, in most cases, are promptly removed by the
spleen.[34] Heinz bodies develop in normal red cells exposed to toxic
agents which induce methemoglobinemia and in red cells of patients
who suffer from enzyme deficiencies (especially glucose-6-phosphate
dehydrogenase deficiency), from genetically determined abnormalities
of hemoglobin structure ("unstable" hemoglobins); and from α-
thalassemia. Heinz bodies are rarely numerous in circulating cells

unless the patient has undergone splenectomy, but in vitro induction of Heinz bodies is a useful diagnostic test for these conditions.

Siderotic granules contain iron but not hemoglobin. Iron-containing granules are normally seen in immature cells actively synthesizing hemoglobin, but as the iron is incorporated, the granules disappear.[45] If hemoglobin manufacture or iron metabolism is abnormal, siderotic granules may accumulate in the cytoplasm of developing cells, having an appearance that has caused them to be called "ringed" sidero-blasts.[11] Iron-containing granules may be seen in circulating cells if the problem is severe. These become visible when cells are treated with the Prussian blue reaction for iron.

ABNORMALITIES OF SHAPE

The term poikilocytosis means irregularity of cell shape, while aniso-cytosis means that the cells vary in size. If all red cells are uniformly large, the condition is known as macrocytosis. More often, however, there is irregularity of both size and shape. In iron deficiency anemia and thalassemia, average cell size is much less than normal (hence the designation microcytosis), but there is also pronounced variation in size, shape, and staining characteristics.[21]

The most familiar abnormality of red cell shape is the sickle cell; this shape change occurs when intracellular deoxygenated hemo-globin S transforms from a soluble molecule to a crystalloid form. Sickling most often occurs in small vessels, leading to cell seques-tration and destruction.[36] It is uncommon to see large numbers of sickled cells on peripheral blood smears, except in very severe crises.

Target cells, also called leptocytes (literally, "thin cells"), have an enlarged central pale zone with a pigmented area like a bull's eye in the middle. Because target cells have less intracellular content than normal, the proportion of surface membrane to cell volume is greater than normal. Target cells characterize both homozygous and hetero-zygous thalassemia and are numerous in hemoglobin C disease and other hemoglobinopathies. They may also occur in liver disease, in disorders of iron metabolism, and in certain disorders of membrane lipid composition.

Spherocytes, conversely, have a smaller than normal ratio of surface to volume. The biconcave shape of normal red cells disappears if membrane area is lost, because the constant volume of cell content must be enclosed by a smaller surface membrane. The sphere is the geometric shape with the lowest possible surface to volume ratio. In spherocytic red cells, hemoglobin is uniformly distributed within the sphere, giving the appearance of more dense concentration than is seen in biconcave cells. The actual hemoglobin content, however, is not increased.

Spherocytes are numerous in hereditary spherocytosis and in hemolytic conditions due to progressive membrane fragmentation. Red cells suffer repeated small losses of membrane as they pass through the spleen,[53] through small blood vessels which contain abnormal fibrin deposits,[9] or through mechanical irregularities in prosthetic heart valves. Spherocytic transformation is irreversible, since lost membrane cannot be restored. Spherocytic cells are less flexible and less deformable than normal cells, and are more liable than normal cells to destruction in the splenic vascular bed.[51]

"Helmet" cells or *schistocytes* are roughly triangular cells of smaller than normal volume that also occur with membrane loss. They are characteristic of microangiopathic hemolytic anemia,[9] of anemia associated with severe uremia and hypertension, and of hemolysis due to physical agents or toxins.

Instead of a smooth, disc-shaped contour, red cells may have irregular spur-like or knobby projections. They are variously called *spur cells, burr cells, echinocytes,* or *acanthocytes.* Different disease states create slightly differing appearances, which some workers claim to be sufficiently distinctive that they can place them in diagnostic categories. *Echinocytes* (from the Greek *ekhinos,* "sea urchin"), whose spicules are of regular size, shape, and distribution, can revert to disc shape if conditions return to normal.[6] High levels of fatty acids, bile acids, barbiturates, salicylates, phenylbutazone, and other chemicals can transform normal cells to echinocytes in vitro. The cells revert to normal when washed and resuspended in normal plasma. *Acanthocytes* (from the Greek *akantha,* "thorn") have irregular spicules and are permanently misshapen. The defect reflects altered proportions of lecithin and cholesterol in the membrane, and occurs in severe liver disease and in abetalipoproteinemia.[37]

Stomatocytes and *ovalocytes* (*elliptocytes*) occur as congenital abnormalities or can be induced by manipulation of membrane composition. There is a severe form of hereditary elliptocytosis in which hemolysis occurs, but 90 percent of patients with this rare disorder have normal red cell survival. Stomatocytes (from the Greek *stoma,* "mouth") are cup-shaped cells whose zone of central pallor has a rectangular or elongated contour. Besides the hereditary disorder, stomatocytosis can be acquired in severe liver disease, malignant disorders, or acute alcoholism. It also occurs in persons whose red cells lack all detectible Rh activity.

PERIPHERAL BLOOD: WHITE CELLS

Circulating blood contains approximately 4,000 to 10,000 white cells per cubic millimeter. Fully mature granulocytes, lymphocytes, and monocytes constitute the normal leukocyte population, but a small number of circulating white cells may be in the penultimate stage of maturation. White cells are in the blood on their way to another location; they perform no physiologic function within the vascular bed.

Techniques

White cells are distinguished from circulating red cells by the presence of a nucleus. Counting procedures enumerate all nucleated cells as white cells. If large numbers of nucleated red cells are present, the white cell count must be suitably corrected, but the *total white count* usually is determined without difficulty. The *differential white count* gives the proportions of different cell types that comprise the total number of white cells. Differential counts are sometimes omitted if the total count is normal and there is no clinical or laboratory evidence of hematologic abnormality. However, many neoplastic, inflammatory, and immunologic conditions alter cellular proportions within a normal level for total white cells.

Like red cell counts, white counts use a small sample of diluted blood and are subject to sampling and dilution errors. Because blood contains far fewer white than red cells, the dilution is less, and a larger volume of blood is examined than in red cell counting. Nearly all large-volume laboratories use automated methods for white cell counting, either by electronic particle counting or by light-scattering principles. Manual dilution and visual examination of hemocytometer counts remain highly reliable when carefully done.

Visual examination of stained blood films remains the mainstay of differential white cell counting, but automated procedures are gaining acceptance. Two different approaches are in use. In one of these, a sophisticated computer program for pattern recognition is linked with a lens that scans the stained blood film; this is fundamentally the same approach as that of the human eye and brain. The count is usually done on 100, 200, or 500 cells. A completely different technology separates the various kinds of white cells by manipulating the chemical properties of the medium in a continuous-flow mode, and then enumerates the individual populations by light-scattering and absorbance techniques. Much larger numbers of white cells are sampled in this approach. Despite impressive advances in speed, accuracy, and reliability, automated differential counting remains expensive and continues to require significant human input to achieve consistent, dependable results.[15,17,47]

Granulocytes

In adults, half or more of circulating white cells are granulocytes, cells whose cytoplasm contains readily visible granules of varying chemical and enzymic composition. The same precursor cells give rise to granulocytes and monocytes. Specific granules are first seen in *promyelocytes*, the next developmental phase after differentiation into a *myeloblast* (from the Greek *myelos*, "marrow"), the earliest cell recognizably committed to granulocytic identity. Maturation occurs only within the bone marrow. Granulocytes normally develop and mature at no other site, and once they are released from the marrow, they cannot reproduce themselves. If there is intense stimulation to increase circulating granulocyte levels, immature cells of this series may appear in the circulating blood. Malignant cellular proliferation or disordered control mechanisms also allow immature or abnormal forms to enter the circulation, sometimes from recrudescent hematopoietic sites in other reticuloendothelial tissues.

NEUTROPHILS

The cytoplasmic granules of neutrophils react with both basic and acidic stains, producing a "neutral" or purple result on Wright-stained preparations, the stain most commonly used. In the mature cell, nuclear chromatin is condensed into discrete lumps, or lobes, connected by thin strands of material. These cells are called *polymorphonuclear leukocytes* because there are so many (*poly-*) possible forms (*morpho-*) that these flexibly linked *nuclear* lumps can assume. Acceptable shortened terms for this polysyllabic description are *PMNs* and "*polys.*" Less mature neutrophils have larger nuclei which are not separated into lobes. The state that precedes maturity is called the *band cell*, because its nucleus is shaped like a curved band, or the *stab cell*, a German term.

Neutrophils are actively motile, and large numbers can congregate at sites of tissue injury within a short time. The process whereby cells move in response to some specific stimulus is called *chemotaxis*. Microbial products, the products of cellular injury, and many plasma protein products can exert a chemotactic effect on neutrophils.

Neutrophils constitute the body's first line of defense when tissue is damaged or foreign material gains entry. Their prompt response to these chemotactic materials makes an efficient attack mechanism. Neutrophils phagocytize and degrade particles of many sorts, and are capable of releasing enzymes into their own cytoplasm or into the surrounding medium. *Alkaline phosphatase* is an enzyme present in late-developing granules of neutrophils, while *peroxidase-reacting enzymes* are present in earlier granules.[12] One way to identify abnormal or ambiguous cells as belonging to the neutrophil series is to elicit these enzyme reactions with cytochemical techniques.

NITROBLUE TETRAZOLIUM TEST

When neutrophils phagocytize and destroy microorganisms or other materials, a complex series of membrane changes and enzyme reactions must occur.[48] The *nitroblue tetrazolium reduction* (NBT) test highlights one of these enzyme-mediated events. The electron transfer that accompanies effective intracytoplasmic lysis is demonstrated histologically when the colorless compound nitroblue tetrazolium undergoes reduction to large, blue-black granules of formazan. Reduction indicates the existence of effective intracellular metabolism such that enzyme release can occur within secondary lysosomes. Failure to reduce NBT to formazan indicates either absence of activation or inability to mobilize appropriate reactions.[12]

Patients with ongoing bacterial infections have many circulating neutrophils already activated for bactericidal events. This is demonstrated by incubating an unfixed blood smear with NBT. Activated neutrophils rapidly acquire large, black formazan granules in their cytoplasm. In normal persons, fewer than 10 percent of PMNs will contain formazan granules. Patients with bacterial infections have granules in up to 45 percent of circulating neutrophils. NBT reduction is less widespread when fever and leukocytosis are due to nonbacterial causes, but the distinction between infectious and nonbacterial leukocytosis is less complete than it initially seemed. The NBT test has not fulfilled its original promise for differentiating the causes of febrile disease. It has, however, provided useful information about normal and abnormal neutrophil activity.

In *chronic granulomatous disease* (CGD) of childhood, an X-linked defect of neutrophil function, neutrophils are morphologically normal and capable of phagocytosis but not of intracellular bacterial killing.[16] This defect correlates with deficiency of the enzyme system that eventuates in NBT reduction. Patients with CGD have cells which do not reduce NBT. Heterozygous female carriers of the condition have two populations of neutrophils: a normal population and a population with deficient NBT reduction corresponding to those cells in which the defective X chromosome remains active.[38]

EOSINOPHILS

Eosinophils are granulocytes with a two-lobed nucleus and moderately large, refractile granules which stain deep red with the acidic dye eosin. These cells are capable of phagocytosis but are not bactericidal. They are classically associated with immune reactions. Antigen-antibody complexes have been shown to exert a chemotactic effect for eosinophils, although the mechanism is unclear.[57] The granules of eosinophils contain histamine, but this probably does not contribute to vascular activity in allergic and inflammatory reactions. In fact, some studies have shown extracts of eosinophils to have an action which counteracts histamine.[55]

BASOPHILS

Basophils constitute less than 1 percent of normal circulating leukocytes. Their large, coarse cytoplasmic granules stain deeply with blue basic dye and are also brilliantly stained by metachromatic dyes. The granules contain acid mucopolysaccharides, hyaluronic acid, and large amounts of histamine. Basophils in the circulation serve no known function. Similar or identical cells are numerous, however, in the superficial layers of skin and of respiratory and alimentary tract mucosa. In the tissues, these cells are called *mast cells*. They are highly instrumental in atopic and anaphylactic immune reactions, which are mediated by IgE antibodies attached firmly to the cell membranes.

Abnormal Morphology

It is abnormal for more than 8 to 10 percent of circulating neutrophils to be band forms or to have any earlier forms at all in the blood. Besides maturational abnormalities, certain constitutional or acquired abnormalities may be observed.

TOXIC GRANULATION

In the neutrophils of patients severely ill with bacterial infections or fevers associated with tissue damage, large, deeply stained cytoplasmic granules often are present. These are thought to be abnormally activated enzyme-containing granules rather than inclusion bodies or phagocytized material. Frequently, the cytoplasm is vacuolated or takes a more basic stain than normal in these stimulated cells. Cytoplasmic vacuolization, by itself, often accompanies bacterial sepsis.

AZUROPHILIC GRANULES

As granulocytes and other leukocytes develop, they may have numerous small, smoothly rounded cytoplasmic granules which contain a variety of lysosomal enzymes. As specific granules develop, these azurophilic granules decline sharply, but a few may persist in the cytoplasm of mature lymphocytes, monocytes, or neutrophils. They have no pathologic significance.

DÖHLE BODIES

The neutrophils of patients with severe infections, burns, malignant disease, or extensive cell lysis sometimes contain large, round, pale blue masses in the periphery of the cytoplasm. These may also occur in normal pregnancy. The masses seem to be aggregated, rough endoplasmic reticulum. Their presence reflects the same metabolic alterations that stimulate rapid neutrophil generation and toxic granulation.

AUER RODS

Granulocytes and monocytes sometimes contain slender, elongated masses of pinkish-red or purple material in the cytoplasm. These Auer rods resemble azurophilic granules of normally maturing cells but indicate abnormal developmental pathways. Auer rods do not occur in normal or neoplastic lymphocytes; their presence sometimes makes it possible to classify undifferentiated leukemic cells as belonging to the myelomonocytic series.

HYPERSEGMENTATION AND MACROPOLYCYTES

Disordered folic acid or vitamin B_{12} metabolism produces many morphologic abnormalities, of which megaloblastic red cell development is the most conspicuous. Other rapidly proliferating cells also undergo abnormal development. Granulocytic cells tend to be abnormally large, especially metamyelocytes in the marrow ("giant metamyelocytes") and neutrophils in the peripheral blood. These neutrophils have nuclei with seven or eight lobes, instead of the normal three to five lobes, and abundant but morphologically normal cytoplasm.

HEREDITARY ABNORMALITIES

The *Pelger-Huet anomaly* is a constitutional abnormality transmitted as an autosomal-dominant trait. Mature neutrophils have bilobed nuclei and rather coarse chromatin, but the cells are functionally normal, and affected individuals remain in good health. The condition is significant largely because inexperienced morphologists may consider that all the circulating cells are immature or band neutrophils.

   Chediak-Higashi syndrome is a rare autosomal-recessive disorder of lysosomal function and structure, leading to accumulation of giant lysosomes containing various hydrolases and other enzymes. This change is most conspicuous in neutrophils, but it also affects many epithelial cells, nerve cells, and melanocytes in the skin, hair, and eyes. Anemia, thrombocytopenia, decreased leukocyte counts, and increased susceptibility to infection characterize the inexorably downhill clinical course. Aleutian mink, prized for the color of their fur, suffer from a similar form of partial albinism and severe susceptibility to infection.

   Several eponymic conditions produce white cells of abnormal appearance but adequate function. In the *Alder-Reilly anomaly,* neutrophils contain giant, dark-staining granules filled with polysaccharides. Although the granulocytes function normally, patients often have systemic abnormalities of mucopolysaccharide metabolism leading to gargoylism, as is the case in Hunter's syndrome, Hurler's syndrome, and other mucopolysaccharidoses. In the *May-Heggelin anomaly,* large blue or pinkish-blue bodies resembling Döhle bodies distort the cytoplasm of myeloid and monocytic cells. Moderate thrombocytopenia and abnormal platelet morphology often accompany the leukopenia of this condition, but the patient characteristically remains in good health.

Lymphocytes

The past 20 years have seen remarkable expansion of our knowledge about lymphocytes, now known to be the keystone of immunologic activity. These considerations are discussed in the section devoted to immunology. Circulating blood lymphocytes constitute a tiny fraction of the total lymphocyte pool, which includes dense concentrations in lymph nodes, spleen, and the mucosa of alimentary and respiratory tracts, and diffuse numbers in bone marrow, liver, skin, and chronically inflamed tissues at any site.

In healthy adults, about 70 percent of circulating lymphocytes are T cells, 25 percent are B cells, and the remainder are "null" (i.e., without features that allow classification). Lymphocytes travel extensively, exchanging continuously between tissue sites, lymphatic fluid, and circulating blood. The fact that draining lymphocytes from thoracic duct fluid eventually depletes whole-body stores of lymphocytes suggests that fixed and circulating lymphocytes together constitute a single population.

ATYPICAL LYMPHOCYTES

Most immune activity occurs outside the blood stream, but altered immune responsiveness sometimes produces characteristic changes in circulating lymphocytes. The "atypical lymphocytes" or "Downey cells" classically associated with infectious mononucleosis are T-lymphocytes in a state of immune activation (Fig. 3). In infectious mononucleosis, the inciting agent is the Epstein-Barr virus, or cytomegalovirus in heterophil-negative CMV mononucleosis. Similar

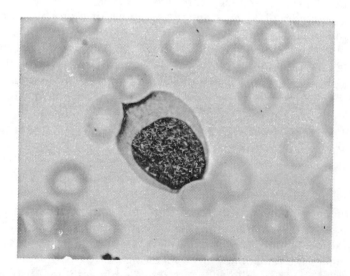

Figure 3. Atypical lymphocyte in blood from a patient with infectious mononucleosis. Note the coarse nuclear chromatin pattern, vacuolated cytoplasm, and cytoplasmic indentation by adjoining erythrocytes.

"atypical" or transformed lymphocytes are seen in patients with hepatitis, viral exanthems, viral pneumonia, and systemic allergic conditions.

Monocytes

Only small numbers of monocytes circulate at any one time. Monocytes constitute 5 to 8 percent of blood leukocytes, but circulating monocytes are a small fraction of the body's total store of these cells. Derived from the same precursor cell as granulocytes, monocytes mature in the bone marrow, circulate briefly, and then enter the tissues to become macrophages. Despite their many names, it appears that "fixed" and "wandering" macrophages, histiocytes, Kupffer cells of the liver, sinusoidal macrophages in spleen and lymph nodes, peritoneal macrophages, and the macrophages that line pulmonary air spaces all belong to the same cell population.[12] Their capabilities include motility, intense phagocytosis, enzyme secretion, particle recognition, and complex interactions with immunogens and with the cellular and protein constituents of the immune system.

Blood monocytes characteristically are large (16–20 μm.), with delicate nuclear chromatin; an elongated, indented, or folded nucleus; and abundant, grayish-blue, translucent-looking cytoplasm. Younger forms, which circulate only under conditions of monocytic stress or abnormal marrow proliferation, have a larger nucleus, sometimes a nucleolus, and more basophilic cytoplasm with more azurophilic granules than the mature forms. It is not clear how peripheral tissue conditions such as tuberculosis or other inflammatory or immunologic events influence monocyte production, but bone marrow response can clearly be demonstrated.[43]

Abnormal Differential White Counts

Since the differential white count is reported in percentages, the total white count must be known in order to understand the pathophysiologic significance of the differential. Proportions can change because there is a true increase in numbers of the preponderant cells (absolute increase) or because a decline in numbers of other cells makes the remaining cells appear increased (relative increase).

Circulating white cell counts are remarkably volatile. Absolute and relative values can change within minutes or hours of stimulation. Perhaps the most dramatic of these effects occur when the adrenal gland is stimulated, either pharmacologically or by physiologic response to stress. Cortical steroids cause lymphocytes and eosinophils to disappear from the circulation within 4 to 8 hours; circulating granulocytes increase somewhat later, probably because of reduced escape from the blood stream. Epinephrine, the hormone of the adrenal medulla, causes granulocytosis within minutes, probably by mobilizing mature neutrophils from "storage" or noncirculating locations.[12] Most of the physiologic stimuli that induce neutrophilic leukocytosis (e.g., exercise, emotional stress, exposure to extreme temperatures) appear to act by stimulating epinephrine output. Still unexplained is how a localized acute inflammatory stimulus influences the bone marrow toward sustained increases of neutrophil production and release. Tables 3 and 4 list conditions that affect neutrophil numbers.

Lymphocyte proportions frequently reflect upward or downward alterations in granulocyte levels, rather than indicating true change in numbers of lymphocytes. Conditions that increase absolute numbers of circulating lymphocytes are shown in Table 5. Relative lymphocytosis is common in acute viral exanthems, in other infectious conditions that cause neutropenia (see Table 4), and in "aleukemic" acute leukemia, when the number of recognizable circulating granulocytes may be very low indeed.

There is no table to show changing basophil levels because these cells are neither numerous nor responsive in the circulation. Tissue basophils are prominent in hypersensitivity reactions, but circulating basophilic leukocytosis is rare. The absolute number of circulating basophils rises in chronic myelocytic leukemia and polycythemia vera, but their niche in the differential count shows little change.

THE "SHIFT TO THE LEFT"

When immature granulocytes become prominent in the differential white count, the condition is sometimes called a "shift to the left." The term derives from early studies which used tabular headings to report the numbers of each cell type. The cell types were listed across the top of the page, starting with blasts on the left and placing mature neutrophils at the right side. Large numbers of immature cells provoked entries in the left-hand columns, normally empty except for a few bands. The results, obviously, were shifted to the left. The causes and significance of altered white cell levels can be presented most economically in tabular form.

Table 3. Conditions Causing Neutrophilia (>8000 PMNs/mm.^{3})

Physiologic response to stress:
  Physical exercise
  Exposure to extreme heat or cold
  Following acute hemorrhage or hemolysis
  Acute emotional stress
  Childbirth

Infectious diseases:
  Systemic or severe local bacterial infections
  Some viruses (smallpox, chicken pox, herpes zoster, polio)
  Some rickettsial diseases (especially Rocky Mountain spotted fever)
  Some fungi, especially if there is acute tissue necrosis

Inflammatory diseases:
  Acute rheumatic fever
  Rheumatoid arthritis
  Acute gout
  Vasculitis and myositis of many types
  Hypersensitivity reactions to drugs

Tissue necrosis:
  Ischemic damage to heart, abdominal viscera, extremities
  Burns
  Many carcinomas and sarcomas

Metabolic disorders:
  Uremia
  Diabetic ketoacidosis
  Eclampsia
  Thyroid storm

Drugs:
  Epinephrine
  Lithium
  Histamine
  Heparin
  Digitalis
  Many toxins, venoms, and heavy metals

CIRCULATING WHOLE BLOOD

Blood Volume

Most laboratory studies are done on small blood samples, and conclusions are drawn from quantities and concentrations in that single
sample. Sometimes it is desirable to evaluate total volume of circu-

Table 4. Conditions Causing Neutropenia (<1500 PMNs/mm.^{3})

Infectious diseases:
  Some bacteria (typhoid, tularemia, brucellosis) `
  Some viruses (hepatitis, influenza, measles, mumps, rubella, infectious
    mononucleosis)
  Protozoa (especially malaria)
  Overwhelming infection of any kind

Chemical and physical agents:
  Dose-related, universal marrow depressants (radiation, cytotoxic drugs,
    benzene)
  Idiosyncratic drug reactions (numerous)

Hypersplenism:
  Liver disease
  Storage diseases

Other disorders:
  Some collagen-vascular diseases, especially lupus erythematosus
  Severe folic acid or vitamin B_{12} deficiency

---

lating blood or of red cells or plasma as, for example, in suspected dehydration or edema or in patients with defective renal function, cirrhosis, or congestive heart failure.

Total volume is not measured directly; it is calculated by means of the dilution principle. If a known quantity of completely diffusible material is added to an unknown volume of diluent, one can calculate the volume of diluent by measuring the quantity of indicator substance in a carefully measured aliquot of the final mixture. For example, two drops of intense red dye will produce a deeply colored solution (high concentration of indicator) if added to a cup of water, but a much paler solution (low concentration of indicator) if added to a pail full of water.

Measuring blood volume is, of course, more difficult than adding dye to a pail of water. The indicator must be easy to measure; it should diffuse completely through the body compartment being measured without missing sequestered areas or pooling in accessible sites; it should not enter other body compartments or be degraded or metabolized into something else; it should not be excreted before measurement is complete or be toxic to the patient. The indicators that meet these requirements best are ^{131}I-labeled human serum albumin, for measuring plasma volume, and ^{51}Cr-labeled red cells, for measuring red cell volume.[25]

Radioactive chromate attaches selectively to the β chain of hemo-

Table 5. Conditions Affecting Lymphocyte Counts

Lymphocytosis (>4000 lymphocytes/mm.^{3} in adults; >7,200/mm.^{3} in children)
  Infectious diseases:
    Bacterial (whooping cough, brucellosis, sometimes tuberculosis, secondary syphilis)
    Viral (hepatitis, infectious mononucleosis, mumps, many exanthems, cytomegalovirus)
    Other (infectious lymphocytosis, toxoplasmosis)
  Metabolic conditions:
    Hypoadrenalism
    Hyperthyroidism (sometimes)
  Chronic inflammatory conditions:
    Ulcerative colitis
    Immune diseases (serum sickness, idiopathic thrombocytopenic purpura)

Lymphocytopenia (<1000 lymphocytes/mm.^{3} in adults; <2500/mm.^{3} in children)
  Immunodeficiency syndromes:
    Congenital defects of cell-mediated immunity
    Immunosuppressive medication
  Adrenal corticosteroid exposure:
    Adrenal gland hyperactivity
    ACTH-producing pituitary gland tumors
    Therapeutic administration of steroids
  Severe, debilitating illness of any kind:
    Congestive heart failure
    Renal failure
    Far-advanced tuberculosis
  Defects of lymphatic circulation:
    Intestinal lymphangiectasia
    Disorders of intestinal mucosa
    Thoracic duct drainage

---

globin. Since only red cells contain hemoglobin, and red cells are normally present only inside the circulatory tree, ^{51}Cr provides a highly specific indicator for red cell volume. ^{131}I-labeled albumin is good, but not perfect, for plasma volume determinations. It requires approximately 15 minutes for albumin to diffuse evenly throughout the circulation, but even in this short time, some albumin leaves the plasma to enter the extravascular fluid compartment. Vascular permeability tends to be increased in precisely those patients with illnesses that make volume measurements important, so the test must be done quickly and accurately.

Table 6. Conditions Affecting Other Circulating White Cells

Monocytosis (>800 monocytes/mm.^{3} in adults)
   Infections (tuberculosis, subacute bacterial endocarditis, hepatitis, rickettsiae, syphilis)
   Granulomatous diseases (sarcoid, ulcerative colitis, regional enteritis)
   Collagen-vascular diseases (lupus, rheumatoid arthritis, polyarteritis)
   Many cancers, lymphomas, and myeloproliferative disorders

Eosinophilia (>450 eosinophils/mm.^{3})
   Allergic diseases (asthma, hayfever, drug reactions, allergic vasculitis, serum sickness)
   Parasitic infections (trichinosis, echinococcus, hookworm, schistosomiasis, amebiasis)
   Skin disorders (some psoriasis, some eczema, pemphigus, dermatitis herpetiformis)
   "Hypereosinophilic" syndromes (systemic eosinophilia associated with pulmonary infiltration and sometimes cardiovascular disturbances)
   Neoplastic diseases (Hodgkin's disease, extensive metastases or necrosis of solid tumors)
   Miscellaneous (collagen-vascular diseases, adrenal cortical hypofunction, ulcerative colitis)

Basophilia (>50 basophils/mm.^{3})
   Chronic hypersensitivity states in the absence of the specific allergen (exposure to the allergen triggers cell lysis and rapid drop in basophil count)
   Systemic mast cell disease
   Myeloproliferative disorders

EVALUATION OF RESULTS

Results of blood volume measurement are given as proportion of body mass in terms either of weight or surface area. Adipose tissue contains relatively less blood than muscle or parenchymal tissues. Since adult men tend to have higher hematocrit and a higher proportion of lean tissue to fat than adult women, normal values both for plasma and red cells are higher in men than in women. Mean normal figures for red cell volume are about 30 ml./kg. in men and about 24 ml./kg. in women; plasma volume runs about 44 ml./kg. in men and 43 ml./kg. in women.[55] This gives blood volume figures of about 7.5 percent of body weight for men and 6.5 percent for women.

   Total red cell mass increases in both polycythemia vera and the polycythemia of chronic hypoxia, but plasma volume and whole blood volume tend to increase much more in polycythemia vera than in reactive erythrocytosis. Red cell volume is sometimes measured to evaluate the extent of acute blood loss or the degree of erythropoietic response to chronic blood loss. Plasma volume measurements, along with estimates of total body water or of extracellular fluid, help to characterize the circulatory problems in chronic edema, congestive heart failure, or severe derangement of electrolyte and acid-base metabolism.

Erythrocyte Sedimentation Rate

Although its name spotlights the red cell, the erythrocyte sedimentation rate (ESR) really reflects the composition of plasma and the relation of red cells to plasma. Anticoagulated blood placed in a vertically oriented small-bore tube exhibits settling of red cells at a rate determined largely by the surface to volume ratio of the red cells. The rate of settling increases as cell weight increases, but decreases with enlarged cell surface. Small cells settle more slowly than clumps of cells because, as cells clump together, the weight of the aggregate mass increases more than does the surface area.

In normal blood, relatively little settling occurs because the gravitational pull of individual red cells is almost balanced by the upward current generated by displacement of plasma. If plasma is extremely viscous, or cholesterol levels are very high, the upward trend may virtually neutralize the downward pull of individual or slightly clumped cells. On the other hand, anything that encourages red cells to aggregate or stick to one another will increase the rate of settling. A high concentration of asymmetrical macromolecules in the plasma reduces the mutually repellent force that separates suspended red cells and thus enhances the formation of *rouleaux*. Rouleaux are clumps of red cells joined, not by antibodies or covalent bonds, but merely by surface attraction. If the proportion of globulin to albumin increases, or if fibrinogen levels are especially high, rouleaux formation is enhanced and the sedimentation rate increases.

TECHNIQUES

In the Wintrobe method for ESR, undiluted, anticoagulated blood is allowed to stand for 1 hour in a tube 100 mm. tall and 2.8 mm. in diameter. The Westergren technique uses a 200 mm. column in which the anticoagulated blood, diluted 4:1 with saline or sodium citrate, is allowed to settle for 1 hour. The Wintrobe technique is easier to perform and appears to be more sensitive to relatively minor departures from the normal.[55] The Westergren technique, which requires meticulous attention to achieve reproducible results, does a better job of differentiating ESR values at the severely abnormal end of the scale. Wintrobe results cannot reliably distinguish among ESR readings greater than 50 mm./hour, whereas the Westergren method, if properly done, allows realistic evaluation of highly abnormal observed rates.

A mechanical technique has been developed, known as the Zeta Sedimentation Rate, in which red cell aggregation is accelerated by controlled, brief bursts of centrifugation at different angles. This method gives very rapid results (5 minutes instead of an hour) and, according to its proponents, is not affected by changes in hematocrit level. Not enough data have been accumulated to allow for a full evaluation of this approach.

INTERPRETATION

Nonspecific increase in globulins and increased fibrinogen levels occur when the body responds to injury, to inflammation. or to pregnancy. A rise in ESR accompanies most acute inflammatory disease, whether localized or systemic, and occurs when smoldering or chronic inflammatory processes flare up. The ESR is especially useful in monitoring the course and therapy of chronic conditions such as rheumatoid arthritis or tuberculosis. It can also help to document whether organic disease is truly present in patients with vague symptomatology or noncontributory physical findings. Multiple myeloma and other dysproteinemias cause a very high ESR; a less marked increase often accompanies solid tumors, especially if necrosis or tissue reaction is widespread.

The observed rate of settling varies as the concentration of red cells in plasma changes. Controversy exists over reporting ESR results in a "corrected" form that takes hematocrit level into account. Formulas are available for correcting Wintrobe results. The Westergren technique, on the other hand, is somewhat less affected by hematocrit because the blood is substantially diluted to run the test.

HEMOLYSIS

Red cell destruction involves loss of membrane integrity and release of hemoglobin. Destruction of developing cells prior to release from the bone marrow is called *ineffective erythropoiesis*. When mature circulating cells are destroyed before the end of their expected 120-day life span, the process is called *hemolysis*. Ineffective erythropoiesis always reflects some inborn or acquired defect in cellular development. Hemolysis, on the other hand, may reflect either accelerated destruction of intrinsically defective cells or the lethal effect of some extrinsic process on normal red cells.

Both hemolysis and ineffective erythropoiesis require the system to dispose of the hemoglobin released from damaged cells and to replace or restore oxygen-carrying capacity (i.e., to prevent or correct anemia). When hemolysis causes reduced tissue oxygenation, the erythropoietin response tends to be pronounced. Red cell regeneration is brisk and dramatic after acute or chronic hemolysis, but reticulocytosis alone is not pathognomonic for hemolysis. The laboratory diagnosis of hemolysis requires demonstration of shortened red cell survival and increased hemoglobin turnover.

Red Cell Survival

Red cell life span can be measured in either of two ways. In the *cohort method*, one introduces a label that tags permanently those cells in production at the moment and then follows the labeled cells from birth to death. In the *random method*, the label is attached randomly to red cells of all ages, and the rate at which the label disappears corresponds to the progressive destruction of an unselected cell population. The cohort method is rarely used clinically, because the observation time must be 120 days in normals and several weeks at least in most abnormal states. With random labeling, the usual end point is the half-disappearance time, which, under normal conditions, is 28 to 35 days; with accelerated destruction the end point may be hours or less than a week.

CHROMIUM HALF-LIFE

Radioactive chromate ($^{51}CrO_4^=$) is an effective red cell label because it binds specifically to hemoglobin. Its biologic half-life is not excessively long; it emits an easily counted high-energy gamma ray; and it does not affect the survival of the cell that incorporates it.[33] Chromium labeling can be used to measure the survival time of the patient's own cells or that of the transfused isologous cells in the patient. After introduction of labeled cells, the baseline radioactivity level indicates the proportion of the total circulating cells that bear the label. This figure is necessary for later comparisons, and, with suitable calculation of dilution, it demonstrates the patient's current red cell volume (see p. 36).

Survival is measured by observing blood samples at intervals in order to determine the amount of radioactivity remaining in the circulation. Normally, half of the initial dose will have disappeared in 28 to 35 days. This figure is often used inaccurately as the "half-life of the red cells." The *half-life* of normal red cells is 60 days; the ^{51}Cr *half-disappearance time* is less because 1 percent or more of the radioactive label elutes from the red cells every day and is lost to counting. A ^{51}Cr half-time (T½) of less than 25 days indicates accelerated destruction. This can be as low as 3 to 5 days in severe intrinsic hemolytic conditions, or be measured in minutes or hours if there is antibody-mediated destruction.

With markedly accelerated destruction, the ^{51}Cr label from hemolysed cells accumulates at the site of cell damage. It has been shown that the spleen conducts most hemolysis in intrinsic hemolytic conditions, whereas it is the liver that accumulates radioactivity when cells are lysed while circulating in the vessels themselves. Intravascular hemolysis occurs with strong complement-binding antibodies such as anti-A and anti-B, or with toxic, chemical or physical damage to cells.

PROBLEMS OF INTERPRETATION

An aliquot of constant volume is used to measure radioactivity under the assumption that as labeled cells are removed from the circulation, new, unlabeled red cells appear to take their place. If red cell replacement is slowed or absent, labeled and unlabeled cells disappear at the same rate, but no new cells appear to change the proportion of labeled to unlabeled cells. If the proportional radioactivity changes very little, the red cell "survival" will appear prolonged. The fact that total red cell mass is declining cannot be detected by examining an aliquot. Conversely, if new red cells enter the circulation with unusual speed (transfusion is more likely to be the culprit than massive erythropoiesis), the proportion of labeled cells to total cells will decline, and survival will appear to be shortened. With blood loss, labeled cells are permanently lost and total available radioactivity declines. In a sample of constant volume, there will be fewer labeled cells, and the half-disappearance time of the isotope is considerably shortened. The loss of as little as 20 ml. of red cells per day can result in the spurious reduction of "survival" figures by one half.[55]

Hemoglobin Release and Degradation

FREE HEMOGLOBIN

When red cells are destroyed within the blood stream, hemoglobin enters the plasma. Here it combines with *haptoglobin*, an α_2-globulin normally present at concentrations of 30 to 190 mg./dl., a quantity sufficient to dispose of up to 100 mg. of free hemoglobin/100 ml. of plasma. Reduction or loss of measurable haptoglobin is one laboratory sign of intravascular hemolysis. Haptoglobin may also drop when the reticuloendothelial system is the site of hemolysis, since hemoglobin may leak from the spleen or other sinusoids into the blood stream. Haptoglobin levels are measured either chemically or, more easily, by radial immunodiffusion or electrophoresis.

Once the binding capacity of haptoglobin has been exceeded, *hemoglobinemia* occurs. In a healthy state, hemoglobin circulates only inside red cells. Provided that the process of venipuncture has not damaged red cells, the presence of hemoglobin in plasma is a sure indication of pathologic red cell destruction. Free hemoglobin crosses the glomerular filter from plasma into the urine with surprising ease for such a large molecule. *Hemoglobinuria* occurs when the tubular capacity to reabsorb hemoglobin (1.4 mg./min. in adult males) is exceeded.[55]

HEMOGLOBIN CATABOLISM

The reticuloendothelial system degrades hemoglobin released from cells. First, iron is removed and either returned to the marrow for re-use or placed in storage. The globin chains are broken down into their constituent amino acids and are restored to the pool available for overall protein synthesis. The residual porphyrin ring is degraded first to *biliverdin* and then to *bilirubin*, which cannot be metabolized further and must be transported to the liver for excretion. Traveling from its site of synthesis in the reticuloendothelial system to the excretory pathways of the liver, bilirubin is in the unconjugated or "indirect" form (see p. 309). Increased levels of indirect bilirubin are a reliable sign that abnormal numbers of red cells are being destroyed.

Upon reaching the liver, bilirubin must enter hepatocytes, which conjugate it with glucuronic acid. Unconjugated bilirubin is insoluble in water, but the bilirubin-glucuronide conjugate is water-soluble and passes freely into the biliary tree. If the biliary system is normal, conjugated bilirubin levels do not rise in hemolytic conditions. As it descends through the biliary system and intestinal tract, bilirubin is degraded into a loosely characterized series of compounds called *urobilinogen*.[19] Urobilinogen is water-soluble and some is reabsorbed from the colon back into the blood, which the portal venous system carries to the liver. With increased hemoglobin degradation and increased bilirubin entering the gut, there will be increased fecal urobilinogen, and increased amounts of reabsorbed urobilinogen return to the liver. If the amount of urobilinogen entering the blood stream is really large, some may escape hepatic reprocessing and be carried to the kidneys, where it readily enters the urine. Increased urinary urobilinogen is characteristic of hemolytic conditions and other states of increased hemoglobin turnover.[49] It is much easier to measure than fecal urobilinogen and thus more widely used as a chemical indicator for ongoing hemolysis.

IRON

Elemental iron is absorbed in a ferrous state from the small intestine. It travels through the blood stream bound to *transferrin*, a β_1-globulin whose function is to bind iron for plasma transport and facilitate its entry into hemoglobin-producing erythropoietic cells. About two-thirds of the body's total supply of iron normally exists as the hemoglobin of circulating red cells. Most of the rest remains in the storage compounds *ferritin* and *hemosiderin*. With normal red cell turnover, the amount of storage iron in bone marrow and other reticuloendothelial tissues remains fairly constant, even though individual iron atoms are entering and leaving storage continually. Ferritin is the more labile storage form. Hemosiderin is less water-soluble, has a lower protein content and a coarser, more irregular crystalline structure. Iron stored in hemosiderin is less readily available than that in ferritin.

When abnormally large numbers of red cells are destroyed, increased amounts of iron are released to be placed in storage. The result of hyperhemolysis or of local red cell destruction is that hemosiderin accumulates in reticuloendothelial tissues and in connective tissue. When hemosiderin deposits in tissue outside the reticuloendothelial system, this indicates that there has been destruction of extravasated red cells. This occurs, for example, in the lungs of a patient with congestive pulmonary disease or at the site of tissue bleeding, hemorrhagic infarctions, or thrombus formation.

The quantity of storage iron can be roughly evaluated by examining bone marrow sections for the presence of increased or decreased

hemosiderin. In chronic hemolytic states, large quantities of hemosiderin accumulate in the reticuloendothelial elements of bone
marrow, spleen, and liver. If hyperhemolysis is extreme or long-
standing, especially if also accompanied by ineffective erythropoiesis,
the capacity of the reticuloendothelial system is exceeded and hemosiderin accumulates in parenchymal cells, including liver, pancreas,
and heart.

Ferrokinetic studies with radiolabeled iron indicate that in hemolytic states, iron turnover increases with shortening of plasma half-
life and increased incorporation of iron into total red cell mass.[56]
Ferrokinetic studies are rarely done in evaluating hemolytic anemia,
since the presence of increased tissue iron indicates abnormal iron
metabolism.

Red Cell Fragility

Some metabolic or structural abnormalities make red cells abnormally susceptible to in vitro hemolysis as well as in vivo destruction.
Fragility tests of this sort are less often used than formerly, because
specific techniques are available to diagnose enzyme defects, hemoglobinopathies, and other conditions. Enzyme studies, however, are
not always accessible and are always expensive. Simpler procedures
often permit presumptive diagnosis, although they cannot be definitive. In hemoglobin S disease, hereditary spherocytosis, and several
enzyme deficiencies, red cells withstand mechanical trauma less
well than normal cells, yielding increased free hemoglobin after
exposure to rotatory trauma. This mechanical fragility test is seldom
done, since reproducibility is poor, and comparable or better information is available from other tests.

OSMOTIC FRAGILITY

The test for osmotic fragility exposes red cells to increasingly dilute
saline solutions in order to determine the point at which the in-
migration of water causes red cells to swell and rupture. Normal disc-
shaped cells can imbibe water and swell significantly before membrane capacity is exceeded, but cells with relatively less surface to
volume will lyse after much smaller amounts of fluid enter. Spherocytes and other cells that have undergone membrane damage burst
when exposed to saline solutions not much less concentrated than
normal saline. In hereditary spherocytosis, the increased osmotic
fragility is enhanced still further by incubating the cells at 37°C. for

24 hours before exposing them to hyposmolar saline. Osmotic fragility is increased in autoimmune hemolytic anemia, presumably because the cells are more rigid than normal and undergo gradual membrane loss. In thalassemia, iron deficiency anemia, and sickle cell disease, red cells are more than normally resistant to osmotic damage.

AUTOHEMOLYSIS

Normal red cells readily survive 48 hours of incubation at 37°C. without any exogenous energy source. Red cells with defective ion transport or energy generation tend to hemolyse after spending 48 hours in their own defibrinated plasma with no added nutrients. The autohemolysis test can be used as a screening test for hereditary spherocytosis, since there is markedly increased autohemolysis which is virtually abolished by incubating the cells with glucose or ATP. In glucose-6-phosphate dehydrogenase (G-6-PD) deficiency, autohemolysis is modestly increased, and neither ATP nor glucose has any effect. Cells with pyruvate kinase (PK) deficiency show marked autohemolysis, which is partially alleviated by ATP but not by glucose. For G-6-PD deficiency and PK deficiency, however, better screening tests are readily available.

Enzyme Defects

GLUCOSE-6-PHOSPHATE DEHYDROGENASE

Glucose-6-phosphate dehydrogenase (G-6-PD), an enzyme pivotal in generating NADPH through the pentose phosphate pathway, is remarkably polymorphic. More than 50 structural variants are known in addition to the structurally and functionally normal molecule called type B. The variant called type A migrates slightly faster than B on electrophoresis, but its activity level is virtually normal, and it is considered a nonpathologic alternative form found predominantly in blacks. Many structural variants have normal or near-normal activity.

Clinically apparent dysfunction occurs only when enzyme activity is less than 25 percent of normal. Defective function is uncovered by exposing red cells to an oxidizing stress. G-6-PD acts to generate reducing activity that protects hemoglobin from oxidative denaturation. Cells with normal hemoglobin but severely defective G-6-PD may undergo oxidation with little or no stress. More often, denaturation occurs only with moderate to severe oxidative challenge. The clinical pattern of most symptomatic G-6-PD deficiency is one of episodic hemolysis following a discrete pharmacologic or physiologic challenge.

Specific enzyme assay and electrophoretic characterization permit definitive diagnosis of G-6-PD deficiency. Except in rare cases, or for characterizing unusual genetic variants, screening tests provide all the information needed for clinical diagnosis and treatment. The oldest procedure, now rarely used, is to induce Heinz bodies by incubating blood with acetylphenylhydrazine in an oxygen-rich environment. This test has low sensitivity and poor reproducibility, besides giving misleading "positives" in the presence of unstable hemoglobin. Better screening procedures use chemical end points to demonstrate whether or not there is sufficient G-6-PD to generate protective reducing activity.

In the *methylene blue-methemoglobin test*, muddy brown methemoglobin evolves from the transparent red hemoglobin solution if G-6-PD is severely deficient. This test detects homozygotes for the common defective variants but is not sensitive enough to detect most heterozygotes.

The *ascorbate-cyanide test* challenges hemoglobin with hydrogen peroxide generated from sodium cyanide and sodium ascorbate. Eventually, this will oxidize even cells with normal enzyme activity, but if a 1- or 2-hour end point is used, a brown methemoglobin end point is seen with G-6-PD deficiency, PK deficiency, paroxysmal nocturnal hemoglobinuria, and unstable hemoglobins, while normal blood remains bright red. The ascorbate-cyanide test is sensitive enough to detect the minimally reduced activity that occurs in G-6-PD heterozygotes and in homozygotes with temporarily increased activity levels; it is not, however, specific for G-6-PD deficiency.[7]

The *NADPH fluorescence test* is specific for G-6-PD and its effect on NADP. If dehydrogenase is present, reducing activity is generated, converting NADP to fluorescent NADPH, which appears as a readily visible spot under ultraviolet light. Blood samples up to several weeks old are suitable for use, and the results are moderately sensitive.

INTERPRETATION

Young cells have higher G-6-PD levels than older ones, regardless of the genetic variant which is present. If the enzyme has defective activity, older cells are preferentially destroyed during a mild to moderate hemolytic event. Reticulocytes generated to replace lost cells have high activity levels. False-negative test results often occur if blood is examined just after a hemolytic episode, because the non-hemolyzed remaining cells are, by definition, those with adequate levels. Newly generated reticulocytes have still higher levels, and this can affect the results for 3 to 10 days after the episode. The ascorbate cyanate test is usually sensitive enough to detect reduced activity under these circumstances, but the test should be repeated after red cell production has stabilized.

PYRUVATE KINASE

Defects of pyruvate kinase (PK) activity are less common and less diverse than variants of G-6-PD. PK deficiency is an autosomal recessive trait exhibiting variably severe, chronic, nonspherocytic hemolysis, which is exacerbated by stresses such as infection. Although fewer than 200 cases have been reported, it constitutes the second most frequent deficiency of a defined red cell enzyme. PK-deficient cells are positive in the ascorbate cyanate screening test. In the specific procedure, normal cells consume fluorescent NADH in converting pyruvate to lactate, while PK-deficient cells, unable to transform the pyruvate, exert no effect on the degree of fluorescence. The test must employ a carefully separated red cell suspension because white cells contribute significant PK activity. Like G-6-PD, PK is higher in reticulocytes and young red cells; falsely normal results occur in samples drawn shortly after an episode of accelerated hemolysis.

Imperfectly Characterized Membrane Defects

HEREDITARY SPHEROCYTOSIS

Osmotic fragility and autohemolysis are the best presumptive tests for hereditary spherocytosis. The specific defect responsible for this rather common familial disease remains unknown, and thus there is no definitive procedure for its diagnosis. The clinical picture of hereditary spherocytosis is detailed in a later section.

TESTS FOR PAROXYSMAL
NOCTURNAL HEMOGLOBINURIA

Paroxysmal nocturnal hemoglobinuria (PNH) is an acquired hemolytic condition in which red cells have decreased levels of the enzyme cholinesterase and are abnormally susceptible to complement-mediated hemolysis. Complement and its interactions with antibodies and membranes are considered in a later section (p. 184). Several effective, extremely simple screening tests for PNH can be done readily on any patient with hemolysis.[44] It has long been noted that PNH cells are hemolyzed by exposure to acidified, complement-containing human serum. Since the serum of a symptomatic patient is often complement-depleted, the test is performed best by incubating the patient's cells with *acidified normal serum*. A pH of 6.5 to 7.0 can be achieved by adding 1 volume of 0.2N HCl to 9 volumes of serum. Normal cells are unaffected, but frank hemolysis occurs with PNH and may be seen with hereditary or acquired spherocytosis or with hereditary dyserythropoietic anemia (HEMPAS cells).

The *sugar water test* distinguishes PNH from hereditary dyserythropoietic anemia. Serum whose complement has been activated by the addition of sucrose solution of low ionic strength hemolyzes PNH cells but not cells with other defects. Heparin or EDTA anticoagulants may cause false negatives, and defibrinated blood may give false positives.

Hemoglobinopathies

Hemolysis is associated with only a few of the more than 100 known abnormal hemoglobins. Of these, the group known as *unstable hemoglobins* or *Heinz body anemias* are numerically insignificant, although biochemically fascinating. Hemoglobin S and hemoglobin C, however, are common among the world's black populations and contribute significantly to worldwide morbidity from all causes.

SICKLE CELL PREPARATION

When hemoglobin S is exposed to low oxygen tensions, the molecules link together as a repeating polymeric configuration called a *tactoid* or *nematic fluid crystal*.[55] This occurs whether the hemoglobin is free in solution or confined within cells. The classic screening test for hemoglobin S is to add sodium metabisulfite, a powerful reducing agent, to a cell suspension. As the oxygen tension falls, cells containing hemoglobin S assume the boat-shaped or crescentic *sickle* form. Sickling is more rapid and complete if hemoglobin S is the only hemoglobin in each cell, but the metabisulfite creates such low oxygen tension that substantial sickling occurs even in cells with large amounts of hemoglobin A or other non-S hemoglobin. The end point is observed microscopically after 15 minutes. The test requires a sizable investment in time, equipment, and personnel, if large numbers of samples must be processed. False negatives may occur if technique is poor, but false positives are extremely rare.

SOLUBILITY TEST

A very quick, moderately effective screening test exploits the fact that polymers of deoxygenated hemoglobin S are insoluble, creating turbidity in an aqueous medium. A dithionite solution is used to reduce the hemoglobin. When 0.02 ml. of blood is added to 2 ml. of reagent and incubated for 3 minutes, polymerized hemoglobin S makes the tube so turbid that black print cannot be read through the solution.[28] Both homozygous and heterozygous hemoglobin S cells give positive results, but because positive results depend on the absolute amount of reduced hemoglobin S present, false negatives may occur in severe anemia. It is helpful to add double the usual amount of blood if the hematocrit is below 30 percent. False positives can occur if the concentrated reagent solution causes myeloma proteins or other abnormal serum constituents to precipitate; if the red cells contain numerous Heinz bodies, or if too much blood has been added. Electrophoresis, the technique for definitive diagnosis, should be done to confirm positive screening results and to evaluate patients with negative screening tests but with clinical history strongly suggestive of sickle cell disease.

ELECTROPHORESIS

Electrophoresis, which separates hemoglobins according to their mobility in an electric field, is usually enough to characterize all hemoglobins present, but occasionally other biochemical and genetic studies are needed for complete delineation. Electrophoresis easily distinguishes between homozygous and heterozygous hemoglobin S, which screening procedures cannot do. It also detects hemoglobin C, for which there are no biochemical screening tests. Increased amounts of HgbA$_2$ or HgbF have diagnostic significance in the thalassemias and can be demonstrated with electrophoresis.

Antibody-Mediated Destruction

The evaluation of autoimmune and isoimmune processes that cause hemolysis is discussed in Chapter 8.

SPECIAL LEUKOCYTE STUDIES

Histochemical Studies

White cells on a freshly made blood film retain enzyme activity and can alter added substrates. This is most useful when cells are morphologically so abnormal that it is difficult to detect what cell line they came from. Enzyme studies also are useful in assessing cellular maturation and evaluating departures from normal differentiation.

ALKALINE PHOSPHATASE

Among the enzymes in neutrophilic granules is a phosphatase capable of hydrolyzing phosphate-containing substrates into a product that binds to highly colored dyes. Leukocyte alkaline phosphatase (LAP) can be roughly quantitated by scoring the size and intensity of the stained granules. Normal levels fall between 13 and 130 out of a maximum of 400. LAP increases in polycythemia vera and myelofibrosis, and decreases in chronic granulocytic leukemia. It is normal or elevated in leukemoid reactions to infections. Since all these conditions have increased numbers of immature circulating neutrophils, LAP scores can be helpful in distinguishing them. Hypoplastic or ineffective marrow activity is often accompanied by decreased LAP, as, for example, in pernicious anemia, aplastic anemia, and thrombocytopenia. Values are often low in paroxysmal nocturnal hemoglobinuria and infectious mononucleosis. Women on oral contraceptives often have higher than normal values. Leukocyte alkaline phosphatase is completely independent of serum alkaline phosphatase.

LEUKOCYTE PEROXIDASE

During maturation, young neutrophils and eosinophils and, to a lesser extent, monocytes contain an enzyme that transfers hydrogen from a donor compound to hydrogen peroxide. Immature lymphocytes do not have this enzyme. The peroxidase test is useful in identifying cells with few or no visible granules. The blasts of acute leukemia can often be classified in this way.

SUDAN BLACK B

Sudan black B stains neutral fats and reacts intensely with lipid elements in cytoplasmic granules and Auer rods. In acute leukemias, myeloblasts tend to be moderately or heavily stained and may have small, discrete sudanophilic granules, while lymphoblasts remain unstained.

Philadelphia Chromosome (Ph¹)

Granulocytes cultured from the peripheral blood or bone marrow in chronic granulocytic leukemia consistently contain an abnormal G group chromosome (chromosome 22) called the *Philadelphia chromosome* (Ph¹). Half the long arm of this already small chromosome is absent, a feature whose significance is more diagnostic than constitutional. Granulocytes in Ph¹-positive chronic leukemias consistently have low levels of leukocyte alkaline phosphatase, but the two observations may not be causally related. The Philadelphia chromosome is an acquired abnormality found only in hematopoietic cells during active disease. During complete remission, the abnormal chromosome disappears from peripheral blood cells but persists in the marrow.[55] Ph¹ remains present during the terminal blast crisis of chronic granulocytic leukemia but does not occur in the blastic presentation of acute granulocytic leukemia. There is some suggestion that the relatively few CGL patients negative for Ph¹ have a poorer prognosis than do Ph¹-positive cases.[12]

REFERENCES

1. Akun, S. N., Miller, I. F., and Meyer, L. M.: *Vitamin B₁₂ absorption test.* Acta Haematol. 41:341, 1969.
2. Allen, R. H.: *Human vitamin B₁₂ transport proteins.* Prog. Hematol. 9:57, 1975.
3. Beck, W. S.: *Folic acid deficiency,* in Williams, W. J., Beutler, E., Erslev, A. J., and Rundles, R. W. (eds.): *Hematology.* ed. 2. McGraw-Hill, New York, 1977.
4. Beck, W. S.: *Vitamin B₁₂ deficiency,* in Williams, W. J., Beutler, E., Erslev, A. J., and Rundles, R. W. (eds.): *Hematology.* ed. 2. McGraw-Hill, New York, 1977.
5. Berlin, N. I., and Berk, P. D.: *The biological life of the red cell,* in Surgenor, D.MacN. (ed.): *The Red Blood Cell.* Academic Press, New York, 1975.
6. Bessis, M., and Lessin, L.: *The discocyte-echinocyte equilibrium of the normal and pathologic red cell.* Blood 36:399, 1970.
7. Beutler, E.: *Energy metabolism and maintenance of erythrocytes,* in Williams, W. J., Beutler, E., Erslev, A. J., and Rundles, R. W. (eds.): *Hematology.* ed. 2. McGraw-Hill, New York, 1977.
8. Beutler, E.: *Red Cell Metabolism: A Manual of Biochemical Methods.* ed. 2. Grune & Stratton, New York, 1975.
9. Bull, B. S., and Kuhn, I. N.: *The production of schistocytes by fibrin strands (a scanning electron microscopic study).* Blood 35:104, 1970.

10. Bunn, H. F.: *Erythrocyte destruction and hemoglobin catabolism.* Semin. Hematol. 9:3, 1972.

11. Cartwright, G. E., and Deiss, A.: *Sideroblasts, siderocytes, and sideroblastic anemia.* N. Engl. J. Med. 292:185, 1975.

12. Cline, M. J.: *The White Cell.* Harvard University Press, Cambridge, Mass., 1975.

13. Committee for Clarification of the Nomenclature of Cells and Diseases of the Blood and Blood Forming Organs: *Condensation of first two reports.* Blood 4:89, 1949

14. Cooper, R. A.: *Destruction of erythrocytes,* in Williams, W. J., Beutler, E., Erslev, A. J., and Rundles, R. W. (eds.): *Hematology.* ed. 2. McGraw-Hill, New York, 1977.

15. Cotter, D. A., and Sage, B. H.: *Performance of the LARC classifier in clinical laboratories.* J. Histochem. Cytochem. 24:202, 1976.

16. *Disorders of neutrophil function.* Lancet 1:438, 1974.

17. Dutcher, T. F., Benzel, J. E., Egan, J. J., et al.: *Evaluation of an automated differential leukocyte counting system. I. Instrument description and reproducibility studies.* Am. J. Clin. Pathol. 62:525, 1974.

18. Ebbe, S.: *Thrombopoietin.* Blood 44:605, 1975.

19. Elder, G., Gray, C. H., and Nicholson, D. C.: *Bile pigment fate in gastrointestinal tract.* Semin. Hematol. 9:71, 1972.

20. England, J. M., and Fraser, P. M.: *Differentiation of iron deficiency from thalassemia trait by routine blood count.* Lancet 1:449, 1973.

21. England, J. M., Ward, S. M., and Down, M. C.: *Microcytosis, anisocytosis and the red cell indices in iron deficiency.* Br. J. Haematol. 34:589, 1976.

22. Erslev, A. J., and Silver, R. K.: *Compensated hemolytic anemia.* Blood Cells 1:509, 1975.

23. Finch, S. C.: *Granulocytopenia,* in Williams, W. J., Beutler, E., Erslev, A. J., and Rundles, R. W. (eds.): *Hematology.* ed. 2. McGraw-Hill, New York, 1977.

24. Finch, S. C.: *Granulocytosis,* in Williams, W. J., Beutler, E., Erslev, A. J., and Rundles, R. W. (eds.): *Hematology.* ed. 2. McGraw-Hill, New York, 1977.

25. Freeman, L. M., and Blautox, M. D.: *Hematological studies with radionuclides.* Semin. Nucl. Med. 5:1, 1975.

26. Gansome, A. M., Oakes, R., and Hillman, R. S.: *Red cell aging in vivo.* J. Clin. Invest. 50:1371, 1971.

27. Glaser, K., Limarzi, L. R., and Poncher, H. G.: *Cellular composition of the bone marrow in normal infants and children.* Pediatrics 6:789, 1950.

28. Greenberg, M. S. Harvey, H. A., and Morgan, C.: *A simple and inexpensive screening test for sickle hemoglobin.* N. Engl. J. Med. 286:1143, 1972.

29. Haurani, F. I.: *Vitamin B_{12} and the megaloblastic development.* Science 182:78, 1973.

30. Hillman, R. S.: *Acute blood loss anemia,* in Williams, W. J., Beutler, E., Erslev, A. J., and Rundles, R. W. (eds.): *Hematology.* ed. 2. McGraw-Hill, New York, 1977.

31. Ingram, M., and Preston, K., Jr.: *Automatic analysis of blood cells.* Sci. Am. 223:72, 1970.

32. International Committee for Standardization in Haematology: *Recommendations for haemoglobinometry in human blood.* Br. J. Haematol. (Suppl.) 13:71, 1967.
33. ISCH Panel on Diagnostic Applications of Radioisotopes in Hematology: *Recommended methods for radioisotope red cell survival studies.* Br. J. Haematol. 21:241, 1971.
34. Jacob, H. S.: *Mechanism of Heinz body formation and attachment to red cell membrane.* Semin. Hematol. 7:341, 1970.
35. Kelly, A., and Munan, L.: *Haematological profile of natural populations: red cell parameters.* Br. J. Haematol. 35:153, 1977.
36. Klug, P., Lessin, L., and Radice, P.: *Rheological aspects of sickle cell anemia.* Arch. Intern. Med. 133:577, 1974.
37. Lessin, L. S., and Bessis, M.: *Morphology of the erythron,* in Williams, W. J., Beutler, E., Erslev, A. J., and Rundles, R. W. (eds.): *Hematology.* ed. 2. McGraw-Hill, New York, 1977.
38. MacPherson, B. R.: *The clinical and laboratory diagnosis of chronic granulomatous disease of childhood.* CRC Crit. Rev. Clin. Lab. Sci. 8:81, 1977.
39. Naets, J. P., and Wittek, M.: *Erythropoiesis in anephric man.* Lancet 1:941, 1968.
40. Osgood, E. E., and Seaman, A. J.: *The cellular composition of normal bone marrow, as obtained by sternal puncture.* Physiol. Rev. 24:46, 1944.
41. Pearson, H. A., and O'Brien, R. T.: *Sickle cell screening in newborns.* Am. J. Dis. Child. 130:799, 1976.
42. Phillips, M. J., and Harkness, J.: *Plasma and whole blood viscosity.* Br. J. Haematol. 34:347, 1976.
43. Robinson, W. A., and Mangalik, A.: *The kinetics and regulation of granulopoiesis.* Semin. Hematol. 12:7, 1975.
44. Rosse, W. F.: *Studies for paroxysmal nocturnal hemoglobinuria,* in *Williams, W. J., Beutler, E., Erslev, A. J., and Rundles, R. W. (eds.): Hematology.* ed. 2. McGraw-Hill, New York, 1977.
45. Roth, E. F., Elbaum, D., and Nagel, R. L.: *Observation on the mechanical precipitation of oxy-Hb S and other mutants.* Blood 45:377, 1975.
46. Silver, R. K., and Erslev, A. J.: *The action of erythropoietin on erythroid cells in vitro.* Scand. J. Haematol. 13:338, 1974.
47. Simmons, A., and Elbert, G.: *Hemalog-D and manual differential leukocyte counts: a laboratory comparison of results obtained with blood of hospitalized patients.* Am. J. Clin. Pathol. 64:512, 1975.
48. *Testing neutrophil function.* Lancet 2:1391, 1976.
49. Todd, D.: *Diagnosis of haemolytic states.* Clin. Haematol. 4:63, 1975.
50. Vaughn, S. L., and Brockmyre, F.: *Normal bone marrow as obtained by sternal puncture.* Blood (special issue) 1:54, 1947.
51. Weed, R. I.: *The importance of erythrocyte deformability.* Am. J. Med. 49:147, 1970.
52. Weiss, L., and Chen, L.-T.: *The organization of hematopoietic cords and vascular sinuses in bone marrow.* Blood Cells 1:617, 1975.
53. Weiss, L., and Tavassoli, M.: *Anatomical hazards to the passage of erythrocytes through the spleen.* Semin. Hematol. 7:372, 1970.

54. Williams, W. J., and Schneider, A. S.: *Examination of the peripheral blood,*
    in Williams, W. J., Beutler, E., Erslev, A. J., and Rundles, R. W. (eds.):
    Hematology. ed. 2. McGraw-Hill, New York, 1977.
55. Wintrobe, M. M., Lee, G. R., Boggs, D. R., et al.: *Clinical Hematology.* ed.
    7. Lea & Febiger, Philadelphia, 1974.
56. Yamada, H., and Gabuzda, T. G.: *Erythroblast ferritin: synthesis, structure,
    and function in developing erythroid cells.* J. Lab. Clin. Med. 83:478, 1974.
57. Zucker-Franklin, D.: *Eosinophil function and disorders.* Adv. Intern. Med.
    19:1, 1974.

CHAPTER 2

HEMOSTASIS AND TESTS OF HEMOSTATIC FUNCTION

Hemostasis is the collective term for all the mechanisms the body uses to protect itself from blood loss. Holes in the cardiovascular system must be prevented or repaired to avoid excessive blood loss. In order to flow, blood must remain fluid; under conditions requiring hemostasis, fluid blood becomes solid. This affects local circulation and can affect the rest of the circulatory system as well. Several interrelated systems affect both hemostasis and the maintenance of fluidity and circulation.

Failure of hemostasis leads to *hemorrhage*; failure to maintain fluidity leads to *thrombosis*. Both hemorrhage and thrombosis are extremely common and dangerous clinical problems. It is easier to identify and treat hemorrhage than to prevent or treat thrombosis. Characterizing the defects that cause hemorrhage is, at present, incomparably easier than characterizing potentially treatable conditions that predispose to thrombosis.

HEMOSTASIS

Hemostatic mechanisms are organized into three categories: vascular activity, platelet function, and coagulation. Blood vessels have one or several layers of smooth muscle surrounding endothelial lining cells. When vessels are damaged, muscle constricts, narrowing the path through which blood flows and sometimes halting blood flow entirely. This *vascular phase* of hemostasis affects only arterioles and their dependent capillaries; large vessels cannot constrict sufficiently to prevent blood loss. Even in small vessels, vasoconstriction provides only the briefest sort of hemostasis.

Permanent repair requires that breaks in the vessel wall be plugged; the effective hemostatic plug consists of platelets and the gel-like protein *fibrin. Platelets* are non-nucleated fragments of cell cytoplasm, but they are living entities with complex structure, active metabolism, and a reactive biological constitution. *Coagulation* is a chemical process whereby plasma proteins interact to convert the large protein molecule *fibrinogen* into the stable gel called fibrin.

Platelet Activity

Platelets are essential to protect vascular surfaces from the countless "microtraumas" of everyday life. Patients whose platelets are deficient either in number or function experience innumerable tiny hemorrhages. It is not clear how platelets prevent these tiny leaks from occurring. In some way, platelets protect endothelial surfaces or cell junctions and repair incipient damage before it becomes apparent.[31]

ADHERENCE AND RELEASE

Damage to vessel walls exposes flowing blood to basement membrane, collagen, elastic fibrils, and other elements of the wall that are usually inaccessible. Within a second or two, platelets adhere lightly to injured areas where these materials are exposed. The initial phase of adherence is a surface phenomenon, and participating platelets retain their original shape and appearance. The interactions of adherence, however, stimulate platelets to release their intracellular adenosine diphosphate (ADP) into the immediate environment.[17] As ADP builds up in the environment, platelets undergo a shape change, becoming less disc-like and more irregular and intertwined. The accumulation of ADP and of irregularly shaped platelets recruits additional platelets from the passing blood stream into the adherent mass.

IRREVERSIBLE CHANGES

As additional ADP is released, the platelets undergo irreversible aggregation and release additional material from their cytoplasmic granules. ADP, serotonin, and other vasoactive amines accumulate within and around the platelet mass. This release phenomenon results partly from stimulation by ADP and partly from the lytic effects of *thrombin*, a proteolytic enzyme generated when the coagulation system is activated. Platelet activity and coagulation enhance each other, since aggregated platelets contribute phospholipid (platelet factor 3) to the coagulation sequence. Local slowing of blood flow, local chemical changes, and alterations of the vascular surface stimulate the coagulation system, so that thrombin is generated. Thrombin cleaves fibrinogen to generate fibrin, and fibrin strands surround and strengthen the platelet plug. It is this combined mass of platelets and fibrin that constitutes the *hemostatic plug* which is effective in sealing the vascular break and preventing further blood loss.

PLATELET PHYSIOLOGY

Platelets derive from the cytoplasm of *megakaryocytes* — large, multinucleated cells found in the bone marrow. After platelets bud from the megakaryocyte, their structure includes an outer membrane, numerous granules, mitochondria, contractile proteins, and a "microskeleton" of cytoplasmic tubules that allows the platelets to change shape. Normal blood contains approximately 150,000 to 450,000 platelets/mm.[3] Of these, about one tenth are required to maintain endothelial integrity,[2] and the remainder are available for hemostasis.

Platelets survive only 9 or 10 days in the circulation, but their fate is somewhat mysterious. Abnormally large spleens sequester and destroy platelets with unusual rapidity, but in normal circumstances, it is not clear what happens to unused platelets. Platelet production is apparently controlled by a humoral activity which, by analogy with erythropoietin, is called *thrombopoietin*; no specific substance, however, has been found or characterized.[10] When thrombopoietic stimulation occurs, megakaryocyte numbers increase, and platelets are processed more rapidly from inception through maturation to release. Platelets which are released early are larger than normal. An increase in the mean size of circulating platelets tends to indicate either specific stimulation of the megakaryocytes or generalized bone marrow hyperactivity.[20]

Coagulation

Fibrin, the visible end product of coagulation, is a gelatinous protein easily identified in tissues or test tubes. Conversion of fibrinogen to fibrin is the last step in a highly complex series of protein interactions which can best be described schematically (Fig. 4). Official nomen-

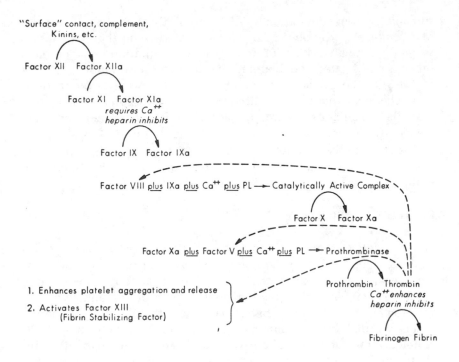

PL = Phospholipid

Figure 4.   A schematic representation of the sequential interactions that cause blood to coagulate (i.e., that convert fibrinogen to fibrin). Pictured is the intrinsic system of plasma procagulants. In the extrinsic system, the product of tissue thromboplastin and Factor VII interaction directly activates Factor X; the remaining reactions are the same for both systems. (Reproduced with permission from Widmann, F. K.: *Pathobiology: How Disease Happens.* Little, Brown, Boston, 1978.)

clature uses Roman numerals to identify coagulation factors;[35] some have descriptive or eponymic names as well. Almost all these factors are present in circulating blood in an inactive, precursor form. The activated form which participates in the sequence is designated by an "a" after the number.

THE COMMON PATHWAY

Activation of Factor X (Stuart factor) initiates the terminal phase of coagulation; the several events that can activate Factor X are described below. Activated Factor X cleaves the glycoprotein *pro-*

thrombin to produce the proteolytic enzyme *thrombin*. The reaction of Xa with prothrombin requires calcium ions and phospholipid and is markedly enhanced by association with another plasma protein, *Factor V*.

Thrombin is a proteolytic enzyme of tremendous potency and relatively little discrimination. The quantity of thrombin that evolves from a single milliliter of plasma, if released simultaneously throughout the circulation, could solidify the entire blood stream. Under normal hemostatic conditions, only small amounts of thrombin develop at a time. Besides converting fibrinogen to fibrin, thrombin also enhances platelet release reactions (see preceding section), and augments the activation of Factor V and Factor VIII (see below). Under pathologic conditions, thrombin can cleave fibrin into fragments and split the peptide bonds in a wide range of proteins.

Fibrinogen becomes fibrin when thrombin removes the tips of two pairs of peptide chains. The resulting molecule, which consists of 97 percent of the original fibrinogen molecule, is a fibrin monomer. Fibrin monomers polymerize spontaneously to form a loosely adherent gel which quickly depolymerizes if exposed, in laboratory conditions, to a 5 M. urea solution or 1 percent monochloroacetic acid. In vivo, the fibrin monomer constitutes a bulky but fragile clot. Irreversible polymerization occurs when activated Factor XIII causes the peptide bonds to cross-link. Thrombin is also responsible for activating Factor XIII.

THE INTRINSIC PATHWAY

Everything necessary to activate Factor X exists in normal plasma but in inactive form. A suitable initiating stimulus sets into motion the cascade of activating events. This sequence is called the *intrinsic pathway* because all constituents are already in the blood. The *extrinsic pathway* also activates Factor X, but elements from outside the blood must be present as well. The proteins that induce Factor X activation are called *plasma procoagulants*.

Intrinsic coagulation begins with activation of *Factor XII* (Hageman factor). Materials or surfaces characterized by rigidly spaced negative charges will activate Factor XII. In the laboratory, contact with glass, kaolin, or ellagic acid activates Factor XII, but exposure to "nonwettable" surfaces such as silicone or some plastics will not do so. In physiologic settings, activation of Factor XII follows contact with altered vascular surfaces, with antigen-antibody complexes, or with other biologically active proteins such as those of the complement or kallikrein systems. Another coagulation protein, *Fletcher factor,* participates in activation of Hageman factor, but the mechanism remains obscure.[32]

Activated Factor XII converts *Factor XI* to XIa. Persons congenitally deficient in Factor XII or Fletcher factor suffer no apparent hemostatic deficiency, and thus the significance of contact activation remains mysterious. Absence of Factor XI, however, does cause bleeding problems. In the presence of ionized calcium, Factor XIa converts *Factor IX* to its active form, which then interacts with *Factor VIII.* Small amounts of heparin inhibit this interaction. Full physiologic action of Factor VIII requires ionized calcium and phospholipid, and is enhanced by thrombin. What activates Factor X is the combined product of IXa, VIII, calcium, phospholipid, and possibly also thrombin. Absence or inactivity of Factor IX or Factor VIII causes severe bleeding disorders.

THE EXTRINSIC PATHWAY

Products of damaged tissue induce coagulation of fluid blood. Although the nature of the *tissue factor* is not entirely clear, it seems to involve both lipid and protein elements. Another name for this ill-defined, clot-promoting principle is *tissue thromboplastin.* Tissue juices alone, however, are ineffective. Also needed are calcium ions and the plasma protein called *Factor VII.* Just how Factor VII, tissue thromboplastin, and calcium combine to activate Factor X is not understood. Indeed the physiologic significance of the entire extrinsic system is unclear. It seems to be an alternate route to the common goal of Factor X activation, but in a clinical sense, the extrinsic and intrinsic pathways are not substitutes for one another. Factor VII deficiency by itself is very rare but can cause severe bleeding. The hemorrhagic diathesis of Factor VIII or Factor IX deficiency, however, is far more severe.

In the laboratory, Factor X also can be activated by exposure to snake venom (e.g., that of the Russell's viper) or to trypsin. This appears to be direct proteolytic cleavage which does not require Factor VII.

THE CLOTTING FACTORS

Factor I. Factor I, always called *fibrinogen*, is a glycoprotein weighing 330,000 daltons and is composed of three pairs of polypeptide chains. Synthesized in the liver, it has a half-life of about 3.5 to 4 days. Fibrinogen levels increase with hemostatic stress and also with nonspecific stresses such as inflammation, pregnancy, or autoimmune illnesses. Normal plasma concentration is 150 to 400 mg./dl.

Factor II. Factor II, usually called *prothrombin*, is a glycoprotein with a molecular weight of 70,000 daltons, which is closely related to Factors VII, IX, and X. All are manufactured in the liver and require fat-soluble vitamin K for synthesis. All four of these "liver factors" are heat-stable, retain their potency in stored blood or plasma, and remain present in serum after plasma has clotted. Prothrombin has a half-life of 2.5 to 3 days.

Factor III. Factor III is the term assigned to *tissue thromboplastin*, but the numerical designation is never used. The clot-promoting activity of tissue products is too poorly characterized to be described as a specific factor. The most active tissues are brain, lung, and placenta, but all tissues have some clot-promoting activity.

Factor IV. Factor IV, or *ionized calcium*, is necessary for activation of Factor IX, for activation of Factor X by the IXa-VIII-phospholipid complex, for conversion of prothrombin to thrombin by Xa, and for polymerization of fibrin monomers. There must be at least 2.5 mg./dl. of calcium before coagulation can occur in vivo or in vitro. Hypocalcemia never causes clinical bleeding difficulties, however, because the heart stops beating when calcium levels decline to values still well above 2.5 mg./dl. Citrate, oxalate, and EDTA are anticoagulants because they chelate calcium and prevent it from participating in coagulation.

Factor V. Factor V, also known as *proaccelerin* and *labile factor*, is a poorly characterized protein, which is synthesized in the liver and may be low in patients with liver disease. Its activity disappears rapidly when anticoagulated blood or plasma is stored in liquid state. It also disappears rapidly from circulating blood and has a half-life of only 15 hours.

Factor VI. This term is not used.

Factor VII. Factor VII is variously called *proconvertin, autoprothrombin I, serum prothrombin conversion accelerator,* and *SPCA.* The multiplicity of names reflects uncertainty about its structure, origin, and function. It is usually referred to by number. One of the vitamin K-dependent liver factors, it has a half-life of 5 hours and is the first clotting factor to decline after administration of vitamin K antagonists.

Factor VIII. Factor VIII is also known as *antihemophilic factor, AHF,* and *antihemophilic globulin.* The site and manner of its production remain unclear. Factor VIII has a biologic half-life of 10 hours and disappears rapidly from stored liquid blood or plasma. Congenital deficiency of Factor VIII causes hemophilia A or classical hemophilia, the commonest of the constitutional bleeding disorders. Many Factor VIII-deficient patients manufacture a protein that has antigenic properties of normal Factor VIII but lacks procoagulant activity.

Factor IX. Factor IX, also called *Christmas factor, plasma thromboplastin component,* and *PTC,* is another vitamin K-dependent liver factor. Unlike II, VII, and X, Factor IX deficiency exists fairly commonly as an isolated constitutional defect. The disease hemophilia B, or Christmas disease, closely resembles Factor VIII deficiency in laboratory aspects. The factor has a physiologic half-life of about 24 hours but remains at high levels in stored liquid plasma. It is also present in serum.

Factor X. Factor X, often referred to as *Stuart factor* or *Stuart-Prower factor,* is another of the vitamin K-dependent liver factors and is the key protein in all activation pathways. Isolated congenital deficiency does occur, though rarely, causing moderately severe clinical bleeding. Factor X has a biologic half-life of about 40 hours.

Factor XI. Factor XI is also known as *plasma thromboplastin antecedent* or *PTA.* Probably synthesized in the liver, this factor does not diminish in liver disease and is not vitamin K-dependent. It is stable in stored blood or plasma and is present in serum. Isolated deficiency occurs as an autosomal-recessive trait. After Factor VIII and Factor IX deficiencies, it is the least uncommon congenital deficiency state, but the bleeding diathesis is rather mild. The biologic half-life is about 2 days.

Factor XII. Factor XII, commonly called *Hageman factor,* is a real mystery. Its source and physiologic function are unknown. It exists at very low concentrations in plasma and remains present in serum. Isolated deficiency does not cause bleeding manifestations, and the first patient found to have Factor XII deficiency subsequently died of thrombosis at a fairly ripe age. The biologic half-life is about 2 days.

Factor XIII. Factor XIII is the *fibrin stabilizing factor.* Both liver and megakaryocytes appear to be implicated in Factor XIII production. More than half of blood XIII levels exist in platelets. It has a long biologic half-life (5 to 10 days) but disappears when plasma is converted to serum.

SERUM VS. PLASMA

Plasma is the liquid part of fluid blood. Outside the vascular system, blood can be kept fluid either by removing fibrinogen or by adding anticoagulants, most of which prevent coagulation by chelating calcium ions. *Citrate, oxalate,* and *EDTA* are anticoagulants of the chelating agent category. *Heparin* prevents coagulation by directly inhibiting thrombin; it prevents conversion of fibrinogen to fibrin without affecting calcium concentration. Freshly drawn plasma contains all proteins present in circulating blood; as plasma is stored, Factor V and Factor VIII activity gradually decline.

Serum is the fluid remaining after blood coagulates. Coagulation converts all fibrinogen into solid fibrin and consumes Factor VIII, Factor V, and prothrombin in the process. The other coagulation proteins, and proteins not related to hemostasis, remain in serum at the same levels as in plasma. Normal serum lacks fibrinogen, prothrombin, Factor VIII, Factor V, and Factor XIII, but contains Factors XII, XI, IX, X, and VII. If the coagulation process proceeds abnormally, serum may contain residual fibrinogen, fibrinogen cleavage products, or unconverted prothrombin.

Absorbing plasma with barium sulfate or aluminum hydroxide removes the vitamin K-dependent "liver factors" (i.e., Factors II, VII, IX, and X). Barium-absorbed plasma contains fibrinogen, Factor XIII, the labile Factors VIII and V, and Factors XII and XI. It does not coagulate because prothrombin and Factor X are absent, as are Factor VII, which is needed for extrinsic activation, and Factor IX, which is needed for intrinsic activation. Factors XII and XI are stable in stored plasma, are not absorbed by barium, and are not consumed in the coagulation process.

ANTAGONISTS TO HEMOSTASIS

Both platelet activation and coagulation are self-perpetuating processes. As interaction products accumulate, they initiate further activation, a sequence that could, if unchecked, cause massive coagulation and interference with blood flow. Circulatory dynamics help to prevent uncontrolled activation. Local conditions of platelet activation and fibrin deposition dissipate if newly entering blood dilutes activated coagulation factors or disperses aggregated platelets. Partially activated coagulation factors are carried to the liver and reticuloendothelial system where they are degraded. Briskly flowing blood also brings in antagonists to specific coagulation products.

Fibrinolysis

Stable polymerized fibrin is dissolved and gradually removed by a fibrinolytic system somewhat analogous, in its stepwise activation, to the coagulation system. Fibrin is cleaved into progressively smaller fragments by *plasmin*, a proteolytic enzyme which, like thrombin, acts potently against many protein substrates and does not circulate in active form. Normal plasma contains 10 to 20 mg./dl. of the precursor substance, *plasminogen*.

Plasminogen is converted to plasmin by several *plasminogen activators*. Tissues of the genitourinary tract contain *urokinase*, an activator which has full activity at the time it enters the circulation. Endothelial cells and plasma contain a precursor product that remains inactive until contact with injured tissue converts it into a plasminogen activator. An intrinsic system of plasminogen activation also exists which cascades into action when Factor XII and Fletcher factor are activated. *Streptokinase*, a streptococcal product, also has plasminogen-activating capability.

PLASMIN AND ITS ANTAGONISTS

Once generated, plasmin exerts rather indiscriminate proteolytic activity. Besides digesting fibrin, it also cleaves fibrinogen into peptide fragments that are incoagulable and prevent coagulation of normal fibrinogen.[21] Plasmin also degrades Factor VIII, Factor V, and Factor XIII. Normally, very little plasmin accumulates. Plasma contains two agents that neutralize plasmin: a rapidly acting *antiplasmin* and a slower acting antagonist, *alpha-1-antitrypsin*. Under physiologic conditions, plasmin is protected from these antagonists because it is sheltered by its close proximity to fibrin.

Plasminogen adsorbs to fibrin as fibrin deposits, and bound plasminogen is gradually activated by contact with endothelial elements, a process which, under normal conditions, generates just the right amount of plasmin to prevent excessive fibrin accumulation. Excessive accumulation of activated plasmin can cause proteolysis directed locally at proteins other than fibrin. Systemic activation of plasmin may also occur, or plasmin antagonists may be exhausted. The section on disseminated intravascular coagulation (p. 168) discusses some of the consequences.

Antithrombin Activity

Various substances and interaction products that inhibit thrombin have been assigned Roman numerals from I through VI; only two have merited much attention. "*Antithrombin I*" is not a substance. The term refers to the adsorptive capacity of fibrin, which blots up and inactivates large quantities of thrombin. Adsorbed thrombin retains proteolytic potential, but its physical confinement by fibrin prevents it from exerting enzymatic activity.

HEPARIN AND ANTITHROMBIN III

Antithrombin III is an α_2-globulin, synthesized by the liver, which causes slow but irreversible neutralization of thrombin. One milliliter of normal plasma contains enough antithrombin III to neutralize 300 NIH units of thrombin; the fibrin that develops from 1 ml. of plasma can adsorb 1000 units of thrombin. Antithrombin III acts earlier in the coagulation process than fibrin does, and it also inhibits the activated forms of Factors XI, IX, X, and VII. Its actions thus affect both intrinsic and extrinsic coagulation systems. There is increasing evidence that antithrombin III is an important physiologic monitor that prevents inappropriate or pathological clot formation.[33] Heparin greatly augments the actions of antithrombin III; this action may well be heparin's major anticoagulant mechanism. Antithrombin III appears to be the material formerly described as *heparin cofactor*.

TESTS OF PLATELET ACTIVITY

Patients with too few platelets, or with platelets that function poorly, experience numerous, pinpoint-sized hemorrhages (*petechiae*) and multiple small, superficial bruises (*ecchymoses*). Frequently there is generalized oozing from mucosal surfaces, especially the gastrointestinal tract, and from venipuncture sites or other small, localized injuries. Large, deep hematomas and bleeding into joints are not characteristic of thrombocytopenia. *Thrombocytopenia*, the presence of too few platelets, occurs a great deal more often than *thrombopathias*, or disorders of function. Many laboratory procedures reveal defects of platelet number or function, but most have proved difficult to standardize or to adapt to general clinical application.

Bleeding Time

The single best indication of platelet deficiency is prolonged bleeding after a controlled, superficial injury. The bleeding time is prolonged in thrombocytopenia of any cause, in von Willebrand's disease, in most dysfunctional conditions, and after aspirin exposure. The bleeding time test is somewhat difficult to standardize and to use repeatedly for evaluation of changing conditions. Every operator performs it differently; the nature of the "standard" injury differs each time it is inflicted; and results differ with different skin sites and external conditions. In addition, it is unpleasant for patients to be subjected to a standard skin incision time after time.

GENERAL TECHNIQUES AND INTERPRETATION

Capillaries subjected to a small, clean incision bleed until the defect is plugged by aggregating platelets. If blood accumulates over the incision, coagulation occurs and the overlying fibrin prevents additional bleeding. Welling blood must be removed, but gently so as not to disrupt the fragile platelet plug. After the incision is made, oozing blood is removed at 15-second intervals by touching filter paper to the drop of blood without touching the wound itself. As platelets accumulate, bleeding slows and the oozing drop of blood gets smaller. The end point occurs when there is no fluid blood left to produce a spot on the filter paper. Some variation is inevitable; duplicate results on the same individual should agree within 2 to 3 minutes at most.

   Bleeding time is prolonged when platelet counts fall below 100,000/mm.[3] Aspirin prevents platelet aggregation and prolongs the bleeding time for as long as 3 days after a single dose of 300 mg.[4] Patients should be warned not to take aspirin or any over the counter pain remedies for 3 days before the test is scheduled. Congenital absence of fibrinogen and hereditary coagulation defects do not prolong the bleeding time, but acquired fibrinogen problems often do. Bleeding time may be less prolonged than expected in some thrombocytopenic patients if all their circulating platelets are young, since young platelets have enhanced hemostatic capabilities.

IVY AND TEMPLATE TECHNIQUES

The bleeding time is best done on the volar surface of the forearm, a site that is readily accessible, has a reasonably uniform superficial blood supply, is relatively insensitive to pain, and can easily be subjected to mildly increased hydrostatic pressure. The incision should be made at a cleansed site that is free of skin disease and away from obvious underlying veins. A constant pressure of 40 mm. Hg should be applied throughout the test. In the Ivy technique, incisions 3 mm. deep are made freehand with a blood lancet. With the Mielke template it is possible to achieve a reproducible, precise incision every time.[11]

A normal Ivy bleeding time is 3 to 6 minutes. When platelet counts are low, one can calculate the expected bleeding time with the following formula:[11]

$$\text{Bleeding time} = 30.5 - \frac{\text{Platelet count/mm.}^3}{3850}$$

A bleeding time longer than that calculated from platelet numbers alone suggests defective function in addition to reduced number. It is also possible to detect above-normal hemostatic capacity in cases in which active young platelets comprise the entire population of circulating platelets.[10]

DUKE TECHNIQUE

In the Duke technique, the dependent surface of the earlobe is incised. Normal values are 1.5 to 3.5 minutes. The Duke technique is less sensitive to small variations than the Ivy or template test. It is also less satisfactory because the capillary supply to the area varies unpredictably and because there is no way to impose a uniform, gentle increase in hydrostatic pressure.

Platelet Counts

The quickest, simplest, but least accurate way to assess platelet number is to examine a stained blood film. This approach has the advantage of revealing platelet size and morphology but the disadvantage that adherence to glass or uneven distribution within the smear can impose marked differences in the apparent degree of platelet concentration. A rule of thumb is that the platelet count is adequate if the smear contains one platelet per 20 red cells or two to three platelets per oil-immersion field.

CHAMBER COUNTS

The best manual counting method uses phase contrast microscopy on a sample diluted 1:100 in ammonium oxalate. If the platelet count is known to be low, a lower dilution factor can be used. The major problem, besides technical conditions of accurate dilution, adequate mixing, and avoiding adherence or aggregation, arises from sampling error. Very few platelets are seen and counted, and the total count is extrapolated from these limited data.

ELECTRONIC COUNTING

With electronic particle counting, larger numbers of platelets are examined. This technique is subject to error if the white count is over 100,000/mm.[3], if there is severe red cell fragmentation, if the diluting fluid contains extraneous particles, if the plasma sample settles too long during processing, or if platelets stick to one another.

INTERPRETATION

Normal platelet counts are between 175,000 and 400,000/mm.[3]; the mean is about 250,000/mm.[3] The blood must be drawn briskly through a clean, nontraumatic venipuncture, and it must be mixed promptly and adequately with anticoagulant. If the coagulation sequence is minimally activated, platelets clump together and adhere to the walls of the test tube. Excessive agitation should be avoided, because this, too, causes adherence. A properly drawn specimen, mixed with EDTA and kept at room temperature, retains a stable platelet count for as long as 12 hours.[2]

Tourniquet Test

The tourniquet test demonstrates how well small vessels withstand increased hydrostatic pressure. A tourniquet, inflated to pressure midway between systolic and diastolic blood pressure, is applied to the upper arm for 5 or 10 minutes and the forearm examined to see how many petechiae develop. More than 10 petechiae constitute an abnormal result. Petechiae may occur in patients with normal platelets but abnormal degrees of tissue fragility. The tourniquet test provides no information that cannot be obtained more reliably by platelet count or bleeding time. Often it is the occurrence of spontaneous petechiae that makes it necessary to evaluate platelet function; nothing new is gained by using a tourniquet to elicit more petechiae.

Clot Retraction

When blood first clots in a test tube, the entire column of blood solidifies. As time passes, the clot diminishes in size. Fluid (serum) is expressed, and only the red cells remain enmeshed in the shrunken fibrin mass. Platelets are necessary for the fibrin clot to retract and for serum to be expressed.

The speed and extent of clot retraction indicate, roughly, the degree of platelet adequacy. A normal clot, gently separated from the side of the tube and incubated at 37°C., shrinks to about one-half its original size within an hour. The result is a firm, cylindrical fibrin clot that contains all the red blood cells and is sharply demarcated from the clear serum. Patients with thrombocytopenia or abnormally functioning platelets have samples with scant serum and a soft, plump, poorly demarcated clot.

OBSERVING THE CLOT

Clot retraction is a simple test that can be performed repeatedly by individuals without special technical training. Attempts to quantitate the test by measuring size of the clot or quantity of serum do not really enhance its usefulness. The clot is small and serum voluminous if the patient has a low hematocrit. Patients with polycythemia have poor clot retraction because the large numbers of captured red cells separate fibrin strands and interfere with platelet contraction. If fibrinogen levels are low, the initial clot is so fragile that the delicate strands rupture and red cells spill out into the serum when retraction begins. Serum contamination by red cells is especially striking if fibrinolysis is abnormally brisk, as often happens with reduced fibrinogen levels. Sometimes, in these cases, the incubated tube contains only cells and plasma with no fibrin clot at all.

PLATELET ANTIBODIES

The clot retraction test can be modified to demonstrate the inhibitory effect of antiplatelet antibodies, especially those associated with drugs.[15] Clot retraction is abolished if more than 90 percent of platelet activity is neutralized. Serum suspected of containing antibodies can be added to known normal blood to see if retraction is inhibited. It is essential to have a control tube containing normal serum added to the normal whole blood. Both normal and patient serum should be ABO-compatible with the red cells used. When drug-antibody complexes are thought to be involved, the suspect serum can be incubated with the drug before adding it to the normal whole blood.[36]

Platelet Aggregation

Platelet aggregation can be measured by bringing platelet-rich plasma into contact with known inducers. Most inducers, such as collagen, epinephrine, or thrombin, act through the effects of ADP that the platelets themselves release. Adding exogenous ADP causes aggregation directly. Aggregation is quantitated by determining whether turbid, platelet-rich plasma becomes clear as evenly suspended platelets aggregate and fall to the bottom of the tube. "Aggregometers" are spectrophotometers adapted to record changes in light transmission while maintaining constant temperature and gentle agitation of the platelet suspension.

INTERPRETATION

Once a normal curve of light transmission is obtained, the test platelets can be exposed to various agents and varying conditions. Aspirin, other anti-inflammatory agents, and many phenothiazines markedly inhibit the aggregating effect of collagen and epinephrine, but do not interfere with the direct action of added ADP.[17] Constitutional disorders of platelet function differ from one another in the nature of the agents that fail to elicit aggregation. It is essential that patients suspected of these disorders abstain from all medications for at least a week before testing.

An excellent diagnostic test for von Willebrand's disease (see pp. 159 and 168) exploits the fact that these patients lack a normally present plasma factor that causes platelets to aggregate after exposure to ristocetin, an antibiotic.[13,29] Ristocetin is no longer used therapeutically because of this aggregating property, which occurs in vivo as well as in the laboratory.

It is difficult to prepare a good sample of platelet-rich plasma because platelets tend to aggregate spontaneously. If the sample is collected through a plastic syringe, with good venipuncture technique and prompt but not over-vigorous mixing, it can be kept up to an hour at room temperature before the test is done. The platelet-rich plasma should contain between 200,000 and 300,000 platelets/mm.^{3} This is achieved by mixing centrifuged, concentrated platelets with platelet-poor plasma until the desired concentration is reached.

Platelet Retention

Platelets must adhere to an altered or wettable surface before they undergo release and aggregation. The adhesive qualities of platelets can be measured by allowing platelet-rich plasma to percolate through a column of glass beads. The difference between platelet count in the original plasma and that in the plasma leaving the column reflects the degree to which the platelets adhere to a wettable surface. Normally, between 30 and 80 percent of platelets remain trapped in the column. This test is difficult to standardize since it varies with such factors as the caliber of column or tubing, the rate of plasma flow, and the size and composition of the beads or particles.

In von Willebrand's disease, platelet retention is much reduced. Other qualitative platelet disorders produce variably reduced retention values, but the test has much less diagnostic specificity than the aggregation tests mentioned above.

COAGULATION TESTS

Innumerable tests have been devised to diagnose inherited, acquired, or iatrogenic deficiencies of coagulation. Some of these require specialized techniques or rare reagents available only in laboratories that do many such tests. Other tests are less precisely diagnostic but more available and more readily applicable to immediate clinical situations. The following discussion concentrates on tests that are widely available.

Lee-White Clotting Time

The oldest but least accurate test of coagulation is to measure how long it takes whole blood to clot in a test tube. The Lee-White clotting time employs three tubes incubated at 37°C., each containing 1 ml. of whole blood. These are gently tilted at 30-second intervals to enhance the contact between blood and glass surface and to see when clotting occurs. Normal blood clots firmly within 4 to 8 minutes.

INTERPRETATION

The Lee-White test is unsatisfactory for many reasons. The sensitivity is so low as to make it almost worthless as a screening technique. For many factors, deficiency must fall to 1 percent or less of normal levels before clotting time is consistently prolonged; problems of mild or moderate severity will not be apparent. Heparin prolongs the clotting time, and the test is commonly used to monitor heparin therapy so as to keep the clotting time at about 20 minutes. Rare indeed is the clinical service with enough personnel to perform well-standardized 20-minute clotting times every 6 or 8 hours on every patient receiving heparin. Variations in technique produce variations in test results that are as large as, or larger than, the variations induced by medication. Hasty tilting, careless temperature control, and observations missed because of other responsibilities are the rule, not the exception, in most services. The result is that clinical judgment or scheduled medication rounds dictate the dosage, rather than a careful set of physiologic measurements.

ACTIVATED COAGULATION TIME

Some centers have found that adding celite, a finely divided clay, shortens the whole blood clotting time, reduces test variability, and allows more precise correlations between heparin dosage and laboratory results. Normal blood clots in less than 100 seconds when added to a tube containing celite. With heparin, the goal is to achieve an activated coagulation time (ACT) of 300 to 600 seconds. The ACT has found greatest use in monitoring heparin therapy given during extracorporeal circulation.[5] Repeated bedside determinations can be correlated with the patient's clinical status and heparin or its antagonist given to induce changes in the desired direction. The ACT is less suitable for intermittent checks on heparin dosage, partly because it must be done immediately after the blood is drawn and therefore cannot be done on specimens submitted to a central laboratory. Many laboratories have found the activated partial thromboplastin time (see below) to be the most satisfactory test for hospital-wide monitoring of heparin therapy.[3]

Prothrombin Time

Reagents for the prothrombin time (PT) are tissue thromboplastin and ionized calcium. When added to citrated plasma, these substitute for the extrinsic coagulation pathway to activate Factor X directly, without involving platelets or the procoagulants of the intrinsic pathway. To give a normal prothrombin time result, plasma must have at least 100 mg./dl. of fibrinogen and adequate levels of Factor X, Factor VII, Factor V, and prothrombin. Brain extract is the tissue most often used, in a reagent form standardized to elicit a firm fibrin clot in 11 to 13 seconds. Test results are sometimes given as "percent" of normal activity, comparing the patient's results against a curve that shows how rapidly clotting occurs in diluted plasma. "Percent" results have little clinical value, since dilution affects all the coagulation proteins and also changes the ionic composition. Prolongation of PT occurs in patients whose plasma contains normal levels of most factors but lacks only a few specific factors. It is far preferable to report PT results as the actual time in seconds and also to give the normal or control value. The PT should be performed within 4 hours of venipuncture. Excessive room temperature storage can allow Factor V to deteriorate and thereby prolong the PT. Refrigerated storage can activate Factor VII, which causes the PT to become shorter.

MONITORING COUMARIN THERAPY

Coumarin anticoagulants act by inhibiting hepatic synthesis of the vitamin K-dependent factors: II, VII, IX, and X.[19] The goal of anticoagulant therapy is to prevent intravascular thrombosis without inducing a dangerous hemorrhagic tendency. Coumarin, in proper dosage, is an effective long-term anticoagulant, but patients differ markedly in their response to this drug. Even a single patient may react differently at different times. Because individual metabolism, alcohol intake, and the presence of other drugs significantly affect response to coumarin, any therapeutic regimen must be carefully monitored. The PT is a simple, effective, and inexpensive test for monitoring coumarin therapy. Drug dosage can be adjusted to keep the patient's prothrombin time at the desired degree of prolongation. Barbiturates and oral contraceptives antagonize coumarin, while salicylates, anabolic steroids, quinidine, disulfiram (Antabuse), and many other agents enhance its anticoagulant effects.

CONGENITAL AND ACQUIRED BLEEDING DISORDERS

Because it bypasses the plasma procoagulants, the prothrombin time cannot detect the two commonest congenital disorders: deficiencies of Factor VIII and Factor IX. Congenital deficiencies of Factors X, VII, V, or fibrinogen are very rare, but these will prolong the PT if deficiency exists. Acquired coagulation disorders, however, are very common. The commonest condition that prolongs the PT is liver disease, in which manufacture of Factors II, VII, IX, and X declines and the PT gets longer. Administration of vitamin K does not help, since parenchymal cell function is deficient.[28] Factor V levels also decline in patients with liver disease, but the degree to which this affects the PT is not clear. Thrombocytopenia, by itself, does not prolong the PT.

If platelets are diminished because of widespread intravascular coagulation, the PT becomes abnormal because other factors are also consumed. The products of inappropriate fibrinolysis actively inhibit clot formation and additionally prolong the PT in many cases of intravascular coagulation/fibrinolysis. Patients given heparin for any reason have an abnormally long prothrombin time.

Partial Thromboplastin Time

The intrinsic coagulation system can be activated by the addition to plasma of phospholipid reagents similar to thromboplastin reagent but less potent. A fibrin clot evolves from normal plasma 60 to 85 seconds after addition of the "partial thromboplastin" reagent and ionized calcium. Factors XII, XI, IX, and VIII must all be present at adequate levels to have a normal partial thromboplastin time (PTT), as must Factors X, V, prothrombin, and fibrinogen. Factor VII is not required for the PTT, because the test bypasses the extrinsic system. The PTT is more sensitive in detecting minor deficiencies than the PT. As a general rule, factor levels below 30 percent of normal prolong the PTT.[33]

ACTIVATED PARTIAL THROMBOPLASTIN TIME

The intrinsic coagulation sequence begins when contact with glass or other surface-active agents activates Factor XII and Fletcher factor. In the laboratory, this activation step is both time-consuming and unpredictable. The partial thromboplastin test can be made more rapid and more reliably reproducible by standardizing this contact phase. The modified test is called the *activated partial thromboplastin time* (aPTT). For the aPTT, the thromboplastin reagent includes either particulate matter (kaolin or celite) or a chemical reagent (ellagic acid) that rapidly activates the contact factors. The aPTT is usually standardized so that normal is between 35 and 45 seconds. The aPTT is more reproducible than the unmodified PTT and just as sensitive in detecting minimal deficiencies.

HEPARIN AND OTHER ACQUIRED INHIBITORS

Many workers use the aPTT to monitor heparin dosage. Although there is not a directly parallel dose/response relationship, the aPTT changes in a manner that reflects fairly sensitively the changes in heparin level. The best approach is to determine a desired level for the aPTT and then adjust dosage to maintain the test results in this range.[23]

Anything that prevents conversion of fibrinogen to fibrin prolongs all the tests that use fibrin formation as the end point. In addition to heparin, common inhibitors are circulating products of fibrin and fibrinogen degradation. If the PTT or PT is prolonged, it is not difficult to distinguish whether the problem is simple factor deficiency or presence of an inhibitor. Simple factor deficiency can be corrected by adding normal plasma to the deficient sample, often one part of normal plasma to one to four parts of patient plasma. If the patient's plasma contains an inhibitor, it will prolong the previously normal PTT of the normal plasma to which it is added.[25]

FACTOR DEFICIENCIES

It is possible to infer which factors are deficient by comparing PT with PTT results. A normal PT with prolonged PTT points to Factors XII, XI, IX, and VIII, and to von Willebrand's disease. Normal PTT with prolonged PT occurs only with Factor VII deficiency. Congenital isolated deficiency of Factor VII is extremely rare, but the combination of normal PTT and prolonged PT occurs fairly often in patients with liver disease or coumarin therapy. This is because Factor VII has such a short half-life that it is the first of the liver factors to decline when hepatic synthesis falters. As coumarin dosage is changing or as hepatic disease is first developing, Factor VII may be the only liver factor to decline significantly.

Both PT and PTT are prolonged with severe liver disease or established coumarin therapy. Prolongation of both tests also occurs with disorders of Factors X, V, or prothrombin; with acquired complex deficiencies or inhibition; with high heparin levels; and with congenital or acquired fibrinogen defects. Neither test measures Factor XIII activity. Plasma deficient in Fletcher factor has a normal PT and prolonged PTT. If the plasma is incubated with kaolin or celite, or allowed to stand in glass for several hours, the PTT returns to normal.

CROSS-CORRECTION PROCEDURES

Once a tentative diagnosis is reached by observing abnormal screening results, presumptive confirmation is possible by adding different agents to the patient's plasma to see what corrects the abnormality. The usual diagnostic dilemma lies in separating Factor VIII from

Factor IX deficiency. The clinical findings are indistinguishable: both have prolonged PTT with normal PT, both occur in males with sex-linked inheritance pattern and both are reasonably common in a general population. Treatment, however, differs significantly. It is often desirable to refer the newly diagnosed hemophilic to a specialized center for factor assays and family studies, but a nonspecialized laboratory can make the qualitative diagnosis fairly easily.

Normal serum contains levels of Factors XII, XI, IX, VII, and X which are virtually equal to those of plasma, but lacks Factors VIII, V, fibrinogen, and prothrombin. Fresh plasma contains all the clotting factors, but Factors II, VII, IX, and X can be removed by absorbing the plasma with barium sulfate or aluminum hydroxide. Absorbed plasma contains Factors XII, XI, VIII, V, and fibrinogen. Once the patient is known to have an abnormal PT or PTT, or both, the laboratory can repeat each test on a mixture of the patient's plasma and added materials that contain clotting factors. If the patient's PTT is corrected by serum but not by absorbed plasma, then Factor IX is the culprit; if absorbed plasma corrects and serum fails to correct, the problem is Factor VIII deficiency. If serum and plasma both correct the PTT, the problem involves Factor XII or XI. These usually can be distinguished clinically by the fact that Factor XII-deficient patients have no hemorrhagic symptoms or history of bleeding.

If both PT and PTT are prolonged, it is important to rule out fibrinogen deficiency or circulating inhibitors by performing a thrombin clotting time (see below). If the TCT is normal, prolongation of PT and PTT together suggests deficiency of Factor X, Factor V, or prothrombin. Adding serum to the patient's plasma corrects Factor X or prothrombin deficiency, while absorbed plasma compensates for Factor V deficiency. The commonest cause of prolonged PT and PTT is liver failure in which Factors II, VII, IX, and X decline together and in which Factor V may be depressed as well.

FACTOR ASSAYS

Assays of specific factor levels require a high degree of technical expertise and, often, a bank of frozen rare plasma. These procedures are best done at referral centers, rather than by an eager but inexperienced general laboratory staff. Factor assays are used to discriminate between mild, moderate, and severe deficiency patterns and to follow the course of acquired factor inhibitors.

Thrombin Clotting Time

Preformed thrombin, usually of bovine origin, can be added to plasma to convert fibrinogen directly to a fibrin clot. Deficiencies in intrinsic or extrinsic systems do not affect the thrombin clotting time (TCT), which is performed only to evaluate the last phase of coagulation. Thrombin-induced clotting is very rapid, and the test can be standardized to any desired normal, usually between 10 and 15 seconds. The TCT is prolonged if fibrinogen levels are below 100 mg./dl., if there is an inhibitor, or if the fibrinogen present is functionally abnormal. In all these conditions, the PT and PTT are prolonged as well. Fibrinogen deficiency can be distinguished from inhibitory conditions by adding small volumes of normal plasma to the patient's plasma and repeating the TCT.

FIBRINOGEN "TITER"

It is possible to estimate plasma fibrinogen levels by performing the TCT on serial dilutions of plasma. If the initial fibrinogen level is more than 100 mg./dl., thrombin produces a firm, visible clot after incubation with plasma diluted 1:32. With normal plasma, a good clot develops at dilutions of 1:64 or 1:128. Plasma that is significantly deficient in fibrinogen may clot after 15 minutes of incubation but cannot support dilution past 1:2 or 1:4. This semiquantitative approach can be useful for quick estimation when quantitative tests are not available. More accurate and reasonably rapid tests for fibrinogen have superseded this procedure in most laboratories.

Fibrinogen Measurement

Fibrinogen is unique to plasma. Once clotting has occurred, serum should contain no residual fibrinogen. To measure plasma fibrinogen, it is necessary to make one of several assumptions. *Classical procedures* depend on the assumption that adding thrombin will convert all the available fibrinogen into fibrin. What is actually measured is the amount of protein in the resulting clot; the quantity of precursor fibrinogen is extrapolated from this value. In *immunologic techniques*, the assumption is that any plasma constituent that reacts with antifibrinogen antibodies is, indeed, fibrinogen. Plasma levels are determined by comparing plasma reactivity against a curve derived from known fibrinogen concentrations. *Heat-precipitation tests* proceed on the comparable assumption that all the material responsive to the precipitation technique really is fibrinogen.

Measuring protein in a precipitate or a clot gives an objective, quantitative result, but the techniques are time-consuming and require experienced, careful performance. Immunologic techniques, in which antifibrinogen antibodies are adsorbed to inert indicator particles, use visible agglutination as the end point, and quantitation depends on the results observed with successively diluted samples. Reliability depends on the purity of the antibody and the accuracy of the original standardization done by the manufacturer of the kit. The test is quick and easy, but the user is entirely dependent upon the quality of the kit.

DEFECTS OF FIBRINOGEN

A variety of fibrinogen disorders exists. Rare individuals have *constitutional* fibrinogen deficiency; these patients have low values on all tests for fibrinogen. *Acquired* fibrinogen deficiency is usually a complex state of defibrination, intravascular coagulation, and fibrinolysis. The plasma contains little or no clottable fibrinogen, but there is usually a variable amount of heat-precipitable or immunologically reactive material. Congenital and acquired *dysfibrinogenemias* have been identified in which there are fibrinogen-like molecules in the plasma, but coagulation is either absent, delayed, or peculiar. The physicochemical and immunologic reactivity of these molecules varies with the nature of the disorder.

Fibrinogen Split Products

Plasmin degrades fibrin as its physiologic substrate, but it readily cleaves fibrinogen as well, if disproportion develops between plasmin, fibrin, and fibrinogen.[21] The fragments that remain after plasmin digestion not only fail to clot, they interfere with clotting of whatever fibrinogen has escaped proteolysis. High concentrations of fibrinogen cleavage products also interfere with formation of the hemostatic platelet plug. Whenever fibrin undergoes fibrinolysis, low levels of degradation products enter the circulation, but these are normally cleared by the liver and reticuloendothelial system.[30] With excessive plasmin activity, fibrin and fibrinogen degradation products (FDPs)— also called fibrin or fibrinogen split products—can circulate in levels high enough to cause serious hemostatic difficulties.

Tests for FDP are done on serum. Since FDPs do not coagulate, they remain in the serum after fibrinogen is removed through clotting. Their presence is documented immunologically so as not to require biologic activity from these functionally abnormal molecules. Antifibrinogen antibody is used, since it is neither desirable nor possible to generate antibodies against individual degradation fragments. One simple and widely used procedure employs antibodies adsorbed to inert indicator particles;[8] such techniques as agglutination inhibition and immunodiffusion can also be used.

INTERPRETATION

Because normal serum contains neither fibrinogen nor FDP, there should be nothing present to react with antifibrinogen antibodies. In patients with widespread bleeding or brisk hemostatic activity, small quantities of FDP may circulate, enough to react at a low level with the reagent antibody. Very high levels of FDP are seen if the fibrinolytic system is inappropriately active or if there is widespread intravascular coagulation. Patients with these disorders have blood that clots poorly or not at all. Even if clotting occurs, fibrinogen and FDP remain in the serum at high concentrations.[6]

Fibrinolysis

The combination of severe fibrinolysis with intravascular fibrin deposition can so deplete fibrinogen and generate so much inhibitory activity that clotting does not occur. More often, thrombin induces some degree of clotting, but the fibrin undergoes rapid dissolution. Several qualitative tests are useful for documenting that there is excessive fibrinolytic activity. A normal control should be run in parallel with the patient's sample to provide some relative indication of the seriousness of the problem.

EUGLOBULIN LYSIS TIME

Euglobulins are proteins that precipitate from acidified dilute plasma; these include fibrinogen, plasminogen, and plasminogen activator but very little antiplasmin activity. Thrombin added to a euglobulin solution converts fibrinogen to fibrin and activates plasminogen. In euglobulins prepared from normal blood, the initial clot undergoes dissolution in 2 to 6 hours. Even with excessive fibrinolysis, there is usually sufficient fibrinogen to form a clot when thrombin is added, but its appearance is often abnormal from the start. Lysis may take place in minutes; if the process is less severe, complete dissolution may occur in 60 to 90 minutes. The euglobulin lysis time is abnormally short in blood with normal fibrinolytic activity but reduced fibrinogen, because only a little fibrin is present to be lysed.

DILUTE BLOOD CLOT LYSIS TIME

The whole blood clot lysis test is simpler than the euglobulin test, but the end point is more equivocal and takes longer to reach. Whole blood is added directly to a solution of buffer and thrombin to give a 1:10 dilution. The resulting clot normally undergoes fragmentation within 6 to 10 hours; with excessive fibrinolysis, fragmentation occurs much earlier. The presence of red cells makes it difficult to observe the changing clot, and it may be difficult to distinguish fragmentation from retraction or from a clot that forms poorly at the beginning.

Factor XIII

Deficiency of Factor XIII is an uncommon cause of severe, lifelong hemorrhagic tendency. The diagnosis should be considered in a patient with a well-documented bleeding tendency but without abnormal results on any of the tests described above. Factor XIII promotes stable cross-linkage between individual fibrin monomers. Without Factor XIII, fibrin forms, but the clot disintegrates easily.[32] The screening test for Factor XIII deficiency is very easy. A fibrin clot is generated by adding ionized calcium to plasma. Once the clot is firm, 1 ml. of 5 molar urea solution is added to the tube, which is incubated at 37°C. for 12 hours or overnight. Normally stabilized fibrin remains firm, but a Factor XIII-deficient sample will be completely reliquified. A 1 percent solution of monochloracetic acid can be used instead of urea, or both can be used in parallel tubes. Normal control plasma should always be tested simultaneously.

REFERENCES

1. Abramson, N., Eisenberg, P. D., and Aster, R. H.: *Post-transfusion purpura: immunologic aspects and therapy.* N. Engl. J. Med. 291:1163, 1974.
2. Aster, R. H.: *Production, distribution, life-span and fate of platelets,* in Williams, W. L., Beutler, E., Erslev, A. J., and Rundles, R. W. (eds.): *Hematology.* ed. 2. McGraw-Hill, New York, 1977.
3. Basu, D., Gallus, A. S., Hirsh, J., and Cade, J.: *A prospective study of the value of monitoring heparin treatment with the activated partial thromboplastin time.* N. Engl. J. Med. 287:324, 1972.

4. Bick, R. L., Thompson, A., and Schmalhorst, W. R.: *Bleeding times, platelet adhesion, and aspirin.* Am. J. Clin. Pathol. 65:69, 1976.
5. Bull, B. S., Huse, W. M., Brauer, F. S., et al.: *Heparin therapy during extracorporeal circulation. II. The use of a dose-response curve to individualize heparin and protamine dosage.* J. Thorac. Cardiovasc. Surg. 69:685, 1975.
6. Cooper, H. A., Bowie, E. J. W., and Owen, C. A., Jr.: *Evaluation of patients with increased fibrinolytic split products (FSP) in their serum.* Mayo Clin. Proc. 49:654, 1974.
7. Cowan, D. H., and Graham, R. C., Jr.: *Studies on the platelet defect in alcoholism.* Thromb. Diath. Haemorh. 33:310, 1975.
8. Garvey, M. B., and Black, J. M.: *The detection of fibrinogen/fibrin degradation products by means of a new antibody-coated latex particle.* J. Clin. Pathol. 25:680, 1972.
9. Goodnight, S. H., Jr.: *Bleeding and intravascular clotting in malignancy: a review.* Ann. N.Y. Acad. Sci. 230:271, 1974.
10. Harker, L. A.: *Control of platelet production.* Annu. Rev. Med. 25:383, 1974.
11. Harker, L. A., and Slichter, S. J.: *The bleeding time as a screening test for evaluation of platelet function.* N. Engl. J. Med. 287:155, 1972.
12. Hirsh, J., and Gallus, A. S.: *The activated partial thromboplastin time.* N. Engl. J. Med. 288:1410, 1973.
13. Jenkins, C. S. P., Meyer, D., Dreyfus, M. D., and Larrieu, M. J.: *Willebrand factor and ristocetin. I. Mechanism of ristocetin-induced platelet aggregation.* Br. J. Haematol. 28:561, 1974.
14. Levine, P. H.: *Delivery of health care in hemophilia.* Ann. N.Y. Acad. Sci. 340:201, 1975.
15. Miescher, P. A.: *Drug-induced thrombocytopenia.* Semin. Hematol. 10:311, 1973.
16. Morrison, F. S.: *Disorders of primary hemostasis,* in *Hemostasis for Blood Bankers: A Technical Workshop.* American Association of Blood Banks, Washington, D.C., 1977.
17. Mustard, J. F., Perry, D. W., Kinlough-Rathbone, R. L., and Packham, M. A.: *Factors responsible for ADP-induced release reaction of human platelets.* Am. J. Physiol. 228:1757, 1975.
18. O'Brein, J. R.: *Anti-thrombin III and heparin clotting times in thrombosis and atherosclerosis.* Thromb. Diath. Haemorrh. 32:116, 1974.
19. O'Reilly, R. A.: *Vitamin K and the oral anticoagulant drugs.* Annu. Rev. Med. 27:245, 1976.
20. Paulus, J. M.: *Platelet size in man.* Blood 46:321, 1975.
21. Pizzo, S. V., Schwartz, M. L., Hill, R. L., and McKee, P. A.: *The effect of plasmin on the subunit structure of human fibrin.* J. Biol. Chem. 248:4574, 1973.
22. Rosner, F.: *Hemophilia in the Talmud and rabbinic writings.* Ann. Intern. Med. 70:833, 1969.
23. Salzman, E. W., Deykin, D., Shapiro, R. M., and Rosenberg, R.: *Management of heparin therapy: controlled prospective trial.* N. Engl. J. Med. 292:1046, 1975.
24. Scher, H., and Silber, R.: *Iron-responsive thrombocytopenia.* Ann. Intern. Med. 84:571, 1976.
25. Shapiro, S. S.: *Acquired anticoagulants,* in Williams, W. J., Beutler, E.,

Erslev, A. J., and Rundles, R. W. (eds.): *Hematology*. ed. 2. McGraw-Hill, New York, 1977.

26. Shaw, S. T., Jr.: *Assays for fibrinogen and its derivatives*. CRC Crit. Rev. Clin. Lab. Sci. 8:145, 1977.

27. Soloway, H. B., Cornett, B. M., and Grayson, J. W., Jr.: *Comparison of various activated partial thromboplastin reagents on the laboratory control of heparin therapy*. Am. J. Clin. Pathol. 59:587, 1973.

28. Stenflo, J.: *Vitamin K, prothrombin, and γ-carboxyglutamic acid*. N. Engl. J. Med. 296:624, 1977.

29. Switzer, M. E., and McKee, P. A.: *Evidence that von Willebrand's factor and Factor VIII activities are contained on a single molecule with a covalent subunit structure*. Clin. Res. 23:407A, 1975.

30. Verstraete, M., Vermylen, J., and Collen, D.: *Intravascular coagulation in liver disease*. Annu. Rev. Med. 25:447, 1974.

31. Weiss, H. J.: *Platelet physiology and abnormalities of function*. N. Engl. J. Med. 293:531, 1975.

32. Williams, W. J.: *Biochemistry of plasma coagulation factors*, in Williams, W. J., Beutler, E., Erslev, A. J., and Rundles, R. W. (eds.): *Hematology*. ed. 2. McGraw-Hill, New York, 1977.

33. Williams, W. J.: *Control of coagulation reactions*, in Williams, W. J., Beutler, E., Erslev, A. J., and Rundles, R. W. (eds.): *Hematology*. ed. 2. McGraw-Hill, New York, 1977.

34. Williams, W. J.: *Life-span of plasma coagulation factors*, in Williams, W. J., Beutler, E., Erslev, A. J., and Rundles, R. W. (eds.): *Hematology*. ed. 2. McGraw-Hill, New York, 1977.

35. Wright, I. S.: *The nomenclature of blood clotting factors*. Thromb. Diath. Haemorrh. 7:381, 1962.

36. Zucker, M. B., Ley, A. B., Borelli, J., et al.: *Thrombocytopenia with a circulating platelet agglutinin, platelet lysin and clot retraction inhibitor*. Blood 14:148, 1959.

CHAPTER 3

DISEASES OF
RED BLOOD CELLS

ACUTE BLOOD LOSS

Acute, massive blood loss does not cause immediate anemia. Rapid hemorrhage threatens life by reducing circulatory volume and deranging cardiovascular adjustments. Enough hemoglobin may remain to sustain life, but if circulatory mechanisms fail, hemoglobin cannot get to the tissues and oxygenation is impaired. After acute blood loss, the body adjusts by maintaining circulation through the most vital vascular beds, by speeding up heart rate, and by expanding circulatory volume at the expense of the extravascular fluid. It is this volume adjustment that causes anemia. As extravascular fluid enters the blood stream, it dilutes the remaining cells, and the hematocrit drops over the next 48 to 72 hours.

Hematologic Responses

Acute blood loss stimulates the bone marrow immediately. Platelet count and the number of circulating granulocytes increase before hematocrit falls. Thrombocytosis between 600,000 and 800,000/mm.³ and leukocytosis between 10,000 and 30,000/mm.³ may occur within a few hours, accompanied, in more extreme cases, by outpouring of immature platelets and neutrophils. Erythropoietin levels rise within 6 hours, and reticulocytosis becomes apparent within 24 hours, reaching a peak at 7 to 10 days.[32]

If iron stores are normal, the rate of red cell production increases two- to threefold. Iron-deficient patients cannot increase hematopoiesis as adequately when hematocrit falls. Patients who receive therapeutic iron to supplement an already adequate or borderline supply may show four- to sevenfold rises in erythropoietic activity.[63] Reticulocytosis ceases when lost red cells are restored, usually within 30 days if no further bleeding occurs. Persistently elevated reticulocyte counts suggest continuing blood loss or red cell destruction.

If blood is shed into the body cavities, the lumen of the alimentary tract, or the soft tissues, nonviable red cells and hemoglobin accumulate and must be degraded. These changes cause elevation of blood urea and bilirubin levels. Blood loss to the exterior does not, of course, have this effect.

CHRONIC BLOOD LOSS AND DEFECTS OF IRON METABOLISM

Repeated small hemorrhages and continuous low-level bleeding do not disrupt blood volume, since fluid adjustments occur automatically. However, as red cells leave the body, they take their iron with them. The pathophysiologic result of chronic blood loss is *iron-deficiency anemia*. Iron deficiency can result from problems other than chronic blood loss, but, as the commonest cause of iron deficiency, bleeding should be carefully sought and ruled out before other, less common problems are pursued. The second commonest cause is impaired absorption of oral iron due to mucosal defects. Inadequate dietary intake, by itself, rarely causes whole-body deficiency but may accentuate other problems or become important at times of special stress. Genetic or acquired defects of iron metabolism are rare.

Iron Absorption and Excretion

The newborn infant begins life with 350 to 500 mg. of iron; all further increment comes from the diet. Iron requirements are greatest in the first year of life, when expanding red cell production requires daily intake of 1 mg./kg. to keep pace with growth. Adolescence, pregnancy, and lactation also impose severe erythropoietic stress. Normally, only 5 to 10 percent of ingested iron is absorbed. If body stores are low, absorption may increase to 2 or 3 times normal, but the body can never absorb more than a third of the iron present.

DIETARY INTAKE

Iron is largely absorbed across the mucosa of duodenum and proximal jejunum. Gastric juice plays an important but poorly understood role in promoting absorption. The low pH of gastric juice makes iron more available from hemoglobin-containing meat in the diet, and it affects the valence and chemical configuration of iron in other foodstuffs. Some iron-rich foods never become a useful source for absorption, despite contact with gastric juice; milk and egg yolks are prime examples.

Disorders of the digestive tract interfere with iron absorption. Patients with achlorhydria, surgical resection of stomach or proximal small intestine, abnormally rapid intestinal transit time, or malabsorption syndromes may gradually become iron-deficient, a process much accelerated if they are also bleeding from the alimentary tract or some other site. Iron is excreted very slowly. Only 1 mg. of iron leaves the body each day, largely by desquamation of epithelial cells. Total body iron is between 35 mg./kg. (in women) and 50 mg./kg. (in men). Since some iron absorption occurs even with gastrointestinal disease, it takes a long time for iron deficiency to develop from impaired absorption or from inadequate total dietary intake.

The commonest victims of inadequate dietary intake are small children whose diet consists largely of milk during the first few years of increasing body size and red cell production. In the United States, fortified food products and generally varied diet make poor intake alone a rare cause of iron deficiency in older children and adults. A borderline intake may, however, become inadequate under conditions of increased requirement, such as rapid growth spurts, onset of menstruation, or repeated pregnancies.[34] Adult males and postmenopausal women almost never become iron-deficient, no matter how poor their diet, unless other problems coexist. In less developed countries, the combination of poor diet, frequent parasitic infestations, and repeated pregnancies makes iron-deficiency anemia a widespread and severe health problem.

BLOOD LOSS

Chronic bleeding, often unnoticed, occurs more often from the gastrointestinal tract than from any other site. Peptic ulcer, gastritis, hiatal hernia, diverticulitis, and neoplasms are the usual causes. In many cases, the patient is asymptomatic or, at the very least, unaware that he is losing blood. Heavy use of alcohol or salicylates may cause painful gastritis, but the patient may not notice the small, continuous blood loss.

Excessive menstrual loss is a common cause of iron deficiency in females. Adolescence, repeated pregnancies, and excessive menopausal flow are conditions of special risk. In adolescent girls with their frequently erratic diet and often irregular, heavy menstrual periods, the pubertal growth spurt may tip iron balance into a deficiency state. Every pregnancy drains the mother of 600 to 900 mg. of iron, a substantial loss even if body stores were adequate initially. If an iron-depleted adolescent has several pregnancies within a few years, the results can be disastrous. Pregnancies exert a cumulative effect, and the often profuse loss that accompanies menopause accentuates the imbalance that pregnancies have imposed.

The urinary tract is another avenue of loss. Tumors, stones, or inflammatory disease affecting kidneys, ureters, or bladder may cause blood loss in the urine. A rare cause of urine-related iron deficiency is excretion of large amounts of hemosiderin in patients with chronic hemolytic states.

Iron Deficiency

A person can have reduced body iron without being anemic. Many individuals with normal hemoglobin levels are chronically iron-depleted[23] but do not get into trouble until some stress (e.g., increased demand, repeated blood donation, or acute or chronic hemorrhage) demands more erythropoiesis than the iron level can handle. In a largely white population of middle to lower income status,[15] 20 percent of menstruating females were found to be iron-deficient, but less than half of these women had iron-deficiency anemia. Of the anemias found in the entire study population, about half were due to iron deficiency alone.

LABORATORY FINDINGS

In the anemia of established iron deficiency, red cells are small, irregularly shaped, and contain scant hemoglobin. The cells are described as hypochromic and microcytic.[35] The patient has decreased levels of serum iron and increased total iron-binding capacity. There is increased erythropoiesis in the bone marrow, but decreased red cell survival, and total absence of stainable iron in bone marrow sections. The signs of developing iron deficiency are irregularity of red cell size and shape, despite normal hemoglobin levels, and less than normal saturation of iron-binding protein—16 to 30 percent saturation, instead of the normal 30 percent or more.[23] More severe iron deficiency becomes apparent as hemoglobin and hematocrit decline, mean red cell size and hemoglobin content decrease, and transferrin saturation drops to 15 percent or below.

THERAPY

The iron-deficient patient who receives therapeutic iron develops reticulocytosis within 2 or 3 days. This peaks at 7 to 10 days, and hemoglobin levels begin rising within several weeks. If iron, given in an accessible form, fails to produce reticulocytosis and rising hemoglobin, the diagnosis of iron deficiency anemia was incorrect. Diagnosing iron deficiency is often insufficient by itself. The cause of the deficiency should be sought, especially since occult blood loss so often signifies a potentially dangerous underlying condition. In milk-fed infants, adolescents, and pregnant women, nutritional counseling is important for future health.

Sideroblastic Anemias

In the sideroblastic anemias, the body has adequate, even abundant, iron but is unable to incorporate it into hemoglobin. The iron enters the developing red cell but then accumulates in the perinuclear mitochondria of normoblasts.[12] These siderotic granules are seen, on bone marrow smears stained for iron, as a ring around the nucleus. Cells with this appearance are called "ringed sideroblasts." The mature, non-nucleated red cells are hypochromic. They often vary significantly in size and shape. In many cases, a dimorphic pattern exists, with one population of fairly normal cells and another population of hypochromic, irregularly shaped, generally small erythrocytes. There is increased erythropoietic activity in the bone marrow, and thus the marrow is hypercellular, but circulating reticulocyte levels are not elevated.

This condition of inefficient hemoglobin manufacture is apparent in the increased excretion levels of hemoglobin degradation products, namely urobilinogen and bilirubin. Serum iron levels are high, with increased transferrin saturation and increased plasma iron turnover. Storage iron is increased in the marrow. The presence of severely excessive iron stores can cause parenchymal cells of liver and other organs to accumulate large amounts of hemosiderin. [47]

CLINICAL PATTERNS

The physiologic defects that cause sideroblastic failure of iron incorporation are not well understood. One form of severe sidero-blastic anemia is constitutional, with strong but not conclusive linkage to the X chromosome, but many are acquired. Some patients, of both the constitutional and the acquired types, improve significantly when given massive doses of pyridoxine (50 to 200 mg./ day); some show modest improvement, and some are not helped at all.[55] Folic acid has been beneficial in some patients, especially those whose red cell precursors have megaloblastic nuclear changes as well as siderotic granules.

When sideroblastic anemia accompanies other hematologic diseases, lymphomas, connective tissue diseases, or metabolic disorders, the defect in hemoglobin manufacture tends to correct itself when the underlying disease is treated. Acquired primary sideroblastic anemia occurs in older people, and no therapeutic regimens have given consistent success. [55]

Lead Poisoning

Anemia and disordered heme synthesis accompany lead poisoning and provide the major diagnostic clues for this common, prevent-able disorder. In adults, lead exposure is usually occupational. In children the most common cause is *pica*, a tendency to consume in-edible materials. Lead-containing paint may be consumed in quan-tities sufficient to cause anemia and, if prolonged, neurological symptoms. Children are also sensitive to lead levels in polluted atmospheres. The pathways to neurologic damage and depressed hemoglobin synthesis are not fully understood.[61] It is thought that lead damages sulfhydryl groups in several enzyme systems, espe-cially at the early steps in porphyrin manufacture.[8] Insertion of iron into protoporphyrin is also defective. In many lead-related anemias, ringed sideroblasts are prominent.

LABORATORY FINDINGS

Anemia is mild to moderate in adults and moderate to severe in children with excessive lead exposure. Because pica usually occurs in children who are iron-deficient to begin with, the lead-induced derangement of heme synthesis exerts an especially profound effect. The anemia is somewhat hypochromic and microcytic. As in iron deficiency, there is erythropoietic hyperplasia but relatively little reticulocytosis. Basophilic stippling may be prominent, resulting from aggregation of ribosomes in cells with defective hemoglobin manufacture. Membrane function also is abnormal. Circulating red cells have shortened life span, decreased osmotic fragility, and increased mechanical fragility.

The biochemical markers of abnormal heme synthesis are increased, especially urinary excretion of δ-aminolevulinic acid (ALA), the earliest porphyrin precursor. Urine levels of coproporphyrin and uroporphyrin are moderately and slightly increased respectively. Urine porphobilinogen levels are normal. This distinguishes lead poisoning from the constitutional defect of *acute intermittent porphyria,* in which both ALA and porphobilinogen are excreted in excess. Red cell protoporphyrin levels are high, indicating, in addition, aberration of the last step in heme synthesis—insertion of iron into the porphyrin ring.

HEMOGLOBINOPATHIES

Globin Chain Synthesis

The hemoglobin molecule consists of four moieties of heme, a porphyrin, and four globin chains, which are polypeptides. Four different globin chains are involved in hemoglobin synthesis—α, β, γ, and δ—but in any one molecule only two kinds of chains are present. All normal hemoglobins have a pair of α chains. The identity of the hemoglobin type rests with the identity of the remaining pair—either β, γ, or δ. The notation for hemoglobin structure gives the number and the type of chains present. Thus hemoglobin A, with two α and two β chains, is written $\alpha_2^A \beta_2^A$. A$_2$, which has two α chains and two δ chains, is $\alpha_2^A \delta_2^{A_2}$; and hemoglobin F, which has two α chains and two γ chains is $\alpha_2^A \gamma_2^F$. This notation makes it easy to designate the presence of abnormal chains, as for example, in hemoglobin S, which has characteristically abnormal β chains and is written $\alpha_2^A \beta_2^S$.

There are 141 amino acids in the α chain and 146 in the β, γ, and δ chains, all of which have been identified and sequenced. Amino acid sequence, the primary structure of the polypeptide, is controlled genetically. Changes in DNA base sequence produce alterations in polypeptide sequence. The globin chains of hemoglobin exhibit an extraordinary array of structural abnormalities, more than any other known protein. In addition to structural genes, there are genes which regulate the rate of globin chain synthesis, and these, too, can behave abnormally.

Both the structural and the regulatory genes for α chain synthesis reside on chromosome 2, while control of the remaining genes has been localized to the B group chromosomes, either 4 or 5.[46] For some reason, the β chain seems more vulnerable than the other chains to both structural and regulatory abnormalities. Constitutional defects of β chain structure or rate of manufacture are among the commonest genetically determined diseases and cause extraordinary morbidity and mortality. Since the α chain is vital for all the hemoglobins, it makes sense, from a teleologic standpoint, that maladaptive α-chain mutations have not multiplied in human populations. Hemoglobin F ($\alpha_2^A \gamma_2^F$) is the predominant hemoglobin throughout intrauterine development; a conceptus with severely malfunctioning hemoglobin F would succumb in utero. Very few δ chain variants have been identified. Hemoglobin A_2 ($\alpha_2^A \delta_2^{A2}$) contributes only 1 to 2 percent of the hemoglobin in normal red cells and no more than 8 to 10 percent in any known disease; thus genetic abnormalities of the chain would not, it seems reasonable to assume, cause clinical problems. Nevertheless, δ chain variants are rare in all the world's populations.

PHYSIOLOGIC ACTIVITY

The physical and the physiologic properties of a polypeptide result from its primary amino acid sequence. Secondary, tertiary, and quaternary structures result from the interactions of specific amino acids in specific locations, and these, of course, depend on the DNA-determined selection of amino acid sequence. In hemoglobin, the three-dimensional properties of the molecule depend upon the relationships of the α and other chains to each other. These relationships affect, and are affected by, the state of oxygenation of each iron-containing heme moiety. Altered amino acid sequence affects the secondary and other structural events that determine net physicochemical function.

For example, hemoglobin F, which has two γ chains instead of two β chains, releases oxygen from its iron sites at much lower tissue oxygen levels than does hemoglobin A. When one oxygen attaches to one iron, the surrounding globin chains react to the changed internal milieu with position shifts which, in turn, affect the relationship of one globin chain to the next. Releasing the oxygen causes the chains to readjust again. In hemoglobin A, the presence of oxygen on two or more hemes causes a significant positional shift at the point where one α and one β chain come in contact. If primary amino acid sequence is abnormal, this position shift has different effects than if all four chains are normal.

MATURATIONAL CHANGES

In the earliest embryonic stages, unique hemoglobins are produced by yolk sac derivatives. By 6 weeks, fetal red cells begin producing hemoglobin F, which dominates the oxygen-carrying mechanism until birth.[21] By the sixth intrauterine month, however, β chain production can be detected.[42] At birth, about 30 percent of the hemoglobin in each red cell is hemoglobin A, and the change from fetal to adult hemoglobin progresses rapidly. By 6 months, 80 to 90 percent of hemoglobin is A, and from 1 year onwards, hemoglobin F constitutes less than 2 percent of the total.[37] Delta chain production is insignificant before birth. Adult red cells contain 1 to 2 percent hemoglobin A_2, a level achieved at about 1 year. Every red cell in a given individual contains the same proportions of hemoglobins as every other.

Types of Abnormal Hemoglobin

The most common abnormal hemoglobin is hemoglobin S, or sickle hemoglobin, which has valine instead of glutamine at the sixth position in the β chain. On a weight basis, hemoglobin S in the human population outweighs, by several orders of magnitude, all the other abnormal hemoglobins put together. The number six position occurs at the outer surface of the richly intertwining globin chain configuration, at the area where α and β chains shift positions during oxygenation and deoxygenation. The consequences of this abnormality are discussed in the section on sickle cell disease (p. 96). Other substitutions can and do occur within the folded globin chain, at the contact points between globin chains, or near the heme moiety. Each substitution determines a different abnormal hemoglobin, of which several hundred have been discovered.

Substitutions within the globin chains may cause altered solubility, altered ability to withstand oxidation, increased propensity to methemoglobin production, or increased or decreased oxygen affinity.[21] There even are hemoglobins consisting of four α chains, four δ chains, four γ chains (hemoglobin Bart's), or four β chains (hemoglobin H).

Genes determining globin chain structure are codominant; this means that gene product is detectible no matter which allele is on the opposite chromosome. Heterozygotes, with two different genes for globin structure, will have two kinds of hemoglobin. Usually one is hemoglobin A and the other is a substituted variant, but people who have two different abnormal alleles have red cells which contain two different abnormal hemoglobins and no normal hemoglobin A at all. If the same abnormal allele is present on both chromosomes, the individual is homozygous for that hemoglobinopathy, and all his hemoglobin has the same abnormality.

Most abnormal hemoglobins have little more than curiosity value in general hematology, although protein chemists, geneticists, and individual patients and physicians have great interest in specific molecular peculiarities. Only two hemoglobinopathies are sufficiently common to warrant detailed consideration here. *Hemoglobinopathy* means the presence of hemoglobin with abnormal primary structure. The existence of a hemoglobinopathy is demonstrated by electrophoresis of the patient's hemoglobin. For the common hemoglobin abnormalities, no further diagnostic proof is needed. More detailed study becomes necessary with hemoglobins of rare structure, electrophoretic mobility, or physiologic behavior.

Hemoglobin S

When hemoglobin A releases its oxygen, one α and one β chain change their relative position, moving through a distance of 0.7 nanometer.[63] The chains resume their previous positions when reoxygenation occurs. Hemoglobin S has the hydrophobic amino acid, valine, in place of the hydrophilic amino acid, glutamine, at the 6 position. In the deoxygenated configuration, this substitution assumes critical importance. The valine residue presents a key-like surface structure that just fits into a complementary site on adjacent deoxygenated molecules. As one molecule locks into the next, the deoxygenated hemoglobin forms filaments, which intertwine into elongated, cable-like polymeric masses that are insoluble at high concentrations. The shape change is reversible. If oxygen is restored, the adjacent sites unlock, the β chain returns to the oxygenated configuration, and solubility resumes.

It need not be another molecule of hemoglobin S that links with the key-like surface that valine creates. Deoxygenated hemoglobin S can link with adjacent molecules of hemoglobin A or of other abnormal hemoglobins, but the association is not long-lasting. Temporarily linked molecules do not intertwine into dense, cable-like masses without copolymerization of numerous hemoglobin S molecules. Whether or not insoluble aggregates will form depends on the proportion of hemoglobin S to other hemoglobins, on the absolute concentration of hemoglobin S, and on the degree of deoxygenation. The presence of hemoglobin A guards to a modest extent, against polymerization; hemoglobin F exerts a very strong protective effect.

CELLULAR CONSIDERATIONS

Within the red cell, hemoglobin exists in a concentrated solution. If hemoglobin S comprises most or all of the intracellular hemoglobin, polymerization readily occurs as oxygen tension drops, resulting in the development of rigid, solid masses called *tactoids*. These cause the cell to assume an elongated, pointed form conventionally described as sickle-shaped. Although polymerization and tactoid formation occur reversibly in a solution of pure hemoglobin, affected red cells may undergo irreversible changes.

It is probable that the cells of patients with sickle cell disease undergo intravascular sickling and unsickling many times as they circulate. Repeated shape change, however, stresses the cell membrane and causes the loss of small membrane fragments. This reduces the ratio of surface to volume, making the cell less flexible and less responsive to physical changes. Some cells gradually lose their mechanical and osmotic resistance and undergo intravascular dissolution, while others withstand individual stresses but are destroyed at an above-normal rate by the reticuloendothelial system. Red cells in hemoglobin S disease experience a chronically shortened life span.[37]

Internal conditions interact with environmental changes to elicit or prevent sickling. Persons heterozygous for hemoglobin S and hemoglobin A have only 30 to 40 percent hemoglobin S in each cell. The high concentration of hemoglobin A is a powerful deterrent to sickling. Except in nonphysiologic conditions of extreme deoxygenation (e.g., in laboratory testing), the cells do not sickle, even though individual molecules undergo the shape change. High intracellular levels of hemoglobin F can protect even homozygous hemoglobin S cells from sickling. A gene common in blacks but not linked to the hemoglobin S locus causes hemoglobin F production to persist throughout life. Patients with two hemoglobin S alleles and the persistence gene have about 70 percent hemoglobin S and 30 percent hemoglobin F in each cell, and rarely experience in vivo sickling.[21]

The likelihood of sickling increases with low oxygen tensions, lowered pH, or increased body temperature. In those parts of the circulation where blood flow is slow or tissue oxygen levels are low, or where metabolic waste products accumulate, sickling is a danger. Sickled cells pass poorly through tiny vessels. This causes blood viscosity to rise, and the rate of flow to slow, which in turn aggravates the problems of poor tissue perfusion, increased acidity, and decreased oxygenation. Systemic conditions that cause fever, acidosis or reduced oxygen uptake or release similarly enhance the danger of sickling.

CLINICAL CONSIDERATIONS

The gene for hemoglobin S occurs in about 8 percent of American blacks, but only 0.2 percent are homozygous for hemoglobin S. Heterozygotes, with one hemoglobin S gene and one hemoglobin A gene, have *sickle cell trait* but no clinical disease. Although the trait can be detected easily by laboratory tests, affected individuals have no hematologic symptoms and have normal life expectancy and normal patterns of morbidity and mortality.[37] The heterozygous hemoglobin S/A state appears to offer significant protection against malarial infection with *Plasmodium falciparum*. This apparently beneficial effect goes far toward explaining why this otherwise deleterious gene has persisted with such high incidence in a population living where malaria is endemic.

Homozygotes for hemoglobin S suffer from *sickle cell anemia,* a lifelong, variably severe hemolytic anemia punctuated with superimposed episodes of hyperhemolysis, bone marrow aplasia, and pain crises. Continuous hemolysis causes erythropoietic hyperplasia of such magnitude that bones may be deformed by the mass of marrow. Hemolysis also induces hypermetabolism, which aggravates the growth retardation, susceptibility to infection, and cardiovascular deficiencies caused by the anemia. Inexplicable episodes of marrow aplasia occur, during which hemolysis continues and erythropoiesis ceases, leading rapidly to dangerous levels of anemia. Perhaps the most frequent and difficult complications occur in small blood vessels, probably precipitated by intravascular sickling and consequent problems of blood flow. Leg ulcers, pain crises, bone infarcts, and CNS symptoms have all been attributed to vaso-occlusion by altered cells.

Sickle cell anemia rarely becomes apparent before 6 months of age, because protective amounts of hemoglobin F remain in each cell. Intrauterine development is not affected because hemoglobin F is not affected by abnormalities of β chain production. Infants with unsuspected sickle cell anemia sometimes come first to medical attention because of sudden, overwhelming bacterial infections.[52]

LABORATORY FINDINGS

Homozygotes for hemoglobin S have positive screening tests and no hemoglobin A on electrophoresis (see p. 51). Hemoglobin levels usually range between 5 and 9 gm./dl. with marked reticulocytosis. Spleen size and function are markedly reduced because repeated vascular occlusions cause infarction, scarring, and involution of this organ. The spleen ordinarily removes red cell inclusions and abnormally shaped cells from the circulation. Since these patients are functionally asplenic, inclusion bodies and bizarrely shaped cells may be numerous. Increased serum bilirubin and urinary urobilinogen testify to ongoing hemolysis. Red cell survival is shortened. The general level of bone marrow hyperactivity causes white cell and platelet counts to be chronically somewhat high. Moreover, serum iron, transferrin saturation, and storage iron levels are all high.

Erythrocyte sedimentation rate (ESR) is lower than normal because the abnormally shaped red cells interact peculiarly with the surrounding plasma. An ESR in the middle or upper end of the normal range should be considered suspicious for intercurrent inflammatory disease. Leukocytosis of 15,000 to 20,000/mm.[3], on the other hand, may be a patient's normal level and should not, by itself, provoke ill-considered appendectomy or other potentially dangerous treatments. Abdominal pain crises may simulate surgical emergencies, but every episode of pain must be considered individually. Patients with sickle cell disease can also suffer appendicitis, perforated ulcer, or other surgical emergencies.

It is difficult to screen newborns for hemoglobin S disease, even when both parents are known to be carriers, because high levels of hemoglobin F interfere with sickling, and only small amounts of β chain-containing hemoglobin are present. Special methods of electrophoresis have been adopted in populations severely at risk for infectious complications and other associated diseases,[52] and intrauterine diagnosis has been successfully attempted.[33,42]

Hemoglobin C

MOLECULAR CONSIDERATIONS

Hemoglobin C resembles hemoglobin S in having a substitution at the 6 position on the β chain; it has lysine in place of normal glutamic acid. On starch gel electrophoresis, hemoglobin C migrates more slowly than either hemoglobin A or S, at about the same rate as A_2. Under intracellular conditions, hemoglobin C is less soluble than hemoglobin A, because the positive charge on the lysine interacts with adjacent negatively charged groups. It is not clear whether in vivo crystallization occurs, but red cells with hemoglobin C as the predominant molecule are more rigid and more liable to fragmentation than are normal red cells.

CLINICAL CONSIDERATIONS

About 2 to 3 percent of American blacks carry the hemoglobin C gene. The heterozygous state does not cause anemia or shortened red cell life span. Although target cells may be seen on blood smears, there is no anemia and no shortening of red cell survival.

One in 6,000 American blacks is homozygous for hemoglobin C. This causes a mild hemolytic anemia with striking morphologic abnormalities. There are numerous target cells, microspherocytes, and intracellular crystals, but hemoglobin levels remain in the range of 8 to 12 gm./dl. The biochemical findings of hemolysis exist to a modest extent. Since the disease has few intrinsic complications and does not interact adversely with other diseases, patients often remain unaware of their condition until detected during hemoglobin screening programs or during medical care for some other condition.

THE HETEROZYGOUS STATE
OF HEMOGLOBIN S/HEMOGLOBIN C

Because the genes for hemoglobin S and hemoglobin C are allelic and are concentrated in the same population, it is not uncommon to find hemoglobin S/C heterozygotes with no hemoglobin A. Hemoglobin C is significantly less protective against sickling than is hemoglobin A. S/C heterozygotes suffer from a mild to moderate level of sickling and hemolysis, worse than homozygous hemoglobin C disease but milder than homozygous hemoglobin S disease.[37]

THALASSEMIAS

The term *thalassemia* derives from a combination of the Greek words *thalassa* (sea) and *haima* (blood). An early name for the severest form of the disease was *Mediterranean anemia*, because Mediterranean populations were the first ones known to be afflicted. Since this condition was first described by Cooley in 1925, it has become apparent that a number of red cell conditions share a common etiology but have variably severe manifestations. The thalassemias are characterized by decreased production rate of one or more globin chains. All chains have normal structure; this sharply distinguishes thalassemias from the hemoglobinopathies.

Molecular Biology

The genes controlling α chain synthesis are on a different autosomal chromosome from the closely linked loci that control β, γ, and δ chains. There are two α chain subloci on each chromosome, providing normal red cell precursors with a total of four α chain genes.[57] The β and δ loci are adjacent to one another, on a single B-group chromosome, and may have joint or individual abnormalities. The γ locus, on the same chromosome, is rarely involved in abnormalities of synthesis.

RNA LEVELS

DNA, the genetic material of the nucleus, determines production of RNA, which in turn carries out protein synthesis. Without a DNA sequence, no RNA and no protein are produced. This direct proportionality between DNA segment and RNA production can be clearly demonstrated for the α chain genes.[57] Deletion of all four α chain loci causes complete absence of mRNA for α chain synthesis; deletion or severe abnormality of three genes causes mRNA levels to be severely deficient; deletion of one or two α chain genes causes slightly reduced levels of mRNA and mild or no reduction in chain synthesis.

Genes for the β chain are more variable. One form, called β^+ thalassemia, results in markedly deficient but still measurable levels of mRNA, while the β^o thalassemia gene produces no mRNA at all. Both of these are genes that are present on the chromosome and determine defective activity. Still a third possibility can affect chain production: deletion of the gene itself, with absence of any DNA to code for either β or δ chains, hence absence of mRNA for both β and δ chains.

HEMOGLOBIN PRODUCTS

Defective α chain production affects all the hemoglobins except those yolk sac-derived embryonic hemoglobins with unique, separately regulated chains. In red cell precursors with grossly deficient α chain supplies, four γ chains or four β chains may unite as a unit. The results are hemoglobin Bart's (four γ chains) or hemoglobin H (four β chains). In persons with defective α chain production, hemoglobin Bart's is conspicuous during fetal existence, when γ is the dominant non-α chain. Hemoglobin H becomes predominant in postuterine life, when β chain production takes over.

The fetus suffers very little if β chain genes are defective, since hemoglobin F ($\alpha_2^A \gamma_2^F$) is perfectly normal. In extrauterine life, inadequate supplies of β chains cause excess α chains to accumulate. Synthesis of γ or δ chains may rise to compensate for deficiency of hemoglobin A, and increased amounts of hemoglobins A$_2$ ($\alpha_2^A \delta_2^{A2}$) and F ($\alpha_2^A \gamma_2^F$) support oxygen transport to some extent. The level of compensatory hemoglobin F depends on how completely the "switch" from γ to β chain production occurs. Massive compensatory δ chain production never occurs. No matter how desirable its presence might be, hemoglobin A$_2$ never constitutes more than 7 to 10 percent of total hemoglobin.[58]

Clinical Findings

α-THALASSEMIAS

Complete absence of α chain production causes stillbirth in midpregnancy. The fetus can survive on embryonic hemoglobins until the second trimester. Once γ chain production occurs, hemoglobin Bart's evolves from all the unpaired γ chains. This has such high oxygen affinity[21] that, although blood reaches the tissues, almost no oxygen is released, and the fetus dies from anemia and congestive heart failure (hydrops fetalis).

Nonfatal but symptomatic abnormalities of α chain genes occur more commonly in Thailand and in certain Oriental Jewish populations than anywhere else.[58] Persons whose cells have only one (of a possible four) functioning α chain locus have hemoglobin H disease, or *thalassemia intermedia.* Adult cells have 4 to 30 percent hemoglobin H, along with inefficient erythropoiesis and moderately severe anemia. Cord blood has up to 25 percent of hemoglobin Bart's.[43]

Heterozygotes for α-thalassemia have two or three functioning α chain genes, and suffer virtually no clinical disability. In certain American black populations, as many as 2 percent may be heterozygotes for α-thalassemia.[52] The diagnosis is best made on cord blood, which has up to 5 percent hemoglobin Bart's. Adult blood, in α-thalassemia heterozygotes, does not contain hemoglobin H, and the hematologic findings are mild and nonspecific. The only problem is that anemia and morphologic changes may arouse suspicion of iron deficiency, and cause the patient to undergo a hematologic workup that he doesn't need.

HOMOZYGOUS β-THALASSEMIA

When both β chain genes are defective, patients suffer a severe, lifelong anemia called *thalassemia major,* Cooley's anemia, or Mediterranean anemia. Hemoglobin ranges from 2 to 6 gm./dl. Red cells are small, pale, and misshapen, with enormous hemolysis and inefficient erythropoiesis. Reticulocytosis runs 15 percent or more. Nucleated red cells are numerous, and severe splenomegaly and moderate jaundice are present. As α chains are produced normally, there is a huge excess of α chains that have nothing with which to pair. These accumulate and form intracellular inclusions (Heinz bodies) which interfere with intramedullary maturation and induce intrasplenic destruction of those cells that do enter the circulation. Splenectomy can permit somewhat enhanced red cell survival but leads to increased risk of sudden, overwhelming bacterial infections.[43]

The severe anemia retards growth and causes generalized debility unless transfusion therapy augments oxygen-carrying capacity. Striking skeletal abnormalities occur because of overwhelming marrow hyperplasia induced by exaggerated erythropoietin levels. Anemia is not the only stimulus to erythropoietin secretion. Hemoglobins F and A$_2$, produced to compensate for absent hemoglobin A, yield oxygen to the tissues less readily than does hemoglobin A. This leads to tissue hypoxia greater than would occur if normal hemoglobin were present at the same concentration. Because there is such brisk erythropoiesis, large quantities of iron are absorbed from the gut. Iron utilization, however, is poor, and large quantities of storage iron accumulate, first in the reticuloendothelial system and later in parenchymal cells, especially those of the heart.

Transfusion therapy ameliorates the anemia and supresses marrow hyperplasia by diminishing erythropoietin production, but each unit of red cells adds 250 mg. of iron to the body's already excessive supply. Careful transfusion therapy can restore patients with thalassemia major to relatively normal existence, but death usually occurs before age 20 because iron overload causes myocardial failure.[58] Therapy with chelating agents and other drugs to mobilize iron excretion gives promise of delaying or preventing this complication, but no presently available regimen is satisfactory.

The syndromes caused by the β^+ and the β^0 thalassemia genes are similar clinically, although on electrophoretic analysis, they differ in the existing proportions of hemoglobins A_2 and F.[57] Thalassemia caused by complete deletion of the gene segment controlling both β and δ chain production is somewhat less disastrous. Absence of the $\delta\beta$ segment seems to allow compensatory γ chain production.[57] These patients have hemoglobin F as virtually their only hemoglobin, and their less severe clinical syndrome is called *thalassemia intermedia*.

HETEROZYGOUS β-THALASSEMIA

Patients with one normal and one abnormal β chain gene have relatively few clinical problems. The laboratory findings vary depending on which abnormal gene is present. Both β^+ and β^0 heterozygotes have hemoglobin A_2 levels raised to about 7 percent of total hemoglobin, and hemoglobin F is variably increased. Heterozygotes for $\delta\beta$-thalassemia have normal A_2 levels, but hemoglobin F may constitute 5 to 20 percent of the total. All three types of heterozygotes manifest the syndrome of *thalassemia minor,* characterized by abnormally small, hypochromic red cells with numerous target cells, basophilic stippling, and increased resistance to osmotic lysis. Anemia, however, is mild (hemoglobin: 10 to 12 gm./dl.), and erythropoiesis is only mildly inefficient. If the spleen is removed, Heinz bodies become apparent in circulating red cells. Serum iron and transferrin saturation are normal or high.[58]

The biggest problem with thalassemia minor comes in distinguishing it from iron-deficiency anemia. Both conditions cause hypochromic, microcytic anemia, often of comparable degree.[35] Measuring serum iron levels, or examining the bone marrow for storage iron, allows the distinction to be made. Patients with thalassemia minor can be iron-deficient simultaneously. When iron levels are low, the characteristic increase in hemoglobin A_2 tends to disappear. This removes the distinctive clue for thalassemia, and the patient seems only to be iron-deficient. After iron repletion, total hemoglobin fails to achieve normal levels, but the abnormal A_2 levels return,[58] and more complete diagnosis can be made.

HETEROZYGOTES WITH HEMOGLOBINOPATHIES

Genes for globin chain structure and for rate of chain synthesis occupy virtually the same locus. It is not clear how functional distinction occurs. The result, however, is that thalassemia genes and hemoglobinopathy genes behave as alleles. The individual with a β^S allele on one chromosome and a β-thalassemia allele on the other will have no hemoglobin A, but often has more A_2 and F than is seen in homozygotes for hemoglobin S. Still another allele, which causes γ chain production to continue throughout adult life, can be paired with normal, thalassemia, or hemoglobinopathy genes.[21] Because the heterozygous state of sickle hemoglobin and hereditary persistence of fetal hemoglobin protect the cells against many hemoglobin S-related problems, the absence of hemoglobin A causes surprisingly little difficulty.

INTRINSIC RED CELL DEFECTS

Glucose-6-Phosphate Dehydrogenase Deficiency

A gene on the X chromosome determines the structure of *glucose-6-phosphate dehydrogenase* (G-6-PD), an enzyme essential in the hexose monophosphate pathway which generates NADPH. NADPH is an electron donor which is active in many biologic systems. This reducing capacity is important for the red cell's glutathione system, which protects hemoglobin against oxidative stress and irreversible denaturation. The G-6-PD molecule exhibits remarkable polymorphism in human populations; the B variant (considered as the "normal" against which others are measured) and the A variant (found in 30 percent of American blacks) have comfortably adequate activity levels. G-6-PD function is assessed clinically by subjecting red cells to oxidative stress (see p. 47). Specific variants can be characterized by their electrophoretic mobility, thermal stability, and pH optimum, as well as by measuring their activity in the pentose phosphate cycle.

SEX DISTRIBUTION

The commonest defective G-6-PD variant is A⁻; this gene occurs in 9 to 13 percent of American blacks. Since it is on the X chromosome, its activity is unopposed in males, who have only one X chromosome. Females, having two X chromosomes, are likely to have, in addition, a normal allele to counterbalance the defective one. About 11 percent of black males have the deficiency. The amounts of normal enzyme and deficient enzyme vary in heterozygous females, because the degree of X chromosome inactivation varies.[20] Nearly all heterozygotes have functionally adequate red cells. Because the gene is a common one, a few females have defective alleles on both X chromosomes.

CLINICAL PATTERNS

Patients with the A⁻ enzyme experience no difficulty under normal conditions. Most remain unaware that hematologic abnormality exists, since the A⁻ enzyme has about 15 percent of normal activity—enough for most purposes. Red cell number, function, and survival are normal unless and until some acute oxidative stress occurs. G-6-PD activity declines as red cells age, no matter what variant is present.[39] When the enzyme is defective, the effects of this decline become more noticeable. Aging red cells are especially susceptible to oxidative challenge by drugs, systemic infection, metabolic acidosis, and other stresses. Oxidative stress induces rapid intravascular destruction of susceptible cells, leading to hemoglobinemia, hemoglobinuria, and a sudden drop in hematocrit. The hemolytic crisis is self-limited, however, because eventually the only cells left are those with sufficient enzyme levels to withstand the stress. Prompt erythropoietic response results in reticulocytosis and the introduction of still more young cells which are well-supplied with active enzyme.

Drugs that hemolyze G-6-PD-deficient cells are those that either act as direct oxidants themselves or produce peroxide activity.[20] Primaquine, an antimalarial drug, is notable in this respect; an older term for the red cell defect of G-6-PD deficiency is *primaquine sensitivity*. Many sulfa drugs, quinine derivatives, nitrofurans, and antipyretic-analgesic drugs can induce hemolysis in G-6-PD-deficient patients. Susceptibility seems to vary among different individuals. The presence of coexisting fever, metabolic disease, or hepatic or renal failure increases likelihood that symptoms will emerge.

THE MEDITERRANEAN VARIANT

Another G-6-PD variant is the *Mediterranean enzyme*. This occurs in Caucasians, especially in those of Greek and Italian extraction and in some small, inbred Jewish populations.[20] The Mediterranean variant has severely reduced activity, so that even very young cells have little capacity to generate NADPH. Hemolytic episodes are more severe, are triggered by a greater variety of stimuli, and are less likely to be self-limited than in patients with the A⁻ variant.[7] Infants with the deficiency may suffer severe neonatal jaundice. *Favism*, a susceptibility to massive hemolysis after exposure to the fava bean, occurs especially in persons with Mediterranean-type G-6-PD deficiency. Serum factors and immune mechanisms also are involved, though in a manner not clearly understood.

At least 100 other variants of G-6-PD have been characterized but have limited clinical implications.

Other Glycolytic Enzymes

Assiduous investigations of hemolytic conditions have uncovered "several thousand"[27] individuals with defects in glycolytic enzymes other than G-6-PD. Of these, about 95 percent have defective *pyruvate kinase*; the rest are metabolic curiosities involving the entire range of available enzymes. Red cells generate 90 to 95 percent of their ATP through the very efficient, aerobic Embden-Myerhoff cycle, which generates 38 molecules of ATP per molecule of glucose. Remaining energy comes from the hexose monophosphate shunt, which delivers only two molecules of ATP per molecule of glucose but generates metabolically important NADPH as a vital by-product. Failure to generate sufficient ATP results in defective control of ions, so that excessive Na^+ and Ca^{++} enter the cell, and membrane phospholipids may sustain damage.

Defective glycolytic enzymes induce hemolytic anemia characterized by increased autohemolysis after incubation, normal white cell and platelet metabolism, normal hemoglobin economy, normal immunologic findings, and normal liver function tests but increased indirect (prehepatic) bilirubin.

Hereditary Spherocytosis

Hereditary spherocytosis (HS), a fairly common hemolytic condition which is transmitted as an autosomal-dominant trait in persons of northern European ancestry, has defied massive attempts to find the molecular defect.[16] In the United States HS affects about 2.2 per 10,000 Caucasians, but the anemia is relatively mild and sometimes goes undiagnosed until late adulthood. Patients with HS, like those with other chronic hemolytic conditions, have marked susceptibility to formation of bilirubin stones in the gallbladder. Often, it is the gallbladder, not the blood problems, that causes patients to seek medical attention.

CELLULAR CHANGES

Hereditary spherocytosis inflicts a host of physiologic abnormalities upon the red cell, but no one enzymatic defect can account for all the changes. Although spherocytes comprise only 2 to 4 percent of circulating cells, all red cells have accelerated glycolytic activity and defective transmembrane "pump" activity.[59] This means that more Na^+ than normal enters the cell. To maintain normally low intracellular Na^+ concentration, membrane systems work extra hard to pump the excess out. Extra energy is consumed in this process, but the result is to maintain normal intracellular conditions as long as adequate energy sources are available. A problem with Ca^{++} transport causes HS cells more difficulty. All membrane transport systems are ATP-dependent and are influenced by Ca^{++} concentrations. HS cells are unusually sensitive to changes in the ratio between intracellular Ca^{++} and ATP.[5] In addition, Ca^{++} may interact adversely with spectrin, the contractile protein on the inner surface of the red cell membrane.[59]

Normal red cells, despite their diameter of 8 μm., readily traverse sinusoids and membrane pores whose diameter averages 3 μm. HS red cells are slightly smaller (diameter: 6 to 6.5 μm.) but have much reduced flexibility. They cannot pass through diameters smaller than 4 μm., and to achieve even that, increased pressure must be applied.[16] Membrane rigidity increases as intracellular Ca^{++} increases or as pH and oxygen tension of the surrounding medium decrease. HS cells have increased intracellular Ca^{++} and consequent increased rigidity at all times. As red cells pass through the spleen, they encounter every possible adverse condition: flow channels have tiny diameters; flow is slow, so pH and oxygen tension drop; hydrostatic pressures are low and thus inadequate to push cells through channels of marginally adequate diameter. It is not surprising that HS cells, whose ^{51}Cr half-life is 4 to 8 days, are destroyed while attempting to traverse the splenic circulation.

LABORATORY FINDINGS

The patient with HS characteristically has a mild hemolytic anemia (hemoglobin: 9 to 12 gm./dl.) with erythropoietic hyperplasia, reticulocytosis between 5 and 20 percent, mildly increased indirect bilirubin, increased urine urobilinogen, and normal immunologic studies. Circulating red cells vary in size. Spherocytes may constitute only 2 to 4 percent of total circulating cells, and some erythrocytes are somewhat larger than normal. The mean red cell volume tends to be normal or only slightly low, but mean intracellular hemoglobin concentration is often increased to 37 or even to 39 percent. Osmotic and mechanical fragility are increased, and a 24-hour period of sterile incubation without glucose causes osmotic fragility to increase still more. After 48 hours of sterile incubation without glucose, up to 50 percent of HS cells hemolyse spontaneously, without osmotic challenge.[63] Adding glucose to the incubation mixture abolishes the hemolytic tendency.

CLINICAL PROBLEMS

Since HS cells are destroyed in the spleen, splenectomy prolongs survival of HS cells to nearly normal levels, even though the cellular defects continue undiminished. Unfortunately, splenectomy seems to leave the patient somewhat more susceptible than normal to systemic infections. This is especially serious in young children. A lessened, but still significant, increase in liability accompanies splenectomy in adults.[16] Infection, a problem for anybody, is especially dangerous for patients with chronic hemolysis because it affects erythropoietic activity adversely. Aplastic crisis is a serious complication of infection in HS patients, with or without spleens. HS patients also are highly sensitive to folic acid deficiency. Alcoholism, poor diet, pregnancy, neoplasms, or intestinal disorders all predispose to folic acid deficiency and may provide the critical event that precipitates anemia in an HS patient.[63]

Paroxysmal Nocturnal Hemoglobinuria

Unlike the red cell defects just described, paroxysmal nocturnal hemoglobinuria (PNH) is an acquired disease. Red cell composition and behavior become defective relatively late in life. Half of PNH cases develop between ages 20 and 40.[18] The defect sometimes occurs in conjunction with other hematologic diseases such as leukemia, myelofibrosis, or aplastic anemia, or it may occur as a primary condition. Exposure to drugs, iron therapy, or infection are common preceding events. Despite the descriptive name, episodic urinary excretion of hemoglobin after a night's sleep occurs in only 25 percent of cases.[50]

CELLULAR DEFECTS

The pathognomonic feature of PNH is strikingly increased liability to complement-mediated red cell lysis. Not every circulating cell is equally affected. Blood from PNH patients contains cells with three different degrees of complement sensitivity: 25 to 30 times normal, 3 to 5 times normal, and normal.[49] The relative proportions of these populations determine how severely the patient is affected. Severity differs markedly from patient to patient but tends to follow an episodic, gradually worsening course in the majority of affected individuals.

The membrane of PNH cells has both morphologic and chemical abnormalities. Scanning electron microscopy reveals strange pits and protuberances on the red cell surface. Analysis reveals deficient acetyl cholinesterase activity and the presence of abnormally constituted glycoproteins.[53] It is probable that both acetyl cholinesterase deficiency and complement sensitivity are manifestations of some underlying, still undefined, causal phenomenon, rather than having a cause and effect relation.

LABORATORY FINDINGS

PNH is diagnosed by demonstrating that red cells experience excessive hemolysis when exposed to complement-containing serum at low pH (Ham's acid hemolysis test) or placed in a medium of low ionic strength (sucrose or sugar-water hemolysis). The acid hemolysis test is less sensitive but more specific than the sugar-water test.[50] PNH patients usually have a chronic compensated hemolysis; however, unlike most patients with ongoing hemolysis, they have low iron stores and may be frankly iron-deficient. Iron depletion occurs because hemoglobin and hemosiderin are excreted in the urine after complement-mediated intravascular hemolysis releases hemoglobin into the plasma.

Bone marrow aplasia is a common presenting event in PNH, causing leukopenia and thrombocytopenia along with depressed red cell production. Of patients with aplastic anemia, as many as 15 percent have PNH red cells.[53] Thrombotic or infectious manifestations are other common presenting events, and, like aplastic crises, they may occur episodically throughout the disease. Reticulocytosis remains disproportionately low for the degree of hemolysis, even between frankly aplastic episodes. Hemolysis may be exacerbated during sleep or by drug or dietary exposure; however, no clear pattern of inciting substances can be described. Transfusion of blood products containing even small amounts of plasma precipitates hemolysis reliably. If red cell transfusions are necessary, washed or deglycerolized frozen cells should be used.[50]

HEMOLYSIS FROM EXTRACELLULAR CAUSES

Nonimmune Destruction

Red cells of normal composition will be destroyed if exposed to various physical and chemical stresses introduced into the cardiovascular environment.

PHYSICAL TRAUMA

Red cells that encounter physical obstacles within the vascular bed lose bits of membrane and undergo progressive reduction in surface to volume ratio.[8] Cracks or other defects in *prosthetic heart valves* induce a chronic hemolytic condition, probably by introducing surface conditions hazardous to passing red cells. Patients whose capillaries are partially occluded by tiny fibrin strands and clots may experience an acute hemolytic process, *microangiopathic hemolytic anemia,* in which red cells show morphologic evidence of fragmentation and distortion. In both conditions, bizarre cells called *schistocytes* are noted on peripheral smears. Plasma haptoglobin declines and plasma free hemoglobin accumulates. The urine contains hemoglobin and sometimes hemosiderin.

Severe burns cause thermal damage to red cells circulating at the time of injury. As many as 20 to 30 percent of the red cells may be lysed within the first 24 to 48 hours,[63] leading to massive hemoglobinemia and hemoglobinuria. Clinically, this may be disastrous, because it contributes to the renal damage initiated by blood pressure changes, fluid loss, and circulation of other cellular breakdown products.

Acute hemolysis and hemoglobinuria sometimes follow massive physical exertion. Both patient and physician may be alarmed at the acute urinary findings, but no permanent harm is done. Not enough cells are destroyed to cause anemia, and the conditions surrounding the hemoglobinemia and hemoglobinuria do not induce renal damage.

INFECTIONS

Malaria is the most dramatic and most common infectious cause of intravascular hemolysis. The protozoon ruptures red cells as part of its life cycle. The periodic chills and fever that characterize the disease occur as parasitized red cells burst to release a new generation of organisms.

Toxins, especially of clostridial origin, may disrupt the lipids of red cell membranes and lead to the massive hemolysis which sometimes complicates fatal septic episodes. The bite of the *brown recluse spider* causes acute hemolysis of a milder sort, possibly mediated through a hypersensitivity reaction.[9]

DRUGS AND CHEMICALS

Most drug-related hemolysis has an immune basis, but some agents damage red cells directly. Accidental introduction of *distilled water* into the circulation causes rapid osmotic lysis. *Arsine gas*, sometimes generated during industrial processes, causes severe hemolysis, as do *copper salts*.

Oxidizing drugs, notably nitrites, nitrates, and aromatic amino and nitro compounds, cause methemoglobinemia and, in severe cases, red cell destruction as well.[8]

SPLENOMEGALY

The normal spleen destroys normal red cells as they age at the rate of 1/120th of the circulating cells each day. Abnormal red cells undergo accelerated destruction in passing through a normal spleen. An abnormally large spleen tends to destroy excessive numbers of red cells, even perfectly normal cells. Any condition that increases spleen size can cause shortened red cell survival; white cells and platelets may also be affected. Liver disease with portal hypertension, chronic congestive heart failure, leukemias, lymphomas, and protozoal infections may all produce increased spleen size, leading to increased red cell sequestration and decreased red cell survival.

Antibody-Mediated Destruction

ISOANTIBODIES

Isoimmunity means activity directed against material from another member of the same species. The commonest example of isoimmunity in humans is antibody production after blood transfusions, although organ transplantation is becoming increasingly important. Antibodies can be directed against antigens of red cells, white cells, platelets, or protein constituents. These antibodies are harmless to the individual, whose own tissues lack the specific antigens involved. Another exposure to the same isoantigens, however, provokes an immune reaction. The second or later exposure occurs when additional transfusions are given. These need not be from the original donor; many people have the same cell and protein antigens (see Chapter 8).

In a *hemolytic transfusion reaction,* antibodies in the recipient's circulation rapidly destroy the transfused cells as they enter the blood stream. Antibodies against A and B antigens usually cause prompt intravascular hemolysis with rapid liberation of free hemoglobin. Rh and many other antibodies attach to the surface of circulating red cells, causing the antibody-coated cells to undergo splenic destruction. Clinical complications from both types of hemolysis can include shock, coagulation abnormalities, and renal failure, but the severity of clinical response varies astonishingly among different patients exposed to the same immunologic situation. Diagnosis depends upon documenting that the transfused cells possess an antigen for which the patient has a specific antibody and that the cells are being destroyed.

AUTOANTIBODIES

Autoimmune hemolytic anemia (AIHA) is a broad category of conditions in which red cells have shortened survival because the patient has antibodies active against his own cells. The reasons for this autodestructive phenomenon are not understood. In many cases, something seems to change cell surface properties sufficiently that they appear "foreign" to the host's immune system.[22] Autoimmune phenomena often accompany other diseases, notably chronic lymphocytic leukemia, lymphomas, lupus erythematosus, and such viral diseases as infectious mononucleosis and hepatitis. These are called *secondary* autoimmune conditions; *primary,* or *idiopathic,* autoimmune hemolytic anemia occurs without any apparent inciting cause. Many patients with primary AIHA later develop signs of other hematologic or immunologic diseases.

It is customary to classify AIHA by the thermal optimum of the antibody, as determined by serologic testing. *Warm* antibodies work best, or only, at 37°C. *Cold* antibodies have a thermal optimum below 37°C.—sometimes in the 20s, sometimes as low as 4°C.

Antibodies reactive only at low temperatures cause no clinical problems in warm, living people. Cold antibodies that cause clinical illness may work best at 25°, 18°, or 4°C., but must retain some activity at 37°C. Most cold antibodies initiate the complement sequence when they combine with antigen, and it is complement that actually damages the circulating cells. Very rarely, powerful cold-reacting antibodies cause agglutination of red cells circulating in the cooler, superficial parts of the vascular bed, such as the fingers and toes. This produces vascular problems of the type called *Raynaud's phenomenon*, and often causes hemolysis as well.[48] Cold antibody-induced hemolysis may be chronic or episodic, but hemoglobin levels rarely fall below 8 or 9 gm./dl. and often remain within the normal range. Symptomatic cold AIHA is relatively rare, usually occurring after mycoplasmal or viral pneumonia or in company with hematologic or other malignancies. Spontaneous, or idiopathic, cold agglutinin disease sometimes occurs in elderly people. It may be necessary for them to wear gloves or move to warmer climates, but the disease is not life-threatening.

Warm AIHA is more common and causes more severe problems than the cold variety.[45] Intravascular lysis does not occur; instead, cells circulate which are coated with antibody, and the spleen removes them from the circulation. The rate of splenic destruction varies with the specificity and concentration of the antibody, the presence or absence of complement attachment, the functional capacity of the spleen, and various imponderables.[22] Autoimmune hemolysis can range from a mild compensated condition with normal hemoglobin levels to cell destruction so inexorable that life is threatened. If erythropoiesis falters as red cell destruction increases, anemia develops more rapidly. Warm AIHA, often idiopathic, occurs without any apparent provocation, especially in younger to middle-aged women.[17] As a secondary phenomenon, warm AIHA may accompany collagen-vascular diseases or lymphomas, or, rather uncommonly, colon or breast carcinoma, tuberculosis, or viral infections.[14]

Diagnosis depends upon demonstrating the presence of antibody or complement on the circulating red cells (see Antiglobulin Testing, in Chapter 8), and the occurrence of accelerated destruction. Anti-body sometimes exists free in the serum, but this is not necessary for diagnosing AIHA.

DRUG-ASSOCIATED HEMOLYSIS

Innumerable drugs have elicited antibodies in patients who receive them, but relatively few do so with great regularity. Probably the commonest offender is the anti-hypertension agent *alpha-methyldopa*. Between one-fifth and one-third of patients who take this drug for more than 6 months develop antibody which attaches to, and seems to be directed against, the red cell membrane itself. The reactive material behaves like an anti-red cell antibody rather than like an anti-drug antibody.[14] Despite the undoubted presence of immuno-globulin on red cell surface, very few such patients have significant hemolysis, and fewer still become anemic. Why the antibody de-velops, why it fails to cause hemolysis more often, and what role the drug plays are questions that remain unresolved.[17]

In most other drug-related hemolytic conditions, antibody is di-rected against drugs rather than against cells. Three types of cell alteration have been described. In the *penicillin* type, the patient develops a circulating anti-drug antibody which causes no ill effects unless the patient receives such large doses of the drug that it attaches to and coats the red cells. When the drug is on the red cell mem-brane, combination with specific anti-drug antibody causes the anti-body to attach to the cells, which then undergo splenic destruction. Penicillin antibodies of this type are demonstrated by inducing agglu-tination of drug-coated reagent red cells in vitro. Hemolysis may be mild or modest and ceases promptly when the drug is discontinued.

A more dangerous type of red cell destruction is the *"innocent bystander"* reaction. The circulating drug combines with circulating antibody to form relatively insoluble immune complexes. The immune complexes settle out on red cell surfaces and attract complement to the scene. It is the complement, not the drug or the antibody, which hemolyzes the cell. Hemolysis is rapid and may be massive. Drugs that fairly often elicit this reaction includes the quinine derivatives, *p*-amino salicylic acid, phenacetin, sulfonamides, and various insecti-cides. Many others have caused problems in individual, idiosyncratic cases. Repeat exposure to even small amounts of the drug can rapidly precipitate hemolysis of the same type and intensity. Diagnosis may be difficult, since the antibody-drug complex often detaches from the red cells, leaving only the complement attached.

Cephalosporins in high doses alter the red cell membrane in some way to allow all sorts of proteins to adhere to the surface. This is not immune attachment, and the attached proteins can include any or all the plasma proteins, even albumin. The antiglobulin test becomes strongly positive, but there is no immunohemolytic activity or impairment of red cell survival or function.

MACROCYTOSIS AND MEGALOBLASTIC ERYTHROPOIESIS

Nearly all conditions with megaloblastic nuclear development have circulating red cells that are larger than normal, but macrocytosis does not infallibly indicate megaloblastic marrow changes. Young red cells and reticulocytes are larger than normal red cells, thus patients with rapid cell production may have high mean cell volume. Macrocytic anemias are seen in many patients with compensated hemolytic conditions; in those recovering from acute blood loss; in those with liver disease, hypothyroidism, or sideroblastic anemia; in many patients with excessive alcohol intake; and in some with aplastic or hypoplastic anemia.[3] Increased cell size in an anemic patient demands bone marrow examination to determine whether or not megaloblastic changes exist.[13]

Megaloblastic Hematopoiesis

In megaloblastic cellular development, DNA production is impaired but not absent. At the same time, because RNA production progresses normally, nuclear and cytoplasmic maturation gets out of phase. DNA and RNA production occurs in all replicating cells; megaloblastic changes are not confined to red cells or even to blood cells. The changes are most dramatic, most clinically apparent, and most easily diagnosed, however, in red cell precursors, and anemia is a common presenting complaint. Diagnostic investigation usually centers around the red cell, but other hematopoietic cells and rapidly reproducing epithelial cells may also have morphologic and functional abnormalities. Both vitamin B_{12} and folic acid are necessary for the intermediary steps that provide raw materials and enzymes for DNA synthesis.

MARROW MORPHOLOGY

Cells in which DNA synthesis is slowed but RNA is developing normally are large and show greater cytoplasmic maturity than would be expected for the stage of nuclear maturity. Nuclear chromatin condenses in a loose, lacy, or sieve-like pattern. (Fig. 5) Cell division can be impaired, but many cells that begin the processes of replication and maturation simply fail to survive. The megaloblastic marrow is inefficient. Because more cells are begun than are completed, there is an excess of mitotic figures and a preponderance of young forms. The entire marrow is hyperplastic, and the red cell series usually is preponderant. If there is infection or other granulocytic stress, white cell precursors may outnumber red cells. Not numerically striking, but pathognomonic when present, are "giant metamyelocytes," which are huge myeloid cells with enormous cytoplasm and chromatin abnormally dispersed in the large nucleus.[3]

CAUSES OF MEGALOBLASTOSIS

The two most common problems leading to megaloblastosis are *vitamin B₁₂ deficiency* and *deficiency of folic acid* (see sections below). Sprue and other enteropathies often depress absorption of both these substances. Many drugs cause megaloblastosis by interfering with DNA synthesis, some as antagonists of folic acid or inhibitors of

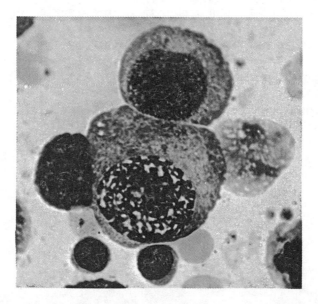

Figure 5. Megaloblasts in the bone marrow of a patient with pernicious anemia. Note the large, immature, atypically clumped nucleus and abundant cytoplasm.

purine or pyrimidine synthesis,[54] and others, especially alcohol, through less clearly defined pathways. Several rare, genetically determined enzyme defects (e.g., Lesch-Nyhan syndrome, orotic aciduria) cause megaloblastosis in addition to other signs and symptoms. In an interesting study of 100 consecutive patients with megaloblastic anemia McPhedran and his colleagues[40] found that 50 were deficient in B_{12} or folic acid or both, 24 had received cytotoxic drugs for treating neoplasms, 15 had liver disease, and 11 were severe alcoholics. Other much less common causes are myxedema, sideroblastic anemia, and multiple myeloma. Widespread neoplastic disease can cause systemic megaloblastic effects. The local presence of tumor cells in the marrow induces megaloblastic change in adjacent hematopoietic cells, suggesting some sort of direct competition for metabolites or inhibition of normal reactions.[3]

LABORATORY FINDINGS

Whether or not anemia exists, megaloblastic conditions provoke increased mean red cell size, involving mean corpuscular volumes of up to 125 or 130 μ^3. Anemia may be profound; levels of 3 or 4 gm./dl. are not uncommon in untreated pernicious anemia. Reticulocyte counts are disproportionately low for the degree of marrow hyperactivity and anemia, but nucleated red cells may be present in peripheral blood. Granulocyte and platelet counts are often below normal. Some neutrophils are strikingly large. Many have nuclei with five or more lobes and are called *hypersegmented neutrophils.*

Serum iron and transferrin saturation are normal or high, unless iron deficiency coexists with the megaloblastic condition. Marrow iron stores are also normal or increased. The inefficient erythropoiesis causes indirect bilirubin levels to rise slightly and urine urobilinogen excretion to increase severely. Lactic dehydrogenase (LDH) levels rise to striking levels with isoenzyme 1 predominating. Total LDH rises in any hemolytic condition, but in most cases, isoenzyme 2 exceeds 1.[3] Vitamin B_{12} and folate assays are diagnostic for these deficiency states but cannot indicate the cause of the deficiency.

Vitamin B_{12} Deficiency

ABSORPTION

Vitamin B_{12} occurs in nature as the product of specialized microorganisms which grow in, or serve as food supply to, animals located below humans in the food chain. Virtually all identifiable dietary B_{12} comes from animal products. Strict vegetarians sometimes develop mild deficiency syndromes, but eggs and dairy products protect less thoroughgoing vegetarians from this problem.[4] The daily requirement for adults seems to be 5 μg., and the "average, Western" diet contains 5 to 30 μg. daily. Pregnancy, rapid growth, hypermetabolism, and decreased absorption serve to increase the daily need.

In the stomach, ingested B_{12} combines with intrinsic factor (IF), a glycoprotein secreted by the parietal cells of gastric mucosa. Gastric acidity enhances the binding process, the product of which is a complex that attaches to a receptor site in the ileal mucosa. Once through the ileal wall, B_{12} combines with a transport protein which carries it to the liver where large quantities are stored. Unbound B_{12} can cross the ileal mucosa by simple diffusion if there is enough of it in the intestinal lumen.

PERNICIOUS ANEMIA

Classical or "Addisonian" pernicious anemia is a chronic disease with familial incidence. The disease complex includes atrophy of gastric mucosa, megaloblastic blood cell changes due to vitamin B_{12} deficiency, a high incidence of autoimmune phenomena, and neurologic manifestations of uncertain origin. Dysplastic changes in oral mucosa and tongue also are common. Because the atrophic gastric mucosa secretes neither intrinsic factor nor hydrochloric acid, diagnostically significant achlorhydria and defective B_{12} absorption are observed. The Schilling test (see p. 18) is the foundation of laboratory diagnosis, once megaloblastic anemia has been established. In most cases, measuring plasma or red cell B_{12} levels is unnecessary.

Pernicious anemia becomes apparent in middle adulthood or later. Incidence is highest in persons of northern European extraction. No clear pattern of genetic transmission exists, but blood relatives of an affected patient are at severe risk for part or all of the disease complex. Patients with pernicious anemia, as well as their hematologically normal relatives, frequently have autoantibodies related to the stomach and, often, related to the thyroid (see p. 223). It is not clear whether autoimmune phenomena produce the mucosal changes or whether mucosal disease so alters the cells that autoantibodies are induced.[25] Antibodies can exist against parietal cell elements, against intrinsic factor (IF) itself, or against both. Some few patients have anti-IF antibodies in gastric juice as well as in serum. These patients fail to absorb B_{12} properly, even when given supplementary intrinsic factor.[31]

Therapy for pernicious anemia is simple and effective. Vitamin B_{12} is given by injection, bypassing the absorption defect and permitting resumption of normal hematopoiesis.[30] Injected B_{12} corrects the neurologic symptoms but affects neither the patient's achlorhydria nor his increased liability (about three times normal) to develop gastric carcinoma. Thyroid and adrenal hypofunction are more prevalent in these patients than in the general population.[4]

OTHER CAUSES OF IMPAIRED ABSORPTION

Gastrectomy, either total or partial, causes intrinsic factor deficiency and may lead, in months or years, to vitamin B_{12} deficiency. Prolonged deficiency of IF can cause such severe atrophy of the ileal absorption site that therapeutic administration of IF takes some time to promote adequate B_{12} absorption. Resection of the ileum or ileal diseases such as gluten-sensitive enteropathy and regional enteritis removes the site of absorption. Organisms within the intestine occasionally deflect luminal B_{12} stores for their own use. This can occur with bacterial overgrowth due to altered intestinal flow patterns ("blind loop" syndrome) or with infestation by the fish tapeworm, *Diphyllobothrium latum*. The tapeworm problem is largely confined to northern Scandinavia, where incompletely cooked fish is consumed by a population with high genetic predisposition to pernicious anemia.

Folic Acid Deficiency

DIETARY CONSIDERATIONS

Folates are abundant in yeast, in many vegetable foods, and in organ meats such as liver and kidney. Leafy vegetables, lemons, bananas, and mushrooms are especially good sources, but ample folate intake occurs in most well-balanced diets. Enormous excess, however, does not exist in most dietary intake, and prolonged boiling can inactivate some accessible folates. The body stores relatively little folic acid— only enough to last through 2 to 4 months of zero dietary intake. Requirements increase with growth, pregnancy and lactation, hypermetabolic states, and malignant neoplasms. Absorption diminishes with intestinal diseases and after subtotal gastrectomy.

Unlike B_{12} deficiency, inadequate diet can directly produce folate deficiency. This is especially noticeable in pregnancy, in poorly nourished adolescents during their growth spurt, and in alcoholics. Infants fed predominantly on milk, and elderly persons who subsist on cheap but filling carbohydrates are also severely at risk.

THE EFFECTS OF DRUGS

Alcohol is undoubtedly the commonest pharmacologic cause of folic acid deficiency,[36] but the mechanisms are complex and poorly understood. Alcohol seems to impair absorption and also to interfere with folate-dependent enzymatic reactions.[54] In addition, chronic alcoholics often have defective diets, multiple vitamin deficiencies, reduced hepatic functions, and poor or absent tissue stores of folic acid. Since alcohol also influences iron metabolism and pyridoxine pathways, it is not surprising that alcoholics so often have complex, severe hematologic problems.[10]

Folic acid antagonists are pharmacologic agents given precisely because they interfere with the folate-dependent steps in cell multiplication. Methotrexate and aminopterin are cytotoxic agents widely used for treating leukemias and other malignancies. When used to treat nonhematologic conditions, their depressive effects on the marrow can sometimes be prevented by simultaneous administration of citrovorum factor.

Oral contraceptives, diphenylhydantoin and related *anticonvulsants,* and the antituberculosis drug *cycloserine* seem to reduce folic acid absorption. Patients taking these drugs should be observed for the development of megaloblastic anemia.

LABORATORY FINDINGS

In addition to the changes seen in all megaloblastic anemias, folic acid deficiency produces low serum and red cell folate levels, increased urinary excretion of formiminoglutamic acid (FIGlu), and normal levels of serum B_{12} and urinary methylmalonic acid.

APLASTIC ANEMIA

Bone marrow failure can affect all, several, or only individual cell lines. When platelets, white cells, and red cells are all involved, the condition is called *pancytopenia*. When hypoplasia affects only one cell line, it is usually the red cell. Marrow deficiency due to a drug, infectious agent, or metabolic abnormality is called *secondary aplastic* (hypoplastic) *anemia*. If no predisposing cause coexists, the condition is called *primary*, or *idiopathic*. Most cases of aplastic anemia are *acquired*, developing in previously normal children or adults. A few cases result from constitutional defects.

Bone Marrow Replacement

When neoplastic cells infiltrate the hematopoietic marrow, pancytopenia develops if the process is extensive, but red cell production is depressed before other cell lines are affected. Leukemias, multiple myelomas, lymphomas, and carcinomas of prostate, lung, and breast are the commonest tumor sources.[63] Diagnosis rests on demonstrating the presence of malignant cells, but the presence of bizarre or randomly immature blood cells in the circulation tends to raise suspicion, especially if there are suggestive x-ray changes.

Myelofibrosis is replacement of hematopoietic marrow by connective tissue elements. This is thought to be one aspect of the larger group of *myeloproliferative syndromes*, which also includes granulocytic leukemia and polycythemia vera.[51] Anemia develops gradually, and misshapen, teardrop cells are frequent. As the bone marrow gets squeezed out, other parts of the reticuloendothelial system begin hematopoiesis, especially the spleen. Splenic sinusoids have less ability than bone marrow to regulate release of maturing cells into the blood. Immature red cells and granulocytes are seen in circulating blood when extramedullary hematopoiesis is present.

Childhood Aplastic Anemias

Severe erythroid hypoplasia may be present at birth or in early infancy. In *Fanconi's syndrome,* decreased production of red cells and granulocytes accompanies a constellation of abnormalities that includes dwarfism, skeletal and renal aberrations, and mental retardation. Reticulocytes are present, although reduced in absolute number, along with increased hemoglobin F. Androgen therapy characteristically improves both red cell and white cell production.[61]

Another constitutional syndrome, named for *Blackfan* and *Diamond*, who first described it, affects only the bone marrow. It causes severe anemia with very few reticulocytes but with relatively normal white cells and platelets. Androgen therapy has been disappointing, but some patients have responded to corticosteroids.

Anemias Associated with Other Diseases

Chronic infections, noninfectious inflammatory diseases such as

rheumatoid arthritis and rheumatic fever, slowly progressive neoplasms, and long-standing renal failure all depress bone marrow
function by mechanisms not clearly understood. The laboratory findings are of a normochromic, normocytic anemia, usually of moderate
degree (7 to 11 gm./dl.), with normal or near-normal red cell survival,
reduced serum iron and transferrin levels, and normal or increased
storage iron in the marrow. The bone marrow may be somewhat less
cellular than normal, but those cells that are present have normal
appearance and proportions. Therapy with iron, androgens, and
adrenal steroids does not ameliorate the anemia and may make it
worse. Successful treatment of the underlying disease corrects the
hematologic abnormalities without further treatment.

Bone marrow aplasia sometimes follows viral hepatitis; usually
this resolves spontaneously, but occasionally it may be fatal.[29] Other
viral infections have been implicated in sporadic cases. Tuberculosis
may depress bone marrow function, but its other possible hematologic
effects include pancytopenia due to splenomegaly, or leukocytosis
so severe as to resemble leukemia.

Hypothyroidism classically causes a rather mild anemia through
generalized hypometabolism. Because metabolic activity is low, the
lowered hemoglobin level does not cause tissue hypoxia; thus erythropoietin is not stimulated, and the bone marrow adjusts to lowered
equilibrium.[63]

Drug-Induced Marrow Failure

DOSE-RELATED DRUGS

Certain drugs reliably depress bone marrow activity at a critical dose
level. Benzene, benzene derivatives, and arsenicals are depressant
drugs to which exposure is usually accidental. The cytotoxic drugs
given to suppress neoplasms all produce marrow depression as part
of their intended pharmacologic effect. Ionizing radiation and radio-
mimetic drugs, folic acid antagonists, purine and pyrimidine analogs,
colchicine, the periwinkle derivatives, and the cytotoxic antibiotics
(daunorubicin and adriamycin) affect rapidly multiplying cells of
any kind. The therapeutic usefulness of these drugs depends upon
the clinician's ability to counteract their marrow-suppressive effects
by means of transfusions and antimicrobial therapy.

IDIOSYNCRATIC EFFECTS

An endless list of pharmaceutical agents has been incriminated in aplastic anemia, granulocytopenia, or pancytopenia. Chloramphenicol is probably the most notorious. In laboratory settings, chloramphenicol inhibits protein synthesis and mitochondrial synthetic activity, but its specific effect in vivo remains obscure. A reversible form of marrow depression, associated with cytoplasmic vacuolization and depressed heme synthesis, often follows chloramphenicol administration but is probably a different effect from that which causes permanent marrow aplasia.[44]

Gold compounds, phenylbutazone, aspirin, sulfonamides, and hydantoins have been associated with modest numbers of case reports.[62] Red cell, white cell, and platelet levels should be monitored in patients receiving chronic treatment with these agents. If a downward trend develops, caution dictates discontinuing the drug if at all possible.

Idiopathic Aplastic Anemia

Marrow failure unrelated to any known cause is called primary or idiopathic aplastic anemia. As many as 50 percent of gradually developing cases have no apparent external cause.[38] Diagnosis depends upon excluding other hematologic or nonhematologic conditions. The anemia is usually normochromic and normocytic and is characterized by low reticulocyte counts, low or normal iron and transferrin levels, normal red cell life span, absence of immunologic abnormalities, and normal hemoglobin structure. The bone marrow is usually hypocellular. Platelets and granulocyte numbers decline in parallel with red cell activity. Red cell hypoplasia along with normal development of other marrow elements suggests anemia of chronic illness, and the patient should be examined for occult illnesses such as infection, indolent inflammatory disease, endocrine abnormality, or incipient neoplasm.

Idiopathic aplastic anemia more often ends fatally if the onset is rapid than if it develops slowly.[38] Many patients with chronic aplastic anemia eventually develop leukemia, other myeloproliferative diseases, or lymphoreticular diseases, but some patients continue unchanged for years, and some get better spontaneously. Paroxysmal nocturnal hemoglobinuria is present, initially or eventually, in a modest number of aplastic anemias.

POLYCYTHEMIA

Polycythemia literally means "many blood cells," but usually it refers to increased red cell mass. When red cell production increases to meet a recognizable physiologic stimulus, the condition is called *secondary*, or *reactive, polycythemia*. Spontaneous or seemingly unprovoked increase in red cell production and blood volume is called *polycythemia vera*, or "true polycythemia."

Secondary Polycythemia

Erythropoietin stimulates red cell production. The pattern of erythropoietin secretion determines the body's red cell mass. Either relative or absolute tissue hypoxia stimulates erythropoietin release. If tissue oxygen levels are perceived as inadequate, red cell production will continue, regardless of the actual hemoglobin or red cell levels. In rare cases, usually involving neoplasms, continuous, inappropriate erythropoiesis occurs without relation to changes in tissue oxygenation.

"SPURIOUS" POLYCYTHEMIA

Increased hematocrit does not always mean increased red cell mass. Hematocrit rises to above-normal levels whenever more fluid is lost from the blood stream than red cells. This can occur in dehydration from vomiting, diarrhea, prolonged fever, or heat stroke, and in the massive plasma exudation that follows extensive burns.[60] Dehydration usually can be inferred from elevated levels of serum proteins and electrolytes, especially sodium.

A peculiar syndrome of elevated hematocrit, high serum levels of cholesterol and uric acid, high blood pressure, and predisposition to thromboembolic episodes is sometimes noted in middle-aged men. Total red cell mass is normal, despite venous hematocrits of between 52 and 60 percent, and there is no increase in white cell or platelet levels. These patients often are somewhat obese. If weight, blood pressure, and serum lipid levels are corrected, the red cell problem disappears.[24]

INAPPROPRIATE POLYCYTHEMIA

Elevated hematocrits occasionally occur in patients with renal carcinoma and in those with cerebellar hemangiomas. Erythropoietin production by tumor cells is a tempting hypothesis, but it has not been demonstrated definitively. In populations in which hepatoma occurs frequently, erythrocytosis has been observed in many patients with this carcinoma. Pheochromocytoma and aldosterone-producing adrenal adenomas also have been associated with elevated circulating erythropoietin levels and high hematocrit.[63]

REACTIVE POLYCYTHEMIA

Tissues may get too little oxygen if there is too little oxygen in the inspired air, if oxygen transport from alveolus to blood stream is impaired, if there is inadequate hemoglobin to carry the oxygen, if abnormal blood flow prevents hemoglobin from reaching the tissues, or if hemoglobin fails to release bound oxygen at tissue sites. Inadequate hemoglobin levels constitute anemia. The other events may occur with normal hemoglobin levels, and the result is stimulation to increased hemoglobin production.

Hypoxic polycythemia occurs in normal persons exposed to air with low oxygen content (high altitude accommodation).[26] Patients with pulmonary disease, with heart defects that allow oxygenated and deoxygenated blood to mix, or with defective hemoglobin function have reactive erythrocytosis at normal oxygen partial pressures. Laboratory findings include a hematocrit of 55 to 70 percent with normal or increased mean cell size and an increased absolute number of reticulocytes. Plasma volume is normal or slightly increased, and white cell and platelet levels are normal. Often one can locate the respiratory defect by comparing blood levels of oxygen and carbon dioxide with gas levels in the alveolar air.

Polycythemia Vera

Polycythemia vera (PV) belongs to the group of myeloproliferative syndromes. Erythrocytic proliferation predominates, but other marrow elements also are hyperactive.[51] PV occurs in older adults, in males slightly more often than in females, usually with an insidious onset easily confused with other problems. The skin is ruddy, and physical examination reveals splenomegaly. Patients often complain of generalized itching or of visual or middle-ear symptoms when the disease is active.[28] Thrombosis or hemorrhage or both are common complications, accounting for about 50 percent of deaths.[28]

In about 15 percent of patients, the clinical course eventuates in acute leukemia; in another 15 percent, the marrow becomes fibrotic and extramedullary hematopoiesis (*myeloid metaplasia*) occurs. Many workers believe that radioactive isotopes given as therapy cause the later malignant evolution; others believe that the malignant predisposition is part of the disease and that radiotherapy simply hastens the result.[56]

LABORATORY FINDINGS

Increased red cell mass, in addition to increased hematocrit, is a diagnostic criterion for PV. Plasma volume may or may not be increased, but there is nearly always an increase in white cells (12,000 to 25,000/mm.^{3} and sometimes much more) and platelets (over 450,000/mm.^{3}). Although white cells have normal appearance and function, platelets may be enlarged or misshapen, and aggregation and ADP release tend to be impaired.[6] Although plasma coagulation factors behave normally, whole blood clotting and clot retraction are abnormal because there is so little plasma and platelet activity relative to the mass of red cells. Markedly increased blood viscosity causes significant circulatory problems.

Early in the disease, red cell morphology is normal. If there is myeloid metaplasia or pronounced splenomegaly, blood findings become increasingly abnormal as the disease progresses. The bone marrow shows hypercellularity in all cell lines, unless myelofibrosis supervenes.

Arterial oxygen saturation is normal or slightly reduced, contrasting sharply with the low levels that characterize secondary polycythemia. Leukocyte alkaline phosphatase levels usually are increased. This finding distinguishes the sometimes marked leukocytosis of PV from that of chronic granulocytic leukemia, in which leukocyte alkaline phosphatase is low or absent. Serum uric acid levels are characteristically high, and a minority of patients develop a secondary gout syndrome. Serum vitamin B_{12} levels are above normal, owing to the presence of excessive B_{12}-binding protein. The reason for this change is unclear.

REFERENCES

1. Balcerzak, S. P., and Bromberg, P. A.: *Secondary polycythemia.* Semin. Hematol. 12:353, 1975.
2. Beck, W. S.: *Folic acid deficiency,* in Williams, W. J., Beutler, E., Erslev, A. J., and Rundles, R. W. (eds.): *Hematology.* ed. 2. McGraw-Hill, New York, 1977.

3. Beck, W. S.: *General considerations of megaloblastic anemias,* in Williams, W. J., Beutler, E., Erslev, A. J., and Rundles, R. W. (eds.): *Hematology.* ed. 2. McGraw-Hill, New York, 1977.
4. Beck, W. S.: *Vitamin B₁₂ deficiency,* in Williams, W. J., Beutler, E., Erslev, A. J., and Rundles, R. W. (eds.): *Hematology.* ed. 2. McGraw-Hill, New York, 1977.
5. Bellingham, A. J., and Prankerd, T. A. J.: *Hereditary spherocytosis.* Clin. Haematol. 4:139, 1975.
6. Berger, S., Aledort, L. M., Gilbert, H. S., et al.: *Abnormalities of platelet function in patients with polycythemia vera.* Cancer Res. 33:2683, 1973.
7. Beutler, E.: *Glucose-6-phosphate dehydrogenase deficiency,* in Williams, W. J., Beutler, E., Erslev, A. J., and Rundles, R. W., (eds.): *Hematology.* ed. 2. McGraw-Hill, New York, 1977.
8. Beutler, E.: *Hemolytic anemia due to chemical and physical agents,* in Williams, W. J., Beutler, E., Erslev, A. J., and Rundles, R. W. (eds.): *Hematology.* ed. 2. McGraw-Hill, New York, 1977.
9. Beutler, E.: *Hemolytic anemia due to infections with microorganisms,* in Williams, W. J., Beutler, E., Erslev, A. J., and Rundles, R. W. (eds.): *Hematology.* ed. 2. McGraw-Hill, New York, 1977.
10. *Blood in the alcohol stream.* Lancet 2:806, 1977.
11. Brewer, G. J.: *A view of the current status of antisickling therapy.* Am. J. Hematol. 1:121, 1976.
12. Cartwright, G. E., and Deiss, A.: *Sideroblasts, siderocytes, and sideroblastic anemia.* N. Engl. J. Med. 292:185, 1975.
13. Chanarin, I.: *Investigation and management of megaloblastic anaemias.* Clin. Haematol. 5:747, 1976.
14. Chaplin, H.: *Autoimmune hemolytic anemia* (Grand Rounds, edited by L. V. Avioli). Arch. Intern. Med. 137:346, 1977.
15. Cook, J. D., Finch, C. A., and Smith, N. J.: *Evaluation of the iron status of a population.* Blood 48:449, 1976.
16. Cooper, R. A., and Jandl, J. H.: *Hereditary spherocytosis,* in Williams, W. J., Beutler, E., Erslev, A. J., and Rundles, R. W. (eds.): *Hematology.* ed. 2. McGraw-Hill, New York, 1977.
17. Dacie, J. V.: *Autoimmune hemolytic anemia.* Arch. Intern. Med. 135:1293, 1975.
18. Dacie, J. V., and Lewis, S. M.: *Paroxysmal nocturnal hemoglobinuria: clinical manifestations, haematology, and nature of the disease.* Sem. Haematol. 3:3, 1972.
19. Das, K. C., and Herbert, V.: *Vitamin B₁₂-folate interrelations.* Clin. Haematol. 5:697, 1976.
20. Desforges, J. F.: *Genetic implications of G-6-PD deficiency.* N. Engl. J. Med. 294:1438, 1976.
21. Desforges, J. F.: *Hemoglobin—a working molecule.* N. Engl. J. Med. 295:164, 1976.
22. Engelfriet, C. P., Borne, A. E., Beckers, D., and Van Loghem, J. J.: *Autoimmune haemolytic anaemia: serological and immunochemical characteristics of the autoantibodies; mechanisms of cell destruction.* Ser. Haematol. 7:328, 1974.
23. England, J. M., Ward, S. M., and Down, M. C.: *Microcytosis, anisocytosis, and the red cell indices in iron deficiency.* Br. J. Haematol. 34:589, 1976.
24. Erslev, A. J.: *Secondary polycythemia,* in Williams, W. J., Beutler, E.,

Erslev, A. J., and Rundles, R. W. (eds.): *Hematology*. ed. 2. McGraw-Hill, New York, 1977.

25. Fisher, J. M., and Taylor, K. B. *The significance of gastric antibodies*. Br. J. Haematol. 20:1, 1971.

26. Frisancho, A. R.: *Functional adaptation to high altitude hypoxia*. Science 187:313, 1975.

27. Glader, B. E., and Nathan, D. G.: *Haemolysis due to pyruvate kinase deficiency and other glycolytic enzymopathies*. Clin. Haematol. 4:123, 1975.

28. Glass, J. L., and Wasserman, L. R.: *Primary polycythemia*, in Williams, W. L., Beutler, E., Erslev, A. J., and Rundles, R. W. (eds.): *Hematology*. ed. 2. McGraw-Hill, New York, 1977.

29. Hagler, L., Pastore, R. A., and Bergin, J. J.: *Aplastic anemia following viral hepatitis: report of two fatal cases and literature review*. Medicine (Baltimore) 54:139, 1975.

30. Havrani, F. I.: *Vitamin B_{12} and the megaloblastic development*. Science 182:78, 1973.

31. Herbert, V. L.: Laboratory aids in the diagnosis of folic acid and vitamin B_{12} deficiencies. Ann. Clin. Lab. Sci. 1:193, 1971.

32. Hillman, R. S.: *Acute blood loss anemia*, in Williams, W. J., Beutler, E., Erslev, A. J., and Rundles, R. W. (eds.): *Hematology*. ed. 2. McGraw-Hill, New York, 1977.

33. Kan, Y. W., Golbus, M. S., Trecartin, R. F., and Filly, R. A.: *Prenatal diagnosis of β-thalassemia and sickle-cell anemia*. Lancet 1:269, 1977.

34. Karp, R. J., Haaz, W. S., Starke, K., and Gorman, J. M.: *Iron deficiency in families of iron-deficient inner-city school children*. Am. J. Dis. Child. 128:18, 1974.

35. Klee, G., Fairbanks, V. F., Pierre, R. V., and O'Sullivan, M. B.: *Use of electronic erythrocyte measurements in the diagnosis of iron deficiency and thalassemia trait*. Am. J. Clin. Pathol. 66:870, 1976.

36. Lane, F., Goff, P., McGuffin, R., et al.: *Folic acid metabolism in normal, folate deficient, and alcoholic man*. Br. J. Haematol. 34:489, 1976.

37. Lehmann, H., Huntsman, R. G., Casey, R., et al.: *Sickle cell disease and related disorders*, in Williams, W. J., Beutler, E., Erslev, A. J., and Rundles, R. W. (eds.): *Hematology*. ed. 2. McGraw-Hill, New York, 1977.

38. Lynch, R. E., Williams, D. M., Reading, J. C., and Cartwright, G. E.: *The prognosis in aplastic anemia*. Blood 45:517, 1975.

39. Marks, P. A., Johnson, A. B., Hirschberg, E., and Banks, J.: *Studies on the mechanism of aging of human red blood cells*. Ann. N.Y. Acad. Sci. 75:95, 1958.

40. McPhedran, P., Barnes, M. G., Weinstein, J. S., and Robertson, J. S.: *Interpretation of electronically determined macrocytosis*. Ann. Intern. Med. 78:677, 1973.

41. Meyer, U. A., Strand, L. J., Doss, M., et al.: *Intermittent acute porphyria — genetic defect in porphobilinogen metabolism*. N. Engl. J. Med. 286:1277, 1972.

42. Nathan, D., and Alter, B. P.: *Antenatal diagnosis of the haemoglobinopathies*. Br. J. Haematol. 31:143, 1975.

43. Orkin, S. H., and Nathan, D. G.: *The thalassemias*. N. Engl. J. Med. 295:710, 1977.

44. Petitpierre, M.-P. J., and Beck, E. A.: *Effects of chloramphenicol on heme synthesis*. Clin. Haematol. 4:167, 1975.

45. Pirofsky, B.: *Immune haemolytic disease: the autoimmune haemolytic anemias.* Clin. Haematol. 4:167, 1975.
46. Price, P. M., Conover, J. H., and Hirschhorn, K.: *Chromosomal localization of human haemoglobin structural genes.* Nature 237:340, 1972.
47. Prieto, J., Barry, M., and Sherlock, S.: *Serum ferritin in patients with iron overload and with actue and chronic liver diseases.* Gastroenterology 68:525, 1975.
48. Rollke, D.: *Cold agglutination: antibodies and antigens.* Clin. Immunol. Immunopathol. 2:266, 1974.
49. Rosse, W. F.: *Variation in the red cells in paroxysmal nocturnal haemoglobinuria.* Br. J. Haematol. 24:327, 1973.
50. Rosse, W. F.: *Paroxysmal nocturnal hemoglobinuria,* in Williams, W. J., Beutler, E., Erslev, A. J., and Rundles, R. W. (eds.): *Hematology.* ed. 2. McGraw-Hill, New York, 1977.
51. Rundles, R. W.: *Myeloproliferative disorders—general considerations,* in Williams, W. J., Beutler, E., Erslev, A. J., and Rundles, R. W. (eds.): *Hematology.* ed. 2. McGraw-Hill, New York, 1977.
52. Sexauer, C. L., Graham, H. L., Starling, K. A., and Fernback, D. J.: *A test for abnormal hemoglobins in umbilical cord blood.* Am. J. Dis. Child. 130:805, 1976.
53. Sirchia, G., and Lewis, S. M.: *Paroxysmal nocturnal haemoglobinuria.* Clin. Haematol. 4:199, 1975.
54. Stebbins, R., and Bertino, J. R.: *Megaloblastic anaemia produced by drugs.* Clin. Haematol. 5:619, 1976.
55. Valentine, W. N.: *Sideroblastic anemias,* in Williams, W. J., Beutler, E., Erslev, A. J., and Rundles, R. W. (eds.): *Hematology.* ed. 2. McGraw-Hill, New York, 1977.
56. Wasserman, L. R. *The treatment of polycythemia vera.* Semin. Hematol. 13:57, 1976.
57. Weatherall, D. J.: *Molecular pathology of the thalassemia disorders.* West. J. Med. 124:388, 1976.
58. Weatherall, D. J.: *The thalassemias,* in Williams, W. J., Beutler, E., Erslev, A. J., and Rundles, R. W. (eds.): *Hematology.* ed. 2. McGraw-Hill, New York, 1977.
59. Weed, R. I.: *Hereditary spherocytosis.* Arch. Intern. Med. 135:1316, 1975.
60. Weinreb, N. J., and Shih, C. F.: *Spurious polycythemia.* Semin. Hematol. 12:397, 1975.
61. White, J. M., and Harvey, D. R.: *Defective synthesis of α and β globin chains in lead poisoning.* Nature 236:71, 1972.
62. Williams, D. M., Lynch, R. E., and Cartwright, G. E.: *Drug-induced aplastic anemia.* Semin. Hematol. 10:195, 1973.
63. Wintrobe, M. M., Lee, G. R., Boggs, D. R., et al.: *Clinical Hematology.* ed. 7. Lea & Febiger, Philadelphia, 1974.

CHAPTER 4

DISEASES OF
WHITE BLOOD CELLS

PROBLEMS OF CLASSIFICATION

It is misleading to consider "white blood cells" as a single category of cells. Classifying physiologic or pathologic responses on the assumption that white cells share common origins or functions is also misleading. One way to classify white cell diseases is by cell origin. In this light, granulocytes and monocytes belong together, since these myeloid cells derive from bone marrow, while lymphocytes develop in lymph nodes and related tissues. If the classification considers site and nature of mature activity, granulocytes stand alone as highly mobile cells involved in acute defensive responses, while monocytes, macrophages, and lymphocytes belong together as cells concerned with phagocytic activity and immunologic reactions.

Classifying pathophysiologic events accentuates the problems of systems and functions. Tissue macrophages, though ultimately derived from bone marrow, participate in nonhematologic conditions such as lipid and carbohydrate storage diseases; they participate in lymphoreticular disorders, notably lymphomas; and they play a leading role in certain leukemias, the quintessential hematologic disease. Similarly, lymphocytes and plasma cells, crucial figures in immunologic diseases that involve parenchymal organs and other nonmarrow tissues, are also the culprits in leukemias and multiple myeloma. Granulocytes, whose origins and functions seem straightforward on first inspection, become involved in bone marrow disorders that affect red cells and platelets but leave monocyte-macrophage activity relatively untouched.

Acknowledging the fact that no classification is ideal, we can attempt to schematize white cell disorders into qualitative changes (functional abnormalities), non-neoplastic quantitative changes, and neoplastic quantitative changes, as shown in Table 7.

Table 7. Diseases Affecting White Blood Cells

Disorders of Function
    Granulocytes: Chronic granulomatous disease; Chediak-Higashi syndrome
    Lymphocytes: Immunodeficiency syndromes
    Monocyte-macrophage: Sphingolipidoses ("storage diseases")
Non-neoplastic Quantitative Changes
    See tables for specific cell types in Chapter 1
    Leukemoid reactions; neutropenia/pancytopenia
    Acute infectious lymphocytosis
    Infectious mononucleosis
Neoplastic Disorders
    Myeloproliferative syndromes: Granulocytic leukemia, acute or chronic; monocytic and myelomonocytic leukemia; polycythemia vera; myelofibrosis; myeloid metaplasia
    Lymphoreticular disease, lymphocytes-plasma cells: Lymphocytic leukemia, acute or chronic; multiple myeloma; macroglobulinemia and other dysproteinemias
    Lymphoreticular disease, lymphoid organs: Hodgkin's disease; lymphocytic and lymphoblastic lymphomas; histiocytic lymphomas

---

DISORDERS OF FUNCTION

Neutrophils

Neutrophils are especially effective defenders against particulate agents, principally bacteria. Granulocytes are motile, responding to chemotactic stimuli to accumulate at the site of injury. Their range of offensive action includes phagocytosis, enzymatic reactions inside the cell, and release of enzymes to the extracellular milieu. If some or all of these functions are defective, the patient becomes abnormally susceptible to infection, even if normal numbers of neutrophils are circulating. Specialized techniques are available for concentrating neutrophils, labeling them, and exposing them to controlled challenges by which individual functions can be evaluated.

These investigations have uncovered a host of rare, exotically named, heritable conditions.[54] In the "lazy leukocyte" syndrome, neutrophils have defective motility, and sufferers experience recurrent pyogenic and fungal infections.[60] In "Job's syndrome," intrinsic motility is normal, but the response to chemotactic stimuli is inappropriate. In the Chediak-Higashi syndrome, phagocytosis is defective and enzymes accumulate in big cytoplasmic vacuoles.[17,64] Total absence of G-6-PD activity (see p. 47) also impairs intracellular defenses.

ACQUIRED OR SECONDARY DEFECTS

Before granulocytes can phagocytize particles, they must accumulate in the area and attach to the particles they are about to engulf. Surface adherence is enhanced if antibodies or complement proteins, or both, coat the foreign particles.[62] Patients with constitutional or acquired hypogammaglobulinemia lack antibodies and experience depressed neutrophilic antibacterial activity. Low complement levels, especially of factors 3 and 5, also impair immune adherence and response to chemotactic stimuli.

Hodgkin's disease and cirrhosis often depress neutrophilic function in patients whose chemotactic functions were previously normal.[53] Both of these conditions are characterized by increased incidence of infections. Exposure to alcohol, aspirin, or prednisone reduces adherent properties of granulocytes.[54] Both aspirin and prednisone are potent anti-inflammatory agents, and reduced adherence is only one of their many effects upon the inflammatory process. Other anti-inflammatory effects of alcohol include depression of cell surface activities (notably ciliary motion in respiratory epithelium); impairment, through folate inhibition, of normal hematopoiesis; and vacuolization of red and white cell precursors in the marrow.[59,63]

CHRONIC GRANULOMATOUS DISEASE

The most clearly characterized disorder of neutrophil function used to be called chronic granulomatous disease (CGD) of childhood; as the same defect has been found in older persons, the age-limited description has become less appropriate. Patients with CGD have granulocytes with normal mobility, normal adherence, and normal phagocytosis, but with defective bactericidal activity inside the cell. Everything goes well until the time for discharge of intralysosomal enzymes, and this discharge fails to occur. The defect relates to enzyme-mediated energy relationships, culminating in failure to generate hydrogen peroxide.[12,25] This failure is demonstrated in vitro with the nitroblue tetrazolium test (see p. 29).

The defective enzyme is the result of a gene on the X chromosome.

The usual form of the disease has an X-linked inheritance pattern. Victims suffer from recurrent bacterial infections, to which their tissue response is an indolent, nongranulocytic kind of inflammation. The usual pathogens are staphylococci, gram-negative bacilli, Candida, and aspergilli, while infections with streptococci and pneumococci rarely occur.

MYELOPEROXIDASE

Bactericidal phagocytosis requires, as a last step, interaction of hydrogen peroxide with an intracellular enzyme, *myeloperoxidase*. The syndrome of CGD occurs if myeloperoxidase activity is congenitally absent. Acquired deficiency of myeloperoxidase occurs in granulocytic leukemia, a fact that may contribute to the increased infection rates that occur in leukemia. Severe bacterial infections depress bactericidal efficiency. It may be that toxic granulations, which characterize neutrophils in severe systemic infections, reflect altered conditions of myeloperoxidase metabolism.

Lymphocytes

When lymphocytes are deficient in number or function, the patient suffers from immunodeficiency. Inherited immunodeficiency syndromes are rare but have an importance out of all proportion to their frequency because of the insights they reveal about normal immune functioning. Acquired deficiency states are very common. Anything that impairs cellular proliferation or protein synthesis can depress lymphocyte and plasma cell activity. Cytotoxic therapy for malignant diseases, adrenal cortical steroids, and negative protein balance are frequent predisposing conditions.

Monocyte-Macrophages

Blood monocytes and tissue macrophages are the same cell in different guises.[63] The circulating monocyte is probably a young or undifferentiated form. Once in the tissues, macrophages assume organelles and enzymes that permit phagocytosis and lytic activity. The cells that line sinusoids in spleen, liver, and lymph nodes also derive from the same monocyte-macrophage pool. Tissue macrophages recruit new members both by local cell reproduction and by repletion from bone marrow precursors. Macrophages exist as inconspicuous histiocytes in most tissues, becoming obvious only when they engage actively in phagocytosis. When there is substantial local demand for macrophages, as in tuberculosis and other granulomatous inflammations, bone marrow and blood monocyte turnover increases,[51] and monocytes accumulate in substantial numbers.

Normal macrophages have enzyme systems capable of synthesizing and of degrading *sphingolipids,* compounds important in biologic membranes and especially prominent in the nervous system.[9] Several different inherited defects involve specific enzymes necessary for lipid breakdown; in these deficiency states, lipid products accumulate in those parts of the cells that normally degrade recycled lipids. These diseases are not really hematologic conditions, although the macrophages of marrow, spleen, and liver become affected. Circulating monocytes and marrow precursors have no abnormalities distinctive for these "lipid storage diseases," but it is characteristic to find hepatosplenomegaly and depression of the bone marrow.[24] The reticuloendothelial system becomes involved in Gaucher's disease, Niemann-Pick disease, Fabry's disease, and "sea-blue histiocyte" syndrome.[5] In other defects of lipid catabolism, the lymphoreticular organs are not notably involved.

NON-NEOPLASTIC QUANTITATIVE DISORDERS

Total and differential white counts are useful but nonspecific diagnostic signs in many physiologic and pathologic states. Changing counts indicate that an abnormal condition exists and that the body is responding. Some of the nonhematologic conditions that affect white cell numbers are listed on pages 36 to 39. Some changes in white cell levels reflect conditions that directly affect the blood-forming organs.

Leukemoid Reactions

Reactive leukocytosis sometimes assumes florid proportions, with immature as well as mature white cells flooding the circulation. Because the blood picture resembles chronic leukemia, this event is called a "leukemoid reaction," but it is still a reaction to a nonhematologic condition. Granulocytes are most often involved, but striking monocytosis can occur in tuberculosis, while leukemoid lymphocytosis has been reported in tuberculosis, whooping cough, infectious mononucleosis, and acute infectious lymphocytosis (see below).

Granulocytosis of leukemoid proportions may accompany malignant tumors with or without metastases to bone;[45] severe pyogenic or tuberculous infection; heavy metal poisoning; or severe metabolic disturbances involving kidneys or liver, especially diabetic keto-acidosis.[16] A patient recovering from agranulocytosis may have such intense white cell production that it suggests leukemic proliferation, but leukopoiesis seldom continues at this rate longer than a week.

When leukemoid reaction is secondary to some obvious underlying condition, distinction from leukemia is not difficult. It should be remembered, however, that leukemia can coexist with other diseases. Leukemia and tuberculosis, for example, can occur together, and each exacerbates the other. If the primary condition is inapparent, the blood picture alone may suggest the presence of leukemia. Features that distinguish leukemoid reaction from granulocytic leukemia include absence of anemia, absence of increased blasts in the marrow, presence of normal or elevated leukocyte alkaline phosphatase, normal or increased platelet levels, and absence of Philadelphia chromosome.

Infectious Mononucleosis

Infectious mononucleosis (IM) is discussed at greater length in Chapter 14, but it is mentioned here because of the striking white cell changes. The white count may be low when the disease begins, but by the end of the first week, leukocytosis of 10,000 to 30,000/mm.[3] is usual.[30] There is an absolute increase in lymphocytes, most of which are large and many of which show the "atypical" changes originally thought to be pathognomonic for IM (Downey's cells). These are T-lymphocytes, showing changes suggestive of immuno-blastic transformation.[34,46] Circulating "virocytes" of this appearance are not unique to IM; in other viral diseases, as well, circulating T-lymphocytes manifest these reactive changes to viral infection of other cells or tissues. In IM, atypical lymphocytes are prominent during the second through fourth weeks of the illness.[28]

Acute Infectious Lymphocytosis

This benign disease of young children is probably viral, but no one agent has been incriminated, and "atypical" lymphocytes or "viro-cytes" are not seen.[26] Instead, there is an increase in small, mature lymphocytes, with counts usually between 25,000 and 50,000/mm.[3] Eosinophils also may be increased, but other hematologic values (hemoglobin, hematocrit, platelet count) are normal, and there are surprisingly few symptoms. The heterophil test is negative. Lymphocytosis lasts for 3 to 6 weeks and subsides uneventfully.[44] Epidemics have been reported among closely observed institutionalized children, but the disease is so minimally symptomatic that its incidence in the general population is not known.

Neutropenias

In several rare constitutional conditions, granulocytopenia occurs as part of a spectrum that also may include defective granulocyte differentiation, defective maturation, increased gamma globulins, decreased gamma globulins, presence of inhibitors to granulocytopoiesis, or presence of leukoagglutinating antibodies.[15] Moreover, the range of symptoms is wide. In familial benign chronic neutropenia, the condition may be discovered only by chance, whereas in infantile genetic agranulocytosis, death from infection usually occurs before the first birthday.

Investigation of a suspected constitutional neutropenia should begin with observation of bone marrow cellularity and maturational pattern. There can be either decreased production or increased destruction, or both. Besides evaluating the size of the spleen, one should evaluate the circulatory survival both of the patient's own cells and of transfused normal white cells. The serum also should be examined for the presence of antibodies, agglutinins, or inhibitors.[31] Attention should be given to the mobility, chemotactic responsiveness, and phagocytic properties of the white cells found in the circulation. A search should be made for simultaneous abnormalities of lymphocytes, of immune activity, and of red cell and platelet development.[50] In addition, the patient's family should be studied to detect a possible familial incidence.

Agranulocytosis

More drastic than lifelong neutropenia is sudden disappearance of granulocytes in a previously normal individual. Acquired neutropenia usually is due to drugs, antibodies, or the effects of infection. Drugs sometimes affect granulocyte levels without affecting other marrow elements, but often red cells and/or platelet numbers are reduced as well.[42] Antibodies may affect white cells only,[31] but drug antibodies that damage cells through the "innocent bystander" effect (see p. 113) sometimes affect all three cell types in the blood.

Most of the agents and pathophysiologic conditions that cause anemia also can depress granulocytes. In the late 1920s and 1930s, the analgesic drug *aminopyrine* was shown to induce antibodies that led to severe, highly specific agranulocytosis in older patients.[15] Except for agents clinically similar to aminopyrine, few other drugs cause fulminating destruction of neutrophils alone. Phenothiazines, hydantoins, some sulfonamides, and some antithyroid drugs depress leukocyte production. Neutropenia persists for several weeks after therapy ceases, but granulopoiesis resumes when the drug is stopped.[63] Chloramphenicol-induced marrow depression, on the other hand, may last for months or years.

INVESTIGATION

Diagnosis depends upon careful evaluation of total and differential white counts. If agranulocytosis causes necrotizing mouth infections, prostration, and fever, it may be difficult to distinguish among induced agranulocytosis, acute leukemia, and the granulo-suppressive effects of massive infection. Evaluation must include a meticulous inquiry about drugs and food additives and about exposure to materials involved in industrial, domestic, recreational, or environmental pursuits.

It is important to evaluate red cell and platelet numbers and bone marrow cellularity. With pure agranulocytosis, the total white count is low, and mature lymphocytes are virtually the only leukocytes in the circulating blood. Red cell and platelet levels, both in blood and in bone marrow, are normal. Pure agranulocytosis is relatively rare, since many exogenous agents also tend to depress red cell and platelet production. In leukemias, the marrow usually has increased proportions of blasts and highly immature cells, and marrow is often hypercellular despite low levels of circulating cells.

NEOPLASTIC DISEASES: MYELOPROLIFERATIVE DISORDERS

The category of myeloproliferative disorders includes a range of malignant and potentially malignant conditions involving bone marrow-derived cells. *Granulocytic* and *monocytic leukemias* are the best-known examples, and *polycythemia vera* can be fitted easily into the concept. *Erythroleukemia* (di Guglielmo's syndrome) may be a variant of granulocytic leukemia, but the involvement of red cell precursors is striking and unique to this condition. *Myelofibrosis* and *myeloid metaplasia* are less obviously myeloproliferative since, in both, the marrow cavity exhibits reduced hematopoietic activity. The marrow elements that exhibit increased activity are non-hematopoietic, namely connective tissue and histiocytes.[35] Hematopoietic elements attempt to compensate for excessive growth of other elements, and red and white cell lines may assume abnormal characteristics.

Acute Leukemias

Acute myeloblastic and acute lymphoblastic leukemia can be difficult to distinguish by simple examination of blood films or even of bone marrow smears. In doubtful cases, morphologic and cytochemical differences usually make distinction possible. The two conditions are so different in general epidemiologic and prognostic features that one must distinguish between them in discussing incidence and treatment. Since both conditions are of unknown etiology, distinction cannot be made on this basis.

EPIDEMIOLOGY

Acute lymphoblastic leukemia (ALL) is primarily a disease of children, while acute myeloblastic leukemia (AML) tends to strike adults. Of all the leukemias, ALL has shown the most gratifying long-term responses to therapy; AML, on the other hand, has the shortest post-therapy life expectancy.[23] Only 10 percent of AML is found in children, while 80 percent of ALL occurs in childhood. Older patients with ALL have a much worse prognosis than do children.[27]

The proportion of acute to chronic leukemia has been rising over the past several decades. In 1950, 44 percent of all leukemias were acute, and 56 percent were chronic; by 1965, the figures had risen to 64 percent acute and 36 percent chronic, and this proportion has continued to the present.[19] Acute leukemia has a lower incidence in blacks than in whites. More males than females suffer from leukemia of all sorts. For acute leukemia generally, the ratio is 3:2, but the male preponderance for ALL in children is much smaller—only 5:4.[6]

CLINICAL PRESENTATION

Both ALL and AML begin abruptly. Fatigue and fever are nearly universal. Presenting symptoms usually relate to anemia, bleeding tendency, or infection. These result directly from decreased red cell production, severely reduced platelets, and granulocyte depression to levels below those needed to combat microbial invasion. The actual white count is unpredictable. About 25 percent of patients have white counts above 50,000/mm.[3] Another 25 percent have subnormal counts (below 5,000/mm.[3]). About 15 percent have a normal number (5,000 to 10,000/mm.[3]) of white cells,[63] but these are clearly abnormal. About half the patients with newly diagnosed acute leukemia have high serum uric acid levels. After treatment, uric acid levels always rise precipitously.[8] Lactic dehydrogenase (LDH) levels often are elevated, with isoenzymes 2, 3, and 4 diffusely predominating.[38]

ACUTE MYELOBLASTIC LEUKEMIA

In acute myeloblastic leukemia, the blasts that overrun the marrow have finely dispersed or granular chromatin; several or numerous nucleoli; delicate, regular nuclear membrane; and modest amounts of cytoplasm, although the cell outline usually is regular.[22] Although maturation is minimal, promyelocytes are present and often are numerous. Auer rods often can be seen in the cytoplasm of those cells that mature. Abnormal eosinophils may be conspicuous. Circulating blood cells have low leukocyte alkaline phosphatase scores, and there are substantial numbers of cells positive for the peroxidase reaction and positive with Sudan black stains.[63]

Nucleated red cells and reticulocytosis tend to be more conspicuous in AML than in ALL. Platelet depression is often less extreme than in ALL; nearly half of AML patients present with platelet counts in the 50,000 to 150,000/mm.[3] range.[63] Hemorrhagic complications are more frequent, however, in the subvariant called *acute promyelocytic leukemia,* where a superimposed coagulation disorder complicates the thrombocytopenia.

Another variant presentation is *chloroma,* which literally means "green tumor"; another name is *granulocytic sarcoma.* This is a solid tumor of bone consisting of uniform, primitive cells which are very difficult to distinguish from the cells of primary bone marrow tumors. Chloroma often accompanies, or occasionally precedes, the blood changes of acute myeloblastic leukemia; it appears to be another facet of the same neoplastic process.[8]

Treatment of AML has been discouraging. Fewer than half of all treated patients achieve more than partial remission on the first course of therapy, and complete remission, when it occurs, lasts only a few months.[29] For those who achieve complete remission, survival averages about 17 months after diagnosis. With partial remissions, survival averages 6 months, and if there is no response to treatment, survival is less than 3 months. Until the introduction of intensive combination therapy, employing such agents as daunorubicin, cytosine arabinoside, and other recently developed drugs, remission rates were less than 25 percent. More recent treatment programs have attained complete or partial remission in 40 to 60 percent of AML.[23,29,63] Thus progress has occurred, though not to the extent seen with acute lymphoblastic leukemia (see p. 141).

ACUTE MONOCYTIC AND MYELOMONOCYTIC LEUKEMIA

When monocytic cells proliferate along with granulocytes, diagnostic categories become a bit fuzzy. Proliferating cells have twisted or indented nuclei, PAS-positive granules in the cytoplasm, and Sudan black staining patterns that differ from those seen in pure myeloblastic leukemia. Auer rods are seen in recognizable monocytes, promonocytes, and abnormal granulocytes, all of which are seen in circulating blood. One striking feature is an increase in urinary lysozyme levels, but the significance of this finding is unknown. These leukemias are less frequent than pure AML, but they occur in the same adult age range and have the same dismal response to therapy.[29]

Chronic Myelocytic Leukemia

Leukemia literally means "white blood." In chronic myelocytic leukemia, white counts can be so high that the blood actually assumes a grayish cast. White cell levels characteristically fall between 50,000 and 250,000/mm.[3] but can go even higher. The terms chronic myelocytic leukemia (CML) and chronic granulocytic leukemia (CGL) are used interchangeably for this leukemia, which occurs predominantly in adults and accounts for 20 percent of all leukemias.[6] Incidence usually occurs after age 20, although childhood cases are not unknown. The peak incidence is between ages 40 and 60.[63]

CLINICAL FINDINGS

CML begins insidiously. Often the patient cannot pinpoint the onset of malaise, fatigue, abdominal fullness, or low-grade fever. There is usually only mild anemia, with hematocrit between 25 and 35 percent; thrombocytopenia is uncommon. Red cell and platelet levels vary independently of white cell count.[52] More than half of CML patients have platelet counts above 450,000/mm^3, but there may be abnormal bleeding despite the thrombocytosis. The spleen almost always enlarges, sometimes to such an extent that the spleen virtually fills the abdominal cavity. Hepatomegaly is also common but less impressive. Bone pain is frequent, especially over the sternum; this is probably related to excessive marrow volume and activity.

Serum and urine uric acid levels are high, and there may be urate kidney stones or clinical gout. Serum B$_{12}$ and B$_{12}$-binding protein usually are above normal. Values for serum potassium often are high and glucose levels low, but these are artefactual findings, the result of prolonged contact between serum and the huge numbers of white cells and platelets. If serum is separated promptly, glucose and potassium levels are normal.[63]

WHITE CELL FINDINGS

The blood and bone marrow look much alike in CML. Vast numbers of granulocytes are present in all stages of maturation, but an interesting peculiarity is that often there are more myelocytes than metamyelocytes.[52] CML granulocytes retain bactericidal capacity, and increased susceptibility to infection is rare at the time of diagnosis. Leukocyte alkaline phosphatase is nearly always low, sometimes dropping to zero. The CML patient who is pregnant or is suffering from certain systemic infections usually has normal leukocyte alkaline phosphatase values. In 90 percent of CML cases, the Philadelphia (Ph^1) chromosome (see p. 53) can be found in cultured myeloid cells. Simultaneous existence of CML and significant B$_{12}$ or folate deficiency may suppress leukemic proliferation of white cells. Treating the cofactor deficiency then permits the leukemia to become apparent.[41]

COURSE OF THE DISEASE

Until recently, untreated patients with CML would survive about 3 years and die with an accelerated, blastic, acute clinical picture. Busulfan therapy has caused impressive improvement in cellular proliferation, hypermetabolism, and the clinical symptoms of CML. Survival figures now run about 3 to 6 years after diagnosis, and most patients enjoy virtually disease-free intervals, even though absolute prolongation of life is only moderate.[47] Successful treatment can restore peripheral white counts and leukocyte alkaline phosphatase values to normal, reduce spleen size, allow normal red cell production, and prevent thrombocytosis. The Ph[1] abnormality, however, remains in marrow cells.

When therapy begins to fail, about 10 percent of CML patients develop a terminal "blast crisis" which progresses inexorably to death in 1 to 6 weeks. In about half of treated patients, the terminal event is "acute transformation," in which anemia, thrombocytopenia, and progressively increasing granulocytic immaturity develop over several months. The remaining patients simply become unresponsive to previously effective therapy. Hematopoietic failure, hypermetabolism, bone destruction, soft tissue replacement, and meningeal or solid tumors recur inexorably, and death results from hemorrhage or infection.

LYMPHORETICULAR SYSTEM: LYMPHOCYTES AND PLASMA CELLS

Lymphoreticular cells can be classified conveniently as either fixed or movable. B-lymphocytes and their plasma cell progeny constitute a mobile or potentially mobile population, even though, at any one time, many cells reside quietly in lymphoid tissues. The monocyte/macrophage/histiocyte population is less conspicuous in body fluids, the cells spending most of their active life within the tissues. To some extent, proliferative disorders of mobile cells become clinically apparent as leukemias or dysproteinemias, which are diseases with significant blood abnormalities, whereas tissue diseases, especially lymphomas, arise from the fixed elements. This division is useful but, like all biologic classifications, somewhat flawed. Moreover, it fails to account for disorders involving T-lymphocytes, a large population whose contributions to the group of proliferative disorders remain unclear.

Acute Lymphoblastic Leukemia

Acute lymphoblastic leukemia (ALL) is the major childhood leukemia, accounting for nearly all leukemias before age 4, and for more than half of leukemias through puberty. It is rare in patients over 30.[63] Clinically, acute lymphoblastic leukemia and acute myeloblastic leukemia have similar features, but the onset of ALL tends to be strikingly acute. Almost never is there a "smoldering" or preleukemic phase. Lymph node enlargement and hepatosplenomegaly occur more often in ALL than in AML, as do bone pain and bone lesions.[21] Leukemic meningitis may occur, although usually late in the disease.

BLOOD AND BONE MARROW

Very few recognizable neutrophils circulate in ALL, and even in the bone marrow, normal red and white cell elements may be hard to find. The predominant cell, both in blood and in marrow, is a blast with a large nucleus, one or two nucleoli, and an irregularly contoured nuclear membrane. The scant cytoplasm contains no sudanophilic granules, no peroxidase-reactive granules, and no Auer rods. The few neutrophils that are present have normal leukocyte alkaline phosphatase scores.

The hypercellular marrow contains mostly blasts. No promyelocytes or promonocytes are in evidence, but there may be increased numbers of small lymphocytes. Anemia is usually pronounced, with few reticulocytes and very low platelet counts. Culturing marrow cells reveals numerous, variable chromosomal abnormalities. There is no consistent abnormality; the chromosomal changes are almost certainly the effect, not the cause, of abnormal proliferative activity.

COURSE OF THE DISEASE

Recent therapeutic advances have dramatically improved the short-term prognosis of ALL. Before 1950, 80 percent of children with ALL were dead 8 months after diagnosis. At present, virtually all young children and most older children and adults are alive at 8 months; with intensive combination therapy, the median duration of remission is over 2 years.[21,63,65] As the numbers of 5- and 10-year survivors increase, many workers feel that long-term prognosis has improved to levels worthy of cautious optimism.

The strategy in treating ALL is an attempt to eradicate every malignant cell so that no malignant cells remain to cause recrudescent disease. Combination therapy employs agents that exert different kinds of damage to multiplying cells so that malignant cells of all sorts and conditions can be destroyed.[27] High doses are given initially, followed by consolidation doses and maintenance therapy to reach any cells that might emerge after the first therapeutic barrage.[18] Because ALL cells have a predilection for the nervous system, and the central nervous system is hard to reach with systemic therapy, some regimens employ direct instillation of cytotoxic agents into the spinal fluid.[21]

COMPLICATIONS OF THERAPY

This kind of rigorous therapy brings numerous complications. Bone marrow suppression is profound. Transfusions of red cells and plate-lets combat part of the problem, but replacing normal granulocytes is far more difficult. Infectious complications are numerous and severe, and, while granulocyte transfusions are more feasible than they used to be, their long-term efficacy has not been demonstrated. Despite transfusion therapy, infection and hemorrhage remain the commonest cause of death.[18,21,65] Immunosuppression invariably accompanies long-term maintenance therapy. Various agents used to induce remission produce a range of other side effects including gastritis, cystitis, hair loss, neuropathies, hypertension, and hepatitis.

With advancing age, response to therapy declines. Children under 4 more often achieve 5-year remissions than older children, and adults almost never achieve remissions of this length. Although more than half of ALL cases now survive 2 years after diagnosis, many of these have already had one or more relapses. Recurrences sometimes appear after many years of remission, but, as a general rule, the length of the first, seemingly complete remission is directly related to overall prognosis.[18,27] In terminal recurrences, death usually results from infection, cerebral hemorrhage, or infiltration of me-ninges, central nervous system, or other organs.

Chronic Lymphocytic Leukemia

Chronic lymphocytic leukemia (CLL) differs from the other leukemias in running typically a rather indolent course over many years. It occurs exclusively in adults over 40 and is the only leukemia that has never been shown to follow ionizing radiation.[19] In CLL, the pro-liferating cells are B-lymphocytes, which have normal surface charac-teristics but no detectible immunologic activity.[10,13] Leukemic B-cells survive as long as 5 years, compared with 1-year survival for normal "long-lived" B-lymphocytes.[57] Because the lymphocyte production rate also increases as much as tenfold, the net result is massive cell-ular accumulation. The accumulating cells are immunologically inert, and their presence crowds out normally reactive B cells. Spleen, bone marrow, and lymph nodes are overrun by these cells, which interfere with the movement of granulocytes and monocytes across vascular membranes.

CLINICAL FINDINGS

CLL always develops gradually. Often it is discovered incidentally during a blood count done for other reasons. The white count runs between 10,000 and 100,000/mm.[3]; 95 percent or more of circulating white cells are small lymphocytes of normal or minimally immature appearance. Granulocytes, although sparse in the differential count, are present initially in normal absolute numbers, and there is no increased susceptibility to infection. As lymphocytes overrun the marrow, platelet counts and red cell production may decline, but intrinsic erythropoietic and thrombopoietic capabilities are normal.

CLL adversely affects immune functioning. Half of CLL patients have decreased immunoglobulin levels, especially IgM, at some time during their disease. A third of patients experience a positive direct Coombs test (see p. 241), often associated with hemolysis that stresses the bone marrow beyond its ability to compensate.[56]

COURSE OF THE DISEASE

Some untreated patients coexist for years with their chronic lymphocytic leukemia. Anemia and thrombocytopenia sometimes occur as indications of the presence of bone marrow infiltration severe enough to require cytolytic therapy. If red cells and platelets remain adequate, patients may never need therapy and eventually succumb to cardiovascular problems or other diseases of old age. Many patients, however, experience a progressively more aggressive course. Patients who, at initial presentation, had hemoglobin levels above 11 gm./dl. and no evidence of lymph node and liver involvement are more likely to survive for long periods than those with lymphocyte counts above 50,000/mm.[3 40] Characteristically, the proliferating cells become less mature, more abnormal in appearance, and more damaging to liver, bone marrow, and lymph nodes as the disease worsens. As organ infiltration progresses, CLL and lymphoma become difficult to distinguish.[55] Toward the end, increasing immunologic impairment, anemia, hemorrhagic complications, and liability to infection can be noted. An interesting but unexplained observation is the finding that patients with CLL more often have solid cancers than age-matched controls; skin and colon are especially common sites.[56]

In treating CLL, it is impossible to eradicate all malignant cells because, by the time the disease becomes apparent, leukemic proliferation is widespread and long-standing. Therapy seeks mainly to prevent bone marrow replacement and to alleviate symptoms arising from splenomegaly or lymph node involvement. Agents useful in treating acute leukemia are ineffective in combating the accelerated terminal phase of CLL.[48]

Plasma Cell Dyscrasias

Many things can go wrong with B-cell development and immunoglobulin production. *Chronic lymphocytic leukemia* is a proliferation of B-cells which fail to produce immunoglobulins. In *multiple myeloma*, the proliferating cells are differentiated plasma cells that produce immunoglobulins which lack detectible functional properties. In *Waldenström's macroglobulinemia*, the relatively few abnormal cells present do not cause the clinical problems; it is the excessive production and accumulation of IgM that is the real concern.[33] In *heavy chain disease,* proliferating abnormal cells cause a lymphoma-like syndrome, and there is, in addition, an unbalanced production of heavy chains that are not incorporated into immunoglobulin molecules.[61]

MULTIPLE MYELOMA

Multiple myeloma, which literally means "many bone marrow tumors," is the malignant multiplication of well-differentiated, immunoglobulin-producing plasma cells. It occurs largely in middle-aged and elderly adults, in males more than in females, with an overall incidence of 2 to 3 per 100,000 population.[4] Usually there are multiple discrete masses of plasma cells located largely in bones. Some patients have only extraskeletal plasmacytomas as their presenting finding, while in others, only a single bone may be involved. With progression, additional bones, bone marrow, and other tissues tend to become involved.

In multiple myeloma, only one class of immunoglobulin molecules accumulates abnormally. All the molecules are identical; all are produced by the offspring of a single autonomously multiplying cell.[32] The progeny of a single cell are called a clone. Myeloma proteins are described as *monoclonal* because only one clone of cells is responsible for their production. Electrophoretic examination of this homogeneous protein reveals a well-defined band that becomes a tall, narrow spike on the densitometer tracing (see Fig. 15, Chapter 7). This is called an *M spike*, with M standing for myeloma or for monoclonal; the M does not stand for immunoglobulin M. Theoretically, myeloma immunoglobulin could be any one of the five immunoglobulin classes. In observed fact, over half of multiple myeloma patients have IgG, about a third have IgA, and some have only excessive production of light chains; IgM, IgD, and IgE are very rare indeed.[3,43]

Laboratory diagnosis rests on demonstrating an M spike on serum electrophoresis and the existence of excessive circulating or excreted light chains. Excess light chains in the urine give the physicochemical reactions characterized as Bence-Jones protein[43] (see p. 574). Biopsy of bone lesions reveals aggregates of normal-looking or increasingly abnormal plasma cells. Marrow specimens obtained at random often contain increased numbers of plasma cells, but large aggregates of myeloma cells develop late, after widespread dissemination has occurred.

When plasma contains excessive immunoglobulin, the erythrocyte sedimentation rate increases, and red cells stick to one another in a peculiar artefact called *rouleaux* formation. Rouleaux are a laboratory phenomenon, but in the intact patient there may be excessive blood viscosity or impairment of clot formation or platelet function. Late in the disease, the patient becomes anemic and, because normal antibody levels decline, there is increased predisposition to bacterial infection. Serum calcium rises, partly because of hyperproteinemia and partly from bone destruction. Renal damage is a common late complication from the effects of excessive globulin in the tubular fluid.[66]

OTHER DYSPROTEINEMIAS

New protein dyscrasias have been discovered as protein electrophoresis and immunoassay techniques have blossomed. Much rarer than multiple myeloma, they also affect older adults and run a chronic but accelerating course of protein accumulation and abnormal cellular proliferation. Amyloidosis has been observed in many dysproteinemias, but renal damage is more common in multiple myeloma than in other related conditions. Bleeding manifestations and symptomatic cold agglutinin disease are notable in Waldenström's macroglobulinemia.

LYMPHORETICULAR SYSTEM: THE LYMPHOMAS

Lymphomas are malignant neoplasms of the lymphoid organs, primarily affecting lymph nodes but often involving alimentary tract, nasopharyngeal tissues, lung, and other tissues with a lymphoreticular component. Diagnosis is by tissue biopsy; laboratory data are at best suggestive or confirmatory. Because of their close association with the hematologic and immunologic diseases already considered, it is worthwhile to offer a brief discussion of diagnosis and classification.

Lymphomas fall into two major categories: Hodgkin's disease and the non-Hodgkin's lymphomas. The non-Hodgkin's category includes *lymphocytic, histiocytic,* and *stem cell lymphomas; mixed lymphomas;* and *Burkitt's lymphoma.*[14] *Hodgkin's disease* deserves a category all its own because it manifests such a complex variety of clinical, epidemiologic, and prognostic phenomena. The non-Hodgkin's lymphomas can be schematized as disorders of lymphocytic and phagocytic cells whose maturation or proliferation becomes abnormal at various stages of cellular differentiation.[55] Like chronic lymphocytic leukemia, these occur almost exclusively in the middle-aged or elderly. More difficult to classify are the T-cell neoplasms *mycosis fungoides* and *Sezary syndrome,* which initially affect the skin, and *Burkitt's lymphoma,* which affects children and occurs almost entirely outside the lymph nodes, especially in the facial bones and the ovaries. Burkitt's lymphoma is unique in its sensitivity to chemotherapy. Prolonged remission (cure?) is the rule rather than the exception in several large series.

Hodgkin's Disease

Hodgkin's disease (HD) is a relatively common disease of young adults, with an incidence of 2 to 3 cases per 100,000 between ages 15 and 40.[49] Two incidence peaks exist, one in young adults and a gradual increase in the elderly. The *Reed-Sternberg cell* is pathognomonic for Hodgkin's disease. This is a large histiocyte with bilobed, vesicular nucleus, prominent nuclear membrane, and distinctive eosinophilic nucleoli. Lymph node biopsies are notoriously difficult to interpret. Most workers believe that without Reed-Sternberg cells, the diagnosis of Hodgkin's disease cannot be made.

CLASSIFICATION AND STAGING

Tissue changes in HD can be classified into four major histologic patterns. *Lymphocyte predominance,* which is the least common (5 to 13 percent of all HD) and carries the most favorable prognosis (65 to 90 percent have 5-year survival); *nodular sclerosis,* which accounts for 40 to 50 percent of HD, has a predilection for young females, and carries a very favorable long-term outlook (55 to 70 percent have 5-year survival); *mixed cellularity,* accounting for 35 to 40 percent of all cases and carrying only a 30 to 35 percent 5-year survival; and *lymphocyte depletion,* 5 to 15 percent of all HD, with most examples running an accelerated course which carries only a 15 to

30 percent 5-year survival.[49,63] The nodular sclerosis pattern tends to remain constant if spread or recurrence takes place, but mixed cellularity patterns often deteriorate toward lymphocyte depletion as the disease progresses.

In assessing treatment and planning clinical strategy, it is important to stage the extent to which the disease has progressed at the time of diagnosis. In *Stage I*, disease involves only a single lymph node group or single extranodal site. *Stage II* has disease in two or more lymph node groups or one lymph node group and one extranodal site, but all involvement is on one side of the diaphragm. In *Stage III*, disease involves nodes both above and below the diaphragm and may include the spleen. In *Stage IV* there is disseminated disease involving many lymph node groups and non-lymphoid organs, notably liver, bone marrow, or lung. The presence of constitutional symptoms, such as fever, weight loss, or night sweats, is noted as class B presentation of a particular stage. Patients in class A have morphologic evidence of disease but no clinical symptoms.

Good therapeutic response and good long-term prognosis correlate directly with presentation at an early stage without symptoms. Women seem to do better than men, and patients under 30 do better than those over 30. These sex and age distinctions are due, in part, to the fact that the prognostically favorable nodular sclerosing pattern occurs predominantly in females under 30.

LABORATORY FINDINGS

Few patients with Stage I disease have abnormal blood findings. As disease advances, there is progressive likelihood of anemia and a leukocytosis in which neutrophils and eosinophils are increased and lymphocytes are decreased.[20,53] Coombs-positive hemolytic anemia sometimes accompanies late disease, but other derangements of B-cell function are rare. Cell-mediated immunity is more often defective. *Anergy*, the absence of skin response to new or previously effective immunogens, is common in Stages III and IV. Erythrocyte sedimentation rate rises while disease is active and becomes normal during remission.[63] Some elevation of serum alkaline phosphatase is fairly common. This occurs if disease involves the liver directly, but sometimes it reflects only nonspecific functional derangement. Serum calcium rises if there is bone involvement. Some patients with advanced disease experience a nephrotic syndrome characterized by massive proteinuria, hypoalbuminemia, and elevated serum lipids, even though no tumor exists in the kidney itself.[49]

Non-Hodgkin's Lymphomas

The classification of non-Hodgkin's lymphomas and theories about their etiology are complex and continually changing. The major histologic distinctions rely on differentiating nodular from diffuse growth pattern and characterizing the proliferating cells as well-differentiated or poorly differentiated.[1,14] Prognosis is better for nodular growth pattern, for good cellular differentiation, and for proliferation of a single cell line. Non-Hodgkin's lymphoma affects the middle-aged and elderly. Survival past 5 years is uncommon except for well-differentiated nodular types; many patients succumb within 2 years despite appropriate therapy. Laboratory findings rarely help in diagnosis, although Coombs-positive hemolytic anemia and depressed serum globulin levels are common findings in well-differentiated lymphocytic lymphomas. Many workers believe that chronic lymphocytic leukemia and well-differentiated lymphocytic lymphoma are different clinical aspects of the same basic disease.[2,55]

REFERENCES

1. Aisenberg, A. C.: *Malignant lymphoma.* N. Engl. J. Med. 288:883, 935, 1973.
2. Aisenberg, A. C., and Long, J. C.: *Lymphocyte surface characteristics in malignant lymphoma.* Am. J. Med. 58:300, 1975.
3. Bergsagel, D. E.: *Plasma cell myeloma,* in Williams, W. J., Beutler, E., Erslev, A. J., and Rundles, R. W. (eds.): *Hematology.* ed. 2. McGraw-Hill, New York, 1977.
4. Bergsagel, D. E: *Plasma cell neoplasmas—general considerations,* in Williams, W. J., Beutler, E., Erslev, A. J., and Rundles, R. W. (eds.): *Hematology.* ed. 2. McGraw-Hill, New York, 1977.
5. Beutler, E.: *Lipid storage diseases,* in Williams, W. J., Beutler, E., Erslev, A. J., and Rundles, R. W. (eds.): *Hematology.* ed. 2. McGraw-Hill, New York, 1977.
6. Burbank, F.: *Patterns of cancer mortality in the United States, 1950–1967.* Nat. Cancer Inst. Monogr. 33:594, 1971.
7. Canellos, G. P., DeVita, V. T., Arseneau, J. C., et al.: *Second malignancies complicating Hodgkin's disease in remission.* Lancet 1:947, 1975.
8. Clarkson, B. D.: *Acute myelocytic leukemia in adults.* Cancer 30:1572, 1972.
9. Cline, M. J.: *Biochemistry and function of monocytes and macrophages,* in Williams, W. J., Beutler, E., Erslev, A. J., and Rundles, R. W. (eds.): *Hematology.* ed. 2. McGraw-Hill, New York, 1977.

10. Cohen, H. J.: *Human lymphocyte surface immunoglobulin capping: normal characteristics and anomalous behavior of chronic lymphocytic leukemia lymphocytes.* J. Clin. Invest. 55:84, 1975.
11. Cohen, H. J., and Rundles, R. W.: *Managing the complications of plasma cell myeloma.* Arch. Intern. Med. 135:177, 1975.
12. Curnutte, J. T., Whitten, D. M., and Babior, B. M.: *Defective superoxide production by granulocytes from patients with chronic granulomatous disease.* N. Engl. J. Med. 290:593, 1974.
13. Davis, S.: *The variable pattern of circulating lymphocyte subpopulations in chronic lymphocytic leukemia.* N. Engl. J. Med. 294:1150, 1976.
14. Dorfman, R. F.: *Classification of non-Hodgkin's lymphomas.* Lancet 1:1295, 1974.
15. Finch, S. C.: *Granulocytopenia,* in Williams, W. J., Beutler, E., Erslev, A. J., and Rundles, R. W. (eds.): *Hematology.* ed. 2. McGraw-Hill, New York, 1977.
16. Finch, S. C.: *Granulocytosis,* in Williams, W. J., Beutler, E., Erslev, A. J., and Rundles, R. W. (eds.): *Hematology.* ed. 2. McGraw-Hill, New York, 1977.
17. Gallin, J. I., Klimerman, J. A., Padgett, G. A., and Wolff, S. M.: *Defective mononuclear leukocyte chemotaxis in the Chediak-Higashi syndrome of humans, mink, and cattle.* Blood 45:863, 1975.
18. George, S. L., Fernbach, D. J., Vietti, T. J., et al.: *Factors influencing survival in pediatric acute leukemia.* Cancer 32:1542, 1973.
19. Gunz, F. W.: *The epidemiology and genetics of the chronic leukaemias.* Clin. Haematol. 6:3, 1977.
20. Heier, H. E., and Normann, T.: *Blood lymphocytes in Hodgkin's disease: lymphopenia related to stages and histological groups.* Scand. J. Haematol. 13:199, 1974.
21. Henderson, E. S.: *Acute lymphocytic leukemia,* in Williams, W. J., Beutler, E., Erslev, A. J., and Rundles, R. W. (eds.): *Hematology.* ed. 2. McGraw-Hill, New York, 1977.
22. Henderson, E. S.: *Acute myelogenous leukemia,* in Williams, W. J., Beutler, E., Erslev, A. J., and Rundles, R. W. (eds.): *Hematology.* ed. 2. McGraw-Hill, New York, 1977.
23. Henderson, E. S., Wallace, H. J., Yates, J., et al.: *Factors influencing prognosis in adult myelocytic leukemia.* Adv. Biosci. 14:72, 1975.
24. Hers, S. G., and van Hoof, F. (eds.): *Lysosomes and Storage Diseases.* Academic Press, New York, 1973.
25. Hohn, D. C., and Lehrer, R. I.: *NADPH oxidase deficiency in X-linked chronic granulomatous disease.* J. Clin. Invest. 55:707, 1975.
26. Horwitz, M. S., and Moore, G. T.: *Acute infectious lymphocytosis: an etiologic and epidemiologic study of an outbreak.* N. Engl. J. Med. 279:399, 1968.
27. Karon, M., Weiner, J. M., and Meshnik, R.: *The interaction of disease factors, host variability, and treatment in acute lymphocytic leukemia.* Adv. Biosci. 14:3, 1975.
28. Karzon, D. T.: *Infectious mononucleosis.* Adv. Pediatr. 22:231, 1976.
29. Keating, M. J., Freireich, E. J., McCredie, K. B., et al.: *Acute leukemia in adults, 1977.* CA 27:2, 1977.

30. Lai, P. K.: *Infectious mononucleosis: recognition and management.* Hosp. Practice, August, 1977, pp. 47–52.
31. Lalezari, P., and Radel, E.: *Neutrophil specific antigens: immunology and clinical significance.* Sem. Hematol. 11:281, 1974.
32. Lindström, F. D., Hardy, W. R., Eberle, B. J., and Williams, R. C.: *Multiple myeloma and benign monoclonal gammopathy: differentiation by immunofluorescence of lymphocytes.* Ann. Intern. Med. 78:837, 1973.
33. MacKenzie, M. R., and Fudenberg, H. H.: *Macroglobulinemia: an analysis of forty patients.* Blood 39:874, 1972.
34. Miller, D. J., Dwyer, J. M., and Klatskin, G.: *T cells and the hepatitis of infectious mononucleosis.* N. Engl. J. Med. 295:450, 1976.
35. Modan, B.: *Inter-relationship between polycythaemia vera, leukaemia, and myeloid metaplasia.* Clin Haematol. 4:427, 1975.
36. Niederman, J. C., Miller, G., Pearson, H. A., et al.: *Infectious mononucleosis. Epstein-Barr-virus shedding in saliva and the oropharynx.* N. Engl. J. Med. 294:1355, 1976.
37. Nichols, B. A., and Bainton, D. F.: *Differentiation of human monocytes in bone marrow and blood.* Lab. Invest. 29:27, 1973.
38. Paloheimo, J. A., and Ikkala, E.: *Serum lactic dehydrogenase activity and isoenzyme patterns in some haematological diseases.* Acta Med. Scand. 117:115, 1965.
39. Perrera, D. J. B., and Pegrum, G. D.: *The lymphocyte in chronic lymphatic leukaemia.* Lancet 1:1207, 1974.
40. Phillips, E. A., Kempin, S., Passe, S., et al.: *Prognostic factors in chronic lymphocytic leukaemia and their implications for therapy.* Clin. Haematol. 6:203, 1977.
41. Pierre, R. V.: *Preleukemic states.* Sem. Hematol. 11:73, 1974.
42. Pisciotta, A. V.: *Immune and toxic mechanisms in drug-induced agranulocytosis.* Sem. Hematol. 10:279, 1973.
43. Pruzanski, W., and Orgryzlo, M. A.: *Abnormal proteinuria in malignant diseases.* Adv. Clin. Chem. 13:335, 1970.
44. Putnam, S. M., Moore, G. T., and Mitchell, D. W.: *Infectious lymphocytosis: long-term follow-up of an epidemic.* Pediatrics 41:588, 1968.
45. Robinson, W. A.: *Granulocytosis in neoplasia.* Ann. N.Y. Acad. Sci. 230:212, 1974.
46. Royston, I., Sullivan, J. L., Periman, P. O., and Perlin, E.: *Cell-mediated immunity to Epstein-Barr-virus-transformed lymphoblastoid cells in acute infectious mononucleosis.* N. Engl. J. Med. 293:1159, 1975.
47. Rundles, R. W.: *Chronic granulocytic leukemia,* in Williams, W. J., Beutler, E., Erselv, A. J., and Rundles, R. W. (eds.): *Hematology.* ed. 2. McGraw-Hill, New York, 1977.
48. Rundles, R. W.: *Chronic lymphocytic leukemia,* in Williams, W. J., Beutler, E., Erslev, A. J., and Rundles, R. W. (eds.): *Hematology.* ed. 2. McGraw-Hill, New York, 1977.
49. Rundles, R. W.: *Hodgkin's disease,* in Williams, W. J., Beutler, E., Erslev, A. J., and Rundles, R. W. (eds.): *Hematology.* ed. 2. McGraw-Hill, New York, 1977.
50. Saunders, E. F., Amato, D., and Freedman, M. H.: *Studies on the patho-*

genesis of congenital neutropenia and aplastic anemia. Clin. Res. 22:744A, 1974.
51. Schmitt, H. E., Meuret, G., and Stix, L.: Monocyte recruitment in tuberculosis and sarcoidosis. Br. J. Haematol. 35:11, 1977.
52. Spiers, A. S. D.: The clinical features of chronic granulocytic leukaemia. Clin. Haematol. 6:77, 1977.
53. Steigbigel, R. T., Lambert, L. H., Jr., and Remington, J. S.: Polymorphonuclear leukocyte, monocyte, and macrophage bactericidal function in patients with Hodgkin's disease. J. Lab. Clin. Med. 88:54, 1976.
54. Stossel, T. P., and Boxer, L. A.: Granulocyte disorders—qualitative abnormalities of granulocytes, in Williams, W. J., Beutler, E., Erslev, A. J., and Rundles, R. W. (eds.): Hematology. ed. 2. McGraw-Hill, New York, 1977.
55. Sweet, D. L., Golumb, H. M., and Ultman, J. E.: Chronic lymphocytic leukaemia and its relationship to other lymphoproliferative disorders. Clin. Haematol. 6:141, 1977.
56. Sweet, D. L., Golomb, H. M., and Ultman, J. E.: The clinical features of chronic lymphocytic leukaemia. Clin. Haematol. 6:185, 1977.
57. Theml, H., Love, R., and Begemann, H.: Factors in the pathomechanism of chronic lymphocytic leukemia. Annu. Rev. Med. 28:131, 1977.
58. Tsukimoto, I., Wong, K. Y., and Lampkin, B. C.: Surface markers and prognostic factors in acute lymphoblastic leukemia. N. Eng. J. Med. 294:245, 1976.
59. Vilter, R. W.: Anemias related to nutritional deficiencies other than vitamin B_{12} and folic acid, in Williams, W. J., Beutler, E., Erslev, A. J., and Rundles, R. W. (eds.): Hematology. ed. 2. McGraw-Hill, New York, 1977.
60. Ward, P. A.: Leukotaxis and leukotactic disorders. Am. J. Pathol. 77:520, 1974.
61. Warner, N. L., Potter, M., and Metcalf, D.: Multiple myeloma and related immunoglobulin-producing neoplasms. UICC Technical Report Series. vol. 13. International Union Against Cancer, Geneva, 1974.
62. Wilkinson, P. C.: Surface and cell membrane activities of leukocyte chemotactic factors. Nature 251:58, 1974.
63. Wintrobe, M. M., Lee, G. R., Boggs, D. R., et al.: Clinical Hematology. ed. 7. Lea & Febiger, Philadelphia, 1974.
64. Wolff, S. M., Dale, D. C., Clark, R. A., et al.: The Chediak-Higashi syndrome: studies of host defenses. Ann. Intern. Med. 76:293, 1972.
65. Zippin, C., Cutler, S. J., and Lum, D.: Time trends in survival in acute lymphocytic leukemia. J. Natl. Cancer Inst. 54:581, 1975.
66. Zlotnick, A., and Rosenmann, E.: Renal pathologic findings associated with monoclonal gammopathies. Arch. Intern. Med. 135:40, 1975.

CHAPTER 5

DISORDERS OF HEMOSTASIS

CLINICAL APPROACH

Bleeding problems may come to medical attention (1) because the patient has noticed abnormal bleeding manifestations, (2) because the responsible clinician notices abnormal physical signs or elicits a suspicious history, or (3) because the clinician specifically tests for hemostatic abnormalities before undertaking a surgical, obstetrical, or dental procedure.

History

What the patient says is important. If a patient complains of bruises, bleeding gums, or difficulty in postsurgical healing, it is wise to take this seriously. Bruising is difficult to evaluate by history, since it occurs so commonly, particularly on thighs and upper arms and especially in postmenopausal women. Often the history means little, but the clinician must, at the very least, examine the areas and take a careful history. If the history strongly suggests a personal or familial tendency toward hemorrhage, normal results on screening tests should not preclude further investigation. Factor levels of 20 to 25 percent of normal may be sufficient to give normal test results but insufficient to meet severe hemostatic challenge.

TYPES OF BLEEDING

Especially important in the history are the onset and course of the difficulty and the nature of the bleeding episodes. Repeated episodes beginning in infancy or childhood suggest a severe congenital disorder; adult onset, especially if sudden, points to an acquired problem. Mild congenital defects may remain asymptomatic until some traumatic stress occurs in adult life, but this is rare. Severe bleeding into skin and mucous membranes suggests platelet problems; if episodes are separated by normal intervals, the suspicion of immunologic or drug-induced damage arises. An important distinction is whether obvious trauma or vascular damage precedes bleeding or whether bleeding occurs spontaneously. Careful inquiry about family history, drug therapy, and ongoing or suspected medical problems is extremely important.

Notable categories of bleeding episodes include bleeding into joints (hemarthroses) and into soft tissues (hematomas), especially muscle; diffuse oozing from mucosal surfaces; blood in the urine (hematuria); pinpoint or spreading hemorrhages into skin; profuse menstrual periods; prolonged bleeding after dental work or minor injury; bleeding or bruising specifically associated with aspirin ingestion; and delayed onset of bleeding after initially normal hemostasis.

Screening Tests

For a seemingly normal patient about to undergo an operation, the prothrombin time (PT), partial thromboplastin time (PTT), and informal evaluation of platelet number probably constitute an adequate screening battery. Bleeding time and platelet count are indicated if history or findings on blood film are suggestive. The whole-blood clotting time and variants such as the capillary tube "coagulation time" should be avoided. They are so insensitive that normal results often engender a false sense of security. Patients with abnormalities of platelets, or of PT or PTT, and those with a positive personal or family history should be studied with more sophisticated procedures, including specific factor assays.

Observations

Although acquired bleeding problems are far more common than congenital disorders, characterization and treatment of congenital syndromes are far easier. Congenital deficiency syndromes attract investigators who use these isolated defects as experiments of nature that elucidate fundamental physiologic and pathologic events. Acquired disorders often accompany other diseases. Aside from treating the underlying disease, the clinician may have few options other than to treat the hemorrhagic diathesis empirically with platelets and plasma for factor replacement. Coagulation problems are probably less common than platelet disorders, but the coagulation mechanisms can be studied and manipulated more readily than can platelets. As a result, a disproportionate amount of discussion is devoted to coagulation defects, while other problems are frequently handled more summarily.

Another striking disproportion exists between the number of studies and tests devoted to thrombosis and attendant complications such as infarction and the frequency and morbid significance of these events. Although much interest now centers on the causes, cures, and prevention of thrombosis, there is still much less to say and to investigate about thrombotic diseases than about hemorrhagic tendencies.

In the following discussion we need say very little about bleeding disorders of purely or principally vascular origin. In such cases, tests of platelet and coagulation functions are normal, and it is desirable to investigate possible morphologic, immunologic, metabolic, and infectious etiologies.

CONGENITAL DISORDERS OF COAGULATION

Deficiencies of Factor VIII and Factor IX

Hemophilia, in general parlance, refers to a severe, lifelong tendency toward excessive bleeding, occurring only in males and following an X-linked inheritance pattern. Defects of Factor VIII or Factor IX produce this syndrome. Hemophilia has been recognized for thousands of years. The Talmud states that a male infant should not be circumcised if two or more of his brothers died from post-circumcision bleeding. In the United States, approximately 1 in 10,000 boys has hemophilia of greater or lesser severity;[3] four out of five cases are Factor VIII deficiencies, and the rest are Factor IX problems. Factor VIII deficiency (hemophilia A, or "classical" hemophilia) and Factor IX deficiency (hemophilia B, or Christmas disease) were not differentiated until 1952. Clinical findings and genetic transmission are identical. The conditions can be distinguished by cross-correction procedures available only recently and only in relatively sophisticated laboratories.

CLINICAL FINDINGS

Depending on the level of available circulating factor, clinical severity of both hemophilia A and hemophilia B can range from florid to mild or almost asymptomatic. As a rule, affected males in any one family tend to have comparable factor levels and comparably severe clinical disease. Severely affected patients have less than 1 percent activity; mildly affected ones have levels between 6 and 30 percent.

Excessive bleeding after obvious trauma is only part of the problem, an aspect that usually can be treated successfully. Of more serious, long-term consequence is bleeding into joints, which often occurs without any apparent incitement and is extremely painful. The sequellae are progressive joint deformity and severe crippling, which more often affects the legs than the arms. Before the advent of effective therapy, hemophiliacs who survived early bleeding episodes almost invariably became severely crippled by adolescence or young adulthood. Even though present-day therapy controls most lethal and many disabling symptoms, hemarthroses have not been eliminated; however, their frequency, magnitude, and crippling effect have been much reduced.

Soft tissue bleeding, especially subcutaneous and intramuscular hemorrhages, can cause compressive damage to muscles and nerves. Hematomas into the soft tissues of head and neck may compress respiratory passages and cause death by asphyxiation. Bleeding into the urinary or alimentary tract is common but causes no long-term complications. Intracranial hemorrhage, on the other hand, sometimes occurs without apparent predisposing trauma and can be extremely dangerous.

Hemophiliacs suffer not only from hemorrhage, but also from delayed wound repair. Before adequate therapy was available, dental or surgical procedures were extremely hazardous. Bleeding after an operation or tooth extraction often can be the first sign of disease in mildly affected, previously unsuspected hemophiliacs.

LABORATORY FINDINGS

Initial diagnostic procedures have been discussed in Chapter 2. After a presumptive diagnosis has been made, it is important to determine the level of factor activity and to test whether an inhibitor exists. Anti-Factor VIII antibodies develop in as many as 5 to 10 percent of treated classical hemophiliacs; it is rare to find antibodies at initial diagnosis. Factor IX antibodies are less common, occurring in less than 2 percent[2] of treated patients. When adequate replacement fails to have therapeutic effect, or if the PTT remains severely abnormal after treatment, an antibody should be suspected. The presence of inhibitor is demonstrated by incubating the patient's plasma with a known concentration of Factor VIII and measuring the thromboplastin-generating capacity of the mixture.

ANTIGENIC ACTIVITY

Hemophilic plasma, despite its deficiency in procoagulant activity, usually contains normal quantities of an immunologically active protein that reacts with nonhuman anti-Factor VIII or anti-Factor IX. This protein, antigenically normal but physiologically inactive, has been called *cross-reacting material* (CRM). Most hemophiliacs are CRM-positive. The few who lack CRM tend to have variant clinical signs as well. It is obvious that the X-linked genes for hemophilia A and hemophilia B do not prevent protein synthesis. Perhaps the defect is absence of an enzyme that rearranges the basic protein units or adds some critical material to the basic polypeptide unit. There is evidence[6] that the basic Factor VIII polypeptide has procoagulant effect only when polymerized or cross-linked in certain fashion. With Factor IX, the defect is less clearly characterized; in deficiency states, antigenically reactive protein is present but lacks procoagulant activity, thus suggesting that the defective gene controls for some sort of late-acting product.

TREATMENT

Factor VIII is available as a highly potent concentrate prepared from large pools of plasma and as a moderately concentrated cryoprecipitate prepared from single-donor plasma. Cryoprecipitate gives good results in treating minor or uncomplicated problems. Concentrates are ideal for treating severe hemorrhagic episodes and for elevating Factor VIII levels to 100 percent prior to surgical procedures. In these circumstances, the therapeutic benefits of the concentrates outweigh the moderate risk of hepatitis. Factor IX is not available as a product separate from the other liver factors (prothrombin, Factor VII, and Factor X). The concentrate of these four factors carries a very high risk of hepatitis transmission. Single-donor plasma, either freshly frozen or salvaged from stored liquid blood, contains substantial Factor IX and should be used for treatment of minor difficulties; for major episodes, the concentrate is invaluable.

THE CARRIER STATE

Women, who always have two X chromosomes, almost always have one normal gene to balance the hemophilia gene. A woman who received an abnormal gene from her carrier mother and another from her hemophiliac father would have true hemophilia. Such a case is extremely rare in humans but is easily achieved in inbred strains of dogs. A phenotypically female patient with the XO geno-type of Turner's syndrome could be hemophilic if the single X chrom-osome carried a hemophilia gene.

When there is one normal and one abnormal gene, the woman often has less than the normal level of factor activity. This deficiency is highly variable and usually too mild to be detected on routine PTT. The carrier state cannot be diagnosed reliably by quantitative assays of factor activity. Sufficient variation occurs that a woman can have normal or near-normal assays and still be a carrier. A highly promising approach for ascertaining Factor VIII carriers has been to compare the level of procoagulant activity against the level of cross-reactive material that reacts immunologically with nonhuman anti-Factor VIII. Carrier females often have wider discrepancy be-tween procoagulant levels and CRM activity than do normal women.[17] These findings remain preliminary, and different laboratories report different levels of success in detecting the carrier state. Factor IX carriers have not been studied as extensively.

Fibrinogen

Plasma may contain no fibrinogen or severely abnormal fibrinogen. The 60 reported cases of afibrinogenemia[20] present the paradoxical situation of patients with totally incoagulable blood, who nonethe-less bleed less often and less dangerously than patients with pro-coagulant deficiencies. Bleeding episodes, bruising, and poor wound healing characterize this disorder, which is inherited as an autosomal-recessive trait. In other rare autosomal-dominant conditions, the fibrinogen molecule is structurally or functionally defective. These dysfibrinogenemias cause relatively mild hemorrhagic symptoms[11]; a few patients have a thrombotic tendency.

LABORATORY FINDINGS

Blood that lacks fibrinogen fails to clot in the PT, the PTT, or the TCT, but addition of afibrinogenemic plasma to normal plasma does not inhibit fibrin formation. All the tests that measure fibrinogen register zero. Nothing clots; there is no precipitate to analyze; and nothing reacts with antifibrin/fibrinogen antibodies. The dysfibrinogenemias, on the other hand, show qualitative as well as quantitative abnormalities. When incubated with normal plasma, dysfibrinogenemic plasma inhibits clotting. Discrepancy exists—often a striking one—between the amount of coagulable fibrinogen and the quantity of immunoreactive or precipitable protein.

Other Factors

Except for the hemophilias and dysfibrinogenemias, deficiencies of coagulation factors follow an autosomal-recessive inheritance pattern. All are rare (less than 1 in 500,000), except for Factor XI deficiency, which occurs in up to 1 in 10,000 in certain Jewish populations.[20] Most cause a lifelong tendency toward severe bleeding episodes, but hemarthroses are rare. Factor XI deficiency causes much milder symptoms, often confined to metrorrhagia, nosebleeds, or bleeding after dental or surgical procedures. Factor XII and Fletcher factor deficiencies do not cause any symptoms at all.

Screening test results for all the coagulation factor deficiencies are shown in Table 8.

Von Willebrand's Disease

Von Willebrand's disease (VWD) is transmitted as an autosomal dominant with variable penetrance, which occurs in both sexes. Since Factor VIII levels are low, it earned the name *pseudohemophilia* and created much confusion for early workers studying hemophilia. There is still much confusion relating to work at a molecular level. Besides the low Factor VIII levels, there is prolongation of bleeding time, a phenomenon inspiring the alternate name, *vascular hemophilia*, for this disease.

PATHOPHYSIOLOGY

Factor VIII has at least three different molecular properties. The procoagulant activity and the separable antigenic activity have already been discussed. A third function is interaction with vascular endothelium in a fashion that somehow prevents excessive capillary bleeding and modifies platelet activity. The name *von Willebrand factor* has been applied to the protein properties with these complex

Table 8. Cross-Correction Studies to Diagnose Coagulation Factor Deficiencies

Deficient Factor	Prothrombin Time			Partial Thromboplastin Time			Thrombin Clotting Time
	PT	PT plus serum	PT plus absorbed plasma	PTT	PTT plus serum	PTT plus absorbed plasma	TCT
I (Fibrinogen)	abn	abn	norm	abn	abn	norm	abn
II (Prothrombin)	abn	abn	abn	abn	abn	abn	norm
V	abn	abn	norm	abn	abn	norm	norm
VII	abn	norm	abn	norm	*	*	norm
VIII	norm	*	*	abn	abn	norm	norm
IX	norm	*	*	abn	norm	abn	norm
X	abn	norm	abn	abn	norm	abn	norm
XI	norm	*	*	abn	norm	norm	norm
XII	norm	*	*	abn	norm	norm	norm
XIII	norm	*	*	norm	*	*	norm

abn = abnormally prolonged.
norm = within normal limits.
* If initial test is normal, adding serum or plasma accomplishes nothing.

results. In classical hemophilia, the procoagulant activity of Factor VIII is low, but von Willebrand factor and cross-reactive material are normally active. In VWD, all three aspects are variably abnormal. The degree of abnormality differs not only from family to family, but from patient to patient within a single family and even from time to time in a single individual.[7] This has made case-finding and classification extremely difficult. Most patients have mild clinical symptoms. Small vessel bleeding (such as mucocutaneous bruising), nosebleeds, and menorrhagia are the most common events. Aspirin enhances the bleeding tendency and exaggerates the defective interaction between platelets, plasma, and vessel wall that characterizes von Willebrand's disease.

LABORATORY FINDINGS

Routine tests of hemostatic functions are somewhat unpredictable. The classic findings are prolonged bleeding time and abnormally long PTT due to low Factor VIII levels. Bleeding time varies only moderately in most patients, but there may be marked fluctuation in Factor VIII level. Platelet count and clot retraction are normal, but there exists a characteristic abnormality of platelet activity that provides the best single diagnostic test for VWD. When exposed to ristocetin, platelets from VWD patients fail to exhibit aggregation; when passed through a column of glass beads, they fail to adhere. Infusion of plasma or of Factor VIII-rich cryoprecipitate causes temporary improvement of ristocetin aggregation and glass bead retention tests as well as an increase in procoagulant activity that lasts much longer than the survival of passively administered Factor VIII.

In most VWD patients, there are comparably low levels of antigenic activity and procoagulant activity. A minority of patients have a normal quantity of protein but with aberrant immunologic reactivity. There seem to be several different fundamental mechanisms. Most patients have quantitatively abnormal synthesis of the entire Factor VIII complex, while others have a qualitative defect of synthesis.[8] Not surprisingly, laboratory observations vary more widely among patients with qualitative or structural variants than among those with quantitative deficiency.

PLATELET DISORDERS

Disorders of platelet number or function cause prolonged bleeding time and poor clot retraction. The platelet count allows quantitation of circulating platelets. To evaluate how many platelets are being produced, it is necessary to examine the bone marrow for mega-karyocyte morphology. If platelet counts are normal but clinical symptoms and screening laboratory tests suggest platelet failure, qualitative tests of platelet function are indicated.[12]

Disordered Function

Reduction in platelet number is far commoner than disorders of function. Most dysfunctional syndromes occur as part of other diseases; constitutional defects of platelet functions are very rare. Of these, von Willebrand's disease is the commonest, but it is not primarily a platelet disease.

DISORDERS SECONDARY TO OTHER DISEASES

Severe uremia impairs the release reaction (see p. 58); the patient's own platelets behave abnormally, and transfused normal platelets acquire the abnormality. Oozing and mucocutaneous bleeding often complicate *advanced uremia*. Although dialysis often restores plate-let function to normal, the bleeding problem may remain difficult to control. Platelets experience difficulty in performing normally when there are high levels of abnormal serum proteins, as seen in *multiple myeloma* and other *dysproteinemias*. High-molecular-weight *dextrans* produce the same effect. The presence of fibrin/fibrinogen split products seems to inhibit both aggregation and release. The normal liver clears from the circulation the low levels of degradation products that occur with everyday trauma and repair. Platelet function is diffusely abnormal in *severe liver disease*; failure to clear fibrin split products may contribute to this situation. The high platelet counts that accompany *myeloproliferative syndromes* often pre-dispose, paradoxically, both to bleeding problems and a thrombotic tendency.

EFFECT OF DRUGS

Many drugs impair platelet function; *aspirin* is undoubtedly the lead-ing offender. Once exposed to aspirin, platelets have impaired release reaction for their entire life span. Other anti-inflammatory drugs have comparable effects. *Antihistamines, antidepressants,* and *methyl xanthines* are among the agents that reduce platelet function to levels that may confuse the results of laboratory tests, even though they rarely cause clinical problems. *Ethyl alcohol* inhibits ADP-related aggregation; this probably does have clinical significance, at least in patients whose liver functions also have been damaged by alcohol.

Decreased Number

Thrombocytopenia can result from decreased platelet manufacture or increased platelet loss. Loss may be the result of massive blood loss or may be mediated by direct destruction, excessive utilization, or splenic sequestration.

REDUCED PRODUCTION

Although reduced thrombopoiesis usually is part of a generalized bone marrow problem, thrombocytopenia tends to be an especially prominent and troublesome aspect of drug-induced *aplastic anemia* and *malignant disease* of the bone marrow. Because the *chemotherapeutic regimens* used to treat leukemias and solid tumors cause profound thrombocytopenia, platelet transfusions have become a standard part of all the rigorous treatment programs. Relatively few drugs affect platelet production selectively. *Chlorthiazide* causes mild thrombocytopenia in about one quarter of those taking it, but this rarely causes bleeding. *Alcohol* depresses platelet production; low platelet counts are found in most alcoholics examined during or immediately after acute or continued ingestion. *Viral infections* sometimes impair platelet production and may additionally damage circulating platelets. Influenza, rubella, and infectious mononucleosis are notable offenders.

LOSS WITHIN THE CIRCULATION

The spleen, under normal conditions, contains up to one third of all circulating platelets, although relatively few platelets undergo destruction on any one passage through the spleen. *Massive splenic enlargement* increases the number of platelets removed from active circulation by splenic sequestration and reduces the survival time of all circulating platelets. *Liver disease, portal hypertension,* and the *lymphomas* are common causes of splenomegaly great enough to affect platelet numbers.

Since platelets adhere to damaged endothelial surfaces, platelet counts often drop dramatically in conditions characterized by widespread endothelial damage. *Rocky Mountain spotted fever* and the hemorrhagic rash of *meningococcemia* are outstanding examples. In these cases, the infection and the localized capillary damage cause hemorrhage and thrombocytopenia; it is not the thrombocytopenia that causes the hemorrhagic rash.

Idiopathic Thrombocytopenic Purpura

Idiopathic thrombocytopenic purpura (ITP) is a fairly common disease that can follow either an acute or a chronic course. The designation "idiopathic" means that the low platelet count is not the result of some other identifiable disease. In the differential diagnosis of ITP, every effort should be made to explore other causes of low platelet counts, especially drug reactions, splenomegaly, hematologic disease, and other autoimmune disorders, notably lupus erythematosus. The thrombocytopenia of ITP results from destruction of platelets, not from reduced production. Bone marrow examination is necessary to demonstrate megakaryocyte activity and to rule out other hematologic diseases.

IMMUNE DESTRUCTION

The platelet destruction of ITP affects both the patient's own platelets and transfused normal platelets. Destruction occurs because the plasma contains an IgG protein which acts in the host and also causes prompt thrombocytopenia if transfused into a normal recipient. Although this IgG behaves in many ways like an antibody, it is not clear what its antigen is, or how it destroys platelets. The primary site of platelet destruction is the spleen. It is probable that the immunoglobulin attaches immunologically to platelets, which are then destroyed by sinusoidal reticuloendothelial cells, but this has not been demonstrated as conclusively as have the comparable events in autoantibody-induced red cell destruction. Adrenal steroids reduce splenic destruction, while estrogens enhance it.

CLINICAL FINDINGS

Acute ITP occurs largely in boys and girls below age 6, often several weeks after a viral infection. The onset is sudden and is characterized by a dramatic onset of bleeding manifestations and a rapid decline of platelet counts to levels below 20,000/mm.[3] The disease lasts several weeks, but in more than 80 percent of cases, it remits spontaneously. *Chronic ITP*, on the other hand, begins insidiously, affects mostly adults between ages 20 and 40, and occurs three times as often in women as in men. Preceding infection is rare. Spontaneous remission also is rare, and the disease tends to persist for months or years. Adrenal cortical steroids, splenectomy, or the two in combination are the most promising therapeutic approaches, but these are by no means universally effective. Immunosuppressive drugs have given gratifying results in some cases.

Drug-Associated Antibodies

Innumerable drugs have been reported to cause thrombocytopenia. Many reports involve rare, idiosyncratic reactions or anecdotal accounts with tenuous documentation of direct cause and effect relationships. Several groups of drugs, however, cause severe, reproducible platelet damage by inducing antigen-antibody reactions in sensitive individuals.

Arsenicals, gold salts, several sulfa drugs, PAS, rifampin, digitoxin, and chlorthiazides are among the drugs that induce IgG antibodies which damage platelets and increase splenic sequestration. These drugs attach to the surface of circulating platelets; the antibody reacts with the drug-platelet complex, rather than with platelets or drugs alone. IgG persists for years, but platelet damage occurs only if the drug is present in the circulation. Stopping the drug usually corrects the condition; if thrombocytopenia persists longer than 2 weeks after all traces of the drug have left the body, the problem is probably not simple drug allergy.

QUININE AND QUINIDINE

Very dramatic platelet destruction occurs in patients sensitized to quinine and quinidine, as well as to drugs of the isopropyl-carbamide group (including the sedative Sedormid which has been taken off the market). The antibody is one which activates complement and is directed against the drug itself. Circulating antibody combines with circulating drug to form an immune complex, which then attaches to the platelet membrane. The presence of antigen-antibody complex attracts complement, which proceeds to destroy the platelet. This is an example of the "innocent bystander" mechanism of cell destruction (see p. 113). Neither the antibody nor the complement has specific affinity for the platelet, but it becomes the victim nonetheless.

These antibodies persist for many years and react explosively with very small amounts of the drug. The quinine in bottled quinine water is enough to induce significant purpura.

ACQUIRED COMPLEX BLEEDING DISORDERS

Liver Disease

Patients with severe liver disease nearly always have abnormal results on laboratory tests of hemostatic function and may bleed significantly after liver biopsy or other surgical procedures. Spontaneous bleeding, however, is surprisingly uncommon, unless there is an obvious hemorrhagic lesion such as esophageal varices or hemorrhagic gastritis. The liver manufactures so many coagulation proteins that factor deficiencies are to be expected when hepatic function fails. Platelet problems, excessive fibrinolysis, and low-grade intravascular coagulation are additional complicating events.

THE "LIVER FACTORS"

Deficiency of the vitamin K-dependent factors (II, VII, IX and X) is the most frequent coagulation abnormality. This deficiency affects both prothrombin time and partial thromboplastin time. Early in the disease, Factor VII may be the only depressed factor; this leads to a prolonged prothrombin time with normal partial thromboplastin time.

If liver cells are badly diseased, giving vitamin K does nothing to increase factor levels, but administering parenteral vitamin K can help to distinguish obstructive from nonobstructive jaundice.[1] In biliary obstruction, factor levels are low because fat-soluble vitamin K is not being absorbed; the liver is capable of synthesizing the proteins, but no bile salts reach the intestine to facilitate fat absorption. After vitamin K is injected, PT and PTT should improve within 48 hours if jaundice is due only to biliary obstruction.

When hepatocellular failure has caused coagulation factor deficiencies, albumin production has usually declined as well. It is rare to have hypoprothrombinemia without pre-existing hypoalbuminemia. A prothrombin time more than one and a half times normal correlates with poor clinical prognosis, but it is hepatic insufficiency, rather than hemorrhagic complications, that causes clinical deterioration. When hemorrhage occurs, large volumes of fresh or frozen plasma may correct the coagulation defect temporarily. In severe crises, commercial concentrates of the liver factors can be useful, but clinical improvement often is disappointingly less than the calculated expected benefit.

OTHER ABNORMALITIES

Factor V levels decline unpredictably in severe liver disease, but it is not clear whether this contributes to clinical bleeding. Factor VIII assays, by contrast, may give higher than normal results. Fibrinogen levels are variable, depending on whether or not fibrinolysis occurs. Even when fibrinogen levels appear normal, coagulation may be qualitatively abnormal. There is a defect in polymerization, but it is not clear whether the abnormality lies in the fibrinogen molecules or in fibrin stabilizing factor.[11]

Activated products of both the coagulation and plasminogen systems normally circulate in small quantities and are cleared by the liver. With hepatic failure, activated coagulation and fibrinolytic factors may persist and accumulate. These factors affect laboratory tests for disseminated intravascular coagulation and for the occurrence of fibrin/fibrinogen degradation. Although the test results are abnormal, it is not clear whether this causes significant clinical effects or whether treatment should be attempted.

Severe liver disease impairs both platelet production and platelet function; this is especially marked in alcoholics. Transfusion of platelet concentrates gives disappointing clinical results, although it may be necessary if active bleeding is present.

Inhibitors to Coagulation Factors

In addition to the inhibitory antibodies that develop in repeatedly transfused factor-deficient patients, antibodies have been observed to develop spontaneously. Antibodies to Factor VIII or, very rarely, to Factor V or XIII, occasionally occur in previously normal individuals of either sex. Usually IgG, these antibodies resemble autoimmune red cell or platelet antibodies. They occur without discernible stimulus; they react with tissue or protein from other humans as well as from the patient; and they cause clinically significant disease.

Spontaneous anti-Factor VIII usually occurs in older people, although it has been reported in young patients with chronic immunoinflammatory diseases such as rheumatoid arthritis, lupus erythematosus, and ulcerative colitis. There is also a puzzling association with pregnancy; when it occurs, however, antibody develops after delivery rather than during the pregnancy itself.

A patient with antibody to Factor VIII has bleeding symptoms very like those of constitutional hemophilia, including hemarthroses, soft tissue hematomas without apparent trauma, and excessive bleeding after minor injuries. The patient's plasma has low or absent levels of procoagulant activity and, after incubation, inhibits the coagulation of previously normal plasma. Treatment is extremely difficult; nonhuman Factor VIII concentrates can be used for one-time correction of a crisis, but these products are immunogenic under the best of circumstances.

Disseminated Intravascular Coagulation

The complex disorder variously called *disseminated intravascular coagulation, DIC, consumption coagulopathy,* or *defibrination syndrome* is a common cause of acquired bleeding tendency. DIC usually occurs as a complication of some other life-threatening illness; the superimposed bleeding problem is often the last event in a rapidly deteriorating situation.

PATHOPHYSIOLOGY

The mechanisms that lead to DIC are normal physiologic processes, but the products and proportions become severely abnormal. The coagulation cascade can be activated toward fibrin generation if thromboplastically active material enters the circulation; if endothelial surfaces undergo widespread changes; if activated coagulation proteins or adherent platelets accumulate without disturbance; or if systemic blood flow patterns or acid-base balance become deranged. Once generalized fibrin deposition occurs, a vicious circle becomes apparent. Coagulation proteins are consumed, platelets are activated and entrapped, and fibrinolysis is initiated. Without the checks and balances that normally regulate thrombin and plasmin, both of these powerful proteolytic enzymes meet little resistance to their lytic attack on whatever Factor VIII, Factor V, fibrinogen, and platelets survive the coagulation processes.

CLINICAL FINDINGS

In the full-blown state of DIC, there is severe depletion of all coagulation proteins, especially of Factors VIII and V; platelets are virtually absent; little or no clottable fibrinogen exists; and high levels of fibrin/fibrinogen degradation products circulate and inhibit fibrin formation. The reticuloendothelial system and the liver attempt to clear these abnormal proteins and restore a semblance of normal protein synthesis. Unfortunately, DIC usually occurs in a setting of circulatory stasis, shock, hypovolemia, or increased vascular permeability. These conditions impair circulation and make it very difficult to initiate compensatory activity.

INCITING EVENTS

The classical stimuli to DIC are surgical, obstetrical, or traumatic events that allow thromboplastic materials to enter the circulation. These events include amniotic fluid embolism; large-scale operations, especially those involving the lungs or the genitourinary system; severe burns; and conditions in which blood cells undergo intravascular destruction, such as hemolytic transfusion reactions, bacterial toxemia, or acute promyelocytic leukemia. Generalized sepsis can cause acute or gradually developing DIC. Products of necrotic tissue can initiate DIC, as may malignant tumors or large infarcts of lung or bowel. Circulatory failure may result in DIC, especially if acidosis, increased vascular permeability, and slowed capillary blood flow are prominent.

MANAGEMENT

Once the pathophysiology of DIC was elucidated, it seemed appropriate to interrupt the underlying processes of coagulation and fibrinolysis by giving heparin and antifibrinolytic agents. Although this approach has had variable degrees of success, there is much disagreement over the use of heparin and of inhibitors of fibrinolysis.

The best therapy is to correct or reverse the initial inciting events. With massive trauma, sepsis, cardiogenic shock, and other clinical catastrophes, this tends to be difficult. Most workers advocate massive replacement of plasma and platelets to correct the bleeding diathesis, but controversy remains about giving heparin and agents to counteract fibrinolysis.

THROMBOSIS

A *thrombus* is a mass, derived from blood-borne elements, that forms during life in heart or blood vessels. Blood that clots in a test tube is not a thrombus; neither is shed blood that collects in the soft tissues or body cavities. The hemostatic plug that closes vascular defects is a thrombus of sorts, but *thrombosis* usually refers to a mass that forms at an inappropriate place or time.

Thrombosis causes far more morbidity and mortality than does hemorrhage. Heart attacks, strokes, thrombophlebitis, pulmonary emboli, and many of the cerebral and musculoskeletal symptoms of old age result from the effects of thrombosis. Until fairly recently, however, thrombosis was rather like the weather: everyone talked about it, but no one could do anything about it. The only known treatment consisted of anticoagulant therapy after thrombosis had already occurred. There were few tests that could predict whether thrombi would form and few safe therapeutic agents capable of preventing thrombosis. These areas are still speculative, but some progress has been made in identifying predisposing features and correcting suspected abnormalities.

Predisposing Features

Thrombosis occurs where blood flow is irregular, where vascular surfaces are altered, or when the blood itself is abnormal. Many circumstances affect blood flow patterns: dilatation or distention of veins; arteriosclerotic, aneurysmal, or inflammatory changes in arterial walls; impaired or irregular myocardial contractility; and ischemic, inflammatory, or metabolic events that cause capillary dilatation and increased vascular permeability. Endothelial surfaces can be damaged by arteriosclerosis, inflammation, deposition of immune complexes, or locally reduced pH or oxygen tension. Changes in the blood itself include increased levels of fibrinogen, Factor VIII, or other factors; decreased fibrinolysis; increases in number or reactivity of platelets; increased numbers of red blood cells; presence of abnormal serum globulins; and activation of the interrelated systems of coagulation, complement, and kinins.

Laboratory Studies

Relatively few of these variables can be studied in the laboratory. A "hypercoagulable" state is difficult to document. Fibrinogen levels correlate unreliably with thrombosis. Fibrinogen is an "acute phase reactant," with a rise in plasma concentration occurring not only after hemorrhagic stress, but also after inflammation and other types of systemic stress. While platelet counts of over $500,000/mm.^3$ may predispose to thrombosis, platelet counts below this elevated level have no predictive value. It seems reasonable to measure platelet aggregability or adhesiveness as a predictor of thrombosis, but these functions show no consistent abnormalities before or during thrombosis.

Arteriosclerosis is the most common condition leading to arterial thrombosis. It is beyond the scope of this section to discuss laboratory investigations into cause, prognosis, and prevention of arteriosclerosis.

ANTITHROMBIN III

One promising investigative avenue has been the correlation of decreased antithrombin III activity with increased likelihood of thrombosis. Antithrombin III is present in normal blood; it neutralizes the effect of activated Factor X and also inhibits the action of the thrombin that does form. Heparin is thought to exert its anticoagulant effect by enhancing antithrombin III activity.[19] This is the rationale for "mini-dose" heparin therapy given to prevent expected thrombosis.

Families with inborn deficiency of antithrombin III have a higher than normal incidence of thrombotic disease.[15] Some studies have shown antithrombin III to be decreased in women who take oral contraceptives.[13] There is, however, no conclusive proof that antithrombin III levels and risk of thrombosis are directly correlated in any one individual.

Clinical Management

Although anticoagulant therapy is widely used to treat thrombophlebitis and certain types of coronary artery disease, therapeutic regimens vary from clinic to clinic, and both theory and practice are the objects of passionate controversy.

In preventing thrombotic disease, two avenues show marked promise: heparin therapy and manipulation of platelets. Small doses of heparin have proved highly effective in preventing venous thrombosis, especially in older people and postsurgical patients.[5] These "mini-doses" apparently enhance antithrombin III activity enough to prevent coagulation, but not so much that physiologically necessary hemostasis is impaired.

Attempts to prevent platelet activation or to modify their interaction with vascular surfaces have been less successful. Agents under study include aspirin, other nonsteroid anti-inflammatory agents, prostaglandin inhibitors, antioxidants, and dextrans.[16] These agents cause significant changes in laboratory results but cannot yet be proven to have clinical significance in preventing thrombotic disease.

REFERENCES

1. Ansell, J. E., Kumar, R., and Deykin, D.: *The spectrum of vitamin K deficiency.* J.A.M.A. 238:40, 1977.
2. Biggs, R.: *Haemophilia treatment in the United Kingdom from 1969 to 1974.* Br. J. Haematol. 35:487, 1977.
3. Blatt, P. M., Stuart, J. H., and Roberts, H. R.: *Hemophilia and other hereditary defects of coagulation* (Parts 1 and 2). Bull. Lab. Med. N.C. Mem. Hosp. 19–20, April–May 1977.
4. Bull, B. S., Huse, W. M., Braver, F. S., and Korpman, R. A.: *Heparin therapy during extracorporeal circulation.* J. Thorac. Cardiovasc. Surg. 69:685, 1975.
5. Gabriel, D. A., Blatt, P. M., and Roberts, H. R.: *Subcutaneous minidose heparin: theory and application.* Bull. Lab. Med. N.C. Mem. Hosp. 7, April 1976.
6. Gralnick, H. R. (moderator): *Factor VIII.* Ann. Intern. Med. 86:598, 1977.
7. Gralnick, H. R., Sultan, Y., and Coller, B. S.: *Von Willebrand's disease. Combined qualitative and quantitative abnormalities.* N. Engl. J. Med. 296:1024, 1977.
8. Green, D., and Chediak, J. R.: *Von Willebrand's disease. Current concepts.* Am. J. Med. 62:315, 1977.
9. Griffiths, B. L.: *A sticky proposition.* The Clotting Times (Ortho Diagnostics) 2(2), February 1977.
10. Griffiths, B. L.: *Let's aggregate.* The Clotting Times (Ortho Diagnostics) 1(11), November 1976.
11. Lane, D. A., Scully, M. D., Thomas, D. P., et al.: *Acquired dysfibrinogenemia in acute and chronic liver disease.* Br. J. Haematol. 35:301, 1977.
12. Levine, P. H.: *Platelet-function tests: predictive values.* N. Engl. J. Med. 292:1346, 1975.
13. Meade, T. W., Brozović, M., Chakrabarti, R., et al.: *An epidemiological study of the haemostatic and other effects of oral contraceptives.* Br. J. Haematol. 34:353, 1976.
14. Nachman, R. L.: *Von Willebrand's disease and the molecular pathology of hemostasis.* N. Engl. J. Med. 296:1059, 1977.
15. *Predisposition to thrombosis.* Lancet 2:1430, 1974.
16. *Prevention of thrombosis.* Lancet, 1:127, 1977.
17. Ratnoff, O. D., and Jones, P. K.: *The laboratory diagnosis of the carrier state for classic hemophilia.* Ann. Intern. Med. 86:521, 1977.
18. Saito, H., Ratnoff, O. D., and Donaldson, V. H.: *Defective activation of clotting, fibrinolytic and permeability-enhancing systems in human Fletcher trait plasma.* Circ. Res. 34:641, 1974.
19. Wessler, S.: *Heparin as an antithrombotic agent.* J.A.M.A. 236:389, 1976.
20. Wintrobe, M. M., Lee, G. R., Boggs, D. R., et al.: *Clinical Hematology.* ed. 7. Lea & Febiger, Philadelphia, 1974.

SECTION 2

IMMUNOLOGY

CHAPTER 6

PRINCIPLES OF IMMUNOLOGY AND IMMUNOLOGIC TESTING

The immune system protects the body from invasion by foreign elements; these can range from microorganisms to ragweed pollen, from transplanted organs to subtly altered autologous proteins. An *antigen* is any substance that elicits an immune response in an immunocompetent host to whom that substance is foreign. There are two categories of immune response: the *cell-mediated* response, produced by locally active lymphocytes present at the same time and place as the specific antigen, and the *humoral* response, the manufacture of antibody proteins that enter body fluids for widespread distribution throughout the body.

TYPES OF LYMPHOCYTES

Lymphocytes play the dominant role in immune reactivity. Two categories of lymphocytes exist: *B-lymphocytes*, which give rise to the immunoglobulin-manufacturing cells, and *T-lymphocytes*, which perform cell-mediated immune activities and also assist B-cells to respond to antigenic stimulation. Although indistinguishable on light microscopy, the two types of lymphocytes differ significantly in surface properties.

Derived from the same primordial stem cells, the two populations very early acquire distinguishing features. T-lymphocytes receive developmental instructions from the *thymus*. B-lymphocytes are so named because, in birds, an organ called the *bursa of Fabricius* instructs precursors to differentiate into antibody-producing cells. Mammals lack a bursa; some tissue or organ causes lymphocytes to differentiate along immunoglobulin-producing pathways, but its identity remains elusive.

B-Lymphocytes

B-cells constitute the minority (only 10 to 15 percent) of lymphocytes in the peripheral blood. B-lymphocytes can be identified because they have immunoglobulin molecules on the cell surface, rather like a sample of the product their descendants will manufacture. The surface immunoglobulin probably permits the B-cell to recognize its specific antigen and to interact with it so that immune activity can begin.[22] Other B-cell receptors interact specifically with several elements in the complement sequence (see later section) or with portions of immunoglobulin molecules.[18]

Any one B-cell can produce only one type of immunoglobulin molecule. Contact with its specific antigen stimulates the reactive B-cell to immune activity. Activation causes the lymphocyte to transform into a larger cell, an *immunoblast*, characterized by active DNA replication which initiates many generations of cell division. Progeny of the immunoblast become *plasma cells*. These cells have a round, compact nucleus pushed to one side of the cell by the large amount of ribosomal material that produces enormous quantities of a single protein molecule.

PLASMA CELLS

Plasma cells are found in lymph nodes, in the lymphoid portions of mucous membranes, and in chronically inflamed tissue. Normally, they are not present in peripheral blood or, except in small numbers, in the bone marrow. The protein that plasma cells manufacture rapidly leaves the cell and enters the body fluids. These proteins are *antibodies*, capable of interacting specifically with other aliquots of the antigen that first stimulated their production. Once antibody is secreted into the body fluids, the presence of plasma cell or precursor B-lymphocyte is unnecessary; all antigen-antibody interactions occur independently of lymphoid cells.

T-Lymphocytes

Of lymphocytes in the circulating blood, more than two-thirds are T-lymphocytes. These cells can be identified easily by the fact that fresh red blood cells from sheep cluster around their surface when the two types of cells are incubated together. This property serves no known biologic purpose and has no immune specificity, but it constitutes the basis for the very useful "E-rosette" test to distinguish T-cells from B-cells. T-cells have unique surface specificities, called theta (θ) or T-antigens, which, when injected into nonhuman hosts, elicit an antibody that reacts only with T-lymphocytes. Anti-T-cell antibodies are useful in enumerating lymphocytes and identifying members of a mixed population. Because the antibody injures T-cells lethally in reacting with them, the antibody cannot be used to identify circulating cells in vivo. T-cells perform a variety of biologic activities. Distinctive classes of T-cells perform distinctive functions; T-cells do not constitute a single, pluripotential race of cells.[2]

DELAYED HYPERSENSITIVITY

The best-defined T-cell role is mediation of the delayed hypersensitivity type of tissue reaction, of which the tuberculin skin test is the classic example. In this form of immune response, a tissue reaction appears, 18 to 48 hours after antigenic exposure, which is characterized by increased vascular permeability, interstitial edema, and accumulation of lymphocytes and macrophages. These tissue effects result from the actions of *lymphokines*, which are products secreted by T-cells only after contact with their specific antigen. Lymphokines do not enter the circulation; their effects on vascular permeability, cell movement, interaction with proteins, and activation of other cells are confined to a very limited zone immediately around the T-cell that produces them.

OTHER EFFECTS

Transplant rejection is another T-cell activity, although circulating antibodies also take part. T-cells appear to play a directly cytotoxic, "killer" effect on transplanted tissues; they also elaborate lymphokines that induce other cells to damage the foreign tissue. Under abnormal circumstances, T-cells may attack cells of the host's own tissues, presumably those with surface properties which have been altered enough that T-cells perceive them as "foreign." This T-cell property is important in surveillance against tumor development and in the genesis of autoimmune disease.

A very important but poorly understood T-cell function affects immunoglobulin production.[14] For some kinds of antigen, T-cells must be present as "helpers" before B-cell activation becomes apparent.[16] Conversely, some T-cells appear to serve a "suppressor" function, preventing the production of antibody to certain antigens under various conditions.[19]

IMMUNOGLOBULINS

Immunoglobulins, proteins of B-lymphocyte origin, all have structural properties in common and possess the capacity for specific combination with the eliciting antigen. All immunoglobulin molecules consist of two pairs of polypeptide chains. The longer pair, called the *heavy chains*, have twice the molecular weight of the shorter chains, called *light chains*. Five different types of heavy chains have been identified; immunoglobulins are classified according to the particular heavy chain type that is present. Two types of light chains exist, but immunoglobulins of all five classes have molecules with either kind of light chain.

Common Features

The amino acid sequence of the heavy chain determines the biologic properties of the molecule. Each immunoglobulin class or subclass possesses an unvarying amino acid sequence, comprising 75 percent of the chain, which is the same for all members. Individual specificity — the capacity to combine uniquely with individual antigens — resides in the amino acid sequence in the variable segment, located at the carboxy-terminal end of heavy and light chains.[3] The variable portion comprises about 50 percent of the light chain sequence and 25 percent of the heavy chain.

Immunoglobulins, complex polypeptides with highly structured three-dimensional configuration, can be immunogenic if introduced into hosts of other species. Using as antigen purified preparations of whole immunoglobulin molecules or of individual chains or segments of chains, one can raise antibodies which identify the determining features for each of the five heavy chains and for subclasses within these five classes.[24] Immunoglobulin classes are designated IgA (with two subclasses), IgD (with two subclasses), IgE, IgG (with four subclasses), and IgM (with several subclasses which are not yet fully defined).

BASIC STRUCTURE

Immunoglobulin molecules have longitudinal symmetry, with disulfide bonds linking the four chains together (Fig. 6). Each light chain links only to one heavy chain; the two heavy chains join one another in a "hinge" fashion, producing a Y-shaped four-chain unit. Breaking the disulfide bonds results in liberation of discrete, intact chains. Enzymatic proteolysis divides the molecule into three fragments: two identical fragments that consist of a whole light chain and half a heavy chain, and one fragment that contains the other half of both heavy chains. The variable sequences that confer antibody specificity exist entirely within the two identical fragments, which are called *Fab* fragments (*F* for fragment, and *ab* for antibody activity). The remaining fragment embodies the unvarying, class-specific part of the heavy chains; it can be crystallized reproducibly and is called *Fc* (crystallizable) fragment.

The amino acid sequence of the Fc fragment determines biologic properties common to all antibodies of that class or subclass. These include the ability to cross the placenta, the capacity to initiate complement activation, the capacity to attach to cell surfaces or to remain fixed when injected into the skin, distribution within body compartments, the ability to neutralize toxins and viruses, and the

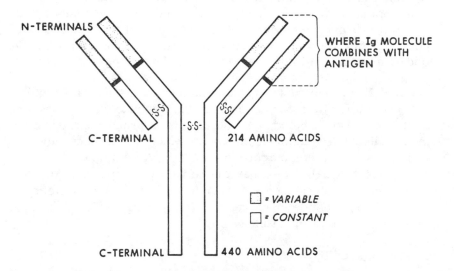

Figure 6. Schematic representation of the basic immunoglobulin structure. The shaded parts of the N-terminal portions of light and heavy chains constitute the individually specific antibody combining site. The remaining three-fourths of the molecule is the same for all examples within a given immunoglobulin class. (Reproduced with permission from Widmann, F. K.: *Pathobiology: How Disease Happens.* Little, Brown, Boston, 1978.)

propensity to unite with antigen in certain predictable physical configurations. Regardless of antigenic specificity, all immunoglobulins of a given class or subclass will have the same behavioral properties.

POLYMERIZATION

The basic immunoglobulin unit consists of two heavy chains and two light chains and has two antibody combining sites. This monomeric unit has a sedimentation constant of 7S when subjected to ultracentrifugation. Immunoglobulins A and M characteristically polymerize; the biologically active IgA or IgM molecule consists of several 7S units joined together in predictable configurations, often with additional short chains or added segments. Not surprisingly, polymerization alters the number of combining sites and/or the manner in which antigen and antibody interact.

IgA

Immunoglobulins with heavy chains described as α are called IgA; they are found predominantly in watery fluids and surface secretions. The lubricating fluids that line the respiratory and alimentary tracts contain high concentrations of IgA antibodies. These surfaces are continually exposed to environmental microorganisms, and IgA antibodies seem to constitute the body's first defense against microbial invasion. IgA is also found in tears, colostrum, and milk.

Circulating blood contains small amounts of IgA with a structure that is slightly different from IgA found in the watery secretions. Except for those in the blood, IgA molecules include a glycoprotein fragment called the *secretory component,* which seems necessary for immunoglobulin secretion outside the blood. A fraction of the small amount of blood IgA also has the secretory component. Another constituent of polymerized IgA, found largely in surface secretions, is a short polypeptide chain called *J* (for joining), which links two basic IgA units into an 11S dimer.

PHYSIOLOGIC ROLE

IgA antibodies develop fairly late in immunologic maturation, appearing no earlier than 6 to 8 months of age and rising rather slowly to adult levels. The major role of secretory IgA antibodies seems to be repelling viral invasion by direct viricidal activity.[21] Their role against bacteria is somewhat unclear, since IgA molecules do not activate complement and do not lyse bacterial cell walls. By attaching to bacterial surfaces, however, IgA antibodies may promote phago-cytosis or interfere with bacterial penetration through mucosal sur-faces.

IgD

The biological functions of IgD remain mysterious. Small amounts circulate in plasma—less than IgA or IgM and much less than IgG, but much more than IgE. IgD is exceptionally sensitive to proteolysis, a trait that makes it difficult to isolate and purify. Substantial amounts of IgD are associated with the surface membrane of B-lymphocytes, especially in cord blood.[22] IgD may serve somehow as antigen re-ceptor or mediator between external molecules and interior B-cell functions, but many steps in these processes remain to be clarified.

IgE

IgE antibodies are responsible for those hypersensitivity reactions described as *atopic* and *anaphylactic*. Examples of IgE-mediated disease include hay fever, asthma, certain types of eczema, and idio-syncratic, potentially fatal systemic reactions to insect venoms, penicillin, and other drugs or chemicals. It is more difficult to identify beneficial effects of IgE activity; clinical correlations suggest that IgE may help to protect mammals against parasitic worms.[11]

Before IgE was characterized, its existence was recognized as an active protein that fixed to cells, caused skin sensitization, and was increased in patients with atopic diseases. The name *reagin* was given to this protein, and IgE antibodies are sometimes described as *reaginic* antibodies.

BIOLOGIC BEHAVIOR

Serum concentrations of IgE are measured in nanograms per milliliter. Low blood levels result partly because IgE is synthesized slowly and has a short half-life (2 to 3 days) but mostly because IgE performs its functions outside the blood stream. Almost all of the body's active IgE is bound to specific tissue cells. The surface membranes of mast cells, which are basophilic granulocytes located in many tissue sites, have Fc receptors with which the IgE heavy chains bind strongly and specifically.[11] Macrophages and neutrophils have surface receptors for Fc portions of IgG molecules, but the affinity is nonspecific and of modest degree.

Mast cells, sometimes called tissue basophils, contain granules rich in histamine and other substances that affect vascular permeability. Interaction of IgE antibody with specific antigen constitutes a stimulus that makes the mast cell release these vasoactive substances. The fact that IgE is fixed to the cell has no effect on the reaction between antibody and antigen. It simply means that the IgE antibodies cannot circulate in search of antigen; they must wait for antigen to enter the area. Once this happens, the Fab portions react with antigen; this produces a conformational change in the Fc portion, which responds by releasing vasoactive amines.

Histamine and other mast cell products are the immediate cause of atopic or anaphylactic symptoms, but the IgE antigen-antibody reaction triggers the clinical sequence.[13] Mast cells are especially numerous in the respiratory tract and in the skin; it is not surprising that hay fever, asthma, and skin rashes constitute the principal symptoms of IgE-mediated syndromes.

IgG

The major immunoglobulin in circulating plasma is IgG, normally present in concentrations of 8 to 15 mg./ml., or 0.8 to 1.5 gm./dl. IgG molecules readily pass from blood stream to extravascular fluid and, alone of all the immunoglobulins, can cross the placenta to enter the fetal circulation. At birth, the infant's IgG antibody levels mirror the mother's. These maternal antibodies are gradually degraded over the first 3 months of life. Independent IgG production begins at 3 to 6 months of age and continues at a high level well into old age.

IgG antibodies develop rather late in the immune response to a newly introduced antigen. IgM antibodies occur first in a primary response, but once specific IgG antibodies appear, production may remain at a high level well after the antigen has been eliminated. Second or later exposure to the same antigen causes IgG antibodies to reappear very rapidly; this constitutes a secondary, or *anamnestic*, response and is another reason that serum levels of IgG are consistently high. IgG also has a half-life much longer than that of the other immunoglobulins.

BIOLOGIC BEHAVIOR

Many, but not all, IgG antibodies activate the complement sequence upon interacting with their antigen. If the antigen is part of a cell surface, the result of antibody-mediated complement activation is membrane lysis and destruction of the cell. This result is beneficial if the antigen is an invading microorganism; it harms the host if the damaged cell is an erythrocyte. Complexes of soluble antigen and IgG antibody may attach to cell membranes or to the walls of blood vessels and attract complement to these surfaces as well.

IgG antibodies are small molecules that can attach to particles without agglutinating them. The bacterium, red cell, or other particle remains freely suspended in blood or tissue fluid, but IgG molecules coat the surface. Granulocytes, macrophages, and B-lymphocytes possess receptors with specific affinity for the Fc portion of IgG molecules. As they circulate, the cells or bacteria that are coated with IgG are far more susceptible to phagocytosis, neutrophilic degradation, or lymphocyte-mediated cytotoxic attack than are uncoated cells. In these circumstances, the antibody itself does not damage the cell, but it sets up its victim for lethal attack by nonspecific agents.

IgM

As the immune system matures, IgM is the earliest immunoglobulin class to be produced. IgM is also the first antibody produced after primary immunizing contact with any previously unfamiliar antigen. IgM production tends to continue as long as antigen remains present and to cease when the antigen has been eliminated.

The biologically active form of IgM is a *pentamer*—five individual 7S units joined together in a 19S macroglobulin. Even though five monomers are present, the active antibody has only five combining sites, rather than 10. Half the combining sites are functionally inaccessible. The 19S macromolecule is highly efficient in agglutinating particulate antigens, in activating complement, and, probably, in neutralizing toxins and extracellular viruses. IgM antibodies do not coat particles without causing an immediate effect such as agglutination or complement activation. There is no special affinity between IgM heavy chains and the membranes of phagocytic or granulocytic cells. Normally, IgM molecules remain confined to the blood stream. They are incapable of crossing the placenta, and they accumulate in extravascular fluid only if vascular permeability is pathologically increased.

THE COMPLEMENT SYSTEM

Complement is a system of protein molecules, the sequential interactions of which produce biologic effects on surface membranes, on cellular behavior, and on the interactions of other proteins. At least 11 different proteins circulate in normal plasma, each inactive by itself but destined to play a specific role once the activation sequence begins.[16] Activation can begin with IgG or IgM antigen-antibody reactions or following contact with aggregated IgA, with certain naturally occurring polysaccharides or lipopolysaccharides, or with activation products of the coagulation or kallikrein systems.

Biologic Actions

Complement proteins are identified by numbers and letters. The activation sequence does not entirely coincide with standard numerical sequence. By convention, the order in which complement factors interact is C1q, C1r, C1s, C4, C2, C3, and then 5 through 9. A bar is placed over factor numbers to indicate that activation has occurred, as, for example, C1qrs or C1423. Activation involves either enzymatic cleavage of large, inactive molecules to leave an active residue or conformational changes without actual cleavage. Calcium and magnesium ions are required for several steps.

Complete activation, from 1 to 9, leads to membrane disruption and irreversible cell damage.[10] Along the way to complete activation, the following activities occur: C2 releases a low molecular weight peptide with *kinin* activity; activation products of C3 and C5 affect mast cells, smooth muscle, and leukocytes to produce an *anaphylactic* effect; other elements of C3 and C5 bind to cell membranes and render them more susceptible to phagocytosis, a process called *opsonization*; fragments of C3 and C4 cause *immune adherence*, in which complement-coated particles bind to cells whose surface membranes have complement receptors; activated C3 and C4 are also capable of *virus neutralization*; and finally, C3 and C5 fragments exert *chemotactic activity* on neutrophils, attracting the in-migration of these motile cells toward the protein fragments. The C5–9 complex influences the *procoagulant activity of platelets,* and, conversely, activation of the procoagulant Factor XII can independently initiate C1 activation. Plasmin (the substance that dissolves fibrin) and thrombin (which converts fibrinogen to fibrin) have proteolytic action that can cleave C3 into its active form.

Activation Pathways

In the "classical pathway" of complement activation, the initial step is activation, by an antigen-antibody interaction, of the q, r, and s components of C1. Because C1q is heat-labile, heating a serum sample can abort the entire complement sequence. Ca^{++} is required for C1qrs association, and Mg^{++} is required for C4 to activate C2. If chelating anticoagulants have been used, plasma lacks available cations, and complement activation cannot take place. After C1qrs activates C4, and C4 activates C2, contact with C2 cleaves C3 into two fragments: a small one, C3a, which disperses into the medium, and a large portion, C3b, which attaches to the cell membrane. C3b is needed to activate C5, but thereafter the remainder of the C5–9 complex assembles itself without other activating enzymes.[15]

The "alternate pathway" of complement activation bypasses C1, C4, and C2 activation, beginning directly with cleavage of C3.[18] Once C3b has been generated, activation of C5 through C9 occurs predictably. The key step in the alternate pathway is activation of *properdin*, a serum protein without biologic effects in its inactive form. Contact with aggregated IgA, with bacterial endotoxins, or with complex molecules such as dextran, agar, or zymosan alters properdin and initiates the sequence that produces C3b.

ANTIGEN-ANTIBODY REACTIONS

Innumerable antibodies exist which are capable of specific reaction with innumerable antigens. The results of antigen-antibody reactions, however, fall into relatively few categories. These effects derive from the physical and spatial characteristics of the antigen molecule and from the physical and biologic properties of the antibody molecule. The laboratory worker can exploit these properties to create readily detectible end points for studies in vitro.

Antibodies are water-soluble proteins, but they can be attached to membranes or other surfaces. They can be incorporated into solid or semisolid mediums. They can be labeled with radioactive, fluorescent, or electron-dense markers. In purified form, they can serve as antigens to induce anti-immunoglobulin serums when introduced into a nonhuman host. Antigens come in many forms: protein, carbohydrate, lipoprotein, or lipopolysaccharide; soluble or particulate; isotopically inert or labeled with radioactive elements; attached to membranes or particles, or existing independently as large or small molecules. The characteristics of the antigen and the antibody determine the physical form that the antigen-antibody reaction will take. Visible end points most often used in laboratory testing include precipitation, agglutination, formation of immune complexes, and initiation or inhibition of biologic activity.

Precipitation

Soluble antigen and soluble antibody are invisible in a fluid medium. When they interact, the intertwining molecules form a three-dimensional complex which often precipitates into a visible, insoluble mass. Precipitation of antigen-antibody complex depends on the proportion between antigen and antibody. When proportions are optimal, antigen and antibody molecules pair off completely, and the resulting precipitate contains all of the previously dissolved antigen and antibody. When antibody is present in excess, insoluble precipitated complexes contain all the available antigen, but unbound antibody remains in the medium. If excess antigen is present, such antigen-antibody complexes that form tend to remain in solution. Since no visible precipitate forms, it is difficult to detect whether or not a reaction has occurred.

GEL DIFFUSION TECHNIQUES

Agar gels are fluids capable of holding proteins in suspension. Molecules of antibody or soluble antigen can travel through the semisolid medium, creating different concentrations in different parts of the gel. In *double diffusion* techniques, antigen and antibody are allowed to move toward each other through the medium. As antigen and antibody diffuse through the agar, they interact in a manner dependent on relative concentrations. In one area, antigen may be in excess, while in another, a superfluity of antibody may exist. In just the right place, optimal concentration of each will allow formation of insoluble precipitate. The location, shape, and intensity of the precipitin line indicates the nature and the concentration of the reacting molecules.

Double diffusion is useful for answering the question, Does this specimen of serum, body fluid, or prepared reagent contain the antigen (or antibody) we are looking for? It is especially useful for determining whether different reacting materials are similar, identical, or unrelated (Fig. 7).

In *single diffusion* techniques, antibody is dispersed uniformly throughout the gel, and antigen-containing material is allowed to diffuse outward from the point of application. Since the antibody is uniformly dispersed, the proportions between antigen and antibody will depend on the rate of antigen diffusion. At the point where proportions are optimal, a line of insoluble precipitate develops. This technique permits accurate quantitation of soluble antigen down to very low concentrations.

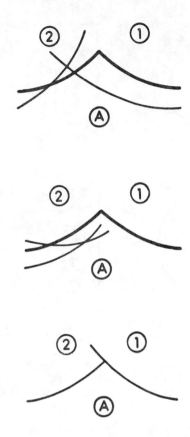

Figure 7. Schematic representation of the double diffusion technique for comparing immunologic identity. In all three panels, well A contains a known mixture of antibodies, and wells 1 and 2 contain unknown specimens. *Top*: Each well has two reactants, as shown by the two arcs. One reactant is common to specimens 1 and 2, as shown by the perfectly symmetrical joined arcs. The other two reactants have no resemblance to each other. *Middle*: Sample 1 contains only one reactant, identical to one of the reactants in sample 2. Sample 2 contains two other, unrelated materials. *Bottom*: Samples 1 and 2 contain related materials that give arcs of similar shape and location. The spur extending past the junction point proves that the reactants are not identical.

In *radial immunodiffusion*, antigen-containing material diffuses outward uniformly around a central well. A circular precipitin line forms where antigen-antibody proportions are optimal. Since the antibody concentration is constant, the radius of the circle depends on the concentration of antigen and the distance it must travel to reach optimal proportions (Fig. 8). At a low initial concentration of

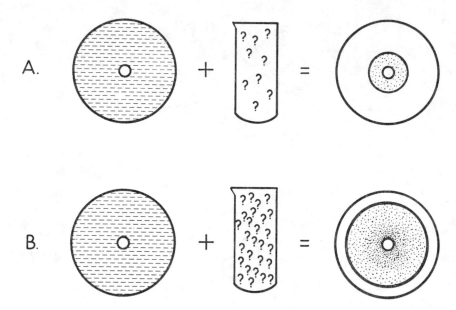

Figure 8. In radial immunodiffusion, antibody concentration is constant throughout the plate. The more concentrated the added antigen solution, the wider the diffusion circle must be before optimal proportions are reached to precipitate the antigen-antibody complex. In panel A, the unknown is of low concentration, and the radius of the precipitin circle is small. In panel B, more concentrated antigen is present, and the precipitin circle has a much larger radius.

antigen, the optimal proportion occurs very near the well. If the test material contains highly concentrated antigen, the proportion optimal for precipitation will develop much farther from the well, after widespread diffusion has occurred. Antigen concentration can be quantitated by comparing the size of the test circle against precipitin circles around known concentrations of the same antigen. This technique is widely used to measure immunoglobulin levels in serum as well as other proteins present in low concentrations.[9]

In *rocket electrophoresis,* an electrical current is passed through the medium to enhance antigen movement; the gel contains uniformly distributed antibody. Proteins move toward the positive electrode at a rate determined by their electrical properties, which depend on primary amino acid composition. The diffusion pattern is not symmetrical; it is parabolic or "rocket" shaped. Electrically enhanced antigen movement occurs rapidly, producing an asymmetrical precipitin arc that is more distinct and easier to measure than the circles achieved in radial immunodiffusion. Immunoglobulins do not migrate rapidly toward the cathode and cannot be measured easily with this technique. "Rocket" electrophoresis gives excellent results with transferrin, haptoglobin, ceruloplasmin, and other nonimmunoglobulin serum constituents.

IMMUNOELECTROPHORESIS

Immunoelectrophoresis is a semiquantitative technique that works well with solutions of mixed antigens, when one wants to identify assorted constituents and to indicate their relative concentrations. It is a two-stage procedure. After electrophoresis is used to separate the constituent proteins according to their electrical behavior, the separated elements are identified by inducing precipitin lines against antibodies of known specificity. Antibody is added after electrophoretic separation has occurred. The number of precipitin lines depends on the number of active antibodies that are used. Antiserum against whole human serum, or against whole classes of human globulins, causes numerous arcs to develop, each representing a different protein in the test serum. With more specific antibodies, there will be fewer arcs. Adaptations of this technique, combined with methods for protein separation and measurement, allow immunoelectrophoresis to be used quantitatively.[23]

Agglutination

When antibody unites with antigen on the surface of suspended particles, the antibody molecules create links between the particles, causing a solid, lattice-like structure to develop. Each antibody molecule must combine with antigens on separate particles so that linkage occurs. This antibody-mediated aggregation of previously distinct particles is called *agglutination*.

For agglutination to occur, the antibody must be specific for the particle-bound antigen; the particles must be sufficiently close together that the immunoglobulin molecule can bridge the distance between them; antigenic sites must be sufficiently numerous that antibody combining sites stand a reasonable chance of finding antigen on nearby particles; and the antibody molecules must not be so numerous that they get in each other's way. The first condition—specificity—provides the basis for many different types of laboratory test. The other conditions of antigen-antibody interaction can be manipulated to elicit new information or expand initial impressions derived from simple agglutination procedures.

SPECIFICITY OF ANTIGEN AND ANTIBODY

In most laboratory tests, either the antigen or the antibody is of known specificity. (In blood transfusion and some circumstances of tissue immunology this may not be the case. These special categories are considered in Chapter 8.) If antibody specificity is known, agglutination tests answer the question, Do these cells (particles) have this antigen on their surface? This is especially useful in classifying blood cells and identifying bacteria and other microorganisms. Staphylococci, for example, will not be agglutinated by antipneumococcus antibodies; antibodies for one strain of salmonella will not agglutinate salmonellae of other strains. Group A red cells will not be agglutinated by anti-B serum (Fig. 9).

With an antigen of known specificity, it is possible to answer the question, Does this serum contain that specific antibody? If antibody is present, the serum agglutinates the antigen-bearing particles; if not, the particles remain in suspension. The serum may contain other antibodies, but these will not be detected without cells or particles that bear the specific antigen. Examples of this application include blood grouping tests, which indicate whether a serum has antibodies

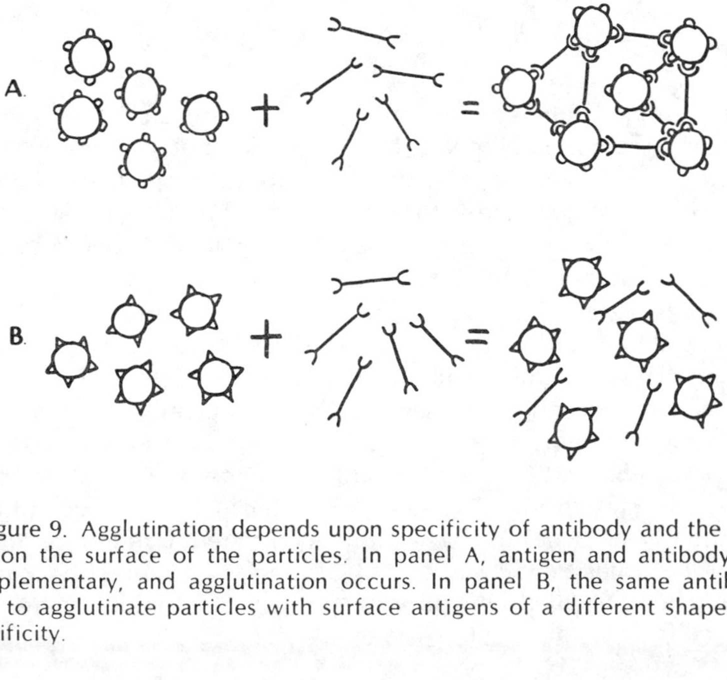

Figure 9. Agglutination depends upon specificity of antibody and the antigen on the surface of the particles. In panel A, antigen and antibody are complementary, and agglutination occurs. In panel B, the same antibody fails to agglutinate particles with surface antigens of a different shape and specificity.

against specific red cell antigens; and serologic tests in microbiology, in which the presence of specific antimicrobial antibodies indicates prior immunizing exposure to the particular organism.

ARTIFICIALLY COATED PARTICLES

Soluble proteins can be rendered particulate by attaching them to a carrier particle, often a latex particle, glass bead, or altered red blood cell. Agglutination is a more sensitive end point than pre-cipitation; it is easier to distinguish and is capable of recognizing lower concentrations of reactants. Converting the soluble protein to particulate form makes it possible to detect antibodies against purified preparations of antigens such as IgG molecules, thyroglobulin, penicillin, and others that are normally soluble. Conversely, known antibodies can be purified and attached to particles so that interaction with a soluble antigen causes the antibody-bearing particles to form a lattice. An example of this technique is adsorption of antifibrinogen antibodies to an inert carrier. When antibody-coated particles are added to fibrinogen-containing serum, agglutination occurs in pro-portion to the fibrinogen concentration in the serum.

QUANTITATION

With agglutination techniques, it is easy to obtain semiquantitative or comparative data about reagent concentration. Once it has been established that specific antigen and antibody are present and that agglutination will occur in the unmodified test system, one can dilute the material that contains either antibody or antigen until the concentration becomes too low to support agglutination. The higher the initial concentration of antibody or antigen, the more the serum must be diluted before agglutination ceases. This value is expressed as the *titer*, the reciprocal of the dilution figure (i.e., if serum diluted 1:64 causes agglutination, but there is no agglutination at 1:128, the antibody titer would be given as 64).

Titration is especially useful in establishing whether an antibody has increased or decreased over a period of time. Although titration is a comparative technique, some idea of absolute concentration can be achieved by comparing the behavior of the material under test to the results obtained when standardized reference material is diluted.

Attachment without Agglutination

Antibodies, especially IgG molecules, sometimes attach to surface antigens without agglutinating the subjacent particles. This occurs if antibody or antigen is in low concentration or if the particles are so widely dispersed that a single molecule cannot bridge the space between two particles.[20] This kind of coating without agglutination occurs both in laboratory testing and in intact biologic systems; red blood cells, platelets, and bacteria are the particles usually affected.

BIOLOGIC EFFECTS

When cells or bacteria are coated by antibody, their biologic behavior changes. Antibody-coated cells display restricted motility and reduced deformability. Deformability is especially important for red blood cells which normally must squeeze through tortuous splenic sinusoids and tiny capillaries; antibody-coated red cells experience mechanical difficulties. The attached immunoglobulins also allow new types of cell-cell interactions. Both neutrophils and macrophages have surface sites that react specifically with parts of the Fc portion of IgG molecules. Bacteria coated with IgG antibody are more readily phagocytized than unmodified organisms, and coated red cells are susceptible to the cytolytic actions of macrophages. IgG-coated bacteria also interact with B-lymphocytes. These cells are not phagocytic or cytotoxic, but they do have Fc receptors on their surface. It may be that the intimate contact between coated organism and antibody-producing cell stimulates especially rapid antibody formation.

This process whereby antibody coats bacteria to enhance phagocytosis is called *opsonization*. Antibodies that induce bacterial coating are called *opsonins,* from the Greek *opsonein*: to buy victuals. An especially effective form of coating involves attaching complement fragments to the cell surface. When a complement-binding antibody reacts with a surface antigen, it sets the complement sequence into motion. The entire sequence need not continue; the significant effect is that C3b attaches to the surface. Many phagocytic cells have membrane sites specific for C3b. The resulting interaction between coated cell and membrane receptor is called *immune adherence*; it markedly facilitates destruction of the affected cell. Antibody-coated red blood cells are caught and attacked by macrophages which ordinarily trap and destroy only those circulating cells too old or inflexible to survive.

ANTIGLOBULIN SERUM

Antibodies, being proteins, can be a highly effective antigen when introduced into a suitable host. Animal antiserums directed against human globulins are extremely useful laboratory reagents.[4] Anti-IgG and anticomplement (especially C4 and C3) are the antibodies most widely used in immunohematology. Adding antiglobulin serum to cells or other particles makes it possible to detect antibodies or complement proteins attached to the surface of suspended particles.

When particles are coated with protein, addition of antiglobulin serum produces visible agglutination of the previously separate cells. The antiglobulin molecules serve as the link between the cells that had been freely suspended in the medium. The usual end point in antiglobulin testing is agglutination (Fig. 10). Other end points can be used by suitably modifying the antiglobulin serum. If a fluorescent or radioactive label is incorporated into the antiglobulin reagent, then residual fluorescence or radioactivity indicates that the antiglobulin serum has found suitable protein on the cell surface.

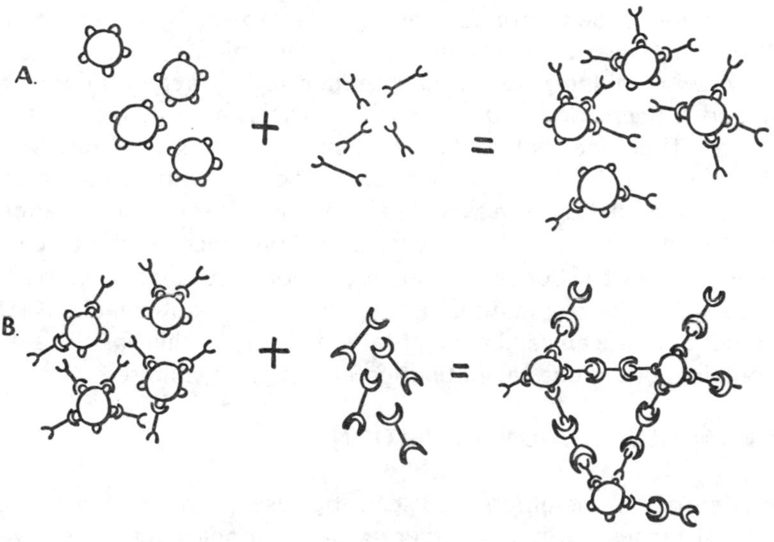

Figure 10. The principle of antiglobulin testing. In panel A, antibody reacts with and attaches to surface antigens, but the properties of antibody, particles, and suspending medium are such that the antibody-coated particles do not agglutinate. In panel B, a second antibody is added, one that reacts with antibody molecules, *not* with surface antigens. When the antiglobulin antibody joins with its immunoglobulin antigen, visible agglutination occurs. Particles without attached immunoglobulin (antibody) molecules would not be agglutinated.

Agglutination Inhibition

Antibodies can recognize and interact with their specific antigens in different physical forms (i.e., soluble, aggregated, or attached to a particle). Antibody formed originally against a surface-bound antigen will unite just as well (indeed, often more readily) with the same antigen in soluble form. This characteristic makes it possible to test for the presence of soluble, otherwise invisible, antigen in a fluid specimen.

For *agglutination inhibition* testing, one must have an antibody of known specificity and cells or other particles that have that specific antigen on their surface. The end point of the indicator system is agglutination of the particles. The test is done in two steps. First, one incubates the fluid under test with the reagent antibody, using conditions that encourage antibody to combine with soluble antigen. In the second step, the indicator particles are added to the incubated antibody-fluid mixture. If the fluid does contain the relevant antigen, incubation allows antibody and antigen to interact, and antibody combining sites become engaged by the soluble antigen. Because very few combining sites, if any, remain to interact with the surface-bound antigen added afterward, the particles are not agglutinated. If the test fluid does not contain antigen, incubation with antibody has no effect. The antibody retains all its activity and agglutinates the indicator particles at the expected level. Thus absence of agglutination is a *positive* test result, indicating the presence of antigen in the specimen tested. Conversely, agglutination of the indicator particles means that the test material is *negative* for the antigen (Fig. 11). The amount of antigen can be quantitated roughly by diluting the antigen-containing fluid until agglutination no longer is inhibited.

HEMAGGLUTINATION INHIBITION

Agglutination inhibition also can be used, under rather special circumstances, to show whether or not antibodies are present. Many viruses and viral products agglutinate human red blood cells by a nonimmune mechanism. Virus-specific antibodies block this capacity for hemagglutination. To test for antibodies against a given virus, one must have an active viral preparation that reliably agglutinates red blood cells. The test then consists of incubating the patient's serum with the viral preparation. If the serum contains the antibody, the incubated mixture of virus and serum will be unable to agglutinate added red cells. Absence of agglutination is a *positive* result. If the

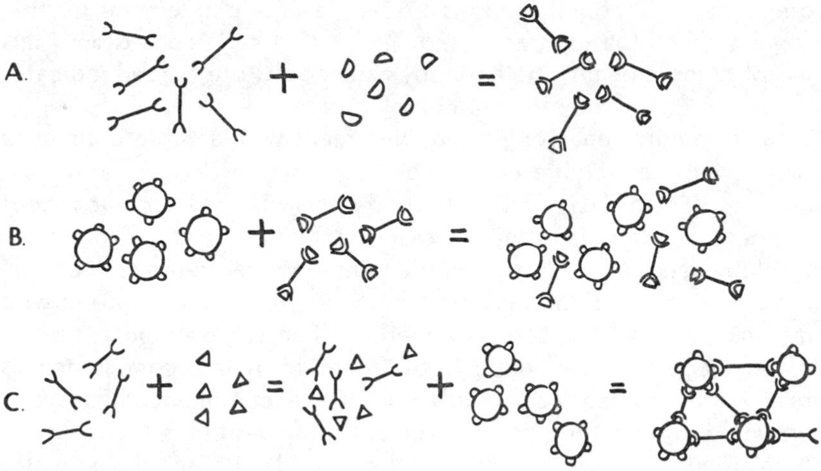

Figure 11. The principle of agglutination inhibition. The unknown antigen in these tests is soluble; particles with known antigen specificity are used as the indicator. In panel A, antibody of known specificity reacts with soluble antigen in the unknown specimen. Panel B shows what happens when indicator particles are added to the antigen-antibody mixture: the particles are not agglutinated, because antibody combining sites are already occupied. In panel C, the unknown specimen contains a different material, which does *not* react with the reagent antibody. In this case, subsequently added indicator particles *are* agglutinated, because the known antibody retains its activity.

serum lacks antibody, the viral preparation retains its ability to agglutinate, and the presence of agglutination is a *negative* test result.

Complement Fixation

Complement is a nonspecific facilitator, active against many biologic products from many different species. Complement derived from guinea pigs or other animals reacts just as effectively as does human complement with human antibodies. Complement of animal origin is used in complement fixation (CF) tests, as part of the indicator system, to demonstrate whether or not a specific antigen-antibody reaction has occurred. The indicator system, in classical CF testing, is complement-mediated lysis of sheep or other animal red blood cells, in a two-step operation. It is possible to coat cells with a specific, complement-activating antibody but to prevent hemolysis by withholding complement. The antibody-coated cells retain the ability to activate complement; if complement is added later, complement fixation progresses and the cells are lysed. Red blood cells coated with this kind of complement-fixing antibody thus constitute a good indicator for the presence or absence of complement.

Many complement-fixing antibodies react with soluble antigen to form nonvisible, soluble complexes that contain antigen, antibody, and complement. It is difficult to detect whether such reactions have occurred, but CF testing allows indirect demonstration. Formation of soluble antigen-antibody-complement complex removes complement from the medium, making it unavailable for combination with any other system. This becomes apparent when, for example, antibody-coated sheep cells are added to the medium. If free complement is present, the indicator cells will lyse. If the complement has been consumed by the original antigen-antibody reaction, there is no complement available to hemolyze the coated cells, and the indicator cells remain unchanged.

CF TESTING

If known antigen is available, complement fixation tests are used to determine presence or absence of a complement-fixing antibody. If the known reagent is antibody, the CF test detects antigen in an unknown specimen. The reagents needed for any CF test include a source of active complement (usually guinea pig) and a suspension of red blood cells (usually sheep) already coated with a complement-activating antibody. It is necessary to eliminate unwanted complement from the test material; if fresh serum is being tested, it must be heated to 56°C. for 30 minutes before testing begins.

To perform the test, one incubates the test material, the specific antibody or known antigen, and a known amount of complement. This allows the antigen-antibody complex to form and to incorporate the available complement. After incubation, antibody-coated indicator cells are added. If the antigen-antibody reaction has occurred, complement will have been bound ("fixed") in the immune complex, and no complement will be available to hemolyze the antibody-coated indicator red blood cells. If the test specimen lacked the antigen or antibody needed to initiate complement fixation, the active complement remains in the medium, able to hemolyze the coated red cells when they are added. Hemolysis, then, is a *negative* test result; failure of hemolysis is a *positive* result, indicating that the relevant antigen or antibody was, indeed, present in the test specimen (Fig. 12).

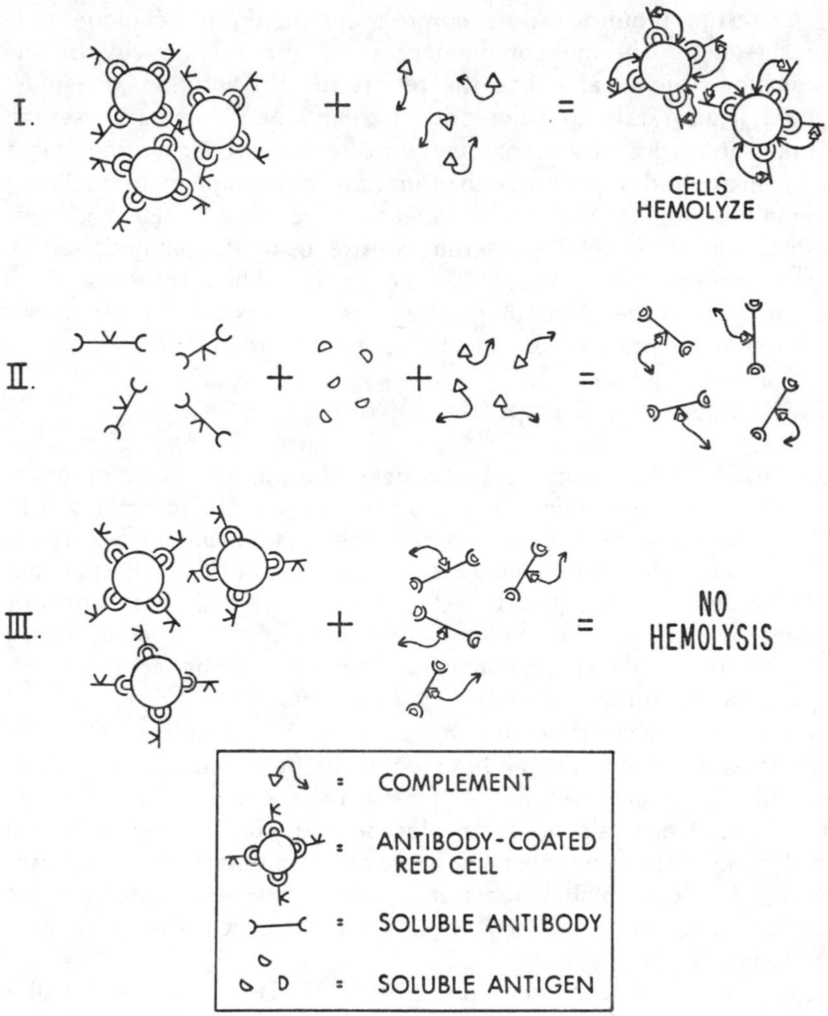

Figure 12. The principle of complement fixation testing. The reagent antibody must be one that fixes complement when it combines with its antigen. The indicator cells are already coated with an antibody that also fixes complement. In panel I, contact between coated cells and complement causes the cells to hemolyze. In panel II, reaction of soluble antibody, soluble antigen, and complement causes complexes to form which bind complement and render it inactive. Subsequent addition of antibody-coated cells (panel III) fails to cause hemolysis because the complement is already bound to soluble antigen-antibody complexes.

CF testing requires careful controls and accurate technique. One must standardize the complement level and the activity of the indicator system each time the test is run. In addition, one must guard against false positives due to "anticomplementary" serum. Some serums inactivate complement directly without an immediate antigen-antibody reaction. Such serums prevent complement-mediated hemolysis, so that every test appears to be positive. Each CF test must be accompanied by a serum control, using the patient's serum, the complement, and the coated red cells, but without reagent antigen or antibody. If the immunologically inert system shows no hemolysis, the seemingly positive test result must be discarded.

Radioassays and Competitive Binding

Remarkably small quantitites of antigen or antibody can be detected by techniques combining the principles of competitive binding with the technology of counting radioisotopes. Radioisotopes are atoms which behave like normal atoms except for emitting radiation that can be detected and quantitated with suitable equipment. Atoms of many elements can be rendered radioactive and then incorporated into complex molecules in place of an inert atom of the same element. Since the quantity of radiation can be measured very precisely, it is possible to measure the number of radiolabeled molecules. Radioactive isotopes of iodine and hydrogen can be introduced into many organic molecules without affecting their chemical or biologic behavior.[7] Since labeled molecules behave exactly like unlabeled molecules of the same substances, one can manipulate the proportions of labeled and unlabeled material so as to infer the quantity of unlabeled material from changes in the measurements of labeled material.

The principle of *competitive binding* holds that if two similar substances compete for attachment to a single binding agent, the initial proportions of the two substances determine the amount of each that ends up bound.[17] Consider, for example, two biologically identical (but physically distinguishable) materials, M-1 and M-2, both equally capable of attaching to B1, a binding substance with limited capacity. If the initial mixture contains equal quantities of M-1 and M-2, the resulting bound mixture will contain half M-1 and half M-2. If the initial mixture is one quarter M-1 and three quarters M-2, then the final bound product will contain one quarter M-1 and three quarters M-2, no matter what the absolute quantities are. It is essential that neither material combine preferentially with B1, because this would upset the principle of direct proportionality.

RADIOISOTOPES IN COMPETITIVE BINDING

Isotopically labeled materials can be measured very precisely; this makes them ideal for use in competitive binding assays. To measure total binding capacity of a system, one allows a pure preparation of radiolabeled material (*M) to interact completely with the binding material (B). After suitable incubation, the amount of *M present defines the amount with which material B can interact. Once the total capacity of B is defined, the quantity of unlabeled material (M) in a test specimen can be determined by competitive binding, using a known quantity of labeled *M.

First, one mixes thoroughly the known quantity of *M with the medium that contains M in unknown amounts. Then one determines the capacity of B, using a pure preparation of *M. Let us say that this amount produces 100 counts when all possible *M is bound. The test step is to incubate B with the mixture of M plus a known amount of *M. In this example, we find that fully saturated B now has 25 counts. Since M and *M attach equally to B, we conclude that the original incubation mixture contained three parts of M and one part of *M. If the final count had been 75, we would conclude that there was much less M in the original mixture—only one part of M to three parts of *M. If the final count were 100, we would conclude that the test material contained no M at all (Fig. 13).

Essential for this technique is a reliable means of removing unbound *M so that the only *M that remains to be counted is bound to B. Some techniques remove the bound materials, consisting of B-M-*M, from the system and count emissions in the removed material. Other procedures wash away excess M and *M, and count emissions in what remains. In either case, two separate products exist when the test is completed: the B-containing fraction that includes all bound M and *M, and a residual fraction that contains unbound M and *M, and has no binding medium at all.

The amount of M in the original material can be calculated either from the radioactivity in the bound product or from the amount of unbound *M present in the residual material. Dilution of radioactive reagents by washing or adding other reagents does not alter the total amount of measurable radioactivity. If the original amount of *M is known, measuring residual, unbound *M permits deduction of the

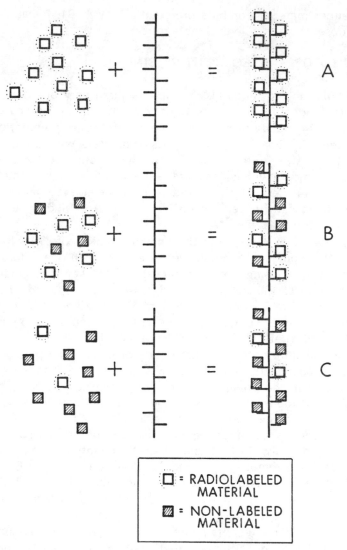

Figure 13. The principle of competitive binding. A binding material of constant, known capacity is used. Labeled (reagent) and unlabeled (unknown) substances attach equally to the binding agent. In panel A, the unknown sample contains none of the material to be measured. Because there is no unlabeled material to compete with the labeled reagent, the final product has 100 percent concentration of labeled material. If the unknown sample contains a moderate amount (panel B) or a large amount (panel C) of unlabeled material, it competes successfully to attach to the binder. The final product has less labeled material, in inverse proportion to the concentration of unlabeled material in the unknown.

amount of unlabeled M that was present in the mixture incubated with B. High residual counts of *M mean that very little *M was bound; thus there must have been a high proportion of M in the reacting mixture. If the residual material contains very little *M, this indicates that the test material contributed very little M to the mixture, and the only material available to combine with B was the added reactant *M.

Antibodies constitute highly specific, readily available binding agents, but other agents, such as biologic receptors or purified transport proteins, also can be used as B. Provided that the binder is specific, that a pure preparation of test material is available for radiolabeling, and that bound and unbound reactants can be separated effectively, the technique can be used to measure all sorts of biologic materials. Antibodies constitute the most specific, the most adaptable, and the most readily prepared reagents. Competitive binding radioassay, using antibodies and their specific antigens, is called radioimmunoassay.

RADIOIMMUNOASSAY

Radioimmunoassay can be used to measure anything that can be sufficiently purified to elict a highly specific antibody in a susceptible host. Either the antibody or the antigen can be labeled for subsequent counting, depending on whether the bound or unbound material is measured as the end point.[12] With radioimmunoassay one can measure hormones, lipoproteins, lipopolysaccharides, and drugs of· all sorts that cannot be measured accurately by chemical means or that exist in such low concentrations that the usual chemical, physical, or immunologic techniques are unreliable. Accurate measurement of nanogram and picogram quantities has revolutionized the study of endocrine physiology and pharmacology. Hepatitis B antigens and antibodies have been studied with radioimmunoassay procedures, unlocking many previously closed doors in the epidemiology and treatment of this disease. Another application of these techniques is the study of circulating antigens associated with neoplasms and other disorders of cell or tissue growth.

Enzyme-Labeled Immunoassays

Enzymes are excellent labels for immunologic reactants because they can be measured specifically and sensitively without expensive radiation-counting equipment. To be a useful label, the enzyme must be available in purified form and must retain its specific activity when cross-linked to complex molecules; glucose-6-phosphate dehydrogenase, alkaline phosphatase, peroxidase, and lysozyme have all proved eminently satisfactory.

Many enzyme-linked immunoassays use the same underlying principles as assays that have radio-isotope labels. The immune reactants must be concentrated, pure, and highly specific. An enzyme label can be attached to antibody, antigen, or partial antigen (hapten), depending on the technique to be used and the material to be quantified. Various names and acronyms have been applied to these techniques; no standard terminology is in use. Generally used terms include enzyme immunoassay (EIA), enzyme-linked immunosorbent assay (ELISA), and enzyme-multiplied immunoassay technique (EMIT).[24]

SEQUENTIAL PROCEDURES

In enzyme-linked competitive binding techniques, labeled reagent antigen and the unlabeled antigenic material under test are reacted with a known quantity of antibody. As with radioimmunoassay, the quantity of bound enzyme labeled antigen in the final, washed preparation indicates the proportion of unlabeled antigen that was present in the original mixture. In other techniques, either antigen or antibody can be prepared in solid phase, bound to the surface of beads, test tubes, or microtiter wells. After complementary material, either antigen or antibody, reacts with the bound material, enzyme-labeled indicators delineate either the amount of material attached to the solid-phase reactant or the amount that remained unbound after all combining sites were saturated. Techniques of this sort require accurate, complete separation of bound and unbound material. It is essential that the enzyme-labeled indicator material enter into predictable, quantifiable immune complexes.

ONE-STAGE PROCEDURES

Unique to enzyme technology are rapid, one-stage assays that exploit biophysical properties of the enzymes. Enzymes sometimes lose or acquire catalytic activity according to the immunologic state of some cross-linked reagent. Some preparations of enzyme cross-linked to antigen or antibody have activity only if the ligand is in uncombined form; others are inactive if the bound material is uncombined and become active only after the antigen-antibody reaction occurs. If degree of enzyme activity and degree of antigen-antibody combination change in parallel, measuring enzyme activity provides quantitative information about the level of immunologically active material present in the test specimen.

This one-stage approach is especially suitable for measuring haptenic antigens, materials which exist in biologic specimens in relatively simple form, but for which highly specific antibodies can be raised. One-stage enzyme assays for anticonvulsant drugs, for drugs of abuse, and for thyroid hormones have found rapid acceptance, because the procedures are sensitive, relatively inexpensive, and far quicker than older methods that require laborious steps for separation and concentration. It is probable that increasing numbers of pharmacologic and physiologic materials will be subjected to this kind of enzyme-linked immunologic measurement.

REFERENCES

1. Alper, C. A., and Rosen, F. S.: *Complement in laboratory medicine*, in Vyas, G. N., Stites, D. P., and Brecher, G. (eds.): *Laboratory Diagnosis of Immunologic Disorders*. Grune & Stratton, New York, 1975.
2. Boyse, E. A., and Cantor, H.: *Surface characteristics of T-lymphocyte subpopulations*. Hosp. Practice 12(4):81, 1977.
3. Capra, D. J., and Edmundson, A. B.: *The antibody combining site*. Sci. Am. 236:50, 1977.
4. Coombs, R. R. A., Mourant, A. E., and Race, R. R.: *A new test for the detection of weak and "incomplete" Rh agglutinins*. Br. J. Exp. Pathol. 26:225, 1945.
5. Foad, B. S. I., Adams, L. E., Yamauchi, Y., and Litwin, A.: *Phytomitogen responses of peripheral blood lymphocytes in young and older subjects*. Clin. Exp. Immunol. 17:657, 1974.
6. Gershon, R. K.: *T-cell control of antibody production*. Contemp. Top. Immunobiol. 3:1, 1974.
7. Gill, T. J., III: *Principles of radioimmunoassay*, in Rose, N. R., and Friedman, H. (eds.): *Manual of Clinical Immunology*. American Society for Microbiology, Washington, D.C., 1976.
8. Götze, D., and Müller-Eberhard, H. J.: *The alternative pathway of complement activation*. Adv. Immunol. 24:1, 1976.
9. Heremans, J. P., and Masson, P. L.: *Specific analysis of immunoglobulins: techniques and clinical value*. Clin. Chem. 19:294, 1973.
10. Humphrey, J. H., and Dourmashkin, R. R.: *The lesions in cell membranes caused by complement*. Adv. Immunol. 11:75, 1969.
11. Ishizaka, K.: *Structure and biologic activity of immunoglobulin E*. Hosp. Practice 12(1):57, 1977.
12. Jaffe, B. M., and Behrman, H. R. (eds.): *Methods of hormone radioimmunoassay*. Academic Press, New York, 1974.
13. Jarrett, E. E. E.: *Activation of IgE regulatory mechanisms by transmucosal absorption of antigen*. Lancet 2:223, 1977.

14. Katz, D. H.: *Genetic controls and cellular interactions in antibody formation*. Hospital Practice 12(2):85, 1977.
15. Mayer, M. M.: *The complement system*. Sci. Am. 229:54, 1973.
16. Müller-Eberhard, H. J.: *Complement*. Annu. Rev. Biochem. 44:697, 1975.
17. Odell, W. D., and Daugherty, W. A. (eds.): *Principles of Competitive Protein-Binding Assays*. J. B. Lippincott, Philadelphia, 1971.
18. Parish, C. R., and Hayward, J. A.: *The lymphocyte surface. II. Separation of Fc receptor, C_3 receptor and surface immunoglobulin-bearing lymphocytes*. Proc. Roy. Soc. Lond. (Biol.) 187:65, 1974.
19. Parker, C. W.: *Control of lymphocyte function*. N. Engl. J. Med. 295:1180, 1976.
20. Pollack, W., Hager, H. J., Reckel, R., et al.: *A study of the forces involved in the second stage of hemagglutination*. Transfusion 5:158, 1965.
21. Roitt, I.: *Essential Immunology*, ed. 3. Blackwell, Oxford, 1977.
22. Rowlands, D. T., and Danielle, R. P.: *Surface receptors in the immune response*. N. Engl. J. Med. 293:26, 1975.
23. Verbruggen, R.: *Quantitative immunoelectrophoretic methods: a literature survey*. Clin. Chem. 21:5, 1975.
24. Wisdom, G. B.: *Enzyme-immunoassay*. Clin. Chem. 22:1243, 1976.
25. World Health Organization: *Nomenclature for human immunoglobulins*. Bull. World Health Org. 30:447, 1964.

CHAPTER 7

SEROLOGY: SELECTED IMMUNOLOGIC TESTS

QUANTITATING NORMAL CONSTITUENTS

As our understanding of immune mechanisms has advanced, measuring specific immune products has become increasingly important. This capacity to quantitate allows sequential study of normal and pathologic responses to immunogens, and makes possible precise diagnosis of immune deficiency states and acquired disorders of immune functioning. Genetically determined immunodeficiency states characteristically affect a single, well-defined element (e.g., T-lymphocytes, individual immunoglobulin classes, or individual complement proteins). Acquired disorders are usually more complex, affecting broad segments of the immune response or reflecting diffuse changes that result from disease in other organ systems. Examples of secondary, acquired abnormalities are the diffuse hyperglobulinemia that accompanies liver disease or the changes in complement activity that occur in renal diseases or arthritis.

Immunoglobulin Levels

SCREENING TESTS

Quantitative disorders of immunoglobulins are found especially in patients who suffer repeated bacterial or fungal infections, experience persistent eczema or asthma, or report a family history of infectious or immunologic diseases. Since IgG contributes between 0.4 and 1.7 gm. of serum protein/dl. in normal adults, deficiency of IgG alone can cause low total globulin levels, as does generalized absence of immunoglobulin. Selective deficiencies of other Ig classes are less apparent from total globulin levels, since IgM levels normally are below 0.2 gm./dl., even in adults, and serum IgA levels are quite variable. Similarly, increased total globulins may result from excess IgG or, less often, IgM but rarely from IgA (except in multiple myeloma) and never from IgE.

Another simple screening test is to observe anti-A and anti-B activity. Except for the 5 percent of persons whose blood group is AB, red cell agglutinins are conspicuous in all normal persons after the age of 6 months. Antibody activity nearly always can be demonstrated in serum diluted 1:8, and most older children and adults have levels above 1:32. Absent or very weak hemagglutinating activity suggests either defective immunoglobulin synthesis or a variant ABO blood group.

Antibodies against specific pathogens such as typhoid or diphtheria-pertussus-tetanus (DPT) can be measured. If a patient has previously received immunizing injections, demonstration of low or absent antibody levels suggests defective immunoglobulin manufacture. A more controlled study is to administer typhoid or diphtheria toxoids and to measure antibody levels before and after immunization.

QUANTITATIVE PROCEDURES

Electrophoresis of serum proteins allows quantitation of total α, β, and γ globulin levels but does not permit subclassification within globulin categories. The volume and shape of protein peaks on a densitometer tracing often suggest specific increase or decrease, or indicate a generalized abnormality (Fig. 14). With *radial immunodiffusion*, specific immunoglobulins can be quantitated precisely. Since this technique measures immunoreactive molecules, antibody levels will appear falsely low if circulating immune complexes of high molecular weight have tied up a specific antibody or immunoglobulin class. Falsely high results occur if IgM is circulating as fragments with low molecular weight or if there is unbalanced production of the heavy chains with which the reagent antibody reacts.[8] Another potential problem is reaction between circulating abnormal antibodies and protein incorporated in the immunodiffusion plate. This can occur if the serum contains rheumatoid factor, which is anti-IgG, or if the patient has antibodies against the animal proteins used to prepare the reagent plate. Animal antibodies of this sort are

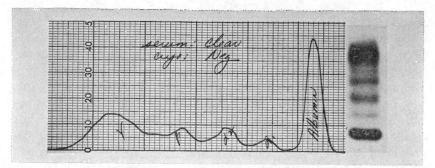

Figure 14. The stained polyacrylamide strip on which the serum proteins migrate is shown at the right. On the left is a densitometer tracing, which translates the stained protein bands into a curve, the contours of which reflect both the intensity and the width of the protein bands. Albumin, the serum protein present in highest concentration, is seen as the dark band at the bottom of the strip and as the tall, symmetrical peak at the right of the densitometer tracing. In this figure, normal quantities and proportions of all proteins are present.

most frequent in patients with selective IgA deficiency; their presence is betrayed by the development of two precipitin rings in the immunodiffusion plate.

Radioimmunoassay is useful in measuring circulating levels of IgE, which is usually present at concentrations too low to be seen by radial immunodiffusion. It is also invaluable in quantitating levels of antibody directed against specific purified antigens.

B-Lymphocyte Studies

Plasma cell progeny of B-lymphocytes produce immunoglobulins. Patients with hypogammaglobulinemia usually have a sparse plasma cell population in bone marrow, lymph nodes, and intestinal mucosa, and their lymph nodes are small, showing poorly developed germinal centers. Since B cells normally contribute only 15 to 30 percent of circulating blood lymphocytes, patients with hypogammaglobulinemia rarely have significantly low total white blood cell counts. They do, however, have markedly reduced numbers of circulating B cells, as can be shown with lymphocyte identification techniques. This is most often done with the sheep cell rosette technique that identifies T cells, or with fluorescent anti-immunoglobulin antibodies that identify the surface immunoglobulin of B cells.

The immunoglobulin class of individual B cells can be demonstrated with fluorescent antibodies specific for one or another heavy chain. In chronic lymphocytic leukemia and in many cases of non-Hodgkin's lymphoma, increased numbers of peripheral lymphocytes circulate, all reacting with a single antibody type. This is considered evidence that all the circulating cells developed from a single precursor, thus representing a single clone of proliferating cells.[32] This type of lymphocytosis differs markedly from that seen in lymphocytosis of infectious origin, in which B cells of all heavy-chain types proliferate. In multiple myeloma, the percentage of B cells in the peripheral blood drops below normal.[19] This helps to distinguish myeloma, a malignant monoclonal gammopathy (see p. 212) from benign monoclonal gammopathy, in which the percentage of circulating B cells remains normal.

T-Lymphocytes and Cellular Immunity

T cells and B cells have unique properties that make it possible to distinguish them in concentrated preparations of peripheral blood lymphocytes. T cells are killed when exposed to animal serum specific for thymocytes, while B cells are unaffected. When lymphocytes are allowed to interact with a suspension of sheep red blood cells, T cells spontaneously cause sheep red cells to cluster around them in rosettes, while B cells do not affect sheep cells. The properties leading to rosette formation are poorly understood, but they appear to weaken in certain disease states. This limits the usefulness of rosette testing in conditions such as Hodgkin's disease. Since T cells normally constitute the bulk of circulating lymphocytes, patients with defects of cellular immunity characteristically have low peripheral lymphocyte counts.

MICROBIAL SKIN TESTS

Many environmental agents induce cell-mediated immunity in normal people without causing any identifiable illness. One way to test whether cell-mediated immune function is normal is to perform intradermal skin tests with several common antigenic materials. Agents commonly used include mumps virus, PPD (purified protein derivative of tubercle bacilli), *Candida albicans*, trichophyton (skin fungi), and the streptococcal product streptokinase-streptodornase. It would be an unusual person who had had no immunizing contact with any of these. Of all these agents, skin tests are most likely to be positive against mumps antigen or streptokinase-streptodornase. The percentage of reactors positive to Candida antigens varies markedly with the injectible preparation used.[30] A person who shows no skin reaction to any intradermal antigen should be suspected of having impaired cellular immunity.

EXPERIMENTAL SENSITIZATION

The integrity of the cell-mediated immune system can be challenged directly by injecting some highly antigenic material to which the patient has had no exposure and measuring the development of delayed hypersensitivity. Halogenated benzenes are useful for this because they reliably elicit cell-mediated reactions in immunocompetent individuals but are not part of the normal antigenic environment, and thus spontaneous immunization does not occur. This test is often done with 2,3-dinitrochlorobenzene (DNCB). When a challenge dose is administered 2 to 3 weeks after the immunizing dose, normal individuals reliably demonstrate a well-defined skin reaction. Failure to become sensitized to DNCB indicates deficient T cell responsiveness.

IMMUNOBLAST TRANSFORMATION

When T cells encounter an antigen to which they are already sensitized, they undergo transformation into *immunoblasts* — large, easily recognized cells with active nucleic acid synthesis and cytoplasm that reacts brilliantly with pyronine. One can demonstrate whether prior sensitization to some antigen has occurred by culturing concentrated lymphocytes with a pure preparation of the antigen in question. If the person has immunocompetent T cells, and if he has previously had experience with that material, contact with the antigen causes his cultured lymphocytes to undergo blast transformation. Transformation is documented by measuring the incorporation of radiolabeled thymidine into the nuclei of the cultured cells. Thymidine is used to synthesize nucleic acids. Absence of thymidine incorporation indicates that there is no increase in nucleic acid synthesis and that the cells have not been transformed. This means either that the lymphocytes have not been sensitized to the antigen or that they lack competence to undergo transformation. If T cell competence can be verified, the technique of culturing lymphocytes with known antigens provides extremely useful information about existing immunity to viral, bacterial, or fungal antigens.

NONSPECIFIC STIMULATION

T cell competence is verified by demonstrating that nonimmun-
ologic stimulation can induce increased nuclear activity in cultured
lymphocytes. Phytohemagglutinin (PHA), a plant derivative, causes
50 to 95 percent of cultured normal T lymphocytes to undergo blast
transformation.[22] Concanavalin A is also effective for T cells; poke-
weed mitogen stimulates transformation of both B cells and T cells.
If T-cell function is seriously defective, less than 5 percent of cells
became blasts after exposure to PHA. PHA transformation is almost
totally absent in congenital T-cell deficiency states such as DiGeorge
syndrome and Swiss-type agammaglobulinemia. It is depressed, to
a variable degree, in acquired immunodeficiency states such as
Hodgkin's disease, chronic lymphocytic leukemia, many viral infections, autoimmune diseases, many nonlymphocyte malignancies,
as well as after severe burns and in conditions of altered metabolism
including uremia, liver disease, and severe malnutrition.

The Complement System

Antibodies can be raised that react specifically with individual proteins in the complement system. With accurately quantitated standards, it is possible to measure the levels of these proteins in the
circulation. In evaluating acquired disease states, it is usually sufficient to measure only C3, or the hemolytic activity of the entire
sequence. Genetic conditions have been found, however, that involve isolated deficiencies of C2, C3, C6 or C7, portions of C1, as well
as the biologic activity of C5 and the inhibitor of activated C1.[1]
These are very rare, and such patients require highly detailed diagnostic evaluation. Acquired changes in complement activity, on the
other hand, are rather common. Tests of complement levels are valuable both in diagnosing and in serially evaluating immune-mediated
diseases.

MEASURING ACTIVITY

The test for total hemolytic activity measures ability of the serum
under test to hemolyze sheep red blood cells already coated with
anti-sheep-cell antibody (see p. 195). The degree of hemolysis reflects
the concentration of complement in the test serum. The end point
most often used is lysis of one-half of the red cells, called the CH_{50}.
·The results are expressed in terms of CH_{50} units, which are extrap-

olated from levels in normal serum known to cause 50 percent hemolysis.

The hemolytic complement assay requires precise standardization of temperature, protein and electrolyte concentrations, pH, and other conditions. Immunodiffusion and electroimmunoassay are easier to perform. These usually use anti-C3 serum, taking C3 levels as representative of complement activity. Immunologic procedures have the usual problems of antibody specificity and reproducibility of test conditions, but an additional problem is that results vary with the age of the serum to be tested. During storage, C3 activation may occur by cleavage of the original molecule. The activated material is a smaller molecule, which travels faster through the medium and gives a wider ring than unmodified C3.

CLINICAL SIGNIFICANCE

Serum complement is consumed by immune events that occur in many systemic diseases. Thus serum CH_{50} values or C3 levels fall during the active phases of lupus erythematosus, especially lupus nephritis; in chronic active hepatitis and subacute bacterial endocarditis; in exacerbations of rheumatic fever; in vasculitis of many kinds; and in severe attacks of rheumatoid arthritis. Serial serum complement levels are especially useful in assessing the clinical course and response to treatment in patients with lupus erythematosus and renal involvement. Synovial fluid normally has complement levels that parallel serum levels. In rheumatoid arthritis, locally affected joints have fluid with significantly reduced complement activity.

ABNORMAL IMMUNOLOGIC PRODUCTS

Abnormal proteins circulate in many immunologic disorders. Usually these are incomplete or abnormal immunoglobulin molecules, or antibodies with aberrant reactivity. The nature of the abnormal protein often points to the nature or location of the immune disorder. The best-known example of a partial globulin is Bence-Jones protein, characteristic of multiple myeloma. Common aberrant antibodies are the cardiolipin-reactive antibodies that give "biologic false positive" results in reagin tests for syphilis (see p. 445) and the heterophile antibody characteristic of Epstein-Barr virus infectious mononucleosis.

Electrophoretic and immunoelectrophoretic techniques make it possible to identify abnormal proteins or normal proteins in characteristically abnormal proportions. It is possible to purify abnormal circulating proteins for use as antigen to raise specific new antiserums; with these antibodies, other patients can be tested for the same or related proteins. These techniques have uncovered and imposed order on many previously puzzling or overlooked immunologic disorders.

Monoclonal Gammopathies

Gammopathy refers to a disease or abnormal state involving globulins; although the term pinpoints the gamma globulins, it covers abnormalities of other immunoglobulins besides IgG. *Monoclonal* means that the abnormal material is produced by a single clone (i.e., one cell and its progeny). Another name given to a protein present in high concentration and purity but abnormal in physiologic function is *paraprotein*. In a monoclonal gammopathy, the densitometer tracing of the electrophoretic bands has a narrow, sharply defined elevation where the protein is concentrated (Fig. 15). This appearance is called an *M spike*, the M standing for myeloma or monoclonal, *not* for IgM. Often the protein can be characterized by its reactions with antiserums against light chains, heavy chains, and heavy chain subclasses. Of all the possible chain classes and allotypic variants, a monoclonal protein has only one type of light chain and one class of heavy chain.

MULTIPLE MYELOMA

In multiple myeloma, the neoplastic plasma cells continue to produce the immunoglobulin for which they are genetically programmed. IgG is the commonest myeloma protein, followed by IgA. IgM is less common, IgD is less common still, and IgE is quite rare.[2] Patients with lymphomas often have M spikes of IgG or IgM; rather small M spikes occasionally result from proteins produced by such epithelial neoplasms as cancer of the breast, lung, or prostate.

If a neoplasm produces heavy and light chains in equal proportions, a complete immunoglobulin molecule can result. In multiple myeloma, light chain production often exceeds heavy chain production. These unpaired light chains are always of one type, either all kappa or all lambda; they can be identified with anti-light-chain antiserum. Serum rarely contains high concentrations of light chains, because the small polypeptide molecules readily enter

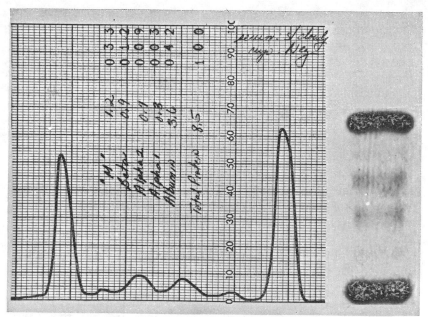

Figure 15. The abnormal protein in multiple myeloma migrates as a single, homogenous front, seen as the dark, sharply defined band at the end of the electrophoretic strip. The densitometer portrays this as a high, narrow peak, often called an "M spike."

the urine. Excess light chains in urine are known as *Bence-Jones protein*.[29] The physical behavior of Bence-Jones protein is unique; it precipitates when heated to between 58 and 60°C. and redissolves at 90 to 95°C. The heat precipitation test is still an excellent screening technique for this protein, which occurs in the urine of 50 to 75 percent of patients with multiple myeloma, but heating does not pick up low urinary concentrations. In questionable cases, or in urines in which excessive albumin obscures the Bence-Jones reaction, electrophoresis of concentrated urine proteins gives a more precise diagnosis.[19]

HEAVY CHAIN DISEASE

Much rarer than light chain overproduction is overproduction of heavy chains, which occurs in several lymphoma-like conditions. Spontaneous heavy chain disease, also called Franklin's disease, usually means overproduction of gamma chains.[8] In lymphocytic leukemia, there may be excessive mu chain production.[10] Lymphomatous proliferation of lymphocytes in the intestinal mucosa sometimes leads to excessive alpha chain production and often to intestinal malabsorption.

Heavy chain paraproteinemia is diagnosed by immunoelectrophoresis. The M spike clearly seen on electrophoretic separation fails to react with either anti-kappa or anti-lambda light-chain serum and does react with specific heavy-chain antiserum.

CRYOGLOBULINEMIA

Cryoglobulins are proteins that precipitate from plasma at 4°C., a category that includes many different materials including antihemophilic factor (Factor VIII). *Cryoglobulinemia* refers to the presence, in the circulation, of abnormal proteins with this thermal property. Monoclonal IgG and IgM sometimes behave in this way, although other examples precipitate or aggregate at higher temperatures. Patients with circulating cryoglobulins that precipitate at temperatures around 30°C. may suffer from capillary occlusion when exposed to the cold (Reynaud's phenomenon).[3] Deposition of globulin-complement complexes is another circulatory problem that occurs in cryoglobulinemia. Symptomatic cryoglobulinemia is liable to occur in lymphoma, myeloma, or Waldenström's macroglobulinemia, a condition of lymphoreticular proliferation associated with excessive IgM production. Occasional patients experience symptomatic cryoglobulinemia and have a monoclonal IgG or IgM spike but show no morphologic evidence of lymphoreticular neoplasm. This is called "essential" cryoglobulinemia because its cause remains obscure.[3]

Polyclonal Increases in Immunoglobulins

Homogeneous, monoclonal protein spikes are a relatively rare occurrence. A far commoner electrophoretic pattern appears when there is a diffuse increase in globulins, imparting a broad, hump-shaped elevation to the densitometer tracing (Fig. 16). Although immunoglobulins contribute most to this diffuse globulinemia, there is often an increase in other proteins that migrate in the globulin range, such as transferrin and ceruloplasmin. Chronic infections and noninfectious inflammatory diseases such as systemic lupus erythematosus or rheumatoid arthritis often have this "broad gamma" elevation; advanced liver disease nearly always produces this pattern. Other causes of diffuse hyperglobulinemia include lymphoreticular neoplasms and sarcoidosis.

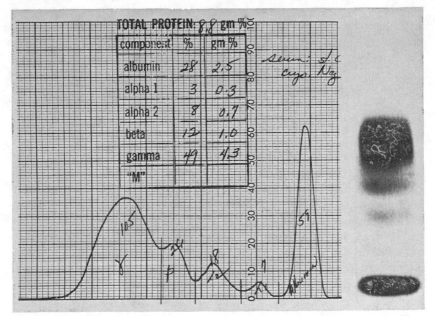

TOTAL PROTEIN: 8.8 gm %		
component	%	gm %
albumin	28	2.5
alpha 1	3	0.3
alpha 2	8	0.7
beta	12	1.0
gamma	49	4.3
"M"		

Figure 16. A heavy, diffuse mass of protein is present at the globulin end of the electrophoretic strip. On the densitometer tracing, this is seen as a broad, irregularly shaped hump.

Specific antibody levels show no consistent rise when generalized hyperglobulinemia occurs. Even when some long-standing inflammatory process induces antibodies to a single causative organism, the specific antibodies contribute relatively little to the total increase. The proteins involved in the "broad gamma" pattern are not structurally abnormal. Because they exist in abnormal proportions and serve no detectible physiologic function, the term *dysproteinemia* can be applied to hyperglobulinemia of this nonspecific type.

AMYLOIDOSIS

Patients who have had increased circulatory levels of monoclonal or polyclonal globulins for a long time often exhibit deposits of abnormal protein in blood vessels, connective tissue, and lymphoreticular tissue. This protein, *amyloid,* shares certain amino acid sequences with immunoglobulin light chains, but amyloid production appears to involve many cells in addition to B-lymphocytes and their plasma cell progeny.[17] Amyloidosis seems to accompany long-standing stimulation of the immune system, since it develops

in patients with chronic infections, autoimmune diseases, parapro-
teinemias, and some kinds of malignant neoplasm.[13] The cause and
the mechanism of amyloid deposition remain obscure. Amyloid
does not circulate; its presence is documented by microscopic
examination of specially stained tissue sections.

Immune Complexes

Immune complexes develop when soluble antibodies react with
soluble antigens. The resulting agglomerates of immunoglobulin
and protein-containing antigen may or may not be soluble. Many
biologically active antigens exist as soluble molecules not part of
membrane, nuclear, or cytoplasmic structures. As free-floating molecules, they interact with antibodies to produce interaction complexes fully capable of initiating immune events such as complement activation, release of vasoactive amines, or activation of neutrophils or platelets. The immune complex may settle out of the
circulation, adhering to vessel walls as a blob of protein which
attracts complement or cells, and localizes the biologic events
initiated by the immune response.

IMMUNE COMPLEX DISEASES

Immune complex deposition is an etiologically important event in
many diseases, especially the glomerulonephritis of lupus erythematosus or of poststreptococcal origin.[5] Other diseases initiated by immune complexes include various kinds of vasculitis, serum sickness,
rheumatoid arthritis, and drug sensitivites of the vasculitis type and
of the cytolytic type that affects red blood cells or platelets. When
immune complexes have deposited onto vascular walls or the lining
of body cavities, it is easy to demonstrate their presence by immunofluorescent examination of biopsied tissue.

LABORATORY DEMONSTRATION

Immune complexes can be identified in body fluids by radioimmunoassay or by ultracentrifugation or column chromatography of serum,
body fluids, joint fluid, or other material. Their presence can also be
shown by immunologic reaction with highly specific antibodies. All
these techniques are highly exacting. The presence of immune complexes can be suspected, however, by observing carefully the patterns
obtained on immunoelectrophoresis or by eliciting a positive test for

cryoglobulins. Immunoelectrophoresis of fluid containing IgG complexes reveals increased total amounts of IgG, and the precipitated material tends to have a broad, trailing contour instead of a clearly defined shape. The association between cryoglobulins and immune complexes is not absolute; often, however, circulating immune complexes lead to a polyclonal cryoglobulinemia.[3]

Miscellaneous Proteins

C-REACTIVE PROTEIN

C-reactive protein (CRP) is a glycoprotein that reacts with the C-mucopolysaccharide of many pneumococci. It was first noted in serum from patients with pneumococcal pneumonia and was considered an antipneumococcal antibody. However, patients experiencing all kinds of inflammatory processes or being subjected to tissue stress, such as pregnancy or certain neoplasms, often develop C-reactive protein in serum and body fluids. CRP is generally described as an "acute phase" reactant (i.e., one of many protein phenomena that occur in response to acute tissue injury).

Tests for C-reactive protein no longer use pneumococcal capsular antigen. The immune reaction uses an animal antiserum raised against C-reactive protein concentrated and purified from human serum. The easiest, most widely used technique is precipitation in capillary tubes; more sensitive or more quantitative studies employ double diffusion in agar or radioimmunodiffusion.

The test for C-reactive protein is used to monitor acute inflammatory activity in rheumatic fever and in rheumatoid arthritis. In these recurrent and often progressive diseases, it is important to detect exacerbations early and initiate treatment before damage progresses. In many patients with rheumatoid arthritis, CRP rises before the erythrocyte sedimentation rate, at the beginning of an inflammatory episode. If anti-inflammatory measures are successful, the CRP returns to normal sooner than does the sedimentation rate. CRP can be detected in the serum of as many as 40 percent of women in the last half of pregnancy and in many women taking oral contraceptives or using an intrauterine contraceptive device.[24] This does not constitute a "false positive" because pregnancy, steroidal contraception, and intrauterine mechanical contraception do, indeed, constitute tissue stress. On this account, however, it may be difficult to interpret CRP results in young women.

HETEROPHILE ANTIBODIES

Humans sometimes develop antibodies that react with red cells of other animals, despite the obvious fact that they have never been transfused with horse, sheep, or bovine cells. Antibodies of this sort are called *heterophilic*, which means that they are reactive with material from some other species. At least two different heterophile agglutinins can be detected, both of which are IgM. One of these, sometimes present in normal serums but usually found at high titers during serum sickness or certain infections, agglutinates sheep and horse red cells and hemolyses bovine cells. Absorption with Forssman antigen, a material prepared from guinea pig or horse kidney, completely removes this antibody from serum. The other, characteristic of EBV infectious mononucleosis, agglutinates sheep red cells, is completely removed from serum by absorption with bovine red cells, but is not affected by attempted absorption with Forssman antigen.

The heterophile antibody that reacts with Forssman antigen can exist in normal serum at titers of 1:28 or even 1:56. After exposure to horse serum or certain poorly understood microbial antigens, it can go as high as 1:224 or 1:448. The heterophile antibody of EBV infectious mononucleosis appears early in the illness and peaks, at levels of 1:224 or above, during the second or third week. It usually disappears at 4 to 8 weeks.[7]

Serologic diagnosis of EBV infectious mononucleosis rests on demonstrating the heterophile antibody that agglutinates sheep or horse red cells, that retains some or most of its activity after exposure to Forssman antigen, but that is completely removed by absorption with bovine red cells. The classic heterophile test is positive in about 70 percent of patients with infectious mononucleosis; 95 percent or more are positive when formalinized horse red cells (Monospot) are used.[17] A patient with signs and symptoms of infectious mononucleosis but without heterophile antibody is probably infected with cytomegalovirus or hepatitis virus. Such patients should have acute and convalescent serum drawn to detect seroconversion to viruses other than Epstein-Barr.

"BIOLOGIC FALSE-POSITIVE" REACTIONS

Reaginic activity often develops in patients with various infections or autoimmune diseases. This causes a positive reaction in nontreponemal tests for syphilis, the phenomenon known as the *biologic false positive* (see discussion on p. 446).

AUTOIMMUNITY

Ideally, antibodies should react only with material foreign to the host who produced them. In disease states, however, both humoral and cellular activity may develop against the host's own tissue. Auto-immune activity is never specific for the host's antigens and no one else's. Autoimmune reactivity recognizes products or components of target tissues present in all or most humans, including the host's tissue. Often the reaction also recognizes nonhuman examples of the antigen. Autoimmunity is an inappropriate response to widely distributed tissue components, rather than an interaction with some tissue product unique to the host.

Classification and Identification

Autoimmune phenomena can be separated into two groups: those that react against a specific organ product or cell type and those that interact with some antigenic configuration shared by many different tissues, organs, or body processes. Organ-specific antibodies include those directed against thyroglobulin, red blood cells, or glomerular basement membranes. Antibodies against DNA, IgG, or mitochondria, on the other hand, react with these materials in many different physiologic or anatomic settings.

Not all autoimmune events cause disease. Some seem to be the result of tissue damage caused by some other agent. Antibodies of this latter type are useful as markers to show that disease exists, but they do not explain what caused the disease. Autoimmunity is probably the primary pathogenetic event in autoimmune hemolytic anemia, in glomerulonephritis due to glomerular basement membrane antibodies, and in some kinds of thyroiditis. The organ-specific reactions that occur in ulcerative colitis, myasthenia gravis, or some kinds of liver disease more likely reflect immune response to pre-existing tissue damage. Once these secondary cellular or humoral autoimmune events take place, however, they may lead to further tissue damage; thus the distinction is not entirely clear-cut.

TECHNIQUES

Organ-specific antibodies can be demonstrated best by indirect immunofluorescent procedures in which serum is incubated with frozen sections of the tissue involved (Fig. 17). It is difficult to prepare tissue-specific antigens in a form that allows a serologic end point

INDIRECT IMMUNOFLUORESCENCE
(TO IDENTIFY ANTIBODY IN UNKNOWN SERUM)

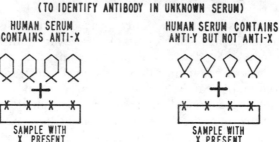

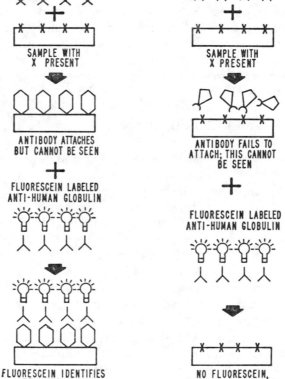

Figure 17. If antibody is present, it attaches to the tissue antigen present on the slide. Fluorescent antiglobulin serum is then added to show where the antibody has attached. Serum that contains no antibody, or that has an antibody against tissue antigens not present on the slide, will not deposit antibody molecules, and the added antiglobulin serum has nothing with which to react.

such as agglutination or precipitation. Autoantibodies against blood cells are an exception, and these techniques are discussed in Chapter 8. Antibodies against specific purified proteins can be demonstrated by competitive binding techniques or by agglutination of particles artificially coated with the antigen.

Thyroid Antibodies

Diagnostically useful antibodies have been found that react with three major thyroid antigens: *thyroglobulin,* the intrafollicular protein that stores thyroid hormone; *microsomal antigen,* which occurs in the cytoplasm of hormone-producing follicular cells; and *the second antigen of the acinar colloid,* an intrafollicular protein product distinct from thyroglobulin. An autoantibody of different kind is *long-acting thyroid stimulator* (LATS). This is an IgG immunoglobulin found in 60 percent or more of patients with thyrotoxicosis (Graves' disease). By interacting with cell-surface receptors, it stimulates hormone production. Immune-mediated thyroid disorders can lead to over-activity, underactivity, or abnormal size or consistency of the gland.

HYPOTHYROIDISM

The most common form of autoimmune hypothyroidism is *Hashimoto's thyroiditis,* also called nonspecific or lymphocytic thyroiditis. Antibodies to thyroglobulin and/or microsomal antigen so regularly accompany this condition that a patient with negative antibody tests almost certainly has some other disease. Positive results do not, however, confirm the diagnosis. These antibodies also can occur in thyrotoxicosis, in some patients with lupus erythematosus and other collagen-vascular diseases, in many patients with pernicious anemia, and in euthyroid relatives of patients with thyroiditis. About 50 percent of patients with carcinoma of the thyroid also have thyroid antibodies, but in titers lower than the 1:5000 or above that occur in Hashimoto's disease.[23] Thyroid antibodies also occur in hypothyroid patients whose gland is not enlarged; this may well represent a variant of the same autoimmune process.[27] Ordinarily, patients with nodular colloid goiter (simple, or nontoxic, goiter) do not have thyroid antibodies.

HYPERTHYROIDISM

Autoimmunity is probably associated causally with thyrotoxicosis (Graves' disease). Long-acting thyroid stimulator (LATS) is an IgG protein with antibody-like properties. Affected patients often have thyroid antibodies and lymphocytic infiltration of the gland. A familial association exists for hypothyroid thyroiditis and thyrotoxicosis. Thyrotoxic patients with significant levels of antithyroid antibodies are more likely than those with low or absent levels to become hypothyroid after treatment.[27]

Gastric Antibodies

In Addisonian pernicious anemia, 80 to 95 percent of patients have circulating antibodies against gastric parietal cells, and 50 to 60 percent also have antibodies to intrinsic factor.[25] The gastric mucosa is atrophic, hydrochloric acid is virtually absent, and there is deficiency of *intrinsic factor*, the parietal cell product with which dietary vitamin B_{12} must combine before it can be absorbed. Impaired absorption of vitamin B_{12} causes megaloblastic changes in both red cell and white cell lines and, in severe cases, neurologic and other symptoms reflecting B_{12} deficiency.

TYPES OF ANTIBODY

Antibodies to intrinsic factor (IF) have either "blocking" or "binding" activity. Blocking prevents the combination of IF with vitamin B_{12}, while binding antibodies interfere with absorption of the IF-B_{12} complex once it forms. Blocking antibodies are more common. They occur alone or in combination with binding antibodies, whereas binding activity rarely exists unless blocking antibodies also are present.[27] Tests for IF antibodies employ radio-cobalt-labeled vitamin B_{12}. Antibodies to intrinsic factor may reach serum levels as high as 1:128.

Antibody to gastric parietal cells is a complement-binding antibody that reacts with a microsomal antigen. Cytoplasmic microsomes of both thyroid and gastric cells may represent a precursor form of the glandular secretory product. Antibody to parietal cell microsomes is demonstrated by immunofluorescent testing, using frozen sections of stomach. Titration is done with a complement fixation technique that uses homogenates of stomach; this test is less sensitive than immunofluorescence but easier to quantitate. Parietal cell antibodies rarely achieve titers above 1:32.

CLINICAL SIGNIFICANCE

Parietal cell antibodies are often found in serum from normal individuals, the incidence increasing with advancing age. Under age 20, 2 percent of normals have these antibodies; between ages 30 and 60, the incidence rises to between 6 and 8 percent and reaches 12 percent in men and 19 percent in women over age 70.[25] Histologic study of the stomachs of these antibody-producing "normal" persons often reveals focal areas of gastric atrophy or lymphocytic infiltrates, even though no gastric or hematologic illness exists.[26]

Patients with simple atrophic gastritis but without anemia often have parietal cell antibodies but lack antibodies against intrinsic factor. Patients anemic from iron deficiency never have anti-IF antibodies and rarely have parietal cell antibodies, unless gastritis also is present. Parietal cell antibodies are rare in patients with gastric ulcers. Pre-adolescent patients with autoimmune pernicious anemia usually lack parietal cell antibodies but nearly always have IF antibodies.[14]

FAMILIAL INCIDENCE

Autoimmune pernicious anemia runs in families. Moreover, seemingly normal first-degree relatives of symptomatic patients are three times as likely to have parietal cell antibodies as is the random population.[4] On testing, many of these relatives prove to have defective gastric acid production. Antibodies to intrinsic factor rarely are found unless hematologic changes also are present.

ASSOCIATION WITH THYROID DISEASE

Immune diseases of thyroid and stomach are closely linked, although the nature of the association is obscure. Of patients with pernicious anemia, as many as 50 percent have detectible thyroid antibodies, sometimes at titers significant for thyrotoxicosis.[25] The converse also holds true. Of patients with Hashimoto's disease, primary hypothyroidism, or thyrotoxicosis, 30 percent have parietal cell antibodies, and as many as 10 percent prove to have impaired IF absorption or outright pernicious anemia. Antibodies to gastric and thyroid antigens sometimes occur as part of an imperfectly understood polyendocrine syndrome of immune etiology. Patients with these organ-specific antibodies do not, however, have an increased likelihood of developing non-organ-specific antibodies such as antinuclear antibodies or rheumatoid factor.

Renal Antibodies

Immune-mediated diseases of the kidney are extremely common and are diagnosed best by direct immunofluorescent study of renal biopsy tissue. Fluorescent-labeled antiserums to IgG, IgM, properdin, and the various components of complement make it possible to differentiate several types of immune complex glomerulonephritis and glomerular damage due to glomerular basement membrane (GBM) antibodies.

Of patients with renal immunofluorescence that suggests anti-GBM glomerulonephritis, 60 to 80 percent can be shown to have circulating antibodies to basement membrane antigens.[34] These were demonstrated originally by the indirect immunofluorescence technique, which is still the most widely used test for anti-GBM in serum. As purified antigens have become available, however, hemagglutination and radioimmunoassay approaches have been adopted. Radioimmunoassay makes it possible to quantitate the level of circulating antibody. It has been known for some time that anti-GBM diminishes and often disappears after the diseased kidneys are removed. Quantitating anti-GBM activity makes it possible to monitor the success of post-nephrectomy therapy and to make rational plans for scheduling subsequent renal transplantation.

Rheumatoid Factors

Several interesting IgG or IgM autoantibodies react specifically with the Fc fraction of human IgG. These are found in the serum of approximately 80 percent of rheumatoid arthritis patients and in other patients as well. First found was an IgM antibody, seemingly diagnostic for rheumatoid arthritis, that agglutinated red cells or other particles coated with IgG; this was called "rheumatoid factor." Since anti-IgG activity occurs in both IgG and IgM immunoglobulins of varying serological and physical behavior, it seems more appropriate to speak of "factors."[18]

AGGLUTINATION TESTS

The commonest tests for rheumatoid factor (RF) are the latex fixation and the sheep cell agglutination tests. Aggregated IgG is adsorbed onto latex particles or the red blood cells of sheep, so that the end point of the antigen-antibody reaction can be agglutination. Because commercially available latex kits vary widely in their reactivity, each laboratory must establish expected activity ranges. Titers above 1:80 usually constitute clear-cut positives; levels between 1:20 and 1:80 may occur not only in patients with rheumatoid arthritis, but also in some with systemic lupus erythematosus, scleroderma, or, less commonly, with immunologically reactive diseases such as tuberculosis, syphilis, infectious mononucleosis, and leprosy.[27]

Serum that has high IgG levels may block the agglutinating activity of IgM anti-IgG, because the endogenous IgG competes with the IgG on the surface of the indicator particles. This sometimes occurs in nonspecific hyperglobulinemia and is also seen when both IgG and IgM rheumatoid factors coexist.

IgG RHEUMATOID FACTOR

Anti-IgG of the IgG class is more difficult to demonstrate than that of the IgM class. All IgG molecules possess the Fc antigen; an IgG antibody against IgG is likely to combine with itself to form immune complexes.[20] In these cases, demonstrating the presence of anti-IgG requires techniques for demonstrating immune complexes. Immunoabsorption is especially useful because the antibody subsequently can be eluted from the complexes and be measured.

CLINICAL SIGNIFICANCE

About 80 percent of patients who fulfill the diagnostic criteria for rheumatoid arthritis have rheumatoid factors in their serum.[20] The 20 percent who are seronegative tend to have less severe illness and less damage to joints and other tissues than those who are seropositive. When seropositivity exists, however, the level of RF correlates poorly with the clinical course; good clinical remissions are often achieved while RF tests remain positive.

In seropositive patients, complexes containing IgG, IgM, and complement often can be found in the tissues and inside phagocytic cells in joint fluid and periarticular tissues. Patients with extra-articular involvement such as subcutaneous nodules, vasculitis, or pulmonary disease are nearly always seropositive, and immune complexes are present in these lesions. Rheumatoid factor, usually IgG, nearly always accompanies Sjögren's syndrome, a form of rheumatoid disease that also involves the eyes and often the salivary glands.[27]

The incidence of RF in normal individuals is fairly low, but it does occur, especially with advancing age. False-positive agglutination tests sometimes occur if complement is inadequately inactivated or if the serum has very high lipid or cryoglobulin levels.

Antinuclear Factors

Antibodies against nuclear constituents develop in many complex immune disorders and occasionally in seemingly normal individuals.

These antibodies react with nuclear material from cells of all types and from many species; a variety of human and nonhuman preparations can be used for diagnostic testing.

The earliest test for antinuclear activity was the LE cell test (see Hematology section); the LE phenomenon results from IgG activity directed against nucleoproteins. The LE cell test is moderately specific but not very sensitive. It is positive in about 50 to 80 percent of patients with systemic lupus erythematosus[21] and in 5 to 8 percent of patients with rheumatoid arthritis.[20] Occasional patients with scleroderma or dermatomyositis have LE cell activity.

FLUORESCENT ANA

The most sensitive screening test for antinuclear activity is the fluorescent antinuclear antibody (ANA) procedure. This is an indirect immunofluorescence test in which patient serum is allowed to react with acetone-fixed substrate cells, and antibody attachment is demonstrated with fluorescent antiglobulin serum. Cells used for testing range from human leukocytes through the red blood cells of chickens (which, unlike human red cells, have nuclei), to mouse kidney or liver. The ANA test is almost always positive in lupus and is positive in many other conditions as well. Serum that gives a positive ANA result can be studied more precisely with other techniques if further quantitation or discrimination is needed.

FLUORESCENCE PATTERNS

Antinuclear antibodies react with different portions of the nucleus. The fluorescence pattern of the ANA test varies according to the particular antibody which is reacting with a given nuclear substrate. The distribution of fluorescence can be peripheral, diffuse, speckled, or nucleolar. If serum contains several different antibodies, the undiluted serum may give several patterns on the same slide. Diluting the sample allows the pattern of the most significant antibody to predominate. Up to 10 percent of normal serums, tested without dilution, give a positive ANA with a finely speckled pattern; only 2 percent remain positive at 1:16 dilution.

The pattern seen in systemic lupus erythematosus is one of peripheral fluorescence; at low dilutions, other patterns also can be seen. In active SLE, the test often remains positive at dilutions of 1:64 or higher.[21] Since 99 percent of SLE patients have positive serum results at dilutions of 1:16, a negative result makes the diagnosis of SLE highly questionable. Peripheral staining also occurs in lupus-like syndromes induced by such drugs as the hydantoin derivatives, procainamide, and apresaline, but titers are low in these conditions, and specific anti-DNA (see below) does not occur.

Sixty percent of patients with rheumatoid arthritis have a positive ANA test[28], usually with a diffuse staining pattern, but titers tend to be low. In scleroderma and in Sjögren's syndrome, a nucleolar pattern is common. Some patients suffer from a condition combining features of both scleroderma and SLE. This "mixed connective tissue" syndrome usually produces a nucleolar or speckled pattern on ANA testing. Some patients with infectious mononucleosis have a shaggy or irregular pattern.

ANTI-DNA

It is difficult to imagine how DNA, an essential part of every nucleus, can be an effective antigen. Except in systemic lupus erythematosus, antibodies to DNA are rare. When they occur, in occasional patients with rheumatoid arthritis, Sjögren's syndrome, or other collagen-vascular diseases, they react only with denatured, single-stranded DNA. Antibodies against the double-stranded native form of DNA occur, for all practical purposes, only in systemic lupus erythematosus.[16]

Levels of anti-DNA activity correlate well with levels of clinical disease, especially of renal damage. Such techniques as agglutination, complement fixation, and counterimmunoelectrophoresis can be used to demonstrate anti-DNA, but the most sensitive and quantitative procedure is radioimmunoassay. In a patient with newly diagnosed SLE, it is useful to determine the baseline level of anti-DNA activity. These levels rise and fall as the disease exacerbates and remits. The success of long-term therapy can be monitored by demonstrating continuing low anti-DNA levels.

OTHER ANTINUCLEAR ANTIBODIES

Antibodies against many specific components of the nucleus, including RNA and various soluble constituents, can be characterized. In research settings, these assist in distinguishing the immunologic features of various collagen-vascular diseases, but they have not yet assumed widespread clinical application.

Other Antibodies

The significance of antibodies against mitochondria and against smooth muscle antigens is discussed in Chapter 12.

REFERENCES

1. Alper, C. A., and Rosen, F. S.: *Complement in laboratory medicine*, in Vyas, G. N., Stites, D. P., and Brecher, G. (eds.): *Laboratory Diagnosis of Immunologic Disorders.* Grune & Stratton, New York, 1975.
2. Bergsagel, D.: *Plasma cell myeloma*, in Williams, W. J., Beutler, E., Erslev, A. J., and Rundles, R. W. (eds.): *Hematology.* ed. 2. McGraw-Hill, New York, 1977.
3. Brouet, J. C., Clauvel, J. P., Danon, F., et al.: *Biological and clinical significance of cryoglobulins: a report of 86 cases.* Am. J. Med. 57:775, 1974.
4. Doniach, D., Roitt, I. M., and Taylor, K. B.: *Autoimmunity in pernicious anemia and thyroiditis: a family study.* Ann. N.Y. Acad. Sci. 124:605, 1965.
5. Dujovne, I., Pollak, V. E., Pirani, C. L., and Dillard, M. G.: *The distribution and character of glomerular deposits in systemic lupus erythematosus.* Kidney Int. 2:33, 1972.
6. Evans, A. S.: *Infectious mononucleosis*, in Williams, W. J., Beutler, E., Erslev, A. J., and Rundles, R. W. (eds.): *Hematology.* ed. 2. McGraw-Hill, New York, 1977.
7. Evans, A. S., Niederman, J. C., Cenabre, L. C., et al.: *Specificity, sensitivity, and persistence of heterophile and EB-virus specific IgM antibodies in clinical and subclinical infectious mononucleosis.* J. Infect. Dis. 132:546, 1975.
8. Frangione, B., and Franklin, E. C.: *Heavy chain diseases: clinical features and molecular significance of the disordered immunoglobulin structure.* Semin. Hematol. 10:53, 1973.
9. Frank, M. M. (moderator): *Pathophysiology of immune hemolytic anemia.* Ann. Intern. Med. 87:210, 1977.
10. Franklin, E. C.: *μ-Chain disease.* Arch. Intern. Med. 135:71, 1975.
11. Garratty, G., Petz, L. D., and Hoops, J. K.: *The correlation of cold agglutinin titrations in saline and albumin with hemolytic anemia.* Br. J. Haematol. 35:587, 1977.
12. Gewurz, H., and Suyehira, L. A.: *Complement*, in Rose, N. R., and Friedman, H. (eds.): *Manual of Clinical Immunology.* American Society for Microbiology, Washington, D.C., 1976.
13. Glenner, G. G., Terry, W. D., and Isersky, C.: *Amyloidosis: its nature and pathogenesis.* Semin. Hematol. 10:65, 1973.
14. Goldberg, L. S., and Fudenberg, H. H.: *The autoimmune aspects of pernicious anemia.* Am. J. Med. 46:489, 1969.
15. Heremans, J. P., and Masson, P. L.: *Specific analysis of immunoglobulins: techniques and clinical value.* Clin. Chem. 19:294, 1973.
16. Inami, Y. H., Nakamura, R. M., and Tan, E. M.: *Microhemagglutination tests for detection of native and single-strand DNA antibodies and circulating DNA antigen.* J. Immunol. Methods 3:287, 1973.
17. Isobe, T., and Osserman, E.: *Patterns of amyloidosis and their association*

with plasma cell dyscrasias, monoclonal immunoglobulins, and Bence Jones proteins. N. Engl. J. Med. 290:473, 1974.

18. Johnson, P. M., Watkins, J., and Holborow, E. J.: Antiglobulin production to altered IgG in rheumatoid arthritis. Lancet 1:611, 1975.

19. Kyle, R. A.: Multiple myeloma: review of 869 cases. Mayo Clin. Proc. 50:29, 1975.

20. Lightfoot, R. W., Jr., and Christian, C. L.: Rheumatoid arthritis, in Miescher, P. A., and Müller-Eberhard, H. J. (eds.): Textbook of Immunopathology. ed. 2. Grune & Stratton, New York, 1976.

21. Nakamura, R. M.: Immunopathology: Clinical Laboratory Concepts and Methods. Little, Brown, Boston, 1974.

22. Oppenheim, J. J., and Schecter, B.: Lymphocyte transformation, in Rose, N. R., and Friedman, H. (eds.): Manual of Clinical Immunology. American Society for Microbiology, Washington, D.C., 1976.

23. Peake, R. L., Willis, D. B., Asimakis, G. K., and Deiss, W. P.: Radioimmunologic assay for antithyroglobulin antibodies. J. Lab. Clin. Med. 86:907, 1974.

24. Pusch, A. L.: Serodiagnostic tests for syphilis and other diseases, in Davidsohn, I., and Henry, J. B. (eds.): Todd-Sanford Clinical Diagnosis By Laboratory Methods. ed. 15. W. B. Saunders, Philadelphia, 1974.

25. Roitt, I. M., and Doniach, D.: Gastric autoimmunity, in Miescher, P. A., and Müller-Eberhard, H. J. (eds.): Textbook of Immunopathology. ed. 2. Grune & Stratton, New York, 1976.

26. Roitt, I. M., Doniach, D., and Shapland, C.: Autoimmunity in pernicious anemia and atrophic gastritis. Ann. N.Y. Acad. Sci. 124:644, 1965.

27. Rose, N. R., and Bigazzi, P. E.: The autoimmune diseases, in Laskin, A. I., and Lechevalier, H. A. (eds.): Handbook of Microbiology. vol. 4. CRC Press, Cleveland, 1974.

28. Rothfield, N. F.: Detection of antibodies to nuclear antigens by immunofluorescence, in Rose, N. R., and Friedman, H. (eds.): Manual of Clinical Immunology. American Society for Microbiology, Washington, D.C., 1976.

29. Solomon, A.: Bence Jones proteins and light chains of immunoglobulins. N. Engl. J. Med. 294:17, 1976.

30. Spitler, L. E.: Delayed hypersensitivity skin testing, in Rose, N. R., and Friedman, H. (eds.): Manual of Clinical Immunology. American Society for Microbiology, Washington, D.C., 1976.

31. Talal, N., and Pillarisetty, R. J.: IgM and IgG antibodies to DNA, RNA, and DNA:RNA in systemic lupus erythematosus. Clin. Immunol. Immunopathol. 4:24, 1976.

32. Theml, H., Love, R., and Begemann, H.: Factors in the pathomechanism of chronic lymphocytic leukemia. Annu. Rev. Med. 28:131, 1977.

33. Weed, R. I.: Membrane structure and its relation to haemolysis. Clin. Haematol. 4:3, 1975.

34. Wilson, C. B., and Dixon, F. J.: Anti-glomerular basement membrane antibody induced glomerulonephritis. Kidney Int. 3:74, 1973.

35. Zlotnick, A., and Rosenmann, E.: Renal pathologic findings associated with monoclonal gammopathies. Arch. Intern. Med. 135:40, 1975.

CHAPTER 8

IMMUNOHEMATOLOGY AND BLOOD BANKING

IMMUNOHEMATOLOGY OF RED CELLS

The red cell membrane contains myriad different proteins and carbohydrates capable of provoking antibody formation and of reacting with those antibodies. More than 300 antigenic configurations have been discovered and classified. For a few, the molecule's biologic role has been inferred;[16,28] for a few others, the chemical composition has been characterized;[13,38,42] but for most, the structure, the function, and the reason for their immunogenicity all remain mysterious.

What does seem straightforward is the genetics. To the best of our knowledge, the genes that determine red cell antigens follow Mendelian laws of inheritance. Most express themselves no matter which other alleles are present, and thus their behavior is described as *codominant*.

ABO System

Discovered in 1900 by the Austrian-born American pathologist Karl Landsteiner, the ABO system is of paramount importance in blood banking. The major antigens are called *A* and *B*; the major antibodies are *anti-A* and *anti-B*. The genes that determine presence or absence of A or B activity reside on chromosome number 9.[3] Normal persons older than 6 months of age almost always have antibodies that react with A or B antigens absent from their own cells.

Antibody presence and specificity are not genetically determined. Instead, antibodies develop after exposure to ubiquitous environmental antigens which share structure and specificity with red cell antigens. Although exposed to both A and B activity in the environment, an individual will not produce antibodies that react with his own red cell antigens.

GENES AND ANTIGENS

The ABO system is not as simple as it first appears. Antigenic activity depends on specific sugar linkages located at the end of a short sugar chain which is attached to a large protein- and sugar-containing molecule called a *glycoprotein*. The backbone of this glycoprotein inserts into the red cell membrane. We do not know the entire glycoprotein composition, but the nature of the short sugar chain has been thoroughly studied. The A antigen results when N-acetylgalactosamine links to a D-galactose moiety. B activity occurs if a D-galactose is present on that terminal D-galactose moiety. The *A* gene determines the presence of the enzyme (transferase) responsible for attaching N-acetylgalactosamine to galactose; the *B* gene produces a galactose transferase.[38]

Before the D-galactose can accept the sugars that determine A or B activity, it must have a fucose sugar already attached. A D-galactose moiety with fucose already attached, but without A-active N-acetylgalactosamine or B-active D-galactose, has antigenic activity described as *H* (Fig. 18). Cells with only the H-active sugar configuration have neither A nor B activity and are called *group O*.

The transferases determined by the A and B genes depend on the presence of precursor H substance for their activity to become apparent. Attachment of fucose to D-galactose provides this precursor. Fucose attachment is mediated by another enzyme, fucose transferase, the presence of which is determined by the *H* gene. The *H* gene is independent of the ABO locus; its chromosomal location is unknown. The *H* gene is extremely common, and nearly everyone has H substance on his red cells. A few people are homozygous for an inactive gene at that site, called *h*. Since persons with two *h* genes cannot generate the enzyme needed to attach fucose, their red cells have no H activity. In the absence of H substance, A- or B-active transferases have nothing to work on; therefore the red cells of these persons lack A or B activity as well. Individuals whose red cells lack A, B, or H activity consistently have strong anti-A, anti-B, and anti-H in their serum.[3] This constitution is called a *Bombay phenotype*, because it was first discovered in that city, and the very rare, inactive *h* gene seems to have its greatest concentration there.

Many alleles exist at the ABO locus. The three commonest are *A*,

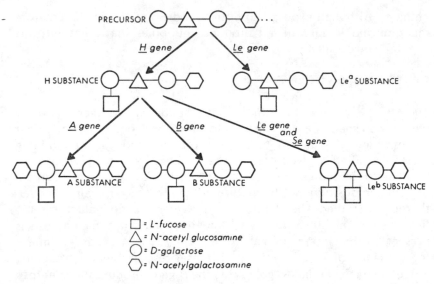

Figure 18. Several sugars, linked together at the end of a much longer glyco-protein chain, determine blood group activity in the interrelated ABO and Lewis systems. Each allelic gene controls a single enzyme, the function of which is to attach a single sugar to the chain. The presence of fucose moieties determines activity of the H, Le^a, and Le^b antigens. A activity arises from N-acetylgalactosamine; B activity exists when D-galactose is present. (Reproduced with permission from the American Association of Blood Banks: *Technical Manual.* ed. 7. A.A.B.B., Washington, D.C., 1977.)

B, and O. A and B produce sugar transferases which alter H reactivity. The O gene has no detectible product; it is called an *amorph*. Persons with two O genes produce no enzymes capable of transforming basic H substance into A or B. Their cells possess only H activity, and their serum contains anti-A and anti-B. A single A or B gene can generate enough enzyme to convert fully the H substance to A or B; the red cells of a person with the genotype A/O do not differ from those whose genotype is A/A. Persons with both A and B genes attach N-acetylgalactosamine to some of their H and D-galactose to the rest of it. These group AB individuals have both A and B activity on their cells, with very little residual H, and their serum contains neither anti-A nor anti-B. Table 9 shows the blood findings and the frequency of the common ABO blood groups.

SUBGROUPS OF A

Two different A genes are common in the general population: A_1 and A_2. The A_2 transferase is less efficient than the A_1 transferase in

Table 9. Antigens and Antibodies in ABO Blood Groups

Blood Group	Antigens on Red Cells	Antibodies in Serum	Frequency (%) in U.S. Population*			
			Whites	Blacks	American Indians	Orientals
A	A	anti-B	40	27	16	28
B	B	anti-A	11	20	4	27
O	neither	anti-A anti-B	45	49	79	40
AB	A and B	neither	4	4	<1	5

*Adapted from data in American Association of Blood Banks: *Technical Manual.* ed. 7. A.A.B.B., Washington, D.C., 1977.

converting H to A. A single A_1 gene produces a transferase that converts nearly all available H to A, but A_2 transferase produces red cells with weaker A activity and more residual H. Persons with genotypes A_2/A_2 or A_2/O have red cells of the A_2 phenotype. Persons with one A_1 gene and one A_2 gene have A_1 red cells. A coexisting *B* gene does not alter A_1 or A_2 activity. About 20 percent of AB persons are A_2B while the majority are A_1B, just as 20 percent of group A persons are A_2.

Still other variant A genes exist, producing progressively less aggressive transferases. These are uncommon or rare, but they occur sufficiently often that a number of weak A subgroups have been identified and classified. Inheritance of these weak variants follows normal Mendelian distribution; the reason for their "deficient" activity is not known. Also unexplained is the fact that variant A transferases exist so often while B variants are so uncommon. Only a few "weak B" genes have been found.[38]

ANTIBODIES

Although anti-A and anti-B react strongly and specifically with the corresponding red cell antigens, the stimulus to anti-A and anti-B production is not exposure to red cells. The same linkages of galactose with N-acetylgalactosamine or with galactose that characterize red cell glycoproteins also exist in bacterial cell walls. Continuous environmental exposure to these widely distributed antigens elicits continuous antibody production in immunocompetent individuals, provided the antigen is not a "self"-constituent of their own red cells. Group A people form only anti-B, and those in group B have only anti-A. Persons of group O have both anti-A and anti-B, while group AB individuals have neither antibody (see Table 9). Infants too young to form antibodies and patients with defective humoral immunity will not have these antibodies.

Environmental bacteria also possess the galactose-fucose linkage that confers H activity. Anti-H, however, occurs very rarely because nearly all red cells possess H antigen in quantities ranging from slight to substantial. A_1 or A_1B persons occasionally develop a weak anti-H, but the only people who form strong anti-H are those with a Bombay phenotype, whose cells are devoid of H activity.

CELL DESTRUCTION

Anti-A and Anti-B are strong agglutinins, easily demonstrated in the laboratory. In the circulation, they cause rapid, complement-mediated destruction of any incompatible cells that chance to enter the blood stream. Except for the few fetal cells that enter the mother's blood stream during pregnancy and delivery, the only way that ABO-incompatible cells get into the circulation is by incorrectly identified transfusions. Incorrect identification of patients, of blood samples, of donor blood, or of clerical notations cause the vast majority of hemolytic transfusion reactions.[3]

Most anti-A and anti-B activity resides in the IgM class of immunoglobulins, which produce immediate agglutination and/or hemolysis. Some activity, however, is IgG, and antibodies of this class attach to the cell surface without immediately affecting their viability. Coating activity due to anti-A or anti-B is difficult to detect in the laboratory, because agglutination occurs first and obscures any other kind of cell-antibody reaction. Anti-A or anti-B of the IgG class readily crosses the placenta and can cause hemolytic disease of the newborn (see p. 259). Group O persons more often have IgG anti-A and anti-B than do A or B individuals. ABO hemolytic disease affects almost exclusively the offspring of group O mothers.

The Rh System

After the ABO system, the Rh system is the group of red cell antigens with greatest clinical importance. Unlike anti-A and anti-B, which reliably occur in normal, unimmunized individuals, Rh antibodies do not develop without an immunizing stimulus. The major antigen of the Rh system, $Rh_o(D)$, is more likely to provoke an antibody than is any other red cell antigen, if cells containing the antigen are introduced into a person who lacks the antigen. $Rh_o(D)$ is present on the red cells of 85 percent of whites and a higher percentage of blacks, American Indians, and Asians. Only 15 percent of whites lack the antigen and are therefore capable of forming the antibody if exposed to $Rh_o(D)$, but 50 to 75 percent of Rh-negative persons exposed to large numbers of Rh-positive cells will form an antibody. No other blood group antigen has comparable immunizing potential.

ANTIGENS

The Rh system includes many different antigens. Persons whose red cells possess $Rh_o(D)$ are called *Rh-positive*; those whose cells lack $Rh_o(D)$ are called *Rh-negative*, no matter what other Rh antigens are present. Besides $Rh_o(D)$, there are four additional Rh antigens of major clinical significance. The genes for the Rh system reside on chromosome number 1.[26] Each allele determines a complex entity, called an *agglutinogen*, which possesses numerous distinct antigenic configurations. Thus each gene controls the presence of several different Rh antigens on the red cell surface. Each allele determines a different combination of two or three major antigens and numerous other antigens of less clinical significance.

Because it so readily provokes an identifying antibody, $Rh_u(D)$ was the first Rh antigen to be discovered. The other four major antigens are rh'(C), rh''(E), hr'(c), and hr''(e); antibodies to these occur less frequently but still fairly often. Many other antigens exist but are either very rare themselves or require rare antibodies to demonstrate their presence.

Two different terminologies are used to identify the Rh antigens, as well as a digital notation best suited for written and computer use. Current formal usage in the United States dictates simultaneous employment of both the Rh-Hr terminology and the CDE terminology, but in common or informal practice, one or the other is usually dropped.

GENES

The Rh genes common in the U.S. population are given in Table 10. It can be seen that all these genes determine the presence of one antigen at the rh'(C)/hr'(c) site and one at the rh''(E)/hr''(e) site. Most also dictate the presence of $Rh_o(D)$, but one common allele does not. The r gene determines a product that lacks $Rh_o(D)$ but possesses hr'(c) and hr''(e). We do not know the specific polypeptides produced by the Rh genes, nor do we know the chemical and spatial composition

Table 10. Rh Genes Common in the U.S. Population

Rh-Hr Terminology	CDE Terminology	Gene Frequency (%)*			
		Whites	Blacks	American Indians	Orientals
R^1	CDe	0.42	0.17	0.44	0.70
r	cde	0.37	0.26	0.11	0.03
R^2	cDE	0.14	0.11	0.34	0.21
R^0	cDe	0.04	0.44	0.02	0.03
r'	Cde	0.02	0.02	0.02	0.02

*Adapted from data in American Association of Blood Banks: *Technical Manual.* A.A.B.B., Washington, D.C., 1977.

that determines antigenic activity. Rh material has a high lipid content and is a more integral part of the red cell membrane than are the ABH antigens.[24]

Since every person has two examples of chromosome 1, everyone has two Rh alleles. These may be either identical or different. If two examples of the same allele are present on the two chromosomes, the red cells will have only one agglutinogen and only one set of antigens. If two different alleles are present, there will be two agglutinogens. Some antigens may be present in both agglutinogens, but some will be part of only one. Of the five common Rh antigens, the minimum number that a normal person could have is two: hr'(c) and hr''(e); this occurs in persons with the r gene on both chromosomes. A single cell tested with the five major antibodies can have a maximum of five different antigens: $Rh_o(D)$, rh'(C), rh''(E), hr'(c), and hr''(e). This occurs with the genotype $R^1R^2(CDe/cDE)$.

Rh-positive cells always have $Rh_o(D)$ as part of at least one agglutinogen. In routine testing, it is not feasible to distinguish cells with a single dose of $Rh_o(D)$ from cells with two agglutinogens that contain $Rh_o(D)$. This distinction sometimes can be inferred from the presence of other antigenic factors that commonly accompany $Rh_o(D)$. Rh-negative cells, which lack $Rh_o(D)$, may have hr'(c) or rh'(C) or both, as well as hr''(e) or rh''(E) or both. Most Rh-negative persons have two examples of the allele r, which determines hr'(c) and hr''(e), but some Rh-negative persons have less common alleles.

ANTIBODIES

Not every Rh-negative person exposed to Rh-positive cells develops anti-$Rh_o(D)$. Transfusion immunizes more consistently than pregnancy, largely because more cells are involved. About 20 percent of Rh-negative mothers develop anti-Rh_o(D) after carrying an Rh-positive infant,[4,45] whereas antibody develops in between 50 and 70 percent of Rh-negatives transfused with Rh-positive blood.[23,38] For this reason, every reasonable effort is made to avoid giving Rh-positive blood to Rh-negative recipients. Antibodies to the other four major antigens occur only sporadically. In routine transfusion practice, no effort is made to match these antigens in donor and recipient. A few people have anti-rh''(E) spontaneously (i.e., without having been exposed to blood, blood products, or pregnancy). Other Rh antibodies almost never develop spontaneously.

When Rh antibodies develop, they are predominantly IgG. Some IgM appears early, but it tends to disappear months or years after the immunizing event, whereas IgG can persist for a lifetime. Rh antibodies seldom activate complement. Their usual biologic effect is to coat the circulating cells and set them up for destruction in the reticuloendothelial system. When antibody attaches to cell-surface antigens, systemic symptoms may occur, such as hypotension, rising temperature, vomiting, or loss of consciousness. The hematologic result is hemolysis, predominantly in spleen or liver, of the antibody-coated cells. Destruction may be complete within a minute or two or proceed slowly over hours or days.[31] In the test tube, Rh antibodies can cause a modest degree of agglutination, but surface coating predominates.

Rh antibodies readily cross the placenta from mother to fetus. Historically, anti-Rh_o(D) has been the commonest cause of severe hemolytic disease of the newborn. Immunosuppressive therapy successfully prevents antibody formation when given to an unimmunized Rh-negative woman just after the birth of an Rh-positive child. Women with anti-Rh_o(D) existing at the time pregnancy begins are very likely to have an affected infant. Other Rh antibodies cause hemolytic disease much less frequently, and pharmacologic means for prevention are not available.

IMMUNOSUPPRESSION

Anti-Rh_o(D) formation is prevented by giving an appropriate dose of preformed anti-Rh_o(D) at the time that Rh positive cells enter the circulation. The administered antibody interferes with the interaction between cell-surface antigen and the recipient's immune system. The cells are not destroyed, but they lose their ability to trigger antibody production. Both the timing and the dosage must be correct. For

15 ml. or less of Rh-positive cells, 20 μg. of Rh immune globulin (RhIG) will prevent immunization. If there are more than 15 ml. of Rh-positive cells, proportionately more RhIG can be given.[3] RhIG can be given effectively at any time during the first 72 hours after Rh-positive cells are introduced. Insufficient data exist to indicate whether this interval can be prolonged safely.

The customary obstetrical dose of RhIG is 20 μg, given in the first 72 hours after delivery or abortion. If more than 15 ml. of fetal cells have entered the circulation, more RhIG can be given. If trauma or fetal-maternal hemorrhage is observed during the pregnancy, RhIG may be given before delivery, but it should be given after delivery as well.

RhIG also is immunosuppressive when given after Rh-positive transfusion to an Rh-negative recipient, but very large doses are needed. Dosage is calculated on the same ratio of 20 μg. of RhIG for every 15 ml. of red cells. The anti-Rh$_o$(D) coats circulating Rh-positive cells and causes somewhat accelerated splenic destruction, but the patient does not experience the cataclysmic effects of a hemolytic transfusion reaction.

Other Blood Groups

Innumerable antigens occupy the red cell surface and are capable of eliciting a variety of possible antibodies. Relatively few, however, have major clinical significance.

"NATURALLY OCCURRING" VS. "IMMUNE" ANTIBODIES

Anti-A and anti-B are the only blood group antibodies regularly found in the serum of unimmunized individuals, but occasional persons with no history of transfusion or pregnancy have antibodies of other specificities. Except in autoimmune disease (see p. 111), these antibodies are directed against antigens absent from the individual's own red cells. We do not know why any one person forms antibody against any particular antigen in the absence of an apparent immunizing event.

Antibodies that occur without a known immunizing event are sometimes called "naturally occurring." They are usually IgM of fairly low titer and react best with saline-suspended cells at temperatures of 30°C. or below. Occasional examples are active at 37°C. and can be dangerous in the clinical setting, but most are predominantly laboratory problems. Being IgM, these antibodies cannot cross the placenta and do not cause hemolytic disease of the newborn.

In contrast to these fairly weak, "spontaneous" antibodies, antibodies that follow transfusion or pregnancy are often high-titered and react best at body temperature. IgM contributes part of their activity, but most are IgG. These "immune" antibodies can cause transfusion reactions and are responsible for hemolytic disease of the newborn. The antiglobulin test (see section below) is the best laboratory technique for their detection and identification.

SPECIFIC BLOOD GROUPS

A blood group system is a series of antigens controlled by allelic genes inherited independently of other genes. Besides the Rh system, the Kell and Duffy systems are most often implicated in immune antibody formation. Anti-Kell (anti-K) and anti-Duffy[a] (written anti-Fy[a]) are, after anti-Rh$_o$(D), the commonest immune antibodies. Other not-uncommon antibodies that develop after transfusion or pregnancy involve Kidd (Jk), Lutheran (Lu), and s antigens. Kidd antibodies (mostly anti-Jk[a]) are especially difficult to identify because they nearly always accompany other antibodies, the activity of which may mask their own. Kidd antibodies are more labile than most, and their activity can drop so low that standard laboratory techniques fail to detect their presence. Transfusion of seemingly compatible Jk[a]-positive blood then triggers a rapid anamnestic response that produces a delayed hemolytic reaction.

Blood groups for which "naturally occurring" antibodies most often develop include the Lewis, MNS, P, and I systems. Lewis antigens are intimately associated with H substance.[13] Lewis antibodies occur sporadically, sometimes appearing and disappearing in a single individual at different times. Their behavior in vitro is unpredictable, and their significance in vivo is controversial. Lewis antibodies are quite common, but transfusion reactions involving the Lewis system are uncommon. Severe problems occur often enough, however, that their presence cannot safely be ignored.

Antibodies against M, P$_1$, and I occur with some frequency but are nearly always cold-reacting and of dubious clinical significance. Anti-I is especially common. It is a cold agglutinin capable of reacting with the patient's own I antigens, but clinically significant red cell damage rarely occurs[15] except with the extraordinarily high titers associated with cold agglutinin disease (see p. 111).

ANTIGLOBULIN SERUM AND ITS USES

Immunoglobulins, the antibody molecules themselves, are antigenic if introduced into a nonhuman host. In 1945, Coombs, Mourant, and Race injected whole human serum into rabbits; the resulting anti-human-serum antibody proved remarkably useful as a laboratory reagent.[8] The term "Coombs serum" is still applied to animal antibodies that react with human globulins. Almost any protein or polypeptide fragment can be used to prepare immunoreactive reagents (see p. 192). Antibodies against the immunoglobulin molecule or various chains or fragments are widely used in immunology. In blood banking, the significant specificities are against IgG and, to a lesser degree, complement (especially C3 and C4).

Principles of Antiglobulin Testing

Agglutination is the easiest immunologic end point to see and to utilize. IgG antibodies often attach to red cell antigens without causing agglutination. Complement-activating antibodies sometimes attach complement components to the cell surface and then depart from the antigenic site without causing agglutination. It is difficult to perceive IgG molecules or complement fragments attached to non-agglutinated cells. If globulin-coated cells are allowed to react with antibody specific for human globulin, however, agglutination occurs. The antiglobulin serum reacts with the attached globulin molecules, not with the red cell membrane or any blood group antigens. Because the globulins are attached to large, easily visible red cells, the interaction of antiglobulin antibody with its globulin antigen causes a highly visible reaction—agglutination of the previously dispersed red blood cells. This provides an obvious indication that antigen-antibody reaction has occurred (see Fig. 10).

Antiglobulin serum also reacts with globulin molecules not attached to surfaces. In fact, reaction with unbound globulin occurs preferentially. If free globulin molecules exist in the same test tube with globulin-coated red cells, antiglobulin serum combines first with the unbound globulins and may not agglutinate the coated red cells at all. In antiglobulin testing, it is essential to remove all traces of unbound antibody before adding antiglobulin reagent.

Antiglobulin serum has many applications in bloodbanking. The direct antiglobulin test answers the question: Does this patient have circulating red cells coated with antibody and/or complement? The antiglobulin antibody screening test answers the question: Does this serum contain IgG antibodies which will coat but not agglutinate red cells of appropriate antigenic composition? Antiglobulin serum used in *red cell typing* answers the question: Do these red cells possess an antigen that reacts with an IgG antibody of known specificity? In *crossmatching*, antiglobulin serum is invaluable in determining whether the particular cells and serum possess matching antigens and antibodies that react with one another without causing immediately visible effects.

The Direct Antiglobulin Test

The direct antiglobulin test detects whether globulin-coated red cells are circulating in the patient's blood stream. It is called "direct" because red cells taken directly from the patient are tested without any intervening manipulation. Before testing, it is important to wash the red cells free of unbound plasma proteins which might preferentially react with the antiglobulin serum. The antiglobulin serum used for screening purposes and in routine blood-bank work is sometimes described as "broad spectrum" because it detects either IgG or complement on the red cell surface. Anti-IgG activity is nearly always stronger and more reliable. Cells found to have a positive antiglobulin test can be tested further, if necessary, with specific anti-IgG and antibodies against different complement components.

CAUSES OF POSITIVE TESTS

The usual cause of a positive direct antiglobulin test is *autoimmune hemolytic anemia* (see p. 111). The patient's antibody reacts with antigens on his own cells, and the circulating cells, coated with protein, undergo accelerated destruction in the reticuloendothelial system. Autoantibody may be IgG or IgM. If it is IgG, the antibody itself coats the cell surface, and anti-IgG serum detects its presence. IgM autoantibodies are less straightforward. The reaction between antigen and antibody causes complement to adhere to the cell surface, but once this has occurred, the IgM antibody does not remain in contact with the membrane.[21] The red cells circulate with the complement fragments attached, but without antibody. These cells will be agglutinated by anticomplement but not by anti-IgG. Autoimmune conditions involve IgG more often than complement, but the direct antiglobulin test should recognize both.[33]

Besides autoimmune disease, other events can produce a positive direct antiglobulin test. In hemolytic disease of the newborn, maternal

IgG crosses the placenta and coats fetal red cells. In transfusion situations, a patient whose serum contains a specific IgG antibody will, if transfused with red cells containing that antigen, develop a positive antiglobulin test that involves only the transfused cells. The crossmatch is supposed to detect the incompatibility and prevent transfusion of such cells, but sometimes the ideal is not achieved. When anti-Rh$_o$(D) immune globulin is given to an Rh-negative patient who has received Rh-positive cells, the Rh-positive cells become coated, while the patient's own cells are unaffected. Inadvertent administration of RhIG to an Rh-positive subject renders all the patient's cells antiglobulin-positive but causes surprisingly little clinical effect. Similarly, transfusing antibody-containing plasma into a patient positive for that antigen induces a positive antiglobulin test but does not harm the recipient noticeably.

The Antibody Screening Test

It is important to know whether transfusion recipients possess unexpected antibodies that might react with transfused cells and whether donor blood has antibodies that might affect the recipient's cells. *Any* antibody other than anti-A or anti-B is considered an unexpected antibody. Screening for unexpected antibodies is vital in transfusion practice and is useful in population testing, genetic studies, and other investigations. The antibody screening test is sometimes called the "indirect Coombs test," an imprecise and misleading term that is better avoided.

In antibody screening, the specificity of the hypothetical antibodies and their immunoglobulin class are unknown. It is necessary, therefore, to subject the serum to conditions optimal for detecting antibodies of various sorts. Group O red cells are used for screening, since anti-A and anti-B do not affect them. Red cells used to screen serums must possess numerous, clearly identified antigens to allow scope for the widest possible range of antibody activity. No one or two screening cells can include every possible antigen to detect every possible antibody. Reagent cells are selected to possess antigens reactive with 95 to 99 percent of clinically encountered antibodies. Very rare antibodies are likely to escape detection.

MULTIPLE TECHNIQUES

The antibody screening test employs different temperatures and suspending mediums to enhance the activity of different antibody classes. For IgM antibodies, saline-suspended cells are incubated with serum at temperatures well below 37°C., usually room temperature. Incubation at 37°C. is necessary for IgG antibodies; many workers add a macromolecular medium such as albumin or a synthetic polysaccharide to enhance agglutination.

Incubation allows antibody to coat the cells or to activate complement; following incubation, antiglobulin serum is added. If antiglobulin serum induces agglutination, it indicates that the serum under test has an antibody that reacts with some antigen on the red cells used. Absence of agglutination means that the serum contains no antibody against the antigens represented. The screening test will be negative if the serum contains an antibody directed against an antigen not present on the reagent red cells.

The screening procedure can be made more sensitive by treating the reagent red cells with various proteolytic enzymes. Enzymes which remove chemically and electrically active surface groups allow antigen-antibody reactions to occur in a different physicochemical environment. This technique enhances the effects of weakly reactive Rh antibodies as well as antibodies in the Lewis and I systems. However, it diminishes activity against M, N, and Duffy antigens.

ANTIBODY IDENTIFICATION

The antibody screening test reveals only that antibody is present. It does not identify the specificity. Antibody specificity is deduced by observing which cells react with the antibody and which fail to do so. Specific antibodies produce a recognizable pattern that depends on the antigenic characteristics of the reagent cells used. For example, a serum that reacts with every Rh-positive cell but not with Rh-negative cells probably contains anti-Rh₀(D). A serum that reacts with all Kell-positive cells but not with Kell-negative cells probably contains anti-Kell. Each reagent cell is typed for many different antigens; testing a serum against a panel of eight or ten fully characterized cells allows identification of most single or combination antibodies. Usually only one antibody is present, but serums fairly often contain a mixture of antibodies. With rare or multiple antibodies, more complicated procedures may be necessary.

The "naturally occurring" antibodies that occur without apparent immunizing event usually react with only one antigen, but a patient who develops antibodies after transfusion or pregnancy may have a serum that reacts with several different antigens. Antiglobulin testing is extremely important in characterizing immune antibodies, because many weak IgG antibodies fail to agglutinate reagent cells and can only be detected by careful attention to their presence coating the cell surface.

Antiglobulin Serum in Crossmatching

The pretransfusion crossmatch attempts to detect potential antigen-antibody reactions before the cells are infused. Transfusion of antibody-containing plasma rarely causes problems, but it is good practice to screen donor units and remove the antibody-containing plasma, leaving only the red cells to be transfused.[2] If the recipient of a transfusion has an antibody, a severe or fatal reaction can occur if the transfused cells possess the relevant antigen. Good blood-banking practice demands that each unit of donor blood be examined individually for compatibility with the recipient's serum, even if the recipient's serum has a negative antibody screening test.

The crossmatch subjects the donor's cells to the recipient's serum under laboratory conditions optimal for antibody activity. The techniques are the same as in the antibody screening test. Again, it is the antiglobulin phase of the test that most sensitively detects red cell antigen-antibody reactions. A negative crossmatch, including room temperature and antiglobulin techniques, does not guarantee a favorable outcome, but it is the best preventive measure presently available against dangerous antigen-antibody reactions involving red blood cells.

TRANSFUSION THERAPY

Circulating blood contains many cellular and noncellular components, each with important physiologic functions. Transfusions should be administered to correct deficiencies of the element(s) needed by the patient.

Red Cell Products

Red cells contain hemoglobin, which transports the oxygen that is necessary to maintain life. In the past, the only indication for transfusion was to replace or restore oxygen-carrying capacity. The bulk of transfusions are still given for this purpose.

WHOLE BLOOD

Circulating blood consists of plasma, red cells, white cells, and platelets. When blood is drawn from the donor, an anticoagulant-preservative solution is added. The resulting product consists of about 450 ml. of blood diluted with 67 ml. of anticoagulant-preservative. Since neither white cells nor platelets survive very long at refrigerator temperatures, stored whole blood consists, functionally, of red cells and plasma. Albumin and most globulins survive throughout storage, but the labile coagulation factors deteriorate unpredictably.

At present, refrigerated whole blood has a shelf life of 21 days.[2] Administering whole blood augments the recipient's total blood volume and oxygen-carrying capacity and is most useful for treating large-scale blood loss. Patients with adequate blood volume but deficient in hemoglobin derive little benefit from plasma of transfused whole blood, and patients whose cardiac function is precarious may suffer congestive heart failure if given whole blood.

RED BLOOD CELLS

Red cells can be separated from the rest of the blood by centrifugation. The resulting red blood cell preparation has all the oxygen-carrying capacity of the original unit without very much plasma to dilute its therapeutic effect.[11] This is especially important for patients with chronic anemia or with problems in regulating blood volume. Red blood cells are more effective than whole blood in raising the recipient's hematocrit. Like whole blood, refrigerated red blood cells have a federally approved shelf life of 21 days. The amount of plasma and white blood cells that remains in refrigerator-stored red cells is not enough to perform physiologically useful functions but is sufficient to induce immunization or precipitate immune reactions in sensitized recipients.

DEGLYCEROLIZED FROZEN RED CELLS

Red cells cannot simply be shoved in a freezer for storage. There must be some cryoprotective agent to prevent damage to the cell membrane. Glycerol is the agent most often used. As red cells are exposed to the glycerol solution, all traces of plasma and nearly all the platelets and white cells are removed. Some workers believe that processing also reduces the infective potential of hepatitis and other viruses from units which originally contained virus.[5] Red cells can be kept in the frozen state for years; upon reconstitution, at least 70 percent of the original cells survive normally, if promptly transfused.

Patients severely immunized to plasma proteins or white blood cells usually tolerate transfusion of deglycerolized thawed red cells without ill effect.[27] Frozen red cells contain very few white cells that could immunize the recipient; it is not clear whether this is an advantage or a disadvantage in patients who will subsequently receive a transplanted kidney.[34] Frozen storage is useful for inventory management, because the red cells have such a long shelf life. It also facilitates stockpiling bloods of rare types needed for patients with difficult antibody problems. Many centers encourage patients wth complex antibody mixtures or antibodies against high-incidence antigens to store their own blood for possible future use.

The cost of processing and storing frozen red cells is very high. Enthusiasm for more general use of this product is tempered, in many settings, by the price tag of $20 to $40 above regular trans-fusion costs. An additional problem is that deglycerolized cells must be used within 24 hours after thawing; this limits the flexibility with which these cells can be handled.

AUTOLOGOUS TRANSFUSION

The safest transfusion product is the patient's own blood. Before an elective operation, many individuals can donate several units of blood for their own later use, under the medical supervision of their own physician and the medical director of the blood bank. With appropriate iron supplementation and clinical surveillance, it is possible to draw two or more units of blood in the 3 weeks before the operation. If frozen storage is available, the time between phlebotomy and autologous transfusion can be extended indefinitely.

Platelet Concentrates

Two kinds of platelet preparations are currently available: a single-unit concentrate, which contains approximately 75 percent of the original platelets suspended in a small amount of plasma, and plateletpheresis concentrates, which contain platelets from the equivalent of six units of blood, all from a single donor. Pheresis procedures make it possible to process large volumes of blood from a single donor, because the red cells and other elements are immediately returned to the donor. Large quantities of plasma, platelets, or white cells can be harvested by means of this technique. Except for small children, adequate platelet therapy always requires infusion of multiple units. With plateletpheresis, all the platelets can come from a single donor, thereby reducing the risks of hepatitis exposure and possible immunization.

PREPARATION AND STORAGE

Platelets have a shorter life span then red cells, surviving only 8 to 10 days in vivo as against 120 days for red cells. Survival in vitro also is much shorter; intense efforts to find preservative solutions or frozen storage techniques have not yet been successful. Platelets have a shelf life of 72 hours, but their postinfusion survival and effectiveness decline severely during storage. Platelet concentrates can be stored either at room temperature or refrigerator temperature. Since different techniques for preparation and maintenance are needed for each temperature, conditions cannot be switched in mid-storage.

Platelets should not be exposed to cold temperatures before separation from whole blood. No matter which storage temperature is planned, separation is carried out at room temperature. At refrigerator temperatures, less plasma is needed to maintain adequate pH levels than when platelets continue to metabolize at room temperature. Minimum plasma volume is 20 ml. for cold concentrates and 50 ml. for the room temperature product.[2] Platelets stored at room temperature must be kept in continuous, gentle agitation to prevent accumulation of metabolites that affect pH and viability. Platelets at refrigerator temperature need not be agitated throughout storage, but they require 30 minutes of equilibration at room temperature and gentle but thorough mixing before they can be infused.

THERAPEUTIC EFFECT

An average single-unit platelet concentrate contains 0.6×10^{11} platelets. Although specific figures vary widely, this is a realistic mean figure when careful techniques of donor selection, phlebotomy, preparation, storage, and shipping have been employed. With optimum technique and in a hematologically stable patient, transfusion of 1.0×10^{11} platelets elevates the platelet count approximately $12,000/mm.^3$ per square meter of body surface.[32]

Active bleeding induces platelets to accumulate at the bleeding site. While performing their hemostatic role, platelets cannot be retrieved or measured as circulating elements. When platelets are given to a bleeding patient, the therapeutic effect is measured by improved hemostasis, not by improved laboratory values. If consumption coagulopathy (see p. 168) has caused the bleeding and low platelet count, transfused platelets suffer the same entrapment and destruction as the patient's own platelets; platelet transfusions cause only slight clinical improvement, if any, in such cases. Patients with large spleens or with autoimmune platelet destruction derive little benefit from transfused platelets. Infection or high fever from any cause also reduces survival of transfused platelets.

PLATELET ANTIBODIES

Tranfused platelets can be destroyed rapidly by isoantibodies in the recipient's plasma. Platelets lack red cell antigens other than A, B, and H, but they share HLA antigens with white cells and other body tissues (see p. 265) and have unique platelet antigens as well. Anti-A and anti-B cause much less damage to incompatible platelets than to incompatible red cells. It is desirable, but not essential, that platelets and patient's plasma be ABO-compatible. HLA antibodies, elicited by past transfusions, damage platelets far more than do ABO antibodies. Isoimmune antibodies to HLA antigens (or, much more rarely, to specific platelet antigens) rapidly destroy transfused incompatible platelets. For the immunized patient who requires platelet transfusions, HLA-typed platelets become a necessity.[3] Difficulties in antibody identification, the expense of HLA typing, and the tremendous range of HLA phenotypes among donors and recipients make it unlikely that routine "type and crossmatch" will precede uncomplicated platelet transfusions in the near future.

Plasma Products

Plasma stored at $-20°C$. or below retains full coagulation potency for at least a year, and the nonlabile proteins remain fully active after 5 years or more at $-20°C$.[2] Freshly drawn plasma contains coagulation proteins, albumin, antibodies of all sorts, and all the other proteins, hormones, and chemical constituents that normally circulate. With commercial processing techniques, immunoglobulins and albumin can be purified and concentrated from large plasma pools. Several coagulation concentrates also are made from large, multidonor pools. Individual blood collection facilities routinely make single-donor products that include freshly frozen whole plasma, cryoprecipitated Factor VIII, and whole plasma which lacks the labile coagulation factors.

FACTOR VIII PRODUCTS

The "unit" for measuring Factor VIII activity is the amount of pro-coagulant activity present in 1 ml. of fresh, normal (pooled) plasma. Plasma from a single donation of whole blood contains approximately 200 units of Factor VIII in a volume of approximately 200 ml. Severe hemophiliacs have less than 1 percent of normal Factor VIII activity; for acceptable hemostasis, 30 percent of normal activity is needed. With large-scale bleeding or complicated problems of trauma, sepsis, or tissue necrosis, much higher levels are preferable. Whole plasma infusions can never raise a patient's Factor VIII concentration very much because they expand blood volume so greatly. The Factor VIII in whole plasma can be concentrated to moderate levels by *cryoprecipitation,* which concentrates 60 to 100 units of Factor VIII into 10 to 15 ml. of plasma. Transfusion of cryoprecipitated Factor VIII raises the recipient's Factor VIII concentration to moderate levels with rather modest volume expansion. Cryoprecipitation also concentrates fibrinogen, though to a lesser degree.

In cryoprecipitation, plasma whose Factor VIII activity has been preserved by quick freezing is slowly thawed at 4°C. After 16 to 20 hours at refrigerator temperature, a gel develops which contains Factor VIII and some fibrinogen. Supernatant plasma is removed, and the cryoprecipitated material is again frozen, for storage. The supernatant plasma can be used as single-donor plasma for patients who have no need of coagulation factors or can be pooled for extraction of albumin, globulins, and other products.

It is difficult to predict how much Factor VIII will be found in any one cryoprecipitate. Even at the best available concentration, it is difficult to achieve massive therapeutic doses by giving cryoprecipitate alone.[22] Cryoprecipitate is most often used for small-scale bleeding problems to prevent their escalating into crippling or life-threatening crises. Because the half-life of transfused Factor VIII is only 12 hours, frequent infusions must be given.

When the Factor VIII level must be increased massively and reliably, it is necessary to use potent concentrates prepared from large pools of normal plasma. These are especially useful in hemophiliacs undergoing an operation or bleeding severely, or in those with antibodies that inhibit Factor VIII activity. Prepared concentrates are assayed for precision in calculating dosage, and huge quantities can be infused if necessary. Both hepatitis risk and expense tend to be fairly high.

FACTOR IX

Factor IX deficiency (Christmas disease) is less common than classical hemophilia, but it is probable that there are between 5,000 and 10,000 males in the U.S. who need Factor IX replacement. Factor IX does not deteriorate in stored plasma; thus bank blood or frozen plasma of any age provides one unit per milliliter of Factor IX activity. This unconcentrated product often suffices to treat mild bleeding in the patient with hemophilia B. No simple means for concentrating Factor IX has been achieved; if a high-potency product is needed, commercially prepared concentrates are the only choice. These concentrates include all the "liver factors" (see p. 166); unfortunately, they include all too often the hepatitis virus as well.[12] The risk of hepatitis transmission is considerably higher for Factor IX concentrate than for Factor VIII.

FIBRINOGEN

Commercial concentrates of fibrinogen carry an unacceptably high risk of hepatitis transmission. Most patients deficient in fibrinogen levels have complex acquired bleeding disorders and require other plasma factors as well. Large doses of fresh frozen whole plasma are both safer and more effective than pooled fibrinogen. If additional fibrinogen is needed, cryoprecipitate can be added to the therapeutic regimen.

FRESH-FROZEN PLASMA

When plasma is frozen within a few hours of phlebotomy, sufficient quantities of coagulation proteins exist to prevent coagulation defects from developing in the much-transfused patient and also to restore most deficits in their early stages. Fresh-frozen plasma is widely used during massive transfusion episodes to prevent exhaustion of coagulation proteins. Stored bank blood may have unpredictably low levels of several factors, and rapid administration of 10 or more units of bank blood may cause coagulation difficulties. Frozen plasma does not, of course, provide platelets.

   The role of fresh-frozen plasma in treating patients with chronic liver disease and other hypoalbuminemic conditions is uncertain. Some centers use this plasma product as a colloid-containing volume expander. It is usually less costly than commercially prepared albumin or plasma-protein solutions, but it carries a higher risk of adverse allergic reactions and of transmitting hepatitis.

The supernatant plasma left after cryoprecipitate is extracted is an excellent transfusion product for many conditions but not, of course, for treating Factor VIII deficiency. It has about 20 percent of the original Factor VIII activity and half the original fibrinogen, along with all the other constituents at normal concentration. When it is available, the cost is much less than that of whole plasma or prepared plasma proteins.

Pretransfusion Testing

DONOR BLOOD

Blood drawn from the donor's vein must be processed for safe transfusion. Regardless of subsequent fractionation, the blood must be found to be free of hepatitis B antigen. Blood found positive for HB_sAg is never transfused. Blood found to have an unexpected red cell antibody is separated into plasma and red cells. The red cells can be used for transfusion, but the plasma is either pooled for large-scale fractionation procedures or saved for reagent purposes.

RECIPIENT BLOOD

Before a patient receives blood, his ABO group and Rh type must be known, and he must be tested for unexpected red cell antibodies. Every blood sample received from each patient undergoes these tests,[2] and the results are compared against previously recorded results. A person's ABO and Rh types do not change, but there is always the danger of incorrectly identified blood samples; comparing present with previous results on the "same" patient has detected many instances of mistaken identity and prevented many transfusion disasters. Antibody screening tests often do change, going from negative to positive in the days, weeks, or months that follow transfusion; it is important to document that immunization has occurred.

It is not essential to test patient's blood samples for HB_sAg, for STS, or for the presence of antibodies on the red cell surface (direct antiglobulin test). Some transfusion services perform some or all of these tests routinely, but many do not.

COMPATIBILITY TESTING FOR RED CELLS

Before blood is transfused into a patient, samples from donor and recipient should be tested for serologic compatibility. The likelihood of incompatibility is much reduced if both patient and donor have negative antibody screening tests, but no screening procedure can ensure against specific rare antigen-antibody interactions. For patients with known antibodies, pretransfusion compatibility testing is crucial.

The *crossmatch* is the final search for incompatibility between a patient's blood and a donor's red cells. Before antibody screening was done routinely on donor blood, a "minor" crossmatch also was performed. The minor crossmatch tests the donor serum against the patient's red cells. It is called minor because the rapid dilution that plasma undergoes on entering the patient's blood stream ensures that problems caused by transfused antibody will be minor at worst. Now that all donor bloods are screened for unexpected antibodies, the minor crossmatch has become an obsolete procedure.

In the "major" crossmatch, a donor's red cells and a patient's serum are combined under conditions designed to elicit both IgG and IgM antibody activity. The cells and serum must be incubated long enough to allow minimally avid antibodies time to react; it is also necessary to add antiglobulin serum after incubation to detect antibodies that coat red cells without agglutinating them. These tests are time-consuming but important. Under emergency conditions, when delaying transfusion jeopardizes the patient's life, incompletely crossmatched blood may be administered, but the crossmatch should be carried to completion.

SELECTION OF BLOOD PRODUCTS

Transfused red cells must lack antigens to which the recipient has antibodies. If anti-A is present, A or AB cells cannot be given; the same applies to B or AB cells in a patient with anti-B. Although antibodies in donor plasma are far less important, occasional units of group O blood contain potent anti-A or anti-B that can damage A, B, or AB cells upon transfusion. The concept of group O as a "universal donor" applies to red cells, not to whole blood. It is good practice to give group-specific blood at all times. When this is impractical, group A or group B recipients can receive O red cells, and AB recipients can receive red cells of any type. An O recipient can receive only group O blood.

Since Rh antibodies are not naturally occurring, no immediate harm results from giving Rh-positive blood to an Rh-negative patient. Subsequently, however, 60 to 75 percent of Rh-negative recipients will develop anti-Rh_0(D),[38] and the practice is considered generally undesirable. It is important to avoid giving Rh-positive blood to Rh-negative girls or women capable of childbearing because hemolytic disease of the newborn is almost certain to occur in any Rh-positive child they might bear.[23]

More flexibility is possible in selecting plasma products and platelet concentrates than in red cell selection. Ideally, all such products should be group-specific; in practice, transfused anti-A and anti-B rarely cause problems except in very small children and rare cases of intensively treated hemophiliacs. Group O plasma is more likely to be dangerous than other groups and should be the last choice for transfusing recipients of blood groups other than O.

The situation with platelet concentrates is awkward. Concentrates stored at room temperature contain at least 50 ml. of plasma, which possesses antibodies that have the potential for injuring the recipient's cells. In addition, platelets have ABH antigenic activity which can react with the recipient's antibody. Group-specific platelets are definitely the product of choice, but nongroup-specific platelets are preferable to none at all.

ADVERSE EFFECTS OF TRANSFUSION

Hemolytic reactions—destruction of donor cells by a patient's antibodies—are the most serious, but fortunately among the rarest of transfusion reactions. Much commoner are uncomfortable, transient problems arising from non-red cell sensitivities that are hard to define. Hepatitis transmission is probably the most frequent of the truly serious adverse effects of transfusion.

Hemolytic Reactions

When anti-A and anti-B destroy incompatible red cells, hemolysis occurs immediately, usually in the circulation itself. Most other antibodies attach to the surface of transfused incompatible cells, coating them and setting them up for extravascular destruction in the reticuloendothelial system. Pretransfusion crossmatching reduces the danger of subsequent hemolysis to the humanly possible minimum. *Most hemolytic transfusion reactions occur because persons or blood samples have been misidentified.* No serologic subtleties are involved when group A blood is given to a group O patient; it is sheer careless-ness. Occasionally, crossmatching fails to demonstrate some very weak or atypical antibody that later causes hemolysis, but hemolytic reactions on this basis are very rare.

CLINICAL EVENTS

Hemolytic transfusion reactions often begin with rising temperature, falling blood pressure, and complaints of palpitations, anxiety, sub-sternal pressure, or flank pain. These events are the result of large-scale, widespread interaction between antibody and antigen. Hypo-tension is almost universal, and sometimes disseminated intravascular coagulation and a generalized bleeding tendency will develop. As red cells are destroyed, hemoglobin is released into the plasma. Although a large protein, hemoglobin readily crosses the glomerular filter, and hemoglobinuria commonly follows hemolysis. Hemo-globinuria by itself, however, does not damage the kidneys. When it occurs, renal failure results from the combined effects of sudden hypotension, massive antigen-antibody reaction, and the presence of hemoglobin in the glomerular filtrate. Damage is especially likely if flow rates are low and the tubular urine is highly concentrated.

To prevent post-hemolysis renal failure, blood pressure should be maintained and brisk diuresis established for the next several hours. Some workers employ mannitol to induce diuresis; others prefer to use furosemide.

IgG-coated cells are destroyed in the reticuloendothelial system, not in the circulation. Plasma hemoglobin levels rise only if cell de-struction is so massive that it overloads the capacity of the reticulo-endothelial system for hemoglobin disposal. If extravascular de-struction occurs gradually, the only sign that there has been a trans-fusion reaction may be a drop in hematocrit or failure to achieve a rise in hematocrit.

LABORATORY EXAMINATION

At the first suspicion of a reaction, the transfusion should be discon-tinued, but the intravenous line or catheter should be kept open. Before beginning laboratory tests, one should check the identity of the patient, the blood, and the forms and labels involved. Mislabeling and misidentification cause most transfusion disasters. Diagnosing this etiology is easy enough, but it may be more difficult to ascertain how and why the mistakes occurred.

Laboratory investigation requires examination of the patient's *post-*

transfusion blood. As soon as possible after the suspected reaction, blood should be drawn and allowed to clot. This sample is examined to see if it contains free hemoglobin in the serum or if antibody-coated red cells are present (i.e., if the direct antiglobulin test is positive). These tests should be done immediately; negative results on both tests make it unlikely that a hemolytic reaction has occurred. If they prove negative, further examination usually can be discontinued; if they are positive, studies must continue to show where and how the problem occurred.

Complete investigation of a hemolytic reaction should include the following: ABO, Rh, and antibody screening on the patient's blood sample used for crossmatching and on the post-transfusion specimen; and ABO, Rh, and antibody screening on the donor blood sample used for crossmatching and on blood from the unit of cells actually transfused. The major crossmatch should be repeated, using both the pretransfusion and post-transfusion specimen against both the donor sample used in crossmatching and the donor blood the patient received. The minor crossmatch, using donor serum and the patient's cells, is sometimes performed. If initial investigation fails to reveal a red cell incompatibility, many laboratories augment the crossmatch procedure with enzymes or other techniques to make antibody detection more sensitive.

The first few urine specimens should be examined for hemoglobinuria, and urine output should be measured. Red blood cells in the urine (hematuria) are not a sign of transfusion reaction. If hemoglobin enters the urine from plasma, it will be in the noncellular supernatant part of a centrifuged specimen. The specimen should be labeled "suspected transfusion reaction" because, in routine urinalysis, only the cellular sediment is examined. Prompt examination is important because red blood cells present in the urine for any reason may lyse and release their hemoglobin if the specimen stands for several hours.

Following transfusion reactions, hemoglobin is converted to bilirubin, peaking at 4 to 6 hours after hemolysis occurs. Measuring bilirubin, however, adds little to the diagnosis or to the treatment of a hemolytic reaction.

Occasionally, all studies are negative, but clinical evidence points strongly to hemolysis. It may be helpful to examine successive blood samples at intervals over the next few days. Very weak antibodies may be missed on initial examination or may be consumed temporarily by the antigen-antibody reaction. The transfusion, however, constitutes a potent reimmunizing stimulus; in samples drawn several days to a week later, high levels of antibody may develop.

Febrile Reactions

If temperature rises 1°C. or more during or after a transfusion, and if there is no other febrile stimulus, the event is considered a febrile reaction. These may be dramatic and uncomfortable, accompanied by shaking chills and other symptoms; more often they are relatively mild. Since rising temperature or pulse rate may be the first indication of hemolysis, it is important to observe the vital signs of every patient who receives blood. Most often, however, these changes in vital signs result from the effects of white cell antibodies and are unrelated to hemolysis.

Many patients, especially multiparous women and the recipients of multiple transfusions, have antibodies against white cell antigens.[19] Such antibodies can be specific for granulocyte antigens or may react with HLA antigens common to nearly all tissues. Circulating antibody can react either with white cells or with nonviable leukocyte debris in the transfused blood; the result is a rise in temperature.

It is not profitable in most cases to attempt matching between donor and patient. A patient who repeatedly experiences febrile reactions, despite symptomatic therapy with antipyretics, should receive deglycerolized frozen red cells or some other red cell product treated to remove most white cells.[30,34] Since platelets cannot be prepared without admixture of white cells, and platelets have HLA antigens, it is necessary to find compatible platelet donors for patients with identifiable HLA antibodies.

Urticaria

Urticarial reactions (e.g., hives or itching) result when a patient has antibodies that react with transfused plasma proteins. Antibodies of this kind usually occur in multiply transfused patients, or in patients with lymphomas, and usually are directed against subgroup determinants of various immunoglobulins. Serologic investigation rarely is fruitful. As with febrile reactions, the patient who gets urticarial reactions despite symptomatic therapy should receive a red cell preparation from which plasma has been removed (i.e., washed red cells or deglycerolized frozen cells).

Occasional patients, congenitally deficient in IgA, have class-specific antibodies directed against all IgA globulins. Such patients may suffer life-threatening anaphylactic reactions if given plasma that contains IgA. Affected patients should receive thoroughly plasma-free red cells or transfusion products prepared from other IgA-deficient individuals.

Disease Transmission

Transmission of hepatitis B is probably the most common severe or fatal transfusion mishap. Accurate figures are hard to find. In transfusion services where careful records are kept, clinical or chemical hepatitis may be found to occur in as many as 0.1 to 1 percent of transfusion recipients,[17,36] despite the best available tests for HB$_s$Ag in donor bloods. Not all post-transfusion hepatitis is hepatitis B. Fairly common after blood transfusion (about 8 percent in one series[1]) is a form of hepatitis called "non-A, non-B." The disease is usually mild, requiring no treatment and presenting no serodiagnostic clues as to the etiologic agent. Its true incidence is unknown, since most transfusion recipients are not followed with liver function tests in the subsequent few months. Blood also can transmit malaria and such viral infections as Epstein-Barr virus and cytomegalovirus.

Circulatory Overload

Whole blood, red cells, and plasma products cause prompt, long-lasting expansion of circulatory volume. This volume increase can push patients with borderline cardiac function into congestive heart failure. Elderly patients and severely anemic infants are at greatest risk. Patients at risk should receive red blood cells, not whole blood, and should be observed for quickening pulse and respiration that may signal incipient pulmonary edema. Circulatory overload sometimes occurs after rapid, massive whole blood transfusion to a patient whose degree of blood loss has been overestimated.

Immunization

Blood transfusion exposes the patient to countless potential immunogens. More than 300 antigens have been identified on red cells alone, not to mention antigenic properties of granulocytes, lymphocytes, platelets, and plasma protein allotypes. Rh$_o$(D) is the most consistently antigenic, eliciting antibodies in 60 to 75 percent of Rh-negative individuals who are exposed to it. It is fortunate that other antigens are less potent. Otherwise, transfusion recipients would produce such a combination of antibodies that subsequent transfusion (other than autologous transfusion) would become virtually impossible. It has been estimated that each transfusion carries a 1 percent risk of immunizing the recipient.[3]

Antibody screening tests and crossmatching detect red cell antibodies. A patient known to have a specific antibody should receive only red cells that lack the corresponding antigen. Some patients develop several different antibodies to antigens in several different systems; it then becomes extremely difficult to find donor blood negative for every one of the relevant antigens.

Immunization to white cell antigens and serum proteins is much harder to characterize, although symptomatic effects may be apparent. Symptomatic treatment with antipyretics or antihistamines is satisfactory for most such patients; if not, deglycerolized frozen red cells are available for use in severely sensitized patients. Type-specific platelet preparations are needed for patients with specific platelet or HLA alloantibodies.

HEMOLYTIC DISEASE OF THE NEWBORN

In hemolytic disease of the newborn (HDN), the mother has antibodies which are harmless to her own cells but which cause damage to the red cells of her fetus. These antibodies cross the placenta, enter the fetal blood stream, and attach to antigen present on the fetal cells. For HDN to occur, the fetus must have an antigen absent from the mother's cells; the mother must have an antibody against that antigen; and the antibody must be IgG, the only immunoglobulin that crosses the placenta. Anti-Rh_o(D) has been, and remains, the commonest cause of HDN, but many other antibodies have been implicated. The pathophysiology and treatment of HDN are the same, regardless of antibody specificity.

Pathophysiology

IMMUNIZATION

IgG antibodies develop when a host is exposed to cells that contain antigens absent from his own cells. Both transfusion and childbearing are routes that introduce foreign cells into the blood stream. With anti-Rh_o(D), pregnancy and childbirth are the immunizing events, since Rh-positive blood almost never is given to Rh-negative females of childbearing age. For other specificities, either transfusion or prior pregnancies (see below) may be the immunizing stimulus.

Fetal red cells enter the mother's circulation throughout the latter half of pregnancy, but usually in insignificantly small numbers. During labor, placental separation and uterine contractions allow larger numbers of fetal cells access to the mother's blood stream. About 20 percent of Rh-negative women with Rh-positive infants subsequently develop anti-Rh$_o$(D).[4,45] If the immunized mother has a subsequent Rh-positive pregnancy, the few fetal cells that enter her circulation during pregnancy become significant as secondary immunizing events. Once antibody production has begun, miniscule later exposures can provoke enormous anamnestic production of IgG antibody.

After anti-Rh$_o$(D), the commonest cause of HDN is anti-A or anti-B. Most anti-A and anti-B are IgM, but group O individuals often have ABO antibodies of the IgG class as well. The reason why IgG antibodies develop in some group O persons but not in others remains unclear. Neither pregnancy nor blood transfusion is needed as an immunizing event. It is also unclear why group A persons do not have IgG anti-B, and vice versa. The fetus of a group O mother will be exposed to her IgG antibodies; if there is substantial anti-A or anti-B, an A or B fetus may suffer red cell damage. It is not feasible to test all group O pregnant women for anti-A and anti-B of the IgG class. Even if such antibodies are shown to be present, it is impossible to predict which few infants will experience clinical difficulties.

CONSEQUENCES TO THE FETUS

If fetal cells lack the antigen, the mother's IgG antibodies can enter the infant's circulation without ill effect. If the fetal cells possess that specific antigen, however, the antibody recognizes the antigen and coats the cell surface. As with IgG-mediated hemolysis in other settings, antibody-coated cells undergo accelerated destruction in the reticuloendothelial system. Often the fetal bone marrow responds to this antibody-mediated hemolysis by increasing red cell production in an attempt to maintain adequate hemoglobin levels and avoid anemia. This increase in erythropoiesis causes many immature, nucleated red cells to circulate prematurely. Another name for HDN is *erythroblastosis fetalis,* emphasizing the prominence of nucleated red cells in the circulation.

As increased numbers of red cells are destroyed, the liberated hemoglobin must be eliminated. Hemoglobin undergoes conversion to bilirubin and other bile pigments that diffuse across the placenta back to the mother's circulation. The mother's liver readily conjugates and excretes the fetal bilirubin. Some bile pigments leak into the amniotic fluid and are not directly excreted.

If the fetal bone marrow cannot compensate for the shortened red cell survival, progressive anemia develops. As hemoglobin drops, tissue oxygenation declines. Hypoxia is most damaging to the heart. In the last 6 or 8 weeks of pregnancy, the severely anemic fetus may go into congestive heart failure and develop systemic edema. Pulmonary edema is no problem because lungs do not function in intrauterine life. The fetus with severe HDN may die of congestive heart failure around the time of delivery. Still another name for HDN is *hydrops fetalis,* which emphasizes the edematous appearance these stillborn infants present.

CONSEQUENCES TO THE NEWBORN

At delivery, the infant severs connections with the mother's circulation and becomes an independent individual. This removes the source of incoming antibody but deprives the infant of an important route for bilirubin disposal. Low hemoglobin, by itself, is rarely the primary problem except for occasional anemic infants born in established or incipient congestive heart failure. The major issue is bilirubin disposition. Antibody-coated cells continue to be destroyed; excessive amounts of bilirubin continue to occur; but now the infant's own liver must dispose of this product.

Before it can be excreted, bilirubin must be conjugated with glucuronic acid. Unconjugated bilirubin is soluble only in organic solvents, not in the aqueous medium of bile. Conjugation requires an enzyme, glucuronide transferase, which develops slowly as the liver matures. Premature infants have very little enzyme, and even full-term infants do not have very much. Faced with excessive quantities of bilirubin, the infant's liver cannot conjugate it rapidly enough to excrete it. The result is that unconjugated bilirubin accumulates in the infant's blood stream.

Unconjugated bilirubin, highly lipid-soluble, tends to be deposited in cells of the developing nervous system. The mature nervous system is not damaged by unconjugated bilirubin, but the infant's neurons can undergo severe, permanent damage. *Kernicterus* is the name given to localized bilirubin deposits in neurons, especially in areas of the midbrain. In the infant severely affected by hemolytic disease, massive kernicterus can cause death in hours or days; with less severe kernicterus, there is permanent mental and physical retardation. The most urgent goal in treating hemolytic disease of the

newborn is to prevent excessive accumulation of unconjugated bilirubin.

Diagnosis

PERINATAL EXAMINATION

Any infant—not just an Rh-positive child of an Rh-negative mother—
can have HDN; conversely, not every jaundiced newborn has HDN.
Sepsis, liver disease, and biliary atresia are important causes of neonatal jaundice, as well as "physiologic jaundice" that occurs in the
first 72 hours of life. Infants with red cell enzymopathies or dys-
erythropoiesis can have many nucleated red cells in their circulation.
To diagnose HDN, one must document that the infant's red cells are
coated by antibody and that the antibody came from the mother.

In the first 36 hours of life, rising bilirubin levels and falling hemoglobin levels alert the clinician that something is amiss. With HDN
of most specificities, the infant's cells have a positive direct Coombs
test; occasional cases of ABO disease may be difficult to document
without augmentation of standard antiglobulin procedures. Free antibody may or may not be found in the infant's serum, depending on
whether or not excess antibody remains after all red cells are coated.
If serum antibody is present, its specificity can be determined by
standard identification techniques. If antibody is present only on
the cell surfaces and not in serum, an eluate can be made from the
coated cells, and the specificity of the eluted antibody is tested.

Identification is easiest on the mother's blood, since she is the
source of the antibody. Unless the antibody is IgG anti-A or anti-B,
the mother will have a positive antibody screening test. In ABO
hemolytic disease, the presence of IgG activity can be unmasked by
inactivating the more potent, agglutinating IgM antibodies. Once
antibody is identified in the mother, it must be shown that it reacts
with an antigen on the baby's cells. Anti-Rh$_o$(D) that crossed the
placenta from an Rh-negative mother to an Rh-negative fetus would
not cause hemolysis in the baby. Once the maternal antibody has
been identified, it is usually easy to test the infant's cells for the
antigen. Occasionally, the antibody may coat the cells so heavily
that there are no antigen sites free to react with the typing serum.
In these cases, antibody must be eluted off and the seemingly negative cells retested.

While serologic examinations are under way, the infant's bilirubin
must be watched. If unconjugated bilirubin rises to dangerous levels,

it becomes necessary to institute symptomatic treatment even if diagnostic procedures are incomplete.

ANTENATAL EXAMINATION

An antibody screening test in the early or middle part of pregnancy detects antibodies likely to cause HDN but does not identify IgG anti-A or anti-B in group O women. Any woman whose earlier pregnancies were affected by HDN must be carefully observed in subsequent pregnancies. ABO hemolytic disease occurs inconsistently in subsequent A or B infants, but with all other antibodies, the disease tends to get worse with each succeeding pregnancy.

Until the mid-1960s, the best way to predict the occurrence and severity of imminent HDN was to titer the maternal antibody repeatedly during pregnancy. If antibody strength increased, it was probable that antigen-positive fetal cells were present and stimulating enhanced IgG production. With rising maternal titers, increasing amounts of antibody could be presumed to be crossing the placenta and injuring fetal cells. Correlation between antibody titers and fetal outcome was fair to good, but sometimes the decision for or against early delivery proved seriously incorrect.

Fetal condition is now best assessed by amniocentesis, a procedure used for many conditions besides HDN. In amniocentesis, amniotic fluid is carefully withdrawn through a needle inserted through the uterine wall. If the mother is known to have IgG blood group antibodies, it is important to determine the extent of fetal hemolysis and the degree to which the fetal bone marrow can compensate. In severe HDN, early delivery often prevents intrauterine anemia and death, but premature delivery carries the risk of hepatic and respiratory immaturity. Accurate fetal evaluation carries important clinical consequences.

The level of bile pigments in amniotic fluid reflects the severity of intrauterine hemolysis. These pigments include, besides bilirubin, all the pigments that absorb light at a wavelength of 540 μ. The same amniotic fluid sample used to evaluate degree of hemolysis can be used to assess respiratory maturity by measuring the lecithin to sphingomyelin (L/S) ratio (see p. 537). Charts are available to correlate the concentration of bile pigments at different gestational ages with likelihood of fetal survival.[25] With this predictive information, and information about maturity of the fetal lung, the obstetrician can decide rationally whether to let the pregnancy continue unmodified, to initiate early delivery, or to perform intrauterine transfusion.

Treatment

INTRAUTERINE TRANSFUSION

Intrauterine transfusion is far more of a risk for the fetus than is amniocentesis. It is done only if anemia is sufficiently severe that the fetus is unlikely to survive long enough to make extrauterine maintenance feasible. Red cells that are group O and compatible with the mother's antibody are instilled into the fetal peritoneal cavity, subject to fluoroscopic observation. Red cells enter the blood stream via the peritoneal lymphatics. Sometimes direct fetal manipulation is performed after fetoscopy or hysterotomy, but all of these procedures carry substantial risk to the fetus. Exchange transfusion is not done on fetuses.

EXCHANGE TRANSFUSION

In exchange transfusion, the infant's blood is gradually removed and replaced by red cells compatible with the mother's antibody. This accomplishes many things. Removing plasma serves to remove unconjugated bilirubin, thus reducing the risk of kernicterus. Unbound antibody, if present, is also removed; this decreases the amount of antibody available to coat new cells as the infant produces them. Antibody-coated cells are removed as well, thus saving them from extravascular destruction and reducing the amount of hemoglobin converted to bilirubin. Adminstering compatible cells improves oxygen-carrying capacity with cells that will not be hemolyzed or contribute to the bilirubin burden. Transfusing red cell concentrates in place of whole blood reduces blood volume and thereby spares the anemic heart additional circulatory load.

Exchange transfusion must be performed with due care for asepsis, regulation of pH and electrolytes, temperature control, and maintenance of total blood volume, but the procedure itself carries no more than a 1 to 2 percent risk to the infant.

Albumin sometimes is infused before exchange is begun. Albumin binds unconjugated bilirubin, functionally removing it from the tissues and holding it firmly in the plasma.[41] Pretreatment with albumin reduces the level of free bilirubin and increases the amount present for removal as plasma is drawn off.

SELECTION OF BLOOD

Cells for exchange transfusion are crossmatched against the mother's serum, in which the antibody is at its strongest; for this reason, laboratory results are as unambiguous as possible. In addition, the mother is more able to spare the few milliliters of blood needed for crossmatching than is the infant. Sometimes the mother and her blood are not available, or her serum contains IgM antibodies that complicate the crossmatch but are not present in the infant. Under such circumstances, the best specimen for crossmatching is an eluate made from the infant's antibody-coated cells. The baby's serum often has so little free antibody that it fails to give clearcut reactions against donor cells. Cells compatible with the eluate, however, should also be tested against the infant's serum, because the mother could have transmitted several IgG antibodies, some of which did not attack the baby's cells.

Exchange transfusion usually uses group O red cells because they will not interact with maternal anti-A or anti-B and will not be destroyed by any anti-A or anti-B that the baby subsequently produces. If the mother and baby are of the same ABO group, it is entirely appropriate to use compatible red cells of that group.

On rare occasions, no compatible donor can be found. If exchange transfusion is essential and the mother is in good health, her cells can be used for transfusion. The plasma, of course, should be fully removed, but the cells are guaranteed to be compatible with maternal antibody. Another alternative, far from ideal but still better than doing nothing, is to use incompatible cells for exchange transfusion. The transfused cells will be coated by any remaining free antibody and will eventually be destroyed, but the exchange procedure does remove bilirubin and antibody and also removes the infant's heavily coated cells. With incompatible cells, it is usually necessary to repeat the exchange procedure a number of times. If compatible cells are used, one unit of blood usually is sufficient. In very severe cases, more than one exchange may be needed to remove the huge load of tissue bilirubin.

Prevention

Rh-negative persons can be protected against antibody production by administering exogenous anti-Rh_o(D) shortly after exposure to Rh-positive cells. Rh immune globulin (RhIG) given within 72 hours after delivery prevents subsequent anti-Rh_o(D) formation if the dose of antibody matches the volume of immunizing cells. Commercially available RhIG preparations contain enough antibody to protect against up to 15 ml. of red blood cells.[3] If more than 15 ml. of fetal cells have entered the mother's circulation, several vials of RhIG can be given.

Large fetal-maternal bleeds are most easily detected by incubating the mother's postpartum blood sample with anti-Rh_o(D) serum and then adding antiglobulin serum. The anti-Rh_o(D) serum does not agglutinate the Rh-positive fetal cells but does coat them sufficiently that antiglobulin serum induces agglutination. A more exacting but considerably more sensitive approach is to determine how many cells in the mother's circulation contain fetal hemoglobin. This is done on a thin film of blood with the Kleihauer-Betke acid elution technique.[3]

Very small numbers of fetal cells can elicit anti-Rh_o(D). Spontaneous or induced abortions in early pregnancy often are accompanied by fetal-maternal hemorrhage. Amniocentesis also can introduce fetal cells into the mother's circulation. The consequences of Rh sensitization are potentially so tragic that most clinicians prefer to administer Rh immune globulin whenever the least possibility of sensitization exists.[9] It should be administered to Rh-negative mothers after known or suspected abortion and after amniocentesis done for any purpose other than monitoring Rh hemolytic disease. RhIG given to a pregnant woman does not harm the fetus, even an Rh-positive fetus, because the quantity of antibody is so small.

HLA ANTIGENS AND ANTIBODIES

All nucleated cells have HLA antigens on their surface membranes. Although sometimes described as "white cell antigens," HLA antigens characterize virtually all cell types except red blood cells. The biologic significance of these membrane characteristics remains unclear. Statistical associations exist between individual HLA antigens and occurrence of certain diseases, but these only deepen the mystery.[40] Mystery surrounds even the name of the system or region. Some sources ascribe to HLA the meaning *histocompatibility locus A*; this implies that other histocompatibility loci, as they are found, would be designated B, C, D, etc. Other sources claim the initial meaning to be *human leukocyte antigens*. Current usage simply employs "HLA" as an independent term, without concern for its linguistic antecedents.

Genes and Antigens

Genes on chromosome number 6 determine the HLA antigens.[3,40] Also in that portion of chromosome 6 are genes controlling the antigenic composition of several plasma proteins, the presence of at least two red cell antigens, and, it seems probable, the degree and extent of overall immunologic reactivity. Because so many diverse functions cluster in this area, the chromosomal segment is referred to as the HLA *region,* not the HLA *locus* or *site.* The easiest cells to study for HLA antigens are blood lymphocytes and monocytes. The discussions below refer largely to lymphocyte or leukocyte antigens, but the reader should remember that other tissue cells share these antigens.

A, B, C, AND D DETERMINANTS

Four different series of antigens have been characterized. Three, designated A, B, and C, react with serum antibodies and are called the serologically defined (SD) antigens. One series, called D, can be identified only by the cytotoxic actions of specifically sensitized lymphocytes; these are called lymphocyte defined (LD) antigens. Terminology in the HLA field has recently been systematized.[44] This chapter will use only the new terminology. Readers who need to translate terms in the older literature should consult more detailed discussions of this topic.

In the A and B series are 20 or more different antigenic specificities; the C series includes six and the D series at least ten. The HLA region of a single chromosome determines one specificity from each of the four series. Individual antigens of each series are allelic to one another. Since each cell has two sets of chromosomes, each cell can have two A, two B, two C, and two D antigens, but no more than two. The combination of HLA antigens that a single chromosome determines is called the *haplotype.* This assortment of one each from the A, B, C, and D series is transmitted as a genetic package. Diploid cells have two haplotypes which, together, constitute the *genotype.*

Antibodies that identify A and B antigens are more widely available than those for the C series. The lymphocyte culture techniques needed to identify D antigens are so exacting that very few laboratories type for these specificities. Because of these technical considerations, most laboratories confine routine HLA typing to the A and B series only. An individual whose two chromosomes each determined the same haplotype would have cells with only one A and one B antigen, but this is uncommon. If there were two different haplotypes but one antigen was common to both, the individual would have one A and two B antigens, or vice versa. Most HLA typing results in a designation of two A antigens and two B antigens.

Numbers have been assigned to antigens of all four series. Table 11

Table 11. Specificities in the HLA System*

A Locus	B Locus	C Locus	D Locus
A1	B5	Cw1	Dw1
A2	B7	Cw2	Dw2
A3	B8	Cw3	Dw3
A9	B12	Cw4	Dw4
A10	B13	Cw5	Dw5
A11	B14	Cw6	Dw6
A25	B15		Dw7
A26	B17		Dw8
A28	B18		Dw9
A29	B27		Dw10
Aw19	B37		Dw11
Aw23	B40		
Aw24	Bw16		
Aw30	Bw21		
Aw31	Bw22		
Aw32	Bw35		
Aw33	Bw38		
Aw34	Bw39		
Aw36	Bw41		
Aw43	Bw42		
	Bw44–54		

*WHO-IUIS Terminology Committee: *Nomenclature for factors of the HLA system—1977.* Transplantation 25:272, 1978.

shows the current numerical terminology. The degree of antigenic characterization varies. Some specificities have not been fully characterized; with these antigens, the letter "w" precedes the number, standing for "workshop." When workshop exchange and discussion conclusively identify all characteristics, the Nomenclature Committee of the World Health Organization can bestow unmodified numerical recognition upon the antigen.

HLA antigens consist of a glycoprotein chain and a globulin chain, together comprising about 1 to 2 percent of cell-membrane weight.[33] Completely different glycoprotein antigens exist on the surface of B-lymphocytes, macrophages, and sperm. These B-cell antigens are intimately associated with immune responsiveness and appear to be controlled by alleles either at, or closely related to, the HLA-D locus. Unmodified reference to "white cell typing" or "HLA antigens" does not include consideration of these B-cell antigens and their antibodies.

LABORATORY TESTING

HLA typing is more complicated than typing for red cell antigens. Now that deliberate immunization is severely restricted, most antibodies come from persons immunized through transfusions or pregnancies, and such immunization usually provokes multiple antibodies. It is difficult and expensive to isolate a strong, specific, single antibody from a multispecific serum. The number of white cell antigens that must be studied on each cell is greater than for red cells, and different examples of a single antigen exhibit different levels of reactivity. Since each cell sample must be examined against a battery of antiserums, all relevant antigens are represented in several different serums. The overall pattern of reactivity determines antigenic interpretation, not just the results of one or a few individual reactions.

Another difference between red cell serology and HLA research is that the relative immunogenicity of different HLA antigens is unknown. After years of transfusion experience and experimental work with the red cell antigens, we can generalize fairly accurately about those antigens that frequently induce antibody formation and those that do not. It is also possible to distinguish the antibodies that are dangerous in transfusion practice from those that are not. This sort of information is not yet available for the white cell antigens.

HLA testing usually uses agglutination or cytotoxicity as end points. Agglutination procedures are easier but are less sensitive, less specific, and more susceptible to false-positive results. Cytotoxicity testing uses complement-binding antibodies which are allowed to attach to the cells during incubation in a complement-free system. Adding active complement to the surface-bound antibody initiates complement fixation that causes lethal damage to the cell. Cell death is most easily demonstrated by adding a macromolecular dye to the medium. Viable cells are able to exclude the large dye molecules. Because a dead cell loses this barrier function, the dye enters and stains the entire dead cell. As the reaction between antibody and cell surface antigen increases in strength and specificity, the number of stained cells in the suspension increases. This permits a degree of qualitative comparison between serum samples that contain different combinations of antibodies.

INTERPRETATION

A two-antigen haplotype consists of one A antigen and one B antigen, transmitted as a package. Even if the same A antigen and B antigen exist in two individuals, it is not necessarily correct to say that they have the same HLA genes. The HLA region of chromosome 6 includes information that codes for many different characteristics, of which only a few are clearly understood. Just because the A antigen and the B antigen are the same in two chromosomes from two different individuals, we cannot assume that the region contains identical genes for all other traits. Within a given sibship, only four haplotypes can circulate—two from the mother and two from the father. Siblings with the same HLA antigens necessarily have the same genetic material; it can be assumed that siblings with identical HLA antigens have identical material at all sites within the HLA region. Unrelated individuals, however, can have the same A and B determinants, but may have quite disparate genetic information elsewhere in the region.

LINKAGE DISEQUILIBRIUM AND ANTIGEN DISTRIBUTION

Certain combinations of HLA antigens are more frequent than others. Some antigens are far commoner or far rarer in one population or race than in others, and some combinations of antigens have strikingly high incidence in specific populations.

The most common B antigens in American whites, for example, are B7, B8, and B12, with frequencies of 23, 20, and 24 percent respectively. In American blacks, the most common of the B series are Bw17 (26 percent), Bw35 (32 percent), and a specificity characterized as 1AG (34 percent); this contrasts with African blacks, whose most common B antigens are B7 (18 percent), Bw17 (33 percent), and 1AG (31 percent).[33]

In American whites, association often exists between A1 and B8, A3 and B7, and Aw25 and B18. American blacks also have frequent association of A1 and B8, but in African blacks, A1 and B8 are, if anything, negatively associated. In American blacks, Aw25 and B18 travel together frequently, as do Aw30 and Bw42. The association between Aw30 and Bw42 also is common in African blacks, but Aw25 and B18 have a negative association in that population. Aw26 and B17 are a common combination in African blacks but have a negative association in American blacks.

Adding further to the confusion is the observation that recombination can occur with a possible frequency of 1 percent.[33] When crossing-over occurs, the C, B, and D loci remain together but separate themselves from the A locus. The portion of the region responsible for extent and intensity of immune responsiveness lies between B and D, most closely linked to D.

Clinical Applications

ORGAN TRANSPLANTATION

HLA typing is only one aspect of donor selection for organ transplantation. Donor's ABO group should be compatible with the recipient, and the recipient should be free of serum antibodies that react, in vitro, with the prospective donor's red or white cells. If there is sufficient time, and viable cells are available from prospective donor and recipient mixed lymphocyte cultures (MLC) are useful in ruling out cell-mediated sensitization between donor and recipient. Transplantation workers are uncertain whether simple "matching" of HLA A and B antigens is important when donor and recipient are unrelated.

When donor and recipient are blood relatives, HLA matching improves the chances of graft survival. Monozygotic (identical) twins, of course, share not only HLA antigens but all their genetic material. Non-twin siblings have only a limited genetic pool from which to receive constitutional attributes. Identity of HLA antigens indicates identity of the entire HLA region, including immune responsiveness genes as well as various red cell and protein allotypes. Since other genes assort independently, siblings are bound to differ significantly, but the more alike the tissues are, the better the graft is likely to survive. In siblings, two-haplotype matches give better results than one-haplotype matches, all other things being equal; one-haplotype matches are better than complete HLA disparity.[33] If no siblings are available with two-haplotype or one-haplotype matches, the patient's parents or children should be considered as potential donors. With parents and offspring, one haplotype necessarily must be identical; the other, of course, will be completely different.

When donor and recipient are unrelated, HLA matching provides much less predictive information. Graft survival is not much improved by using tissue from donors who share one or several A and B antigens with the donor. In patients with preformed HLA antibodies, however, it is important to use tissue negative for the relevant antigen.

TRANSFUSIONS

It is unlikely that antigen matching will become routine for all platelet transfusions for practical reasons, but many workers believe that patients who will need repeated platelet transfusions over a long period should receive HLA-matched platelets. Platelet concentrates are highly immunogenic. Immunocompetent recipients of multiple platelet transfusions frequently develop antibodies, either to HLA antigens or specific platelet antigens, or both. Once antibodies develop, platelets that contain the relevant antigens are rapidly destroyed. Granulocyte transfusions, still an experimental procedure, are also highly immunogenic.

Because platelets and granulocytes survive only a short time, transfusionists need not worry about long-term tissue compatibility. It appears that platelets are less immunogenic if one or several HLA antigens are common to donor and recipient. When blood relatives are available as donors, complete HLA matching may be possible. Even the use of unrelated donors with matching antigens is better than completely random transfusion. Practical considerations do, however, intrude. Technology and reagents exist for typing patients and donors, but the process is expensive, in terms of the reagents needed, and time-consuming. Once donors and patients have been typed, the problems of matching become rather daunting, since the 20 or more A antigens and 20 or more B antigens can assort in any combination. Eventually, it may become obvious which donor-recipient combinations are especially dangerous and which are innocuous, but until then, it seems quixotic to pursue the ideal of matched donors for every recipient.

Antibody development becomes obvious when a patient no longer shows hemostatic improvement or an increment in platelet count after transfusion of unselected platelets. At that point, the antibody must be identified and compatible donors found if further transfusions are to be effective.

The kinds of white cell antibodies that cause febrile transfusion reactions are not necessarily the same as those that destroy platelets. If a patient who repeatedly has febrile reactions is given platelet transfusions, the post-transfusion platelet response should be observed carefully. If platelet survival and therapeutic benefit are poor, the antibody must be identified and compatible platelets given.

DISEASE ASSOCIATIONS

Determining associations between diseases and HLA antigens is difficult because there is such a variety of phenotypes, and so many confounding features obscure observations about disease. Two major approaches are possible. One is to compare the frequency of a given antigen in a group of unrelated patients exhibiting the disease with antigen frequency in a control population. The other is to study families with known haplotypes to see if a particular disease reliably occurs in individuals with a particular haplotype. The latter approach demonstrates whether the disease is associated with events controlled by the HLA region but does not necessarily document association with specific antigens. The former approach documents some genetic marker that travels with the disease in terms of relative risk but gives no information about the disease mechanism.

The best association between disease and HLA involves arthritic disorders and the antigen B27. Ankylosing spondylitis, a clearly defined subcategory of arthritis, is very closely tied to B27. This antigen occurs only in populations native to the northern hemisphere. Worldwide, more than 90 percent of patients with ankylosing spondylitis are positive for B27, compared to 2.8 percent of control populations.[40] Ankylosing spondylitis is virtually nonexistent in populations which lack B27. In populations possessing the antigen, the relative risk that a person having the antigen will also have the disease ranges from 49, in American blacks, to over 300, in Japan. Other arthritic syndromes, notably Reiter's syndrome (urethritis, arthritis, and conjunctivitis), juvenile rheumatoid arthritis, and arthritic complications of psoriasis, show positive correlation with B27 in descending order.[40]

Interesting associations have emerged between diseases of possible autoimmune etiology and antigens at the B and D loci. Myasthenia gravis, Addison's disease, and chronic active hepatitis are modestly associated with Dw3, and Sjögren's syndrome has a fairly strong association.[40] Insulin-dependent diabetes mellitus has been linked with B8 and Bw15 and with Dw3 and 4. The nature of these associations suggests that one or two diabetogenic genes reside somewhere around or between the B and D loci, but their effect does not become apparent unless external influences also coincide. Many workers believe gluten-sensitive enteropathy (celiac disease) to have an immune foundation, and here, too, B8 and Dw3 have been implicated.[40] B8 and Dw3 are also conspicuous among patients with dermatitis herpetiformis.

Future research in disease demography and HLA typing will undoubtedly yield exciting results and tantalizing prospects for greater understanding of disease susceptibility, causation, and prevention.

PARENTAGE ASSIGNMENT

HLA typing is well suited for parentage studies because the antigens are fully developed at birth; they are transmitted in simple codominant fashion; and great phenotypic diversity exists among unrelated individuals. If the HLA phenotypes of a child and one parent are known, it becomes possible to assess fairly accurately whether or not a given individual is the other parent. Up to 75 percent of falsely accused men have been excluded from paternity with HLA testing alone, in jurisdictions that allow HLA results as evidence.[35] Strong (but by no means absolute) statistical support also can be adduced that a given man *is* the father, if the child's haplotype matches that of the putative father. This is true especially if the haplotype is uncommon in the population under study.

REFERENCES

1. Alter, H. J., Holland, P. V., Morrow, A. G., et al.: *Clinical and serological analysis of transfusion-associated hepatitis.* Lancet 2:838, 1975.
2. American Association of Blood Banks: *Standards for Blood Banks and Transfusion Services.* ed. 8. A.A.B.B., Washington, D.C., 1976.
3. American Association of Blood Banks: *Technical Manual.* ed. 7. A.A.B.B., Washington, D.C., 1977.
4. Ascari, W. D., Levine, P., and Pollack, W.: *Incidence of maternal Rh immunization by ABO compatible and incompatible pregnancies.* Br. Med. J. 1:399, 1969.
5. Bayer, W. L.: *The effect of frozen blood on the relationship of cytomegalovirus and hepatitis virus to infection and disease,* in *Clinical and Practical Aspects of the Use of Frozen Blood.* American Association of Blood Banks, Washington, D.C., 1977.
6. Benöhr, H. C., and Waller, H. D.: *Metabolism in haemolytic states.* Clin. Haematol. 4:45, 1975.
7. Capra, D. J., and Edmundson, A. B.: *The antibody combining site.* Sci. Am. 236:50, 1977.
8. Coombs, R. R. A., Mourant, A. E., and Race, R. R.: *A new test for the detection of weak and "incomplete" Rh agglutinins.* Br. J. Exp. Pathol. 26:225, 1945.
9. *Current uses of Rh₀(D) immune globulin and detection of antibodies.* Am. Coll. Obstet. Gynecol. Tech. Bull. 35, January 1976.
10. Dacie, J. V.: *Autoimmune hemolytic anemia.* Arch. Intern. Med. 135:1293, 1975.
11. Dorner, I. M.: *Packed cells—now and in the future,* in *A Seminar on Blood Components: E Unum Pluribus.* American Association of Blood Banks, Washington, D.C., 1977.
12. *Factor IX complex and hepatitis.* FDA Drug Bull. 6:22, 1976.
13. Feizi, T., Kabat, E. A., Vicari, G.,et al.: *Immunochemical studies on blood groups. XLVII. The I antigen complex—precursors in the A, B, H, Leᵃ and Leᵇ blood group system—hemagglutination-inhibition studies.* J. Exp. Med. 133:39, 1971.
14. Garratty, G., and Petz, L. D.: *Drug-induced immune hemolytic anemia.* Am. J. Med. 58:398, 1975.
15. Garratty, G., Petz, L. D., and Hoops, J. K.: *The correlation of cold agglutinin titrations in saline and albumin with haemolytic anemia.* Br. J. Haematol. 35:587, 1977.

16. Gelpi, A. P., and King, M. C.: *Association of Duffy blood groups with the sickle cell trait.* Hum. Genet. 32:65, 1976.
17. Goldfield, M., Black, H. C., Bill, J., et al.: *The consequences of administering blood pretested for HB _sAg by third generation techniques: a progress report.* Am. J. Med. Sci. 270:335, 1975.
18. Goldfinger, D.: *Acute hemolytic transfusion reactions—a fresh look at pathogenesis and considerations regarding therapy.* Transfusion 17:85, 1977.
19. Heinrich, D., Mueller-Eckhardt, C., and Stier, W.: *The specificity of leukocyte and platelet alloantibodies in sera of patients with non-hemolytic transfusion reactions: absorption and elution studies.* Vox Sang. 25:442, 1973.
20. Hollinger, F. B., Bradley, D. W., Dreesman, G. R., and Melnick, J. L.: *Detection of viral hepatitis type A.* Am. J. Clin. Pathol. 65:854, 1976.
21. Hughes-Jones, N. C.: *Red-cell antigens, antibodies and their interaction.* Clin. Haematol. 4:29, 1975.
22. Kasper, C. K.: *Cryoprecipitate and Factor VIII concentrate—aspects of production and use,* in *A Seminar on Blood Components: E Unum Pluribus.* American Association of Blood Banks, Washington, D.C., 1977.
23. Keith, L., Berger, G. S., and Pollack, W.: *The transfusion of Rh-positive blood into Rh-negative women.* Am. J. Obstet. Gynecol. 125:502, 1976.
24. Levine, P., Tripodi, D., Struck, J., Jr., et al.: *Hemolytic anemia associated with Rh_{null} but not with Bombay blood.* Vox Sang. 24:417, 1973.
25. Liley, A. W.: *Liquor amnii analysis in the management of the pregnancy complicated by rhesus sensitization.* Am. J. Obstet. Gynecol. 82:1359, 1961.
26. Marsh, W. L., Chaganti, R. S. K., Gardner, F. H., et al.: *Mapping human autosomes: evidence supporting assignment of Rhesus to the short arm of chromosome No. 1.* Science 183:966, 1974.
27. Meryman, H. T.: *Red cell freezing: a major factor in the future of blood banking,* in *Clinical and Practical Aspects of the Use of Frozen Blood.* American Association of Blood Banks, Washington, D.C., 1977.
28. Miller, L. H., Mason, S. J., Clyde, D. F., et al.: *The resistance factor to Plasmodium vivax in Blacks. The Duffy-blood-group genotype FyFy.* N. Engl. J. Med. 295:302, 1976.
29. Miller, W. J., Provost, P. J., McAleer, W. J., et al.: *Specific immune adherence assay for human hepatitis A antibody. Application to diagnostic and epidemiologic investigations.* Proc. Soc. Exp. Biol. Med. 149:254, 1975.
30. Miller, W. V., Wilson, M. J., and Kalb, J. H.: *Simple methods for production of HLA antigen poor red blood cells.* Transfusion 13:189, 1973.
31. Mollison, P. L., Crome, P., Hughes-Jones, N. C., et al.: *Rate of removal from circulation of red cells sensitized with different amounts of antibody.* Br. J. Haematol. 11:461, 1965.
32. Myhre, B. A., and Nakasako, Y.: *Graphs to facilitate the computation of patient response to platelet concentrates or antihemophiliac concentrate.* Transfusion 17:179, 1977.
33. Payne, R.: *The HLA complex: genetics and implications in the immune response,* in Dausset, J., and Svejgaard, A. (eds.): *HLA and Disease.* Williams & Wilkins, Baltimore, 1977.
34. Polesky, H. F.: *Leukocyte-poor blood, a study in the evolution of component therapy,* in *A Seminar on Blood Components: E Unum Pluribus.* American Association of Blood Banks, Washington, D.C., 1977.

35. Polesky, H. F.: *Paternity Testing.* American Society of Clinical Pathologists, Chicago, 1975.
36. Polesky, H. F., and Hanson, M. R.: *HB₅Ag in donors and transfusion associated hepatitis cases—seven years' experience.* Abstract booklet for the 30th annual meeting of the American Association of Blood Banks, Atlanta, November 1977.
37. Pollack, W., Hager, H. J., Reckel, R., et al.: *A study of the forces involved in the second stage of hemagglutination.* Transfusion 5:158, 1965.
38. Race, R. R., and Sanger, R.: *Blood Groups in Man.* ed. 6. Blackwell Scientific Publications, Oxford, 1975.
39. Reid, M. E., Ellisor, S. S., and Frank, B. A.: *Another potential source of error in Rh-hr typing.* Transfusion 15:485, 1975.
40. Svejgaard, A., and Ryder, L. P.: *Associations between HLA and disease,* in Dausset, J., and Svejgaard, A. (eds.): *HLA and Disease.* Williams & Wilkins, Baltimore, 1977.
41. Tullis, J. L.: *Albumin.* J.A.M.A. 237:355, 460, 1977.
42. Watkins, W. M., and Morgan, W. T. J.: *Immunochemical observations on the human blood group P system.* J. Immunogenetics 3:15, 1976
43. Weed, R. I.: *Membrane structure and its relation to haemolysis.* Clin. Haematol. 4:3, 1975.
44. WHO-IUIS Terminology Committee: *Nomenclature for factors of the HLA system.* Transplantation 21:353, 1976.
45. Woodrow, J. C., and Donohue, W. T. A.: *Rh-immunization by pregnancy: results of a survey and their relevance to prophylactic therapy.* Br. Med. J. 4:139, 1968.

SECTION 3

CHEMISTRY

CHAPTER 9

GENERAL CHEMISTRY

The blood transports a seemingly limitless number of substances, ranging from simple inorganic ions to tremendously complex organic molecules. Most of these substances can be measured fairly precisely by using a variety of techniques which, like the substances involved, range from fairly simple to highly sophisticated. In a book such as this, we can touch only on some of the most frequently measured constituents and comment briefly on problems in measurement and significance of certain abnormalities.

This enormous topic will be approached from several viewpoints. In this chapter the following are considered: glucose; the nitrogen-containing substances in serum, including proteins and the nonprotein elements such as urea, uric acid, ammonia and creatinine; calcium and phosphorus; serum lipids and cholesterol; bilirubin; and a variety of substances of toxicologic importance. In the next chapter (Chap. 10), regulation of acid-base metabolism, fluid balance, and the electrolytes sodium, potassium, chloride, and bicarbonate are discussed. A separate chapter is devoted to serum enzymes of clinical importance (Chap. 11). Certain special topics are discussed in other chapters; thus iodine metabolism is discussed in the section on the thyroid gland (Chap. 15); measurement of serum iron is considered in the hematology section (Chap. 3). Measurement of the plasma proteins that participate in blood coagulation is discussed in the chapter on hemostatic mechanisms (Chap. 2). Normal values for a variety of blood constituents are given in Table 12.

GLUCOSE

The principal fuel for all body activities is glucose, a six-carbon sugar containing, among other side chains, an aldehyde group. Although

Table 12. Normal Blood Chemistry Values for Adults

Substance	Serum, Plasma or Whole Blood	Values	Remarks
Acetone	P or S	0.3–2.0 mg./dl.	
Albumin	S	3.5–5.0 gm./dl.[32]	
Ammonia	WB	102 ± 23 μg./dl.[8] (Seligson-Hirahara method[59])	Patient should be fasting.
Amylase	S or WB	45–50 μg./dl.[8] (Conway method)	Unit is 1 mg. glucose per 100 ml. sample after 30 min. incubation.
		80–150 U/dl.[20]	
Ascorbic acid	P	0.6–2.0 mg./dl.[48]	Heparin as anticoagulant; patient should be fasting.
Bilirubin (total/direct)	S	0.8/0.2 mg/dl.[60]	
Calcium	S	4.25–5.25 mEq./L.[39]	BSP dye interferes; abnormally high or low albumin may raise or lower.
		8.5–10.5 mg./dl.[39]	
CO_2 combining power	S or WB	Arterial: 19–24 mEq./L.[61] Venous: 22–26 mEq./L.[61]	Draw without stasis, under oil or in sealed tube.
content	S or WB	Arterial: 23–27 mEq./L.[61] Venous: 25–29 mEq./L.[61]	
tension (P_{CO_2})	WB	Arterial: 32–45 mm. Hg[61] Venous: 38–53 mm. Hg[61]	Heparin in sealed tube or syringe
Chloride	S	98–106 mEq./L.[64]	
Cholesterol	S		
Total/esters		$220 \pm 50/163 \pm 36$ mg./dl.[74]	
% esterified		50–70%[60]	
Copper	S	Men: 70–140 μg./dl.[65] Women: 80–155 μg./dl.[65]	Estrogens cause rise in ceruloplasmin, hence copper rises in pregnancy and with oral contraceptives.

Test	Specimen	Normal values	Comments
Creatine phosphokinase	S	Men: 5–55 mU./ml.[57] Women: 5–55 mU./ml.[18]	Separate serum promptly. Freeze for storage.
Creatinine	S	Men: 0.6–1.2 mg./dl.[18] Women: 0.5–1.0 mg./dl.[18]	Patient should be fasting. Very wide range occurs with changing metabolic status.
Free fatty acids	S	0.3–1.10 mEq./L.[64] 8–31 mg./dl.	
Fibrinogen	P	200–400 mg./dl.[42]	Serum or plasma value are about 10% higher.
Globulins	S	2.3–3.5 gm./dl.[31]	
Glucose	WB	90–120 mg./dl.[31] (Folin-Wu method) 65–95 mg./dl.[53] (Nelson-Somogyi method) 60–105 mg./dl.[16] (glucose oxidase method) 46–94 mg./dl.[45] (ultra-micro method)	
Iron	S	56–183 μg./dl.[25]	
Iron-binding capacity	S	277–379 μg./dl.[25]	
Lactic acid	P or WB	Arterial: 0.36–0.75 mEq./L.[65] 3.1–7 mg./dl.[65] Venous: 0.5–1.3 mEq./L.[65] 5–20 mg./dl.[65]	Draw without stasis
Lactic dehydrogenase	S	200–450 U./ml.[32] (Wroblewski-LaDue method) 60–120 U./ml.[68] (Wacker method)	Patient should be in completely basal state Unit is decrease in A of 0.001/min./ml. Unit is increase in A of 0.001/min./ml.
Lipase	S	0.1–1.0 U./ml.[66]	Unit is ml. 0.05N. NaOH needed to neutralize fatty acids in 1 ml. serum.

Table 12. Continued

Substance	Serum, Plasma or Whole Blood	Values	Remarks
Lipids (total)	S	450–1000 mg./dl.[21]	Patient should be fasting.
Magnesium	S	1.4–2.2 mEq./L.[3]	
		1.7–2.7 ffig./dl.[64]	
Nitrogen (NPN)	WB	25–40 mg./dl.[4]	Anticoagulant should be free of ammonium salts.
(BUN)	S	5–25 mg./dl.[5]	
Osmolality	S	281–291 mOsm./kg.[30]	
Oxygen tension (PO_2) breathing room air	WB	Arterial: 83–108 mm. Hg[61] Venous (at heart): 40 mm. Hg[61]	Heparin in sealed tube or syringe Keep on ice.
saturation		Arterial: 98%[36] Venous: 55–71%[36]	
pH	WB	Arterial: 7.37–7.42[36] Venous: 7.34–7.39[36]	Heparin in sealed tube or syringe Keep on ice.
Phosphatase, acid	S	0.5–4 U./dl.[10] (Babson-Read method)	Unit is enzyme action that liberates 1 mg. α-naphthol/hr.
		0–0.1 U./dl.[10] (Shinowara method)	Unit is mg. P./hr./100 ml. serum.
Phosphatase, alkaline	S	1.5–4.0 U./dl.[10] (Bodansky method)	Unit is mg. P./hr./100 ml. serum.
		3.7–13.1 U./dl.[10] (King-Armstrong method)	Unit is mg. phenol/30 min./100 ml. serum.
		2.2–8.6 U./dl.[10] (Shinowara method)	Unit is mg. P./hr./100 ml. serum.
Phospholipids	S	To age 65: 175–275 mg./dl.[15] After age 65: 196–366 mg./dl.[15] Pregnancy: 205–291 mg./dl.[15]	
Phosphorus, inorganic	S	2.6–4.8 mg./dl.[14]	Separate serum from cells promptly.
Potassium	S	3.5–5.3 mEq./L.[65]	Specimen must not be hemolyzed.

Proteins (total)	S	6–8 gm./dl.[33]
Electrophoretic partition:		
Albumin		52–68%
α_1-globulin		2.4–5.3%
α_2-globulin		6.6–13.5%
β-globulin		8.5–14.5%
γ-globulin		10.7–21.0%
Sodium	S	135–148 mEq./L.[64]
Transaminase	S	
Glutamic-oxalacetic (aspartate aminotransferase)		12–36 U./ml.[32]
Glutamic - pyruvic (alanine aminotransferase)		6–53 U./ml.[32]
Urea nitrogen (BUN)	S	5–25 mg./dl.[5] For urea, multiply BUN by 2.14.[49]
Uric acid	S	Men: 3.0–7.0 mg./dl.[7] Separate serum from cells promptly Women: 2.0–6.0 mg./dl.[7]

most of the body's glucose comes from dietary carbohydrates, other sources of this necessary compound also are available. Sugars other than glucose can be utilized either by conversion to glucose within the stomach and intestine prior to absorption or by hepatic transformation of such absorbed sugars as galactose or fructose. The liver also can convert fats and proteins into glucose, pathways that become useful in metabolic emergencies. The liver is the clearinghouse for glucose metabolism; it converts excess glucose to storage forms for later use, and it retrieves the stored material for consumption as needed.

The primary storage form of glucose is glycogen, a complex branched molecule consisting of multiple glucose residues. Excess glucose can be transformed into fat and stored in the body's adipose tissues. Through a complicated series of transformations, products of glucose metabolism can be converted into certain amino acids, but this pathway is not routine for glucose storage. The most efficient retrieval of stored glucose is from glycogen. Utilization of glucose from fat or protein sources results in formation of acidic by-products.

Virtually all cells metabolize glucose, and glucose is continually transported to peripheral sites for utilization. The by-products of metabolism—principally carbon dioxide and water under conditions of optimum energy use—are returned in the venous blood for pulmonary or renal excretion. The regulation of blood glucose concentration is a complex process. Peripheral utilization of glucose depends largely on the presence of adequate supplies of insulin, but the secretions of the adrenal cortex, adrenal medulla, and pituitary and thyroid glands all play a part in regulating glucose mobilization and consumption.

Measurement

Measuring the blood glucose concentration aids in assessing the body's overall metabolic state, but any single determination must be related to the individual's dynamic physiologic condition. Blood glucose is measured in either the fasting or postprandial state, depending on the type of information desired. Most so-called normal values are for the fasting state.

The importance of glucose in metabolism has been recognized since ancient times, and many tests have been developed for measuring the sugar content of blood and urine. Two principal methods are now in use. One employs the reducing properties of the aldehyde group in glucose, and variations of this method employ different reactions to indicate the reducing effect. The second method employs the enzyme glucose oxidase which oxidizes the sugar and liberates by-products which then can be measured. Although the reducing methods have the advantage of historical precedent and extensive experience, the enzymatic method is more specific. Both methods require adequate control of physical and chemical variables to prevent distortion of the results.

REDUCING METHODS

The "reducing sugar" tests classically employ copper solutions and measure color change. Two methods are in wide use. For both the reduction methods, and for the glucose oxidase method as well, it is necessary to prepare a protein-free filtrate of the blood sample. For the Folin filtrate, sodium tungstate and sulfuric acid are used, while zinc sulfate and barium or sodium hydroxide are necessary to prepare the Somogyi filtrate. In the Folin filtrate, a proportion of nonglucose reducing substances remains in the filtrate, and these saccharoids give falsely high values in nonspecific tests for glucose. The error introduced remains constant, so that valid comparisons can be made against other determinations made with the same method. Confusion arises if the results from different methods must be compared, so it is advisable to know the particular method in use.

In the Folin-Wu glucose test, application of heat to a mixture of glucose and alkaline copper sulfate solution results in precipitation of cuprous oxide. Addition of phosphomolybdic acid permits the precipitate to dissolve into a colored solution, the intensity of which can be measured colorimetrically. In the Somogyi-Nelson determination, the reduced copper acts upon an arsenomolybdate preparation, and the color of the resulting complex is measured. In one widely used automated technique, the glucose reduces a copper-containing chelate, producing an intensely colored complex that can be measured readily.

ENZYMATIC METHOD

The product measured in the enzymatic reaction is hydrogen peroxide, a by-product of the enzymic conversion of glucose to gluconic acid. The peroxide is measured with a chromogenic indicator in the presence of peroxidase. A number of variables must be controlled with this method, including the temperature, pH, timing, and choice of indicators. Additionally, it is necessary to avoid or remove materials that inhibit enzymic activity. For these reasons, the values reported with the glucose oxidase method may vary from laboratory to laboratory, even though the reaction itself is quite specific.

Significance of Results

Normal values for blood glucose are considered to be 80 to 120 mg./dl. of whole blood for the Folin-Wu method and 65 to 95 mg./dl. of whole blood for the Somogyi-Nelson method. The values with the glucose oxidase method are approximately the same as for the Somogyi-Nelson method, although Fales[16] suggests 60 to 105 mg./dl. as a realistic range for normal fasting blood sugar values. Because the intracellular glucose concentration within red blood cells is lower than the plasma concentration, serum or plasma glucose levels run approximately 10 percent higher than those of whole blood.[16]

ELEVATED LEVELS

Hyperglycemia is the descriptive term for blood glucose concentrations greater than normal, and hypoglycemia describes lower than normal blood concentrations. Diabetes mellitus is the most frequent cause of marked hyperglycemia, but many other conditions may elevate the glucose level. Disorders of the pituitary gland and certain brain lesions may cause markedly elevated levels, and mildly diabetic levels may accompany Cushing's disease and hyperthyroidism. Any condition in which epinephrine is mobilized will be accompanied by hyperglycemia, usually of relatively mild degree. Examples include acute injury, convulsions, mental stress, and the adrenal tumor pheochromocytoma. Shock and severe hemorrhage cause initial hyperglycemia, but this may be followed by dangerous lowering of the blood glucose level. Acute and chronic infections, eclampsia, and hypertension are often accompanied by mild hyperglycemia, and overweight individuals tend to have high fasting blood sugar levels, possibly indicative of impaired insulin activity. Severe liver disease causes generalized alteration of carbohydrate metabolism, so that a glucose load is removed from the blood less rapidly than normal; but hypoglycemia can also occur since glucose is not adequately mobilized in response to falling blood sugar.

DEPRESSED LEVELS

Hypoglycemia is characteristic of hyperinsulinism due either to endogenous pancreatic lesions or to exogenous overdosage. Liver disease may cause episodic hypoglycemia, and some of the congenital deficiencies of carbohydrate-regulating enzymes may cause acute and chronic hypoglycemia. Hormonal deficiency of the adrenal, thyroid, or pituitary glands can cause chronically low blood glucose levels, and prolonged poor nutrition from any cause will lower blood sugar levels and deplete glycogen stores so that acute hypoglycemia cannot be compensated adequately.

The dynamics of carbohydrate metabolism are considered briefly in the chapter on endocrine function.

Urinary Glucose

Glucose levels in the urine often provide valuable clinical information. Glucose is not present in normal urine. Although it passes freely through the glomerular filter, there is virtually complete removal of the sugar from tubular urine, so that none appears in the excreted urine. As long as plasma levels do not exceed 160 to 190 mg./dl. the normal kidney can remove all the glucose from the glomerular filtrate. Beyond this renal threshold, complete resorption is no longer possible, and glucose appears in the excreted urine. Some individuals have congenital or acquired tubular defects, so that glucosuria occurs at much lower plasma glucose levels, but these conditions are readily distinguished from diabetes mellitus by demonstration of normal plasma glucose concentration.

Methods for measuring urinary glucose are similar to those for blood glucose, and both the reducing methods and the enzymatic method are currently used. Commercially prepared "instant" tests are available for screening urine sugars, employing either principle.

NITROGENOUS COMPOUNDS

Proteins constitute the bulk of nitrogen-containing compounds in the blood, their concentration per deciliter being measured in grams, while the remaining nitrogenous constituents are measured in milligrams. Serum proteins and plasma proteins are similar, except that plasma contains fibrinogen, while serum is the fluid portion that remains after fibrinogen has been converted to fibrin. Besides fibrinogen, the principal subdivisions of the protein group are albumin, the α-globulins, and β-globulin, all of which are produced in the liver, and the gamma globulins or immunoglobulins which derive from the lymphocyte-plasma cell system.

FIBRINOGEN

Fibrinogen is a large complex globulin with no known physiologic function except the formation of fibrin. Fibrin is the end product of blood coagulation, and it also participates in localized inflammatory reactions. Fibrinogen is manufactured by the liver, and plasma concentrations range from 200 to 400 mg./dl., tending to be slightly higher in women than in men. During pregnancy, fibrinogen values may go as high as 600 mg./dl. Elevated fibrinogen levels accompany many systemic or local infections and occur in multiple myeloma and nephrosis. A sudden decrease in plasma fibrinogen content may occur in episodes of intravascular clotting or disseminated fibrinolysis. These tend to take place when there is disruption or necrosis of tissue, and acquired hypofibrinogenemia may follow obstetrical accidents or extensive surgical procedures, especially those involving the lungs or urinary tract.

Serum Proteins

In healthy individuals, the serum contains between 6.0 and 8.5 gm. of protein per deciliter. Among the many techniques available for measuring proteins, the Kjeldahl method of measuring nitrogen content is usually considered the standard against which other methods are compared. In this method, the nitrogen is converted to ammonium ion which is measured by titration of ammonia into an acid solution of known strength. Total protein weight is calculated by multiplying the nitrogen content by 6.25, a somewhat arbitrary figure derived from the mean nitrogen content of representative human proteins. The Kjeldahl method is reliable and reproducible but requires an investment of time, space, and equipment that makes it unsuitable for multiple routine determinations.

NONSPECIFIC TECHNIQUES

Several quick methods are available for measuring total serum proteins when a high degree of accuracy is unnecessary. These include measurement of the specific gravity or of the refractive index of serum. Reliance on these methods depends on the assumption that no qualitatively abnormal proteins are present and that such other serum constituents as glucose, urea, and cholesterol are present in normal concentration.

BIURET REACTION

Perhaps the most common method for measuring proteins utilizes the biuret reaction. A blue compound forms when polypeptides of appropriate configuration combine with copper in an alkaline solution. The simplest nitrogenous compound to give this reaction is biuret, for which the prototype reaction has been named. The intensity of the color is proportional to the concentration of polypeptides. The biuret reaction, suitably modified, is used for automated determination of total protein. The accuracy of the determination is impaired if the protein solution is turbid, a problem often encountered with lipemic serum. High concentrations of bilirubin, bromsulphalein, or other pigments may interfere with the procedure, and hemolysis of the sample will falsely elevate the result by liberating normally intracellular hemoglobin into the serum sample.

PROTEIN PARTITION. Although the biuret reaction cannot, by itself, distinguish the various proteins in the sample, it can be used for separate quantitation of albumin and globulin. After the total protein concentration has been measured in a serum aliquot, the globulins can be removed from the sample by precipitation with sodium sulfate, with or without sodium sulfite. If the biuret reaction is repeated on the supernatant material, the albumin alone will be measured. The difference between total protein and albumin is reported as the globulin content. Certain cautions must be observed in the salting-out procedure, including adjustment of the salt concentration. If the serum is shaken excessively, some albumin may be denatured and precipitate with the globulin, while incomplete precipitation of globulins causes falsely high albumin values.

An automated technique for measuring albumin specifically puts to use the affinity between albumin and certain charged molecules. The product measured is a colored complex of albumin and an anionic dye, thereby avoiding the problems of salting-out globulins.

ELECTROPHORESIS

Electrophoresis provides the most generally satisfactory qualitative separation of serum protein. Since different proteins have different amino acid compositions, the isoelectric point of each protein is unique. Migration in an electric field varies with these physicochemical differences, and migration patterns can be plotted for the different groups of proteins. Although more precise work can be done with moving boundary techniques, electrophoresis on fixed media, such as paper, agar, or acrylamide gel, gives excellent separation into a number of protein components. These protein components can be quantitated either by eluting the proteins from the supporting medium and measuring them directly or by staining the preparation and measuring the relative intensity of each segment (see Figs. 14, 15, and 16). Since the staining method offers only comparative figures, the total serum protein content must be measured if the proportions are to be converted into absolute values. Immunoelectrophoresis, ultracentrifugation, peptide mapping, spectrophotometry, and other methods are available for more precise separation necessary in research contexts.

ALBUMIN. Albumin normally occupies between 52 and 68 percent of the total protein value; therefore, changes in albumin content affect total protein value more markedly than do changes in globulins. The more frequent direction of change is down; the albumin concentration is rarely increased except when dehydration and hemoconcentration occur. Disease of the liver, the site of albumin production, depresses serum albumin levels. This does not follow acute liver damage, because albumin has such a long half-disappearance time that several weeks of completely defective manufacture must elapse before pronounced drop occurs. Chronic liver disease is one of the most common causes of hypoalbuminemia. Since albumin contributes approximately 80 percent of the serum colloid osmotic pressure, marked hypoalbuminemia may so depress the colloid osmotic pressure that edema and transudation occur. Albumin production declines in such conditions of poor nutrition as advanced malignancy, malabsorption syndromes, starvation, or beriberi. Albumin levels are low in toxemia of pregnancy and in congestive heart failure, in which both impaired production and hypervolemic dilution may play a part. Low levels of albumin may result from excessive protein loss, either through the kidney as in nephrosis or severe nephritis, through the gastrointestinal tract as in protein-losing enteropathies, or through the skin as with extensive burns.

GLOBULINS. The globulins have been divided on the basis of their electrophoretic mobility into α_1, α_2, β_1, and γ fractions. The gamma globulins are the body's antibodies and are subject to considerable variation in disease states. The alpha and beta globulins change significantly in relatively few states and tend as a group to reflect altered liver function. Patients with constitutionally deficient α_1-antitrypsin (see p. 384) have noticeable reduction of protein in the α_1 band.

Low levels of gamma globulins can occur as a congenital abnormality or as an acquired deficiency. In either case, the patient suffers frequent bacterial infections because the normal immunologic defenses are impaired. Diseases that affect lymphocytes and plasma cells, such as lymphoma, myeloma, or macroglobulinemia, may cause deficiencies of functioning antibody gamma globulin even though there may be an increase in nonfunctional, abnormal globulin fractions.

Chronic infections of any kind—bacterial, fungal, or protozoal— produce high levels of gamma globulins. These specific antibodies often can be identified and measured serologically. Nonspecific elevations of gamma globulin occur in all types of chronic liver disease, in many connective tissue disorders, in far-advanced carcinoma, and in lymphomas and leukemias.

High levels of abnormal globulins occur in the so-called gammopathies, diseases of the lymphocytic and plasmacytic system. These abnormal proteins can be identified in a variety of ways, of which the simplest is electrophoresis. Electrophoresis readily demonstrates the existence of circulating abnormal globulins, but immunoelectrophoresis and other immunologic techniques often permit the identification of their nature and specificity, if any (see below).

A/G RATIO. The ratio of albumin to globulin (A/G ratio) was considered a useful measurement before the development of accurate protein fractionation. It merely gives the proportion of the two types of protein measured in the salting-out procedure described earlier. Since many diseases affect both albumin and globulin, and since the A/G ratio can be affected by changes in either or both, it is an imprecise piece of information at best. Even without the detailed information available from electrophoresis, it is preferable to express albumin and globulin in absolute terms and permit the observer to draw his own conclusions.

IMMUNOELECTROPHORESIS

Electrophoretic separation of proteins derives from differences in size and electrical charge of different categories of proteins. The resulting bands, although susceptible to quantification, tell nothing about their constituent elements. When the separated protein bands are reacted with antibodies against known individual proteins or sub-categories, more detailed partition develops. Thus haptoglobin and ceruloplasmin, both of which migrate as α_2 globulins, can be demonstrated individually as separate precipitin arcs with appropriate antiserums.

The selection of antiserum depends upon the number and nature of proteins sought. Antiserums can be raised against classes of immunoglobulins, against functionally specific proteins, against abnormal protein constituents, or against whole serum or some fraction thereof, which results in a mixture of antibodies. By comparing the patient's results with a normal control or an appropriately quantitated standard, one can observe the number of separate precipitin lines and roughly quantitate the amount of each constituent. This procedure also is used to demonstrate whether a protein-containing solution has one or several different constituents.

Immunoelectrophoresis is especially useful for documenting suspected deficiencies of specific proteins, such as transferrin and thyroid-binding globulin, and for investigating qualitatively abnormal globulins. The electrophoretogram provides a starting point by showing the location of abnormality—a tall, narrow peak indicates a quantity of physically homogeneous material moving at a single rate, while a broader hump results from a heterogeneous group of molecules with various rates of migration.

MONOCLONAL PATTERNS. The single, well-defined peak is usually associated with neoplasms of antibody-producing cells. The unitary nature of the spike and its light or heavy chain class, or both, are identified by immunoelectrophoresis. Immunoelectrophoresis also clarifies possibly confusing patterns; for example, it can distinguish a paraprotein from fibrinogen or from excess lipoproteins, mucoproteins, or glycoproteins arising from carcinomas, or IgG denatured by sample aging or uremia.[34]

The conditions characterized by these electrophoretic spikes are sometimes called monoclonal gammopathies, emphasizing that the offspring of a single cell multiply to form the neoplasm. The term gammopathy, however, is misleading. While approximately 55 percent of myelomas produce globulins of the IgG class, 22 to 28 percent produce IgA, and small percentages produce IgM or IgD globulins.[34] Lymphomas, lymphocytic leukemia, Waldenström's macroglobulinemia, and cold agglutinin disease also can produce paraprotein spikes, while up to 2 percent of the aging population may have paraproteins (usually IgM) without any associated disease.[2]

POLYCLONAL PATTERNS. The increased serum globulin pattern that creates a broad, irregularly contoured hump on electrophoresis is sometimes called a polyclonal gammopathy. These multispecific protein patterns reflect the stimulation of many different cells, producing immunoglobulins of different specificities and different physicochemical characteristics. Even immunization against a single bacterium results in multiple antibodies, since bacteria possess numerous separable antigenic constituents. Antibodies of different immunoglobulin classes, or of different binding constants within the same class, may result from a single immunizing event.

Chronic infections with specific agents, such as parasitic infestations, leprosy, lymphogranuloma venereum, and intrauterine syphilis or viral infections, produce a polyclonal pattern with identifiable reactivity. More challenging are the broad, so-called nonspecific hyperglobulinemias associated with chronic liver disease, sarcoidosis, autoimmune diseases, far-advanced carcinomas, and other long-standing necrotizing processes. Although immunoelectrophoresis or immunoglobulin quantitation by radial diffusion may characterize the relative amounts of increased immunoglobulin, it is not presently possible to draw diagnostic conclusions from these patterns.

Nonprotein Nitrogenous Compounds

THE NPN DETERMINATION

The nitrogen remaining in the protein-free filtrate can be measured by the Kjeldahl method used for determining the amount of protein nitrogen, using materials and equipment for milligram quantities. In practice, however, this is rarely done. Nonprotein nitrogen (NPN) is usually measured as the derived ammonia, which is quantitated by nesslerization or by reaction with alkaline hypochlorite (Bertholet reaction). Normal values for nonprotein nitrogen are approximately 25 to 40 mg./dl. Approximately 55 percent of the nonprotein nitrogen comes from urea, the other components being uric acid, creatinine, ammonia, and free amino acids. Since each of these components, including urea, can be determined separately, the value of the NPN determination is somewhat limited. The nonurea constituents change only within a rather narrow range, and specific measurement provides more sensitive information about these variations. Changing urea values affect the NPN most significantly, although uric acid and creatinine values often are altered by conditions that affect urea concentration.

UREA

Urea, the end product of protein metabolism, is produced only in the liver. From its hepatic origin, urea travels through the blood to the kidneys for urinary excretion. Two general methods are used for measuring urea; in both, the results are expressed as milligrams of urea nitrogen, rather than as total urea. In the monoxime method, urea combines with diacetyl monoxime to give a yellow compound which can be measured colorimetrically. In the enzyme method, urease hydrolyzes urea to CO_2 and NH_3, and the resulting ammonia can be measured by nesslerization or the Bertholet reaction. Although the urease method is indirect, in that a metabolite rather than urea itself is measured, it is probably more reliable than the monoxime method, in which the reaction between urea concentration and colored product may not be linear. The monoxime method has been adapted, with generally satisfactory results, to automated performance.

The normal value for blood urea nitrogen (BUN) ranges from 5 to 25 mg./dl. Values tend to be slightly higher in males than in females, and persons with unusually high protein intake may have BUN levels at the high end of the scale. There is, however, no significant postprandial change. Urea production rarely declines to any measurable extent, except after loss of 80 to 85 percent of hepatic function.[60] Low values for urea concentration usually reflect expanded blood volume rather than diminished production.

UREMIA. The commonest cause of high BUN values (uremia) is renal disease which may be either acute or chronic. All the inflammatory, degenerative, congenital, traumatic, or neoplastic ills that affect the kidney may cause uremia, and the degree of uremia provides a rough index to the severity of the condition. Urinary obstruction at any site can cause uremia. Probably the commonest cause of urinary obstruction is prostatic enlargement, but congenital anomalies, tumors, calculi, pregnancy, or scarring can impair urinary flow. Uremia also can result from conditions not directly related to the kidney or urinary tract. Whenever there is increased protein catabolism, increased urea will be formed; if the same problem also decreases renal blood flow or urine production, blood levels of urea will rise. The list of such conditions includes burns, with subsequent fluid loss; massive hemorrhage into the body cavities or soft tissues; infarction or other accidents to the viscera; pancreatitis; severe diabetic ketoacidosis; and far-advanced carcinoma, with tumor necrosis and cachexia. For

all of these external conditions, appropriate diagnostic and therapeutic measures should be instituted promptly, not because the
uremia itself is life-threatening, but because the primary condition
is dangerous.

URIC ACID

Degradation of nucleic acids leads to uric acid formation, and dietary
and endogenous purines are the principal sources. Two methods are
used to measure blood and urine uric acid. The colorimetric method
measures the blue compound formed by the reducing action of uric
acid upon alkaline phosphotungstate. This approach is used in certain
automated systems.

A more sensitive, reliable method uses spectrophotometric absorption. Uric acid has a characteristic absorbance peak at 292 μ.
The absorbance of the sample is measured before and after treatment with the enzyme uricase, which converts uric acid to allantoin,
which does not absorb at this wavelength. The concentration of uric
acid in the specimen can be calculated from the difference between
pretreatment and post-treatment absorbance.

There is some controversy about the normal range of serum uric
acid concentration. This is sometimes given as 6.9 to 7.5 mg./dl. for
men and 5.7 to 6.6 mg./dl. for women,[72] but many authorities consider as significantly elevated values above 7.0 mg./dl. for men and
6.0 mg./dl. for women.[7] Impaired renal function depresses uric acid
excretion, and the most frequent cause of high serum levels of uric
acid is severe renal disease.

ABNORMAL SERUM URATES. Secondary hyperuricemia is more
common than primary hyperuricemia from gout or other metabolic
diseases involving purine metabolism. In renal failure, the kidneys
cannot excrete nitrogenous wastes, and serum uric acid levels rise,
as do the BUN and serum creatinine levels. Temporary depression of
urate excretion also may elevate serum urates. This occurs with high
circulating levels of lactic acid or ketone bodies, in such conditions
as shock, alcoholism, diabetic ketosis, starvation, or certain glycogen storage diseases. Urate excretion also is depressed by thiazide
diuretics and prolonged low doses of aspirin.[55] Certain x-ray contrast
media and other drugs may increase uricosuria markedly, causing
decreased serum urate level but sometimes producing renal damage
from the urates which precipitate out of the supersaturated urine.
Many drugs cause temporary or spurious elevation of urate results.

L-dopa, alpha-methyldopa, ascorbic acid, thiazides, furosemide, and propylthiouracil may lead to serum urate values high enough to cause clinical concern. Before embarking on a large-scale diagnostic attack, one should repeat the test after the drugs have been discontinued.[58]

A large proportion of patients with gout have relatively impaired urate excretion, but also suffer overproduction. Of primary causes for hyperuricemia, gout is by far the commonest. Whenever nucleic acid turnover is rapid, serum urates rise. In chronic myelogenous leukemia, prolonged hemolytic conditions, and inefficient erythropoiesis, uric acid values are persistently high. Acute elevations, sometimes at dangerously nephrotoxic levels, may follow vigorous cytolytic therapy for leukemia and other neoplasms. Infectious mononucleosis and psoriasis may also produce hyperuricemia, presumably due to impaired renal excretion.

AMMONIA

Ammonia, another end product of protein metabolism, is formed from the action of bacteria on the proteins in the intestinal contents. Some ammonia also derives from hydrolysis of glutamine in the kidneys. Ammonia is detoxified in the liver where it is converted to urea. The small quantity of ammonia in the blood is presumably the material in transit from gut and kidneys to the liver. The ammonia in urine does not arise directly from the blood ammonia, but is rather the result of tubular processes for the excretion of H^+ ions as NH_4^+.

Methods for measuring serum ammonia are only moderately accurate. These depend upon liberating ammonia from the sample and then using titration or colorimetry to measure the quantity liberated. The normal range in whole blood samples is 75 to 200 μg. of ammonia per deciliter, while values for plasma are somewhat lower, ranging from 56 to 122 μg./dl.[59] Blood levels vary with dietary intake of protein, and blood should be drawn when the patient is in a fasting condition.

Blood ammonia determinations are used for evaluating the progress of severe liver disease. Since ammonia is removed by the liver, hepatocellular damage may permit blood ammonia levels to rise. In patients with impaired hepatic function, blood ammonia levels can be lowered somewhat by reducing protein intake and by administering antibiotics to reduce the population of intestinal bacteria.

CREATININE

Creatinine is the anhydride of creatine. Creatine exists in skeletal muscle as creatine phosphate, a high-energy compound that functions in reversible energy reactions involving adenosine triphosphate (ATP) and the enzyme creatine phosphokinase. Conversion of creatine to creatinine is nonenzymatic and irreversible. The serum creatinine level reflects total body supplies of creatine and does not vary significantly with exercise or with diet. Individuals with large muscle mass have higher serum creatinine levels than those with less muscle. Normal values for men are slightly higher than those for women, but the overall normal range is between 0.8 and 1.4 mg./dl.

Creatinine is excreted through the kidneys in quantities proportional to the serum content. Creatinine measurements are most useful in evaluating renal function. By comparing serum creatinine concentration with the total quantity excreted within a given time, one can calculate the *creatinine clearance*. This indicates the efficiency with which the kidneys remove creatinine from the blood, and declining renal function leads to declining values for creatinine clearance. As renal function diminishes, serum creatinine rises, but the rise is less acute than the change in BUN. Serum creatinine may be normal in some cases of acute uremia or mild chronic renal disease, but an elevated serum creatinine value indicates severe, long-standing renal impairment.

CREATINE. Determination of serum and urine creatine is technically more difficult than determination of creatinine, and it is used principally in evaluating muscle disorders. Normally not more than 0.5 to 0.95 mg./dl. of creatine is present in serum. This increases only if degenerative disease of the skeletal muscle releases normally intracellular creatine into the blood. Moreover, creatine normally is not present in urine at levels above 250 mg. per day and is present in significant quantities only in degenerative muscle diseases, notably the muscular dystrophies.

CALCIUM AND PHOSPHORUS

Calcium and phosphorus are discussed together because the two elements are closely associated physiologically. Most of the body's supplies of both minerals exist in the skeleton, but each element has other physiologic functions as well. Calcium ions affect neuro-muscular excitability and cellular and capillary permeability and are necessary for blood coagulation. Phosphorus, in the form of phosphate, is an essential part of energy storage compounds; nucleic acids; intermediary metabolites of carbohydrates and lipids; the enzyme 2,3-DPG, which controls release of oxygen from hemoglobin; and phospholipids that confer structural integrity on cell membranes.[41] Serum inorganic phosphorus levels are measured in terms of the phosphate ions, for ionized free phosphorus does not circulate. The skeleton serves as a storehouse for these elements, and serum values are maintained at the expense of the skeletal minerals.

Physiologic Considerations

Parathyroid hormone promotes phosphate excretion and maintains serum calcium levels. Its secretion is regulated by changes in circulating calcium levels. Since serum calcium and phosphorus levels tend to vary reciprocally, parathormone can raise serum calcium levels by promoting urinary phosphate loss. In addition, it may mobilize calcium from bone directly.

Calcium and phosphorus are absorbed from the small intestine, and adequate supplies of vitamin D are necessary for optimum epithelial transport. Calcium absorption is inhibited if the intestinal contents are too alkaline to permit complete solution of the calcium salts. Malabsorption syndromes, steatorrhea, and prolonged diarrhea lessen absorption by impairing vitamin D absorption and by removing available calcium through soap linkage with fatty acids.

Both calcium and phosphorus are excreted in the urine, the excretion being regulated by active metabolic processes in the tubular epithelium. When renal damage impairs tubular function, rising serum phosphate levels testify to moderate or severe renal disease. This serum phosphate excess depresses serum calcium values, thus stimulating parathormone production in an attempt to increase phosphate excretion.

Measurement

PHOSPHORUS

Laboratory measurement of serum phosphate depends upon the reaction of phosphorus with molybdic acid, giving a phosphomolybdate complex. Subsequent reduction of this phosphomolybdate complex produces a blue compound which can be measured colorimetrically and in automated procedures. Because the reduced compound may reoxidize within a relatively short period, the procedure requires careful timing. The nature of the reducing agent varies in different methods, and a consistent reducing potential must be maintained if determinations are to be consistently accurate. Serum for phosphate determination should be separated rather promptly from the cells to avoid artefactual alteration as a result of continuing glycolytic activity. Normal levels are between 2.5 and 4.5 mg./dl. in adults and between 4.5 and 6.5 mg./dl. in growing children.

CALCIUM

Several methods are employed for measuring calcium, but none is completely satisfactory. The flame photometer can be used, but both positive and negative interference can result from the presence of other inorganic ions. The commonest indirect method involves precipitating calcium ions from solution as calcium oxalate and then measuring the amount of oxalate in the precipitate. In a variation of this method, a calcium phosphate precipitate is used, and the phosphate is measured. In still another method, the presence of calcium ions is signalled by the characteristic color assumed by an indicator substance in the presence of dissociated calcium ions. Titration with a chelating agent, which removes ionized calcium from solution, produces a color change when all the free calcium is bound. This method suffers from interference from other metal ions and from colored compounds, such as bilirubin or hemoglobin, in the serum. There is also some difficulty in obtaining sharp end points. A widely used automated procedure measures the colored complex formed between calcium and an alkaline earth dye. With a fluorescent indicator complex, the end point can be read fluorometrically. Atomic absorption spectrophotometry also is used for calcium determinations.

Normal values for calcium are given in either milligrams per deciliter or milliequivalents per liter. These range from 9 to 11 mg/dl. or from 4.5 to 5.5 mEq./L. Conversion is easily done because calcium's molecular weight and valence of 2 permit rapid calculation. A summary of the chemical features of diseases with disturbed plasma calcium and phosphate is given in Table 13.

Table 13. Summary of Chemical Features of Diseases with Disturbed Plasma Calcium and Phosphate*

Disease	Serum			Urine	
	Calcium	Phosphate	Alkaline Phosphatase	Calcium	Phosphate
Hyperparathyroidism	Increased	Decreased	Normal or increased	Increased	Increased
Paget's disease	Normal	Normal	Increased	Normal	Normal
Hypoparathyroidism	Decreased	Increased	Normal	Decreased	Decreased
Renal insufficiency	Decreased	Increased	Normal or increased	Decreased	Decreased
Osteomalacia	Decreased or normal	Decreased	Increased	Decreased	Decreased
Senile osteoporosis	Normal	Normal	Normal	Normal	Normal
Multiple myeloma	Normal to increased	Normal	Normal	Normal to increased	Normal to decreased
Milk-alkali syndrome	Increased	Normal to increased	Normal	Normal to decreased	Normal to decreased
Vitamin D intoxication	Increased	Increased	Normal	Increased	Decreased
Metastatic carcinoma	Normal to increased	Normal	Normal to increased	Increased	Normal
Sarcoidosis	Increased	Normal to increased	Normal to increased	Increased	Decreased
Hyperventilation (alkalosis)	Normal	Normal	Normal	Normal	Normal

*From Bernstein, D. S., and Thorn, G. W., in Wintrobe, M. M., et al. (eds.): *Harrison's Principles of Internal Medicine*. ed. 6. McGraw-Hill, New York, 1970.

Significant Alterations

HYPERCALCEMIA

Hypercalcemia is most conspicuous in hyperparathyroidism, which may produce calcium values as high as 18 mg./dl. Hypervitaminosis D also causes high serum calcium. In secondary hyperparathyroidism, parathyroid oversecretion occurs in response to an initially lowered calcium level, so the degree of hypercalcemia is rather mild, while the phosphate values are markedly elevated. Hypercalcemia may accompany any condition of bone demineralization, such as multiple myeloma, extensive osseous metastases, or prolonged immobilization leading to bone atrophy. Cancers of breast and lung are the neoplasms most often associated with increased circulating calcium.[47] Sarcoidosis occasionally causes hypercalcemia, and high levels of serum calcium can occur in the milk-alkali syndrome. A problem of differential diagnosis may arise here, because peptic ulceration is a moderately common complication of hyperparathyroidism. Thus the ulcer pain which impels the patient toward overmedication with milk and alkalis may be the presenting symptom of an undiagnosed condition which is the real cause of the hypercalcemia.

HYPOCALCEMIA

Hypocalcemia accompanies hypoparathyroidism and the various conditions described as pseudohypoparathyroidism and pseudo-pseudohypoparathryoidism. In vitamin D deficiency and vitamin D-resistant rickets, low calcium is the rule, and in steatorrhea and pancreatitis, the serum calcium may be low because calcium soaps are formed. In conditions of decreased serum proteins, total serum calcium values will be low, even though the content of ionized calcium may be perfectly normal. Loss of proteins through nephrosis, liver disease, or other diseases removes the binding material for the bound portion of the serum calcium but does not affect the vital physiologic functions served by ionized calcium.

PHOSPHATE ABNORMALITIES

The commonest cause of high serum phosphate levels is renal failure, and values above 8 mg./dl. usually indicate severe renal disease. Hypervitaminosis D and hypoparathyroidism also may cause hyperphosphatemia.

Serum phosphate levels fall if there is massive shift of the ion from extracellular to intracellular fluid. This occurs when rising serum glucose levels provoke increased insulin activity or when large doses of insulin are administered to correct diabetic hyperglycemia.[40] Alcohol abuse causes increased urinary phosphate excretion, a process accentuated by the metabolic acidosis that alcoholics often exhibit. Hospital treatment of alcoholism may convert chronic phosphate depletion to acute hypophosphatemia, with levels as low as 0.5 to 1.0 mg./dl., if rehydration and intravenous nutrients stimulate rapid glycolysis and cause phosphates to enter peripheral cells.[41]

Chronically low serum phosphate levels occur in hyperparathyroidism and vitamin D deficiency. Intestinal malabsorption syndromes deplete body phosphorus and, if steatorrhea is severe, severe calcium loss also may occur. Steatorrhea is one of the few conditions in which both serum calcium and serum phosphate are low. The chronic hypocalcemia may provoke parathyroid hyperactivity, which, in turn, causes additional phosphate excretion.

LIPIDS

Lipid Categories

Although plasma contains many lipid constituents, only cholesterol and triglycerides provide quantitative data useful in clinical management of atherosclerotic disease. *Free fatty acids* contribute little to the numerical total when total lipids are measured—only 25 mg. in the 350 to 800 mg. of total lipids present in 100 ml. of plasma. Free fatty acids can be used as an energy source. Plasma levels and total turnover increase in starvation, in pregnancy, and in poorly controlled diabetic states. *Phospholipids,* notably lecithin and sphingomyelin, are present at concentrations of 150 to 375 mg./dl. Their function in plasma remains unclear, although they are highly significant in membrane structure and function.

TRIGLYCERIDES

Triglycerides consist of three fatty acids esterified to glycerol. Many triglycerides are synthesized by the intestinal mucosa, which absorbs dietary fatty acids and disposes of them in this way. Newly formed triglycerides travel from the intestines to the rest of the body in *chylomicrons,* spherical particles which cause turbidity of the medium when they are evenly dispersed, but rise to the top of an aqueous medium if allowed to settle. Digesting a heavy meal causes a prompt rise in triglycerides and chylomicrons, but normally these are cleared rapidly from the circulation. Triglycerides provide heart and skeletal muscle with much of their energy supply. Excess triglycerides are metabolized by the liver or are stored in adipose tissue. The liver also manufactures triglycerides; most of these reflect secondary metabolic processes rather than direct digestive events. Hepatic triglycerides do not travel as chylomicrons. They form the major constituent of *very low-density lipoproteins* (VLDL), complex molecules with a relative density of 0.93 to 1.006, which also contain cholesterol and several proteins.

CHOLESTEROL

Cholesterol is a complex alcohol essential in cell membrane composition and a precursor for many steroid hormones. Although all cells have the capability of synthesizing cholesterol, nearly all circulating cholesterol derives either from liver, which manufactures it, or intestine, which absorbs it. Cholesterol circulates largely in *low-density lipoproteins* (*LDL*), which transport dietary cholesterol to the liver and other tissues, and hepatic cholesterol to the rest of the body. Dietary intake tends to be 100 to 500 mg. daily, but the level of cholesterol metabolized each day is 2 gm. or more. Some circulating cholesterol is found in *high-density lipoproteins* (*HDL*), which seem to function as the transport medium that carries cholesterol from the periphery back to the liver. The liver is the only known site for cholesterol esterification and excretion.

LIPOPROTEIN CLASSES

Lipids are nonpolar and are immiscible with water. In plasma, an aqueous medium, lipids travel as complex molecules containing several proteins and a variety of lipid components. Lipoproteins fall into several categories. *Chylomicrons,* which comprise the first class, have a relative density of 0.93 or less and a half-life, in the circulation, of about 4 minutes. These consist almost entirely of dietary triglycerides. *Very low-density lipoproteins* (or pre-beta lipoproteins) derive from the liver and carry hepatic triglycerides and cholesterol to the periphery. They have a relative density of 0.93 to 1.006 and a circulatory half-life of 4 to 8 hours. Upon losing their triglycerides, VLDLs become intermediate-density (IDL) and then *low-density lipoproteins* (or beta-lipoproteins). The LDL group consists very largely of cholesterol, synthesized in the liver and traveling to peripheral cells of all types. LDLs have relative density of between 1.006 and 1.063 and have a plasma half-life of 3 days. Membranes of peripheral cells have specific LDL receptors,[17] by means of which the cells ingest cholesterol and protein. Cholesterol is an essential cellular constituent; intracellular levels regulate both intracellular metabolic activity and the surface interaction between membrane receptors and LDL. The heaviest molecules are the *high-density lipoproteins* (HDL), or alpha-lipoproteins, the function of which consists of inbound transportation of cholesterol from the periphery to the liver.

Different lipoproteins migrate electrophoretically at different rates. The *lipoprotein phenotype* establishes, by electrophoresis, the proportion of different classes present. Lipoprotein phenotyping has shown some promise of establishing rational diagnostic categories for different constitutional and acquired diseases. Recent work, however, suggests that measuring only triglycerides, total cholesterol, and the cholesterol present in HDL provides enough information to classify most lipid-related diseases.[29,37]

Measurement

Both cholesterol and triglycerides are measured best by automated enzyme techniques. The cholesterol content in HDL can be measured directly once the HDL fraction has been isolated, either by ultracentrifugation or by precipitation. Analytic methods have reasonably good reproducibility, provided that the techniques are strictly followed. Physiologic fluctuations cause far greater discrepancies than analytic variations. Day-to-day changes in cholesterol level can be as high as 10 percent in the same individual,[27] and triglycerides can vary by 15 to 25 percent. These, it should be noted, are changes occurring when test conditions are strictly standardized.

PREPARATION OF THE PATIENT

Valid lipid determinations require a 12- to 14-hour fast before the specimen is drawn. Because dietary fat intake promptly and directly affects triglyceride level, a fasting baseline is necessary. The patient should be relaxed and seated for at least 10 minutes. Either serum or plasma can be used; EDTA is the anticoagulant of choice if plasma is used. Physical and pharmacologic stress affect lipid levels. If there is more than a casual interest in the results, it is desirable to control conditions for some time before making the determination. If possible, the patient should avoid thyroid medication, steroidal contraceptives, or lipid-lowering drugs for 3 weeks[73] and should not have gained or lost weight in the preceding month. Since myocardial infarction causes an increase in very low-density lipoproteins and a fall in low-density lipoproteins,[73] it is inappropriate to perform lipid studies while a patient is hospitalized for a heart attack.

NORMAL CHOLESTEROL VALUES

Disagreement exists about the lipid levels that should be considered "normal." Most workers believe that the average levels observed in an unselected, seemingly healthy, middle-aged American population are undesirably high. Age-adjusted average values for cholesterol and triglycerides follow an upward trend with increasing age, but this does not necessarily indicate "normal" physiologic processes. In large prospective population studies, cholesterol values are modestly valuable in predicting risk of subsequent coronary artery disease, with risk increasing substantially at total levels above 250 mg./dl. Recent conclusions drawn from the Framingham study suggest that 200 mg./dl. should be considered the upper desirable level for total cholesterol.[37]

HIGH-DENSITY LIPOPROTEINS

Much recent interest has centered on the high-density lipoprotein level as a predictor of coronary disease. High HDL levels seem to signify low risk of coronary disease, while low HDL levels indicate high risk.[26] When HDLs are separated and their cholesterol content measured separately (HLD-C), it has been shown that persons with HDL-C below 35 mg./dl. have a risk of future coronary events eight times that noted in persons with HDL-C levels above 65 mg./dl. Statistically, the biggest dividing line came between the 35 to 44 mg./dl. group, which had a high risk, and the 45 to 54 mg./dl. group, whose risk was much lower. Women have higher HDL-C levels, at all ages, than men of comparable age. High associations occur between low HDL-C values and obesity and diabetes. Levels of physical exercise correlate in direct proportion to HDL-C; the effect of alcohol on HDL-C remains controversial, and cigarette smoking seems to have no effect.

In patients with high total cholesterol, most of the cholesterol resides in the LDL fraction (LDL-C), but there is relatively little direct correlation between LDL-C and risk of coronary events.[26] It is obviously rash to assign to any one cholesterol level the status of "normal." It is probably prudent to consider total cholesterol levels between 250 and 300 mg./dl. to be worrisome and anything above 300 mg./dl. at any age to be excessive.

TRIGLYCERIDE LEVELS

Triglycerides usually are measured indirectly by hydrolyzing the esters and then measuring glycerol. A wide normal range exists, with some increase in observed average values with increased age. One suggested range extends to 150 mg./dl. in persons under age 40 and to 190 mg./dl. in those over age 50,[28] but others consider 300 mg./dl. as the level at which active concern becomes necessary.[27]

Triglycerides exist primarily in chylomicrons and very low-density lipoproteins (VLDL). The triglyceride level can be estimated usefully by observing a refrigerated serum or plasma sample. After 8 to 12 hours at 4° C., serum should be clear. Fasting blood should be free of chylomicrons, since these carry dietary fatty acids. If excessive chylomicrons are present, there will be a creamy top layer; this is always abnormal in a fasting specimen. When VLDL levels are excessive, the refrigerated sample is uniformly turbid. Cholesterol content and LDL levels cannot be estimated by this rough-and-ready approach.

Disease Associations

The reason for studying blood lipids is to assess the likelihood, in individuals or populations, that there will be clinically significant atherosclerotic cardiovascular disease. Blood lipids fall in hyper-thyroidism, malabsorption syndromes, and severe liver disease, and rise with diabetes and hypothyroidism, but lipid evaluation plays only a small role in diagnosing these disorders. Although everyone agrees that blood lipids and atherosclerosis are intimately associated, there is little agreement about direct causal mechanisms and still less agreement about the ways in which therapeutic intervention can affect vascular disease, if it can do so at all.

GENETIC CONSIDERATIONS

Some lipid disorders follow a clearly familial distribution, and the nature of the genetic defect is known. The most common and most thoroughly studied lipid disorder is familial hypercholesterolemia (Type II hyperlipidemia). This monogenic condition occurs in 1 to 5 per 1000 population and causes severe, early atherosclerosis, especially of the coronary arteries. In addition, cholesterol deposits occur frequently in skin and tendons. Homozygotes have cholesterol levels of 600 to 800 mg./dl., or higher, and begin having symptomatic vascular disease by their late teens. Heterozygotes have cholesterol levels between 300 and 600 mg./dl. and suffer accelerated adult-onset atherosclerotic disease. The defect seems to reside, at least in part, in the membrane receptors for LDL, so that intracellular cholesterol metabolism and regulation are disrupted.[6] Triglyceride levels, chylomicron metabolism, and enzyme activities are all normal. Although serum cholesterol can be reduced modestly by treatment with drugs or ileal bypass surgery, it is not clear whether this improves the course of the vascular disease.

Hereditary deficiency of lipoprotein lipase is another clearly characterized disorder, caused by a rare autosomal recessive. Triglycerides and chylomicrons are significantly elevated, and there is pronounced predisposition to crises of abdominal pain and pancreatitis. Restriction of dietary fat intake reduces chylomicron levels, but the compensatory high carbohydrate intake needed to provide calories causes increased endogenous production of triglycerides.

Lipid metabolism reflects not only genetic factors, but also such acquired influences as diet, exercise, hormonal disorders, drugs, and intercurrent diseases. In addition, there is interconversion between carbohydrates and lipids, and instability among proportions of different lipoprotein classes. These factors make it extremely difficult to delineate precisely characterized disease categories, let alone to trace their occurrence in family members.

PROGNOSTIC CONSIDERATIONS

Confusion has long existed in attempts to correlate cholesterol and/or triglyceride levels with vascular disease or coronary morbidity. A general association exists between increasing serum cholesterol levels and increasing risk of vascular disease, but the situation is by no means clear-cut. Both hypertension and impaired glucose tolerance significantly affect disease incidence and seriously confound the significance of cholesterol alone.[37] Triglyceride levels, by themselves, have little predictive value. In association with cholesterol levels, they may clarify the nature of certain genetic predispositions, but many persons with shifting elevations of one or both values are difficult to classify. Recent emphasis on HDL cholesterol carries interesting connotations for future work, but this test is not, as yet, widely available.

Perhaps the most vexing issue of all is treatment. Since no one knows what causes the lipid disturbances, or how the lipid disturbances cause vascular disease, it is difficult to make rational therapeutic decisions. Drugs, diet, and exercise have their passionate proponents and equally passionate detractors. In consequence, it would be foolhardy to attempt to discuss such complex problems in this chapter.

Lipoprotein Lipase Activity

Lipoprotein lipase clears triglycerides from circulating plasma. Its particular target is dietary triglycerides in the chylomicrons. It differs from pancreatic lipase in its sites of production and storage, its site of action, and its diagnostic significance. Pancreatic lipase is found in serum only following damage to its parent organ, but serum lipoprotein lipase activity occurs in normal and many hyperlipidemic individuals following heparin injection. This activity, called postheparin lipolytic activity, or clearing factor, is deficient in patients with Type I hyperlipidemia and may be reduced in nephrotic syndrome, hypothyroidism, severe alcoholism, and following prolonged low fat intake.

BILIRUBIN

Bilirubin is the predominant pigment of human bile which causes the characteristic golden yellow color. Bilirubin is formed from hemoglobin of destroyed erythrocytes by the reticuloendothelial system, including the Kupffer cells of the liver. It is, therefore, found normally at a level of about 0.7 mg./dl. en route to the liver for excretion. The polygonal cells of the liver have nothing to do with the production of this pigment, but they do withdraw it from the blood and excrete it in the bile. In cases of hemorrhage into connective tissue and serous cavities, hemoglobin is converted directly into bilirubin. Following such hemorrhage, hyperbilirubinemia may develop.

The Liver

It should be recognized that there is a difference between the bilirubin before (prehepatic) and after (posthepatic) it has passed through the liver cells. Bilirubin that has passed through the polygonal cells of the liver is more dialyzable, more oxidizable, more readily absorbed by precipitated protein, and is not soluble in chloroform. Within the liver, bilirubin is enzymatically conjugated with glucuronic acid, and the characteristic posthepatic form of bilirubin is actually bilirubin diglucuronide. Because of its ability to cross membranes, only posthepatic bilirubin appears in the urine. Newborn infants, whose livers have inadequate enzyme levels, are poorly equipped to convert bilirubin to the glucuronide. As a result, most of the circulating bilirubin is of the prehepatic type in hemolytic disease of the newborn.

THE DIAZO REACTION

Prehepatic and posthepatic forms of bilirubin are distinguished by the different manner in which they react with diazo reagents. In the van den Bergh reaction, sulfanilic acid and bilirubin—in the presence of nitrous acid—undergo a diazo reaction to form pink azobilirubin, which can be measured colorimetrically. Posthepatic bilirubin, the glucuronide, participates in this reaction in an aqueous medium, while the prehepatic, unconjugated form reacts only after addition of methyl alcohol. This procedural necessity has produced another set of terms to describe the different forms of bilirubin. Since the posthepatic form reacts promptly when the reagents are added, it is called direct-acting bilirubin; the prehepatic form, which requires methyl alcohol as an additional reagent, is called the indirect form. In Table 14, certain features of the two types of bilirubin are listed. Normal total serum bilirubin ranges between 1.0 and 1.5 mg./dl., varying somewhat from laboratory to laboratory. Of this, no more than 0.3 to 0.5 mg. is ordinarily in the posthepatic form.

Differential Diagnosis

The separation of bilirubin into prehepatic and posthepatic forms appears to offer a splendid means of differentiating the various etiologies of jaundice. Jaundice simply refers to the yellow coloration imparted by increased circulating bilirubin. In theory, it would appear that an increase in posthepatic bilirubin must derive from obstruction of the biliary tract, through which conjugated bilirubin must pass on its way from the liver into the intestinal lumen. Conversely, an increase in prehepatic bilirubin implies hepatic inability to keep up with the input of newly formed bilirubin, owing either to hepatic in-

Table 14. The Two Types of Bilirubin

Type of Bilirubin	Synonyms	Characteristics
Prehepatic	Unconjugated Free Indirect-reacting	Does not cross glomerular filter Harmful to neonatal nervous system Formed in reticuloendothelial system (peripheral) Requires organic solvent for diazo reaction
Posthepatic	Conjugated Glucuronide Direct-reacting	Freely crosses glomerular filter Formed by enzymatic activity, in liver Gives diazo reaction in aqueous medium

sufficiency or to the presence of vast quantities of bilirubin, as may occur in severe hemolytic processes.

In clinical situations, the laboratory findings are seldom clear-cut. Hemolysis does, indeed, produce a pure increase in prehepatic bilirubin, but there is usually little difficulty in diagnosing hemolytic anemia on the basis of hematologic findings. Disease of the hepatobiliary tract is almost always complex so that, for example, hepatitis may cause hepatocellular insufficiency and increased levels of prehepatic bilirubin, but the posthepatic form also is increased, owing to increased permeability of the inflamed biliary radicles. Although pure, acute obstruction of the biliary tract causes increased posthepatic bilirubin, persistence of the obstruction for any length of time causes secondary hepatocellular damage with a consequent increase in prehepatic bilirubin.

PREHEPATIC BILIRUBIN

Elevated levels of prehepatic bilirubin occur in autoimmune or transfusion-induced hemolysis and in hemolytic processes due to sickle cell disease, pernicious anemia, various other intrinsic red cell defects, malaria, and septicemia. Hemorrhage into the body cavities or soft tissues is followed by a bilirubin rise within 4 to 6 hours. In hemolytic disease of the newborn, levels of indirect bilirubin may rise to levels above 20 mg./dl. within a few hours, owing to the biochemical immaturity of the infant's liver.

POSTHEPATIC BILIRUBIN

Posthepatic bilirubin is increased in obstructive diseases of the biliary system due to calculi, tumors, extrinsic pressure, or intrahepatic abnormalities. Toxic, infectious, or autoimmune hepatitis results in increase of both fractions, and cirrhosis produces both hepatocellular and biliary tract damage.

Icterus Index

The icterus index is an approximate measure of the degree of jaundice and does not measure bilirubin as such. The serum is compared against standardized solutions of potassium dichromate, a golden yellow compound, and the comparative results are expressed in arbitrary units. The icterus index of normal serum, which has a yellowish tinge, ranges from 2 to 8 units, and clinical jaundice usually is evident at approximately 15 units. Rough quantitation is possible, using a conversion factor of 10 index units to equal 1 mg. of bilirubin. This does not, of course, distinguish between prehepatic and posthepatic forms of bilirubin. The serum must be clear, unhemolyzed, without undue lipemia, and free of other pigments (usually carotene is the only offender).

TOXICOLOGY

Complete discussions of the clinical, legal, and biochemical implications of toxicology are available in specialized monographs. In this chapter, we can address only a few lines to the commoner types of poisoning encountered in clinical practice, especially those for which adequate diagnosis and treatment are available in a general hospital.

Barbiturates

Barbiturates are a group of compounds that depress the central nervous system and the activity of nerves and muscles at all sites. A variety of preparations exists, differing in the duration of their activity. The physiologic effects of any barbiturate vary with the route of administration, the degree of individual tolerance, and the presence or absence of modifying compounds. The combination of alcohol and barbiturates greatly potentiates the depressive effect of each.

According to the dose and nature of the drug, barbiturate intoxications produce nervous system depression, respiratory depression, bradycardia, and circulatory collapse. Clinical staging has been attempted by judging the presence of various reflex responses. Shock, profound respiratory depression, and absence of deep reflexes constitute the most severe intoxication. During therapy, tubular damage from renal ischemia may complicate recovery, and prolonged respiratory depression accounts for serious morbidity.

DIAGNOSTIC PROBLEMS

Diagnosis of barbiturate intoxication may be difficult since a variety of conditions can produce coma, and more than one drug may be involved in accidental or intentional overdosage. Even when barbiturates are known to be involved, prognosis is difficult to estimate because serum levels may not accurately reflect the overall physiologic condition. As a general rule, higher serum levels can be tolerated from long-acting barbiturates, while lower doses of short-acting drugs carry more immediate risk. One scale of potentially lethal serum concentrations starts with 3 mg./dl. for very short-acting preparations and goes up to 10 mg./dl. for the longest-acting preparations such as phenobarbital.[38] Although the dose and other contributing factors may be unknown, clinical course and the changing blood levels over the initial treatment phases may help in prognosis. Opinions vary as to the efficacy of analeptics in treating severe barbiturism. Hemodialysis, when readily available, can be extremely helpful. The most important problems in all patients are respiratory support and the avoidance or correction of shock and hemoconcentration.

A useful screening test gives a colored mercury diphenyl-carbazone complex when any of the common barbiturates, the hydantoins, or glutethimide (Doriden) is present. Although a positive result does not identify the specific offender, a negative result eliminates a large group of potential intoxicants.

The barbiturates are soluble in organic solvents, and methods of determination depend on extraction from blood or urine with chloroform or acid-ether. Quick qualitative identification of barbiturates in urine can be done if color develops when cobalt acetate and isopropyl amine are added to a concentrated acid-ether extract of urine. Intermediate- and short-acting preparations produce a blue-violet compound on addition of cobalt acetate alone, while phenobarbital requires addition of isopropyl alcohol as well. Quantitative methods involve measuring ultraviolet absorption, and paper chromatography can be used for accurate identification.

Bromide

Bromide is a central nervous system depressant which formerly enjoyed widespread medical endorsement but now is found largely in patent medicine preparations and nerve tonics. The gastrointestinal irritant effect usually foils attempts at massive acute ingestion, but chronic bromide intoxication is by no means uncommon, especially in individuals given to self-medication. Symptoms are nonspecific and include emotional lability, impaired intellectual function, motor incoordination, and nodular or acneform dermatitis. Anorexia, constipation, and weight loss also occur with chronic bromide ingestion, and a variety of organic and psychic illnesses may be diagnosed in patients with any or all of the above symptoms of bromism. Because psychic disturbances are fairly common in the population that ingests large quantities of bromide nostrums, the diagnostic problems may become rather complicated.

Bromide excretion occurs through the renal pathways for chloride excretion. The plasma half-life of a moderate dose of bromide is 12 days. Treatment is directed at accelerating urinary excretion primarily by administering mercurial diuretics and copious amounts of chloride ion.

Serum bromide levels above 90 mg./dl. tend to cause toxic symptoms, but there is considerable variation in individual effect. When gold chloride is added to a protein-free filtrate of serum containing bromide, a yellow-orange color results and can be measured colorimetrically. One qualitative method involves silver nitrate precipitation to silver bromide. In another qualitative technique, a mixture of serum and chlorine water causes yellow discoloration of added chloroform if bromides are present; in this procedure, a purple discoloration occurs in the presence of iodides.

Carbon Monoxide

Carbon monoxide is toxic because it combines with hemoglobin to produce carboxyhemoglobin, a physiologically inert compound that damages the victim by reducing the quantity of hemoglobin available for oxygen transport. Because injury occurs from hypoxia, carbon monoxide is especially dangerous to those whose oxygen needs are high or whose oxygen transport system is precarious. Thus children with their high metabolic rate, anemic patients with a low hemoglobin mass, and patients with cardiorespiratory disease are particularly susceptible to carbon monoxide toxicity.

Carbon monoxide, a product of incomplete combustion of carbon-containing compounds, occurs in automobile exhausts, illuminating gas, and the fumes from improperly functioning furnaces. Both accidental and suicidal intoxication occur, and the principal early symptoms are headache and dizziness. Continuing exposure causes increasing quantities of carboxyhemoglobin to replace oxyhemoglobin until carboxyhemoglobin levels of 60 to 80 percent lead to coma and death.[38] Treatment is directed at displacing carbon monoxide from the hemoglobin and is best done by administering high concentrations of oxygen.

Carbon monoxide poisoning usually can be diagnosed from the situation in which the patient is found, although unsuspected chronic intoxication may result from repeated exposure to the fumes of a poorly functioning heating unit. The blood has a characteristic bright cherry-red appearance, and in individuals who have died following carbon monoxide poisoning, the mucous membranes and vascular endothelium may be bright red. Several quick qualitative tests are available for identification of carboxyhemoglobin. When 20 percent sodium hydroxide solution is added to a drop of blood diluted in 10 to 15 ml. of water, normal blood turns straw yellow immediately, while blood with more than 20 percent carboxyhemoglobin remains pink for several seconds before changing color. A normal control should be run simultaneously. Another method involves evaporating 1 ml. of blood to dryness. At carboxyhemoglobin concentrations of 40 percent or above, the residue is brick red, while normal blood produces a brownish black deposit. Quantitative methods are available, using the reduction of palladium chloride, while the most accurate method is gas chromatography. Fatal concentrations range between 40 and 80 percent, while values as high as 5 percent may occur in otherwise normal individuals who are heavy smokers.[38]

Alcohol

Ethyl alcohol becomes a subject of laboratory concern in cases of coma of unknown etiology, or when the amount of alcohol present must be quantified, usually for legal purposes. Qualitative tests for alcohol employ the reducing property common to ethyl alcohol, methyl alcohol, formaldehyde, paraldehyde, acetaldehyde, and acetone. Rapid diffusion techniques and more quantitative distillation techniques use potassium dichromate as the indicator substance. These are not specific for ethanol, but most often clinical circumstances indicate that ethyl alcohol is the reducing substance present.

ETIOLOGIC AGENTS OF COMA

In cases of coma of unknown etiology, it may be necessary to discriminate among these substances. Gas-liquid chromatography is probably the procedure of choice. Specific chemical tests are available when appropriate indications warrant individual testing. Acetone can be identified in blood or urine with sodium nitroprusside. Paraldehyde has a characteristic odor and imparts reducing properties to the urine. Formaldehyde is not usually a clinical problem. The screening and quantitative procedures for methyl alcohol actually measure its oxidation product, formaldehyde. This is produced by preliminary oxidation of the sample, but if the specimen has been taken at autopsy, formalin contamination may present a problem. Since both heparin and EDTA produce false positives,[38] other anticoagulants should be employed.

ETHYL ALCOHOL

Legal considerations often surround tests to quantify ethyl alcohol. Most jurisdictions consider blood ethanol levels of 150 mg./dl. (0.15 gm. percent) as prima facie evidence of being "under the influence," but levels between 50 and 150 mg./dl. exert unmistakable effects on behavior, especially on driving. The blood alcohol levels associated with fatal ethanol intoxication vary over a remarkably wide range depending upon such factors as the individual's prior condition, other drugs present, elapsed time after ingestion, and speed of absorption. Alcohol potentiates the depressant effects of innumerable other substances, so that low blood alcohol levels should not lull the practitioner into a sense of security. Barbiturates, antihistamines, anticonvulsants, morphine derivatives, and tranquilizers are frequently found in association with alcohol and should be considered in cases of accidental or, especially, suicidal poisoning.

Lead

Lead intoxication is usually chronic and unintentional. Lead fumes may be inhaled during repeated exposure to paints, acetylene torches, or combustion products from burning battery casings. Oral ingestion is most common in children who consume lead-containing paint from flaking surfaces or from toys and furniture and in persons who drink whiskey that has been distilled through lead-contaminated equipment. Toxic blood levels are considered to be above 0.10 mg./dl., although symptoms may occur at lower levels. Urinary lead excretion in concentrations higher than 0.08 mg. per liter is suggestive of excessive lead exposure, while values above 0.15 mg. per liter usually indicate toxicity. Accurate measurement of lead levels in blood and urine requires meticulous techniques and scrupulously clean equipment. In cases of suspected lead poisoning, other laboratory determinations usually are done first.

Lead poisoning should be suspected in any anemic child with a history of eating dirt or other nonfood materials or of exposure to battery fumes. Industrial workers in high-risk occupations should be under periodic surveillance. A mild, normochromic, hemolytic anemia is usually found in chronic lead poisoning, and among the early signs are increased urinary levels of delta-amino levulinic acid and coproporphyrin III. Since these compounds can be measured more easily than urinary lead, they constitute effective screening procedures for group or individual studies. In children, severe lead intoxication may cause encephalopathy characterized by clumsiness, irritability, and progressive neuromuscular excitement. Lead encephalopathy is uncommon in adults, who more often suffer anorexia, muscle pains, and constipation. Severe involvement may cause lead colic. Long-continued exposure, especially in children, may result in deposition of lead compounds at the base of the teeth and in bones, but the so-called lead line does not always occur.

Phenothiazines

Severe phenothiazine intoxication, as an isolated phenomenon, is relatively rare. The drugs may cause dermatologic reactions, hypotension, extrapyramidal motor disorders, or jaundice in susceptible patients, but these problems usually constitute side effects of therapeutic administration. The phenothiazines become important in toxicology because they are widely distributed, readily available, and are frequently included in a group of agents taken with suicidal intent. Proprietary drugs in this group include Sparine (promazine), Thorazine (chlorpromazine), Compazine (prochlorperazine), and Phenergan (promethazine hydrochloride), among others. Fatalities due to the phenothiazines alone are exceedingly rare, but this group of drugs potentiates the depressant effects of alcohol, barbiturates, morphine, and meperidine, any or all of which may be used in suicide attempts.

The presence of phenothiazines can be demonstrated best in urine or on tissue samples. The blood level tends to be low, since the material is bound very rapidly in tissue and is slowly excreted in feces and urine. Phenothiazine metabolites may persist in the body and sometimes in the urine for many months following discontinuance of a therapeutic regimen. The simplest urine test for phenothiazines is addition of 6 drops of sulfuric acid and 1 drop of 10 percent ferric chloride to 1 ml. of urine. If phenothiazines are present, a lilac color develops. The simultaneous presence of salicylates does not interfere with this test. Quantitative tests can be done on tissue or urine by measuring ultraviolet absorbance after adding sulfuric acid to a sodium hydroxide-ether extract of the sample. The identity of the particular phenothiazine compound does not affect the results.

Salicylates

Salicylate intoxication is a common medical problem in both pediatric and adult age groups, accounting for as many as one quarter of all accidental intoxications.[49] In children, toxicity may occur through over-zealous therapy or from accidental ingestion by the inquisitive child. In adults, aspirin often is used in suicide attempts, and remarkably large doses of salicylates may be taken by enthusiastic self-medicators. Nonfatal ingestion of 130 gm. of aspirin by an adult has been reported, but adult fatalities occur at doses as low as 10 gm. or 30 to 40 regular-sized tablets.[71] Fatalities more often occur in children, especially if pre-existing fever or infection aggravates the metabolic effects of the drug.

The problems of acute salicylate toxicity arise chiefly from acid-base disturbances. Initial respiratory alkalosis occurs from direct stimulation of the respiratory center. To maintain the blood pH, pulmonary loss of carbon dioxide is compensated by renal excretion of bicarbonate, and the result is carbon dioxide deficit accompanied by loss of sodium and potassium in the urine. A later effect of salicylism is metabolic acidosis from organic acids and salicylic acid derivatives, resulting in still further drain on the body's buffering capacity. Although the effects on pH may counter-balance each other, the effect on the buffer mechanism is cumulative. Renal function may be impaired by dehydration, bicarbonate alterations, and severe potassium depletion, and depressed renal function further complicates the metabolic derangements.

Mild degrees of salicylate intoxication cause headache, audial and visual disturbances, dizziness, hyperventilation, and gastrointestinal irritation. Although salicylates affect platelet function and several procoagulant interactions, overt bleeding is a rare complication of mild or moderate intoxication. Purpuric manifestations may accompany fatal salicylism.

The therapy of salicylism is too complicated to be detailed here. Salicylates are excreted through the kidney, so that toxic renal damage may complicate efforts to reduce blood salicylate level. Exchange transfusion and hemodialysis have been used as life-saving measures when salicylate levels are extremely high.

INITIAL BLOOD LEVEL

The blood salicylate level correlates fairly closely with the serverity of symptoms and prognosis in children, provided that correction is made for the time elapsed after ingestion. Thus a moderate elevation persisting many hours after ingestion may carry a graver prognosis than a higher figure occuring a short time after the drug was taken. The prognosis should be based on calculated initial blood level rather than on the actual level at the time of examination. Done[11,12] gives formulas and a nomogram for calculating initial blood levels and offers the following prognostic data, based on calculated initial serum concentration: up to 50 mg./dl. tends to cause no ill effects; 50 to 80 mg./dl. causes mild symptoms; moderate intoxication follows levels of 80 to 100 mg./dl. An initial salicylate level above 160 mg./dl, almost always carries a fatal outcome. If the blood level is measured within 6 hours of acute ingestion, the actual determination can be used as the initial level. The metabolism and excretion of salicylates occur at a constant rate or may slow as the size of the ingested dose increases. Induced diuresis may speed excretion, but in very severe cases, dialysis has proved useful.[12]

MEASUREMENT

The ferric chloride test on urine is a quick means for demonstrating the presence of salicylates, but positive reactions occur after doses as small as 5 grains (300 mg., or one adult-size tablet).[70] The quantity can be very roughly guessed from the intensity of purple color resulting when 1 ml. of 10 percent ferric chloride is added to 3 ml. of urine. This screening test has its greatest value in the differential diagnosis of coma due to unknown causes. Both glucose and salicylates appear as reducing substances in the urine, and it is often essential to distinguish between diabetes and salicylate intoxication as the cause of acidosis and coma. The urine should be heated gently to drive off acetone bodies, which tend to accompany both conditions and which produce a positive ferric chloride test. More accurate measurement is done on blood samples, according to a variety of colorimetric and spectrophotometric techniques.

REFERENCES

1. Alberti, K. G. M. M., and Hockaday, T. D. R.: *Diabetic coma: a reappraisal after five years.* Clin. Endocrinol. Metabol. 6:421, 1977.
2. Axelsson, U., Bachmann, R., and Hallen, J.: *Frequency of pathological proteins (M-components) in 6,995 sera from an adult population.* Acta Med. Scand. 179:235, 1967.
3. Basinski, D. H.: *Magnesium (titan yellow),* in Meites, S. (ed.): *Standard Methods of Clinical Chemistry.* vol. 5. Academic Press, New York, 1965.
4. Beach, E. F.: *Non-protein nitrogen,* in Seligson, D. (ed.): *Standard Methods of Clinical Chemistry.* vol. 2. Academic Press, New York, 1958.
5. Bretaudiere, J. P., Phung, H. T., and Bailly, M.: *Direct enzymatic determination of urea in plasma and urine with a centrifugal analyzer.* Clin. Chem. 22:1614, 1976.
6. Brown, M. S., and Goldstein, J. L.: *Familial hypercholesterolemia: a genetic defect in the low-density lipoprotein receptor.* N. Engl. J. Med. 294:1386, 1976.
7. Caraway, W. T.: *Uric acid,* in Seligson, D. (ed.): *Standard Methods of Clinical Chemistry.* vol. 4. Academic Press, New York, 1963.
8. Conn, H. O.: *Blood ammonia,* in Meites, S. (ed.): *Standard Methods of Clinical Chemistry.* vol. 5. Academic Press, New York, 1965.
9. *Cooperative Lipoprotein Phenotyping Study: Alcohol and blood lipids.* Lancet 2:153, 1977.
10. Demetriou, J. A., Drewes, P. A., and Gin, J. B.: *Enzymes,* in Henry, R. J., Cannon, D. C., and Winkelman, J. W. (eds.): *Clinical Chemistry: Principles and Technics.* ed. 2. Harper & Row, Hagerstown, Maryland, 1974.
11. Done, A. K.: *Salicylate intoxication. Significance of measurements of salicylate in blood in cases of acute ingestion.* Pediatrics 26:800, 1960.
12. Done, A. K.: *Treatment of salicylate poisoning: review of personal and published experiences.* Clin. Toxicol. 1:451, 1968.
13. Doumas, B. T., Watson, W. A., and Biggs, H. G.: *Albumin standards and the measurement of serum albumin with bromcresol green.* Clin. Chim. Acta 31:87, 1971.
14. Dryer, R. L., and Routh, J. I.: *Determination of serum inorganic phosphorus,* in Seligson, D. (ed.): *Standard Methods of Clinical Chemistry.* vol. 4. Academic Press, New York, 1963.
15. Ellefson, R. D., and Caraway, W. T.: *Lipids and lipoproteins,* in Tietz, N. W. (ed.): *Fundamentals of Clinical Chemistry.* ed. 2. W. B. Saunders, Philadelphia, 1976.
16. Fales, F. W.: *Glucose (enzymatic),* in Seligson, D. (ed.): *Standard Methods of Clinical Chemistry.* vol. 4. Academic Press, New York, 1963.
17. *Familial hypercholesterolemia.* Lancet 1:733, 1977.
18. Faulkner, W. R., and King, J. W.: *Renal function,* in Tietz, N. W. (ed.): *Fundamentals of Clinical Chemistry.* ed. 2. W. B. Saunders, Philadelphia, 1976.

19. Fisher, W. R., and Truitt, D. H.: *The common hyperlipoproteinemias: an understanding of disease mechanisms and their control.* Ann. Intern. Med. 85:497, 1976.
20. Frankel, S.: *Enzymes,* in Frankel, S., Reitman, S., and Sonnenwirth, A. C. (eds.): *Gradwohl's Clinical Laboratory Methods and Diagnosis.* ed. 7. C. V. Mosby, St. Louis, 1970.
21. Friedman, H. S.: *Quantitative determinations of total lipids in serum.* Clin. Chim. Acta 19:291, 1968.
22. Freimuth, H. C.: *Toxicology for the general hospital laboratory.* Hosp. Prog. 47:90, 1966.
23. Gambino, S. R.: *pH and P_{CO_2},* in Meites, S. (ed.): *Standard Methods of Clinical Chemistry.* vol. 5. Academic Press, New York, 1965.
24. Genuth, S. M., Houser, H. B., Carter, J. R., Jr., et al.: *Community screening for diabetes by blood glucose measurement. Results of a five year experience.* Diabetes 25:1110, 1976.
25. Giovanniello, T. J., and Peters, T., Jr.: *Serum iron and serum iron-binding capacity,* in Seligson, D. (ed.): *Standard Methods of Clinical Chemistry.* vol. 4. Academic Press, New York, 1963.
26. Gordon, T., Castelli, W. P., Hjortland, M. C., et al.: *High density lipoprotein as a protective factor against coronary heart disease.* Am. J. Med. 62:707, 1977.
27. Gwynne, J. T.: *Laboratory evaluation of lipid disturbance.* Bull. Lab. Med. N.C. Mem. Hosp. 25, October 1977.
28. Havel, R. J.: *Classification of the hyperlipidemias.* Ann. Rev. Med. 28:195, 1977.
29. Hazzard, W. R., Goldstein, J. L., Schrott, H. G., et al.: *Hyperlipidemia in coronary heart disease. III. Evaluation of lipoprotein phenotypes of 156 genetically defined survivors of myocardial infarction.* J. Clin. Invest. 52:1569, 1973.
30. Hendry, E. B.: *Osmolarity of human serum and of chemical solutions of biologic importance.* Clin. Chem. 7:156, 1961.
31. Henry, J. B.: *Clinical Chemistry,* in Davidsohn, I., and Henry, J. B. (eds.): *Todd-Sanford Clinical Diagnosis by Laboratory Methods.* ed. 15. W. B. Saunders, Philadelphia, 1974.
32. Henry, R. J., Chiamori, N., Golub, O. J., and Berkman, S.: *Revised spectrophotometric methods for the determination of glutamic-oxalacetic transaminase, glutamic-pyruvic transaminase, and lactic acid dehydrogenase.* Am. J. Clin. Pathol. 34:381, 1960.
33. Henry, R. J., Golub, O. J., and Sobel, C.: *Some of the variables involved in the fractionation of serum proteins by paper electrophoresis.* Clin. Chem. 3:49, 1957.
34. Hobbs, J. R.: *Immunoglobulins in clinical chemistry.* Adv. Clin. Chem. 14:219, 1971.
35. Hsieh, K. M., and Blumenthal, H. T.: *Serum lactic dehydrogenase levels in various disease states.* Proc. Soc. Exp. Biol. Med. 91:626, 1956.
36. Ibbott, F. A., LaGanga, T. S., Gin, J. B., and Inkpen, J. A.: *Blood gases and pH,* in Henry, R. J., Cannon, D. C., and Winkelman, J. W. (eds.): *Clinical Chemistry: Principles and Technics.* ed. 2. Harper & Row, Hagerstown, Maryland, 1974.

37. Kannel, W. B.: *Some lessons in cardiovascular epidemiology from Framingham.* Am. J. Cardiol. 37:269, 1976.
38. Kaye, S.: *Handbook of Emergency Toxicology.* ed. 3. Charles C Thomas, Springfield, Ill., 1970.
39. Kessler, G., and Wolfman, M.: *An automated procedure for the simultaneous determination of calcium and phosphorus.* Clin. Chem. 10:686, 1964.
40. Knochel, J. P.: *The pathophysiology and clinical characteristics of severe hypophosphatemia.* Arch. Intern. Med. 137:203, 1977.
41. Kreisberg, R. A.: *Phosphorus deficiency and hypophosphatemia.* Hosp. Practice 12(3):121, March 1977.
42. Langdell, R. D.: *Coagulation and hemostasis,* in Davidsohn, I., and Henry, J. B. (eds.): *Todd-Sanford Clinical Diagnosis by Laboratory Methods.* ed. 15. W. B. Saunders, Philadelphia, 1974.
43. MacDonald, R. P.: *Bilirubin (modified Malloy and Evelyn),* in Meites, S. (ed.): *Standard Methods of Clinical Chemistry.* vol. 5. Academic Press, New York, 1965.
44. MacDonald, R. P.: *Salicylate,* in Meites, S. (ed.): *Standard Methods of Clinical Chemistry.* vol. 5. Academic Press, New York, 1965.
45. Meites, S.: *Ultramicroglucose (enzymatic),* in Meites, S. (ed.): *Standard Methods of Clinical Chemistry.* vol. 5. Academic Press, New York, 1965.
46. Mikkelsen, W. M., Doge, H. J., and Valkenburg, H.: *The distribution of serum uric acid values in a population unselected as to gout or hyperuricemia: Tecumseh, Michigan, 1959-60.* Am. J. Med. 39:242, 1965.
47. Myers, W. P. L.: *Differential diagnosis of hypercalcemia and cancer.* CA 27:258, 1977.
48. Nino, H. V., and Shaw, W.: *Vitamins,* in Tietz, N. W. (ed.): *Fundamentals of Clinical Chemistry.* ed. 2. W. B. Saunders, Philadelphia, 1976.
49. Nobel, S.: *Toxicology in a general hospital,* in MacDonald, R. P. (ed.): *Standard Methods of Clinical Chemistry.* vol. 6. Academic Press, New York, 1970.
50. *Normal laboratory values.* N. Engl. J. Med. 298:34, 1978.
51. Permutt, M. A.: *Postprandial hypoglycemia.* Diabetes 25:719, 1976.
52. Peters, T.: *Serum albumin.* Adv. Clin. Chem. 13:37, 1970.
53. Pileggi, V. J., and Szustkiewicz, C. P.: *Carbohydrates,* in Henry, R. J., Cannon, D. C., and Winkelman, J. W. (eds.): *Clinical Chemistry: Principles and Technics.* ed. 2. Harper & Row, Hagerstown, Maryland, 1974.
54. Pruzanski, W., and Ogryzlo, M. A.: *Abnormal proteinuria in malignant diseases.* Adv. Clin. Chem. 13:335, 1970.
55. Rastegar, A., and Their, S. O.: *The physiologic approach to hyperuricemia.* N. Engl. J. Med. 286:470, 1972.
56. Rice, E. W., Fletcher, D. C., and Stumpf, A.: *Lead in blood and urine,* in Meites, S. (ed.): *Standard Methods of Clinical Chemistry.* vol. 5. Academic Press, New York, 1965.
57. Rosalski, S. B.: *An improved procedure for creatine phosphokinase determination.* J. Lab. Clin. Med. 69:696, 1965.
58. Salway, J. G.: *Drug interference with laboratory investigations.* Lancet 1:483, 1977.

59. Seligson, D., and Hirahara, R.: *The measurement of ammonia in whole blood, erythrocytes, and plasma.* J. Lab. Clin. Med. 49:962, 1957.
60. Sherlock, S.: *Diseases of the Liver and Biliary System.* ed. 5. Blackwell Scientific Publications, Oxford, 1975.
61. Siggaard-Andersen, O.: *Blood gases,* in Tietz, N. W. (ed.): *Fundamentals of Clinical Chemistry.* ed. 2. W. B. Saunders, Philadelphia, 1976.
62. Statland, B. E., and Winkel, P.: *Variations of cholesterol and total lipid concentrations in sera of healthy young men.* Am. J. Clin. Pathol. 66:935, 1976.
63. Sodhi, H. S., and Mason, D. T.: *New insights into the homeostasis of plasma cholesterol.* Am. J. Med. 63:325, 1977.
64. Thiers, R. E.: *Magnesium (fluorometric),* in Meites, S. (ed.): *Standard Methods of Clinical Chemistry.* vol. 5. Academic Press, New York, 1965.
65. Tietz, N. W.: *Electrolytes,* in Tietz, N. W. (ed.): *Fundamentals of Clinical Chemistry.* ed. 2. W. B. Saunders, Philadelphia, 1976.
66. Tietz, N. W., and Fiereck, E. A.: *Measurement of lipase in serum,* in Cooper, G. R. (ed.): *Standard Methods of Clinical Chemistry.* vol. 7. Academic Press, New York, 1972.
67. Valberg, L. S., Corbett, W. E. N., McCorriston, J. R., and Parker, J. O.: *Excessive loss of plasma protein into the gastrointestinal tract associated with myocardial disease.* Am. J. Med. 39:668, 1965.
68. Wacker, W. E. C., Ulmer, D. D., and Vallee, B. L.: *Metalloenzymes and myocardial infarction. II. Malic and lactic dehydrogenase activities and zinc concentrations in serum.* N. Engl. J. Med. 255:449, 1956.
69. Watson, D.: *Albumin and total globulin fractions of blood,* in Sobotka, H., and Stewart, C. P. (eds.): *Advances in Clinical Chemistry.* vol. 8. Academic Press, New York, 1965.
70. Williams, L. A.: *Toxicology,* in Frankel, S., Reitman, S., and Sonnenwirth, A. C. (eds.): *Gradwohl's Clinical Laboratory Methods and Diagnosis.* ed. 7. C. V. Mosby, St. Louis, 1970.
71. Woodbury, D. M., and Fingl, E.: *Analgesic-antipyretics, anti-inflammatory agents, and drugs employed in the therapy of gout,* in Goodman, L. S., and Gilman, A. (eds.): *The Pharmacologic Basis of Therapeutics.* ed. 5. Macmillan, New York, 1975.
72. Wyngaarden, J. B., and Kelley, W. N.: *Gout,* in Stanbury, J. B., Wyngaarden, J. B., and Frederickson, D. S. (eds.): *The Metabolic Basis of Inherited Disease.* ed. 4. McGraw-Hill, New York, 1978.
73. Yeshurun, D., and Gotto, A. M.: *Drug treatment of hyperlipidemia.* Am. J. Med. 60:379, 1976.
74. Zak, B.: *Total and free cholesterol,* in Meites, S. (ed.): *Standard Methods of Clinical Chemistry.* vol. 5. Academic Press, New York, 1965.

CHAPTER 10

ACID-BASE AND ELECTROLYTE REGULATION

ACID-BASE REGULATION

The pH of normal circulating blood ranges from 7.38 to 7.44, while the limits compatible with life are approximately 6.8 to 7.8. The pH is the negative logarithm of the hydrogen ion concentration, a term used because the number of decimal places involved can become cumbersome (i.e., a concentration of 0.000001 hydrogen ions per liter is more effectively expressed as pH 5.0). The pH is a concept rather than a concentration. It is, of course, dependent upon the number of free hydrogen ions in a solution; the larger the number of hydrogen ions, the smaller the pH value. In the blood, free hydrogen ions are present in very small numbers. Complete neutrality is expressed by pH 7.0. The blood contains between 36 and 44 nanoequivalents of free hydrogen ions per liter, at the normal pH range of 7.38 to 7.44. The pH range compatible with life is much greater—approximately 6.8 to 7.8. This rather narrow numerical spread in pH units corresponds to H^+ concentrations between 16 and 110 nanoequivalents per liter.[9]

Fundamental Concepts

ACIDS AND BASES

An *acid* is any substance capable of liberating a hydrogen ion into the solution; a *base* is any substance that can accept a hydrogen ion from the solution. The ability of a compound to donate or to accept a hydrogen ion depends, among other things, on the pH of the medium. Compounds that are commonly called "acids" must be considered as pairs of an acid and a base. A hypothetical acid, HAc, consists of the ions H^+ and Ac^-. The compound acid, when it dissociates, donates an H^+ ion into the medium; the Ac^- ion, in its dissociated state, is a base because it can combine with (accept) a hydrogen ion.

Some compounds that are not, in common parlance, "acids" are in fact hydrogen ion donors under appropriate circumstances. For example, both NH_4^+ and $HPO_4^=$ can liberate a hydrogen ion into a medium relatively low in hydrogen ions. If the medium contains a large number of hydrogen ions, $HPO_4^=$ can act as a base, accepting a hydrogen ion to become $H_2PO_4^-$. The number of anions and cations in a solution must always be equal; therefore, none of the ions just mentioned could exist in a solution without a balancing ion. Some combinations of anion and cation dissociate freely, and each ion floats separately in the medium. Other combinations remain more closely tied to one another. The tendency of a compound to dissociate is described by the terms weak and strong.

STRONG AND WEAK ACIDS

A *strong acid* is one which dissociates to liberate its H^+ under a wide range of conditions, even into mediums with an already high hydrogen ion concentration. A *weak acid* is one which dissociates poorly; that is, relatively few free ions enter the medium, and the positive ion and negative ion remain closely associated with each other. To form the salt of an acid, the hydrogen ion is replaced by a cation which does not affect the pH of the medium. If we replace the H^+ by Na^+ in the acid HAc, we then have two electrically balanced ions, Na^+ and Ac^-. Although the Na^+ ion does not alter the pH, the Ac^- ion remains capable of combining with (accepting) an H^+ ion.

If the acid HAc is a weak acid, it will dissociate into H^+ and Ac^- only if very few H^+ ions are present in the medium; that is, it dissociates at a relatively high pH. The salt NaAc dissociates much more freely, and the Ac^- floats free and is capable of combining with any H^+ ions that might be available. The resultant compound HAc is, as we have said, a weak acid; as long as the medium is moderately acidic, it does not dissociate its H^+ back into the medium. The result of adding the salt of a weak acid to a moderately acid medium is that dissociated hydrogen ions combine with the anions to form undissociated weak acid, and the medium becomes less acid. This is shown in the following equations:

$$NaAc \rightleftharpoons Na^+ + Ac^- \text{ (the salt of a weak acid)}$$

$$HCl \rightleftharpoons H^+ + Cl^- \text{ (a strong acid, freely dissociated)}$$

$$Na^+ + Ac^- \text{ added to } H^+ + Cl^- \text{ gives } HAc + Na^+ + Cl^-$$

BUFFER SOLUTIONS

A solution that contains a weak acid together with the salt of that weak acid is called a buffer solution, meaning that it is capable of assimilating (buffering) added H^+ or OH^- ions with relatively little change in pH. This is true because the ionization of the weak acid varies with the number of H^+ ions in the solution. If additional H^+ ions enter the solution, the Ac^- ion from the dissociated salt combines with the H^+ ion to form the poorly dissociated acid. If OH^- ions are added, the medium becomes much less acidic, and the weak acid dissociates to provide H^+ ions which neutralize the added OH^-. These situations are shown in the following equations, in which strong acid or strong base is added to a buffer solution of the weak acid HAc and its salt NaAc:

$$H^+ \text{ and } Cl^- \text{ added to } HAc + Na^+ + Ac^- = 2HAc + Na^+ + Cl^-$$
$$Na^+ \text{ and } OH^- \text{ added to } HAc + Na^+ + Ac^- = H_2O + 2Na^+ + 2Ac^-$$

In both cases, the pH remains unchanged. Obviously, if more H^+ or OH^- were added, the pH would change when the weak acid or its salt was exhausted. The ideal buffer pair consists of equal quantities of salt (base) and acid, so that dissociation or recombination can occur in either direction without exhausting the supply of either base or acid.

THE HENDERSON-HASSELBALCH EQUATION

The buffering capacity of a salt-acid pair depends upon the number of hydrogen ions already present (i.e., the pH of the solution) and the physical property of the acid (i.e., its inherent tendency to dissociate). These relationships are illustrated in the Henderson-Hasselbalch equation:

$$pH = pK + \log \frac{[A^-]}{[HA]}$$

It is not necessary, for our purpose, to show how this equation is derived. The terms used are as follows: pH is the hydrogen ion concentration in the solution at the time under consideration; pK is a constant specific for each base-acid combination, designating that pH at which the compound is half dissociated and half undissociated; the proportion $[A^-]/[HA]$ refers to the actual concentrations of base (dissociated anion capable of uniting with an H^+ ion) and acid (undissociated form in which the H^+ ions do not affect the pH) in the solution at the time under consideration.

In simple nonmathematical terms, the Henderson-Hasselbalch equation tells us that the pH of an acid-containing medium is proportional to the existing concentration of dissociated salt and combined acid. Different acids have different buffering capacity depending upon their pK (i.e., the pH at which half the acid is undissociated) and upon the pH at which they are required to act. Even the best of buffer pairs can accept only a limited challenge of H^+ or OH^-. Once the acid or the salt has been consumed in the buffering process, additional H^+ or OH^- changes the pH unhindered.

Blood pH

The pH of the blood affects critically the health of the organism; the body must protect itself continually against drastic pH changes. Most metabolic reactions produce acid end products. Vast quantities of carbon dioxide are produced as energy is generated and consumed; CO_2, in hydrated form, is the acid H_2CO_3. However, CO_2 is volatile and can be excreted readily through the lungs once it arrives there from the site of production. In conditions of normal respiratory function, CO_2 is transported and rapidly excreted without affecting the blood pH. Certain nonvolatile acids also are produced; these originate from sulfur- and phosphate-containing compounds and from various incomplete combustion reactions. The nonvolatile acids normally are excreted through the kidneys. Both CO_2 and the nonvolatile acids must be neutralized at the site of production and transported through the blood to the site of excretion.

PHYSIOLOGIC BUFFERS

There are many buffer compounds in the circulating blood that prevent local acid accumulation and permit the transportation of acids through the body. Some available buffer pairs derive from amino acids of the serum proteins, from the phosphate compounds in plasma and red cells, and from the amino acids of intracellular hemoglobin. The most significant of the blood buffers, however, is the bicarbonate-carbonic acid pair. Carbonic acid is weakly dissociated, and large quantities of bicarbonate exist in the plasma. The bicarbonate-carbonic acid system has its pK, hence optimal buffering capacity, at pH of 6.1, far below the pH of normal blood. In addition, the proportion of bicarbonate to carbonic acid is 20:1, far removed from the optimal buffering ratio of 1:1. At first glance, this seems an unpromising combination. The peculiarities of physiology are such, however, that the bicarbonate buffer system is remarkably effective, and the other buffer systems mentioned play a much smaller part in pH regulation.

THE BICARBONATE SYSTEM. As we pointed out earlier, a buffer pair (i.e., the base and the acid form) loses its buffering capacity if either member is totally consumed. In the body, several mechanisms combine to maintain the normal 20:1 proportion between bicarbonate and carbonic acid, thus to maintain the blood at its normal pH. For convenience, let us restate the Henderson-Hasselbalch equation, using the actual compounds involved:

$$pH = pK + \log \frac{[HCO_3^-]}{[H_2CO_3]}$$

Because the denominator is kept low by continuous excretion of CO_2, the accumulation of H_2CO_3 is prevented. The numerator, or bicarbonate portion, can be increased or decreased as necessary through renal excretion mediated by carbonic anhydrase activity. If anything happens to increase the bicarbonate or decrease the CO_2 concentration, the blood pH will rise, and anything that increases the CO_2 concentration or diminishes the bicarbonate will lower the pH. In metabolic balance, however, acids are produced, neutralized, and excreted, and the buffer pair remains constant.

Laboratory Measurement

A variety of derangements can alter the normal condition, and when this occurs, it is necessary to measure the changes in pH and buffering capacity. Blood pH can be measured directly, and under certain conditions this determination is invaluable. If pH change occurs, the body has sustained serious metabolic derangement. The blood pH portrays the end result of the buffering process; measurement of the buffer components provides dynamic information about ongoing processes of compensation. The ratio between bicarbonate and carbonic acid, as stated in the Henderson-Hasselbalch equation, determines the blood pH. Thus the measurement of any two variables permits calculation of the third variable.

pH DETERMINATION

Since changes as slight as 0.01 pH units may have considerable physiologic significance, pH determinations must be highly accurate if they are to be used at all. Titrimetric methods, although potentially quite accurate, are difficult and time-consuming. Electrometric pH measurement is now used almost exclusively in clinical situations. Electrometric methods measure the potential generated across a glass membrane separating two solutions of unequal hydrogen ion concentrations. The sample to be measured is placed on one side of the membrane, and a standard solution of known hydrogen ion concentration is on the other.

SUITABLE BLOOD SAMPLE. For pH determinations, either whole blood or plasma can be used; arterial, venous, or capillary blood may be suitable. Venous blood has a pH approximately 0.03 pH units below arterial blood,[6] owing to accumulation of metabolic acids; if venous blood is used, it should be "arterialized" by warming the site for 15 minutes before venipuncture. To avoid accumulating additional acids, the patient should maintain a relaxed state and not "pump" his fist. A tourniquet, if required, should exert pressure no greater than the mean arterial blood pressure and should remain in place as blood is withdrawn.

ARTEFACTS. Many artefacts can affect the pH of the sample. Ideally, the blood should be maintained anaerobically, and the test should be started within 5 minutes. As time passes, glycolytic activity produces acid metabolites that lower the pH; storage at room temperature accelerates the fall. If the test cannot be done immediately, the sample can be kept safely, anaerobically and in ice, for up to 2 hours. In bloods with high white counts, glycolysis is increased, and the pH drops more rapidly. Sodium fluoride, sometimes used to inhibit glycolysis, introduces artefacts in either direction if the concentration is not rigidly standardized.

WHOLE BLOOD VS. PLASMA. Temperature change also affects the pH by altering protein ionization. Since red cells contain more protein than plasma, whole blood pH is more temperature-sensitive than plasma pH. The measured pH of whole blood is 0.01 units lower than that of plasma, partly because the red cells accumulate at the reference electrode.[6] The pH of whole blood may be altered unpredictably by the carbonic anhydrase activity of the red cells; therefore, if time must elapse between collection and determination, plasma is probably more reliable. The anticoagulant always should be heparin, since oxalate tends to raise the pH, and citrate and EDTA tend to lower it.[6]

RESULTS. Two sets of terms are used to describe the physiologic conditions in which pH change occurs: acidosis and alkalosis, and acidemia and alkalemia. Those who advocate using the latter terms suggest that *acidosis* and *alkalosis* describe pathologic conditions in which buffering action is necessary to prevent pH change, while the terms *acidemia* and *alkalemia* make it clear that actual pH change has occurred. This usage distinguishes between uncompensated conditions, in which the pH does change, and compensated conditions, in which the pH is preserved but at the expense of buffer constituents.

MEASURING THE BUFFER PAIR

The proportion of free bicarbonate to carbonic acid determines the blood pH, the critical proportion being

$$\frac{[HCO_3^-]}{[H_2CO_3]}$$

Both numerator and denominator contain measurable carbon dioxide. At pH of 7.4, the proportion is 20:1, and the dominant carbon dioxide-containing compound is bicarbonate. The denominator, written as H_2CO_3, consists partly of undissociated carbonic acid but mostly of physically dissolved carbon dioxide. The volume of dissolved CO_2 is directly proportional to the partial pressure of carbon dioxide in the alveolar air.

If the concentration of buffer compounds is measured as total CO_2 content, both numerator and denominator are included in one figure without partition. If the partial pressure of carbon dioxide (P_{CO_2}) is determined as well, the proportion can be fully defined. In most cases, especially when the history is clear-cut, CO_2 content alone can indicate the extent of the metabolic derangement. In more complex situations, when more than one mechanism may be operative, the fullest information possible must be obtained.

COLLECTING THE SAMPLE. For all types of test, there is the problem of maintaining the blood sample in the same condition as when the blood was drawn. Since carbon dioxide enters and leaves the blood freely and since the partial pressure of atmospheric carbon dioxide is far lower than in alveolar air, significant escape of CO_2 tends to occur if the sample is freely exposed to the atmosphere. Collection of the blood under mineral oil in a test tube is not entirely satisfactory for preventing loss of CO_2. In addition to the difficulty of handling the oil without spilling, carbon dioxide can diffuse into the overlying oil. It is preferable to seal the blood in the syringe or to collect the blood in a vacuum tube which contains heparin, taking care to fill the tube to capacity.

CARBON DIOXIDE COMBINING POWER. The earliest meaningful test of buffer capacity was determination of the carbon dioxide combining power. In this test, the problem of CO_2 escape was avoided by arbitrarily equilibrating the sample with an atmosphere having a P_{CO_2} of 40 mm. Hg, the normal P_{CO_2} of alveolar air. Using his own alveolar air, the technician restored the dissolved CO_2 to a uniform, arbitrary value which was then subtracted from the final figure. The remaining volume of CO_2 came from the bicarbonate in the sample, so that the test effectively measured only the numerator of the Henderson-Hasselbalch buffer pair. Since the numerator is always much larger than the denominator, and since changes in bicarbonate alone often indicate the severity of the problem, this test has proved clinically useful. It does not, however, measure subtle changes arising from alterations in the denominator.

The CO_2 combining power is reported in milliequivalents per liter (mEq./L.), representing the HCO_3^-. Normal values are 19 to 24 mEq./L. in arterial blood and 22 to 26 mEq./L. in venous blood. Earlier workers expressed their findings as volumes (milliliters) per 100 ml. of serum, and the normal range was 55 to 65 volumes percent. To convert from one set of units to the other, volumes percent is multiplied by 0.45 to give milliequivalents per liter.

CARBON DIOXIDE CONTENT. Total carbon dioxide content measures both elements of the proportion and permits somewhat more accurate assessment of clinical problems. If carbon dioxide content is to be measured, blood must be drawn anaerobically, separated promptly, and stored anaerobically until the test is run. Arterialized venous blood, freely flowing capillary blood, or arterial blood are all suitable for tests of CO_2 content. The quantity of CO_2 is expressed as millimoles per liter. Since H_2CO_3 dissociates into univalent ions, the value in millimoles can be expressed directly as milliequivalents. The normal range for CO_2 content is 23 to 27 mEq./L. in arterial blood and 25 to 29 mEq./L. in venous blood. The CO_2 content gives the total of the numerator and denominator but does not assign values to either. These values can be calculated or derived from a nomogram if the pH and total CO_2 are known.

THE PCO_2

MEASUREMENT IN ALVEOLAR AIR. The denominator in the Henderson-Hasselbalch equation can be evaluated directly by measuring dissolved CO_2, since little of the H_2CO_3 is present as undissociated carbonic acid. Dissolved CO_2 is proportional to partial pressure of CO_2 in the alveolar air, which is the gaseous atmosphere at equilibrium with the blood. If the PCO_2 of alveolar air can be measured directly, this value, in mm. Hg, is used to represent the PCO_2 of arterial blood. Collection of alveolar air requires the patient's active participation, and is often most difficult in the very patients for whom the determination is most important.

THE ASTRUP TECHNIQUE. This technique employs both measurement and calculation. The pH of the patient's blood is first determined directly. Two aliquots of blood are then equilibrated with carbon dioxide, one with 2 percent carbon dioxide and the other with 6 percent carbon dioxide. The pH of these two samples is determined after full equilibration has occurred. With this information, both the PCO_2 and pH of two blood samples are known, so that a graph can be constructed to express the relationship of pH and PCO_2. By locating the pH of the original sample on this line, one can calculate from the graph what the native PCO_2 must have been to give the original pH.

Measuring Blood Gases

BLOOD SAMPLE

Advances in electrometry now make possible very rapid, simultaneous determination of pH, partial pressure of carbon dioxide (PCO_2), and partial pressure of oxygen (PO_2) on small samples of blood. Heparinized blood, either venous or arterial, should be drawn into an airtight syringe and tested within 15 or 20 minutes. EDTA and chelating agents are unsuitable anticoagulants because they derange the pH. Oxygen partial pressure undergoes artefactual changes more rapidly and more significantly than does carbon dioxide tension or pH. Metaboliz-ing white cells utilize oxygen. The number of white cells, the temper-ature of storage and handling, and the time that elapses between ob-taining and testing the sample can all affect the results. The higher the initial oxygen tension, the more rapidly the values will change. Icing the specimen slows oxygen consumption and pH change, but the tests should be run with as little delay as possible.

OXYGEN TRANSPORT

In the blood, oxygen travels in two forms: a small part is physically dissolved, and the vast majority is bound to hemoglobin. Electro-metric blood gas analyzers measure oxygen tension and the partial pressure of dissolved oxygen but not total oxygen or bound oxygen. It is the oxygen partial pressure (P_{O_2}), however, that determines the amount of oxygen that will bind to hemoglobin. Hemoglobin binds oxygen at a rate which is proportional to the oxygen tension and is affected by ambient pH. In most situations, simply measuring the P_{O_2} of blood provides enough clinical information. If total oxygen must be known, this can be calculated from the P_{O_2}, the concentration of hemoglobin, and the pH of the blood. If P_{O_2} remains constant, hemoglobin binds less oxygen at low pH than at higher pH. This characteristic is described as *oxygen dissociation* and is a property determined by the physical and chemical structure of the hemoglobin molecule.

Many conditions affect the quantity of oxygen delivered to the tissues: (1) there must be adequate oxygen in the inspired air; (2) inspiratory effort must be sufficient to bring oxygen to the air-exchanging lung tissues; (3) the lung must possess adequate air-exchanging tissue with adequate blood supply and suitable structural conditions that gas can diffuse from air to blood and back again; (4) the blood must contain enough hemoglobin that it can bind adequate amounts of oxygen; (5) the pH of blood and tissue must be such that oxygen is taken up in the lungs and released at the tissues; and (6) circulation must be sufficiently brisk that all parts of lung and all areas of metabolizing tissue continually receive renewed blood supply.

BLOOD OXYGEN LEVELS

Arterial P_{O_2} reflects the amount of oxygen passing from inspired air into the blood. This level is influenced by respiratory capacity, the area and conditon of pulmonary perfusing surfaces, the distribution of pulmonary blood flow, and the adequacy of pulmonary and systemic circulation. In many conditions of pulmonary and cardiovascular disease, blood oxygen values provide critically important information about these interrelated variables. Of particular importance, if there is diminished ventilation or diffusing capacity, is observation of the way in which arterial P_{O_2} changes with changing P_{O_2} in the inspired air. When tissue perfusion or altered systemic metabolism is a problem, comparing the P_{O_2} of arterial and of venous blood indicates efficiency of oxygen delivery.

BLOOD CO₂ LEVELS

Carbon dioxide, a metabolic end product, enters the blood stream from the tissues and is carried to the lungs for excretion. The partial pressure of CO_2 in the blood (P_{CO_2}) reflects both the amount of CO_2 generated by metabolic processes and the efficiency with which pulmonary excretion occurs. Carbon dioxide diffuses more readily across alveolar surfaces than does oxygen. If diffusing capacity is modestly reduced, arterial P_{O_2} falls before P_{CO_2} changes. The relationship between gases that enter the lung and gases that exist in the blood stream is expressed as the ventilation-perfusion ratio (V/Q). Reduction in diffusing capacity disturbs V/Q relationships and changes the values for P_{O_2} and P_{CO_2}. If there is mild disturbance of V/Q, the body compensates by increasing respiratory effort. This brings more oxygen into the lungs and leads to increased CO_2 excretion. Thus, in mild V/Q disturbance, a slightly decreased P_{CO_2} may be evidence that a seemingly normal P_{O_2} has been purchased at the cost of abnormal respiratory effort. As the V/Q becomes more severely disturbed, P_{CO_2} tends to rise because outward diffusion of CO_2 becomes impaired.

Pulmonary function is not, of course, the only determinant of P_{CO_2}. Systemic metabolism and renal function contribute significantly to total carbon dioxide levels. In order to maintain pH levels, the buffer system compensates for low HCO_3^- by excreting CO_2 and keeping as constant a ratio as possible between numerator and denominator of the Henderson-Hasselbalch equation. With disturbances of overall acid-base metabolism (see section below), the relationship between pH and P_{CO_2} undergoes significant changes. The availability of rapid, accurate measurements of pH, P_{CO_2}, and P_{O_2} makes it much easier to evaluate complex disturbances than was formerly the case.

Effect of Electrolytes

Changes in such serum electrolytes as Na^+, K^+, Ca^{++}, Cl^-, and others do not themselves affect the pH, but the electrolyte changes reflect physiologic derangements which also may affect acid-base balance. Renal excretory pathways are such that, in normal conditions, either Na^+ or K^+ is the primary urinary cation. If a sodium ion is reabsorbed from tubular urine, then a potassium ion is excreted in its place; the reverse occurs if potassium is reabsorbed. Hydrogen ions, either H^+ or NH_4^+, compete with K^+ in this exchange. In conditions of H^+ excess or K^+ deficit, hydrogen ions are excreted to replace Na^+.

The Anion Gap

Since serum is electrically neutral, total anions and total cations must be equal. Sodium and potassium are the major reported cations, while chloride and carbon dioxide provide the major anions. The totals of these two sets of laboratory data are not equal; the sum of sodium plus potassium is always greater than the sum of chloride plus total carbon dioxide. Anions deriving from nonvolatile organic acids and inorganic acids such as sulfates and phosphates account for the difference, sometimes called *anion gap* or *unmeasured anions*. Anion gap, calculated as $(Na^+ + K^+) - (Cl^- + CO_2$ content), is usually about 12 ± 2 mEq./L.

ABNORMAL IONS

Relatively few conditions cause the anion gap to diminish. The major cause is *paraproteinemia,* in which abnormal proteins replace sodium as serum cations. Serum sodium falls, causing a relative hyperchloremia and apparent reduction in unmeasured anions. IgG myeloma is far more likely to cause a reduced anion gap than is IgA myeloma.[4]

When serum bromide is high, chloride values drop, and there is a true increase in unmeasured anions. *Bromism* is by no means rare in those who take over-the-counter medications; it may cause anorexia, constipation, weight loss, irritability, and mental confusion—symptoms commonly attributed to irreversible senility in older people but reversible if due to an exogenous cause such as bromine self-medication.

INCREASED ANION GAP

The level of unmeasured anions is most useful in the differential diagnosis of acidosis. CO_2 levels actively change in response to changing pH and buffering needs; chloride rises as CO_2 declines if no other acidic ions are in the circulation, causing the total chloride plus CO_2 to remain fairly constant. Thus acidosis resulting from diarrheal loss of bicarbonate, renal tubular disorders, or administration of chloride-containing acidifying agents is characterized by low CO_2 levels, high serum chloride concentration, and relatively normal anion gap. If acidosis is due to circulation of ketone bodies, excessive lactate, or toxic metabolites of methyl alcohol, salicylates, or paraldehyde, other anions fill in the gap that occurs as carbon dioxide falls, and chloride levels remain unchanged. Renal failure alone causes a modest rise in unmeasured anions, because the acids normally present from ongoing metabolism are not excreted at normal rates. Acid retention from this cause rarely raises the anion gap beyond 20 to 25 mEq./L. If lactic acidosis or toxin ingestion is superimposed on known renal failure, the rise in anion gap can become very impressive.[10] Anion gap also rises in mixed conditions, when compensatory alkalosis combines with acidosis to produce normal bicarbonate values, but the underlying acidosis is apparent from the presence of circulating unmeasured anions.[5]

THE PRINCIPAL BUFFER SYSTEM

The bicarbonate-carbonic acid buffer system is peculiarly effective because the carbonic acid level can be altered rapidly by pulmonary CO_2 excretion, and the bicarbonate concentration is regulated in the kidney by excretion, reabsorption, and regeneration of the ion. Pulmonary compensation occurs very rapidly, but renal changes require several hours. The kidney also excretes nonvolatile acids by excreting the anion as the salt and disposing of the hydrogen ion. An excess acid load cannot simply be excreted as the hydrogen ion H^+ and the anion Ac^-, for this would lower the urinary pH beyond physiologic tolerance. Instead the Ac^- is excreted with Na^+, K^+, or other cations. Excess H^+ can be converted to NH_4^+ for excretion or may remain in the blood where it must be buffered.

When acid production or retention produces a hydrogen ion load, the body can neutralize the H^+ by conversion of HCO_3^- to H_2CO_3. This produces an increase in blood carbon dioxide, thus stimulating respiratory activity so that the carbon dioxide is blown off and the acid causes no physiologic damage. When the body's supply of HCO_3^- is depleted, this buffering activity must stop, and hydrogen ion accumulates. The ultimate solution, of course, is to reverse whatever process caused the build-up of acids. To consider all the complexities of acid-base and electrolyte interaction and appropriate therapeutic measures is beyond the scope of this discussion. We can, however, consider the main categories of acid-base disturbance, their usual etiologies, and associated laboratory findings.

DISORDERS OF ACID-BASE REGULATION

At this point, let us restate the Henderson-Hasselbalch equation, which describes the relationship between pH and the concentration of the buffer compounds:

$$pH = pK + \log\frac{[HCO_3^-]}{[H_2CO_3]}$$

In subsequent paragraphs, the bicarbonate concentration sometimes will be referred to as the numerator, and the P_{CO_2} (or transported CO_2) as the denominator; both these terms refer to the Henderson-Hasselbalch equation. At the normal pH of 7.4, the normal ratio between numerator and denominator is 20:1.

A pH rise is termed alkalosis or alkalemia. This can result from respiratory CO_2 loss (decrease in the denominator) or from a metabolically induced increase in bicarbonate (increase in the numerator). Acidosis or acidemia is a decrease in pH, which can have either a respiratory origin as carbon dioxide retention or a metabolic origin as loss of bicarbonate. Bicarbonate is lost when nonvolatile acids increase, since the bicarbonate must become H_2CO_3 to buffer the excess hydrogen ion, and the resulting carbon dioxide is lost to the body through respiratory excretion. The direction of pH change cannot be inferred simply from determination of bicarbonate content, as can be seen in Table 15.

Metabolic Acidosis

DIABETIC KETOACIDOSIS

The most dramatic example of metabolic acidosis is diabetic ketoacidosis, in which incomplete combustion of proteins and fatty acids

Table 15. Changes in Carbon Dioxide and pH

	Direction of pH Change	Change in PCO_2	Change in HCO_3^-
Metabolic acidosis			
Early	↓	↓	↓↓
Compensated	toward normal	↓↓↓	↓↓
Respiratory acidosis			
Early	↓	↑↑	↑
Compensated	toward normal	↑↑	↑↑↑
Metabolic alkalosis			
Early	↑	↑	↑↑
Compensated (often poor)	toward normal or ↑	↑	↑↑
Respiratory alkalosis			
Early	↑	↓↓	↓
Compensated	toward normal	↓↓	↓↓↓

produces nonvolatile ketoacids. These acids must be excreted in the urine along with some of the body's cations, and they must be buffered in the blood by conversion of bicarbonate into carbonic acid.[13] In trying to maintain the proportion of bicarbonate to carbonic acid at 20:1, the body continually decreases the denominator by respiratory excretion of CO_2 as the numerator decreases. The result is a tremendous loss of total CO_2 and a reduction in buffering capacity. Massive excretion of glucose and ketoacids leads to dehydration by osmotic diuresis. The osmotic diuresis impairs renal concentrating mechanisms, leading to still further water loss. Hyperventilation accentuates dehydration by insensible water loss. With dehydration, body temperature rises, and the resulting hypermetabolism induces further incomplete combustion and ketoacid production. To balance the excretion of ketoacid anions, massive cation loss occurs in the urine, leading to Na^+ and K^+ depletion.

THE POTASSIUM PROBLEM. Another mechanism for stabilizing blood pH is the exchange of serum hydrogen ions for intracellular potassium ions. When hydrogen ions disappear into the cells, the blood pH is partially protected, but the intracellular pH suffers. Furthermore, potassium ions which enter the blood from their previous intracellular location rapidly leave the body as urinary cations, so that whole-body stores of potassium are seriously depleted. The serum potassium concentration at any given moment may be normal or low but does not reflect the whole-body state.

LABORATORY FINDINGS. Typical laboratory findings in diabetic ketoacidosis include marked reduction in total CO_2 and significant fall in P_{CO_2}, pH drop proportional to the severity of the condition, decreased serum sodium with a variable level of serum potassium, marked increase in unmeasured anions with relatively small change in chlorides, and, of course, tremendously elevated blood glucose levels.

ACIDOSIS OF RENAL DISEASE

Another relatively common cause of metabolic acidosis is severe renal disease, which ordinarily produces a chronic condition rather than a sudden, dramatic episode. Overall metabolism produces approximately 50 to 75 mEq. of hydrogen ion daily, an amount which, if retained, depresses the bicarbonate buffer by approximately 3 or 4 mEq./L. in a 70-kg. individual.[9] This acidosis may develop rapidly in acute renal failure, but more often the hydrogen ion excretion is partially effective and other defects combine to produce a series of problems. As the kidney loses its ability to excrete nonvolatile acids, carbonic anhydrase activity diminishes as well, so that bicarbonate reabsorption and regeneration are severely impaired. The combination of nonvolatile acids and decreased bicarbonate is similar in general outlines to diabetic acidosis. In the chronic state, CO_2 content persists at a low level. Because there is no acute rise in denominator to precipitate hyperventilation, the P_{CO_2} is less depressed than in diabetic ketoacidosis. Cation loss is not significant, and as the renal disease worsens, hyperkalemia may occur. The blood glucose is normal, but there is an increase in unmeasured anions, and high levels of BUN and creatinine are present.

INTOXICATIONS

Acidosis with increased unmeasured anions occurs with certain intoxications, notably from salicylates, methanol, and paraldehyde. Salicylism is an especially complex problem, since there are elements which dispose toward both respiratory alkalosis and metabolic acidosis. Salicylism also causes lactic acid to accumulate (see below).

Lactic Acidosis

Very severe pH drop, with a large anion gap and markedly increased plasma osmolality, occurs in lactic acidosis.

BIOCHEMISTRY

Lactic acid is the reduction product of pyruvic acid. Pyruvic acid is formed early in glycolysis, under aerobic or anaerobic conditions. When oxygen is plentiful, pyruvate enters the mitochondria for further metabolism. Under anaerobic conditions, or when hydrogen ion concentration increases, pyruvate is converted to lactate. Pyruvate also participates in gluconeogenesis, the conversion of amino acids to glucose. Further conversion to glucose or direct entry into the tricarboxylic acid cycle depends upon the presence of plentiful NAD^+, the oxidized form of this electron receptor, and upon adequate functioning of the enzyme pyruvate dehydrogenase.[2]

Pyruvate accumulates if there is insufficient oxygen to allow aerobic energy production or if anything increases protein breakdown and amino acid conversion. Conditions that inhibit pyruvate dehydrogenase or that interfere with restoration of NAD^+ from NADH promote the conversion of pyruvate to lactate. When NAD^+ is plentiful, lactate is converted to pyruvate, which then can undergo oxidative metabolism or be converted into the amino acid alanine.

CLINICAL CONDITIONS

Lactic acidosis occurs under two different sets of circumstances. When there is tissue hypoxia and poor perfusion due to circulatory collapse, hydrogen ion concentration increases and oxygen saturation declines. This inhibits energy-generating oxidation of pyruvate and causes large-scale conversion of pyruvate into lactic acid. The resulting accumulation of acid aggravates hypotension, further slowing perfusion and interfering with release of oxygen from hemoglobin. Rising lactate concentration is the immediate cause of systemic acidosis, but it is the primary condition, such as cardiogenic or endotoxic shock, left ventricular failure, or severe anemia, that causes the lactate accumulation. Alkalinizing therapy may ameliorate part of the problem, but treating the underlying process should be the major consideration.

More complex metabolic derangements cause lactic acidosis of the type unaccompanied by tissue hypoxia. Uncontrolled diabetes mellitus, severe liver disease, and renal failure may produce acute lactate accumulation, owing in part to impaired hepatic clearance of lactate, depleted NAD^+, enhanced protein breakdown, and, in diabetes, to inadequacy of insulin levels so that lactic dehydrogenase activity declines. Leukemias and lymphomas, characterized by large numbers of cells with abnormal carbohydrate metabolism, also may cause lactic acidosis.[3]

Many exogenous agents promote lactic acidosis. The biguanide group of oral antidiabetic agents interferes with the transport of pyruvate across mitochondrial membranes. Nonglucose sugars administered as part of intravenous hyperalimentation regimens undergo rapid conversion to lactate. Ethyl alcohol pushes the $NAD^+ \rightleftarrows NADH$ conversion heavily to the side of NADH, causing lactate to accumulate sharply at the expense of pyruvate. If hepatic metabolism is already impaired by chronic liver damage or acute hepatitis, the lactate-promoting effects of alcohol are multiplied. With these metabolic problems, intensive alkalinization is extremely helpful in combating the vicious circle of lowered pH, lowered lactate conversion, and increased lactate production.

LABORATORY FINDINGS

Normal blood lactate levels are between 0.4 and 1.3 mM./L. If lactate rises above 2.0 mM./L. and pH falls below 7.37, a state of lactic acidosis exists. Renal disease or diabetic ketoacidosis may accentuate the pH drop and the increase in anion gap, but lactate measurements reveal the degree to which lactic acidosis constitutes a separate problem. Additional findings include markedly increased plasma osmolality, increased levels of lactate dehydrogenase and glutamic-oxalacetic transaminase, and, sometimes, increased serum phosphate levels.

Primary Bicarbonate Alteration

Acidosis without increased unmeasured anions occurs when large amounts of bicarbonate are lost, typically from prolonged or severe diarrhea. Distal to the entrance of the alkaline pancreatic juice, intestinal contents contain large amounts of bicarbonate. Excessive fecal excretion seriously depletes this anion. Renal disease, in which bicarbonate reabsorption and regeneration are impaired, may cause a similar situation. This type of renal tubular acidosis results from hereditary or acquired tubular defects or from massive ingestion of a carbonic anhydrase inhibitor or ammonium chloride.

Significant findings in such cases include increased serum chlorides, which rise to compensate the anion deficit caused by bicarbonate loss. Serum sodium and potassium are variably diminished, and total CO_2 content usually is reduced only moderately. If compensatory mechanisms are adequate, the pH change is relatively slight, but if the diarrheal process is catastrophic, as it may be in small children or in any patient with certain bacterial infections, rapid and severe acidosis may occur.

Respiratory Alkalosis

As in metabolic acidosis, CO_2 content diminishes in respiratory alkalosis. The primary defect is increased pulmonary loss of carbon dioxide, which decreases the denominator of the Henderson-Hasselbalch equation and disposes toward pH rise. To prevent this pH change, the body increases bicarbonate excretion and lowers the numerator to maintain the proportion. The net result is depletion of both bicarbonate and carbonic acid, with ultimate loss of buffering capacity and rise in pH. Respiratory alkalosis more often is acute than chronic, and the most usual cause is psychogenic hyperventilation. Salicylate intoxication, early in the disease, causes respiratory alkalosis by directly stimulating the respiratory center. Later, metabolic acidosis supervenes, intensifying the loss of total CO_2 even though the direction of pH change is reversed. Any conditions of high body temperature or hypermetabolism, such as severe febrile illness or thyrotoxicosis, may cause CO_2 loss through increased respiration. Chronic states of hyperventilation are rare but do occur in certain central nervous system lesions.

LABORATORY FINDINGS

In chronic conditions, urinary bicarbonate excretion increases, and excretion of this anion requires the balancing presence of such cations as sodium, potassium, or calcium. Serum chloride rises as bicarbonate levels fall, and serum sodium and potassium values are low. In acute episodes, the only abnormal laboratory findings may be low P_{CO_2} and high pH, since compensatory bicarbonate change requires several hours. Fairly common symptoms of hyperventilation are light-headedness, carpopedal spasm, and muscle tremors. These symptoms are halted dramatically if the patient rebreathes air in a paper bag, thereby raising the P_{CO_2} of the alveolar air and increasing the denominator of the fraction.

Metabolic Alkalosis

In metabolic alkalosis, the total CO_2 increases because the bicarbonate numerator rises. The initial response to an increased numerator is to decrease respiratory effort and conserve CO_2 so that the denominator can increase as well. This compensation is doomed to failure, for respiration can diminish only to a certain point. Beyond that point, the rising P_{CO_2} has a stimulatory effect on the respiratory center. If the respiratory center becomes refractory to CO_2 rise, hypoxia alone can promote respiratory effort.

THE POTASSIUM PROBLEM

The causes of metabolic alkalosis are varied. Excess bicarbonate ingestion, by itself, rarely causes significant alkalosis because the properly functioning kidney can excrete enormous amounts of this ion. If something prevents the suitable excretion of bicarbonate and accompanying cations, equilibrium is disturbed and alkalosis may occur. Prolonged bicarbonate excretion forces the urinary loss of abundant potassium as well as sodium. If potassium loss is not compensated by increased intake, potassium deficiency may occur. In an effort to conserve potassium, the kidney excretes hydrogen ions into the urine, reabsorbing both sodium and potassium. As sodium ions return from the tubular urine into the blood, they carry bicarbonate back with them, thus reversing the direction of bicarbonate flow and defeating the effort to excrete excess bicarbonate. If potassium is lost in the urine, serum levels are supplied from intracellular stores. To replace potassium in the intracellular fluid, hydrogen ions leave the blood stream. This maintains the ionic balance in the cells, but the H^+ loss additionally raises the serum pH. A primary potassium deficit from unbalanced parenteral feeding, drug-induced diuresis, or gastrointestinal loss, can by itself initiate metabolic alkalosis through this effect.

THE BICARBONATE PROBLEM

Loss of gastric contents by prolonged vomiting or gastric suction is the most common cause of metabolic alkalosis. Gastric secretions are acid, containing high levels of hydrogen and chloride ions as well as large amounts of water. Prolonged vomiting leads not only to hydrogen ion deficit, but also to hypochloremia and dehydration. Serum bicarbonate rises to compensate chloride loss. Potassium and sodium also are lost with gastric contents, so that cation deficits may complicate the condition. As the kidney attempts to increase bicarbonate excretion, further sodium and potassium loss occurs in the urine. In its attempt to conserve cations and continue excreting bicarbonate, the kidney may excrete hydrogen ions to balance the bicarbonate anions. The seemingly paradoxical result is an acid urine at a time of increasing alkalosis.

LABORATORY FINDINGS

The laboratory findings in metabolic alkalosis may be complex. The blood pH and total CO_2 content are increased, but P_{CO_2} cannot rise beyond a certain point. Serum chloride values are low, and sodium and potassium levels may be misleading. The serum potassium and sodium concentrations are affected by dehydration. If water loss exceeds electrolyte loss, hemoconcentration may result in normal or even elevated sodium values.

Respiratory Acidosis

The defect in respiratory acidosis is impaired excretion of carbon dioxide, so that CO_2 retention increases the denominator of the fraction. Normally, there is rapid and complete diffusion of carbon dioxide from capillary blood into alveolar air spaces. Only the most severe thickening of the alveolar walls can, by itself, impair gaseous exchange significantly. This may occur in hyaline membrane disease in infants; the presence of intra-alveolar edema fluid or inflammatory infiltrate can exert a similar effect. Gas exchange more often is impeded by a combination of thickened alveolar wall and loss of capillary blood supply, through scarring, vascular disease, or destructive processes.

Respiratory acidosis usually is a chronic problem occurring in patients with long-standing pulmonary or cardiovascular disease. The respiratory center responds to elevated P_{CO_2} levels (hypercapnia) with increased ventilation. This alone can return the P_{CO_2} to normal if the condition is mild. More often, if the pulmonary problem is a chronic one, increased respiratory effort succeeds only in preventing additional CO_2 buildup, but does not return the CO_2 levels to normal. To compensate for this persistently elevated denominator, the kidney retains bicarbonate and sodium and excretes the excess hydrogen ions as NH_4^+. These cations remove chloride through the urine, so that serum chloride falls and bicarbonate rises. Both numerator and denominator increase; if the proportion of 20:1 is maintained, pH remains unchanged.

CHRONIC HYPERCAPNIA

This condition of compensated respiratory acidosis with chronically elevated P_{CO_2} causes the respiratory center to become progressively less sensitive to existing P_{CO_2} elevation. Only an additional rise in P_{CO_2} causes the respiratory center to respond once again to stimulation. This process of accommodation to rising P_{CO_2} levels may reach extreme proportions, so that P_{CO_2} virtually loses its power to affect respiration. At that stage, the effective stimulus to respiratory effort is hypoxia, and well-meaning treatment which suddenly restores oxygen values to normal may remove the only stimulus left for respiratory effort. Treatment of far-advanced pulmonary disease should be planned carefully, and mechanical respirators frequently are advisable during the period of physiologic readjustment.

Respiratory acidosis is the condition in which P_{CO_2} determination has its greatest value, since the pH and the total CO_2 content may not reflect rapid changes in respiratory state. If compensation is successful, of course, the pH does not change at all. Total CO_2 may be misleading if concomitant metabolic problems also affect the bicarbonate level. In pure respiratory acidosis, the potassium and sodium are approximately normal, the chloride is low, and the total CO_2 and P_{CO_2} are elevated.

WATER AND ELECTROLYTES

Approximately 45 to 70 percent of the body's weight is water, and a variety of substances are dissolved or suspended in this medium. The principal electrolytes of the extracellular fluid are sodium, chloride, and bicarbonate; lesser contributions to the anions come from phosphates and organic acids, and to the cations from potassium, calcium, and magnesium. The fluid within cells is quite different, containing potassium as its principal cation, while proteins and bicarbonate markedly affect the anionic content.

Fluid Balance

Body water comes from oral intake and from metabolic processes — the so-called water of oxidation. Water is lost through many routes. Insensible loss, amounting to about 400 ml. per day, occurs from the skin and the lungs. Increase in body temperature or environmental temperature increases this quantity. A minimum of 500 ml. of urine per day is necessary to excrete metabolic end products if the kidneys can exert maximum concentrating power. Fecal losses vary with the state of gastrointestinal physiology, but tend to average about 100 ml. per day. Sensible sweating accounts for a variable fluid loss, depending on activity, environmental temperature, and body temperature.

Regulation of fluid and electrolyte balance occurs largely through the kidney, for the losses from skin, lungs, and intestines are under little physiologic control. The kidney regulates sodium, potassium, hydrogen ion, and bicarbonate excretion to maintain electrolyte balance, while regulation of urinary volume and concentration maintains fluid homeostasis. Renal regulation of volume is directed largely by the pituitary hormone vasopressin (antidiuretic hormone), through the action of which the kidney can secrete small volumes of concentrated urine when water must be conserved. Sodium is retained and potassium excreted under the influence of the adrenal hormone aldosterone. Bicarbonate, ammonium, and hydrogen ions are regulated by chemical reactions in the tubular epithelium. Phosphate excretion is influenced by the parathyroid hormone. These multiple influences on normal fluid and electrolyte regulation can be challenged by a variety of abnormal states, affecting virtually any organ system.

Laboratory Determinations

The flame photometer is used to measure serum sodium and potassium concentrations. Chemical reactions are used for measuring chlorides, phosphates, and, usually, calcium. Measurement of the bicarbonate-carbon dioxide variables was discussed in an earlier section. Total serum osmolality can be measured directly through freezing point determinations.[7] Although sodium chloride is the major normal determinant of serum osmolality, glucose and urea can contribute significantly if these are deranged. Sodium, urea, and glucose are all measured easily, and can be used to calculate expected osmolality, using the formula:[12]

$$SO = 2\,(Na^+) + Glucose/18(or\ 20) + BUN/2.8(or\ 3)$$

where SO is the calculated serum osmolality, Na^+ is expressed in milliequivalents per liter, and glucose and BUN are measured in milligrams per deciliter. Normal osmolality ranges between 280 and 300 mOsm./kg. of serum water and usually is given as 285 mOsm./kg.

ELECTROLYTES AND OSMOLALITY

It must be remembered that normal serum is only 93 percent water. The remaining 7 percent is contributed by solids (i.e., lipids and protein). If dysproteinemia, hyperglobulinemia, or hyperlipidemia exists, the amount of water per volume of serum declines. This affects the measured value of electrolytes, since there is less water in which they are dissolved. These bulky molecules do not notably affect the serum osmolality, as measured by freezing point depression. Comparing the calculated serum osmolality with the measured osmolality can indicate whether water depletion is present. Low serum sodium and, consequently, low calculated osmolality in the presence of normal measured osmolality suggest increased amounts of osmotically inactive solid molecules in the serum.

Conversely, a normal calculated value in the presence of increased measured osmolality indicates the presence of unmeasured molecules that do contribute osmotic activity. Ethanol is a notorious offender in this regard. Elevated serum lactate, either as primary lactic acidosis or secondary to alcohol abuse, also commonly increases measured osmolality. Other osmotically active materials that should be kept in mind include mannitol or sorbitol, methanol, and isopropyl alcohol.

Electrolyte values alone can be misleading unless the overall state of hydration is known. Serum sodium concentration, for example, can be low when edema or congestive heart failure expands the extracellular fluid volume, but the whole-body supply of sodium tends to be greater than normal. In dehydration, the serum sodium concentration may be high, but if both water and electrolytes have been lost, the overall sodium stores may be significantly lower than normal.

In estimating the overall state of fluid and electrolyte equilibrium, a variety of laboratory determinations can supplement serum electrolyte measurements. Examination of urine volume and specific gravity indicates the overall state of hydration, and measurement of urinary electrolyte concentrations may clarify the etiology of the metabolic alterations.

Sodium

WHOLE-BODY DEFICIT

If fluid and sodium are lost in proportions equal to that in plasma, isotonic dehydration results, with relatively little change in electrolyte concentrations. In diagnosing this state, elevated levels of serum proteins and a high hematocrit indicate hemoconcentration. Consideration of the patient's clinical state is essential in diagnosing and treating dehydration. Severe vomiting, hyperventilation, sweating, or diuresis may cause loss of water in excess of sodium loss, resulting in hypernatremic dehydration, even though total sodium supplies are decreased to some extent. In these cases, serum sodium concentration may be normal or high, along with elevated hematocrit and high serum protein values. The urinary sodium load will be very low, indicating a whole-body need for sodium retention despite normal serum values.

WHOLE-BODY EXCESS

In states of increased total body water, the whole-body sodium supply may be high, even though the sodium concentration in a serum aliquot is lower than normal. This occurs in cardiac failure, renal insufficiency, cirrhosis, and other conditions in which hypoalbuminemia reduces plasma colloid pressure and decreases renal plasma flow. Low serum sodium concentration may occur in states of water intoxication, which is often iatrogenic, or in conditions of inappropriate secretion of antidiuretic hormone.

Potassium

WHOLE-BODY DEFICIT

The relation between whole-body potassium and serum potassium concentration is variable as well. Since potassium is primarily an intracellular ion, the bulk of the body's stores cannot be measured in routinely available tests. If there is massive loss of extracellular potassium, normally intracellular potassium may leave the cells to support the serum concentration. This process cannot be measured directly and can only be inferred from an understanding of the clinical state and from such signs as dehydration, muscle weakness, tremors, and changes in the electrocardiographic tracing. Diabetic ketoacidosis is a prime offender in this respect, and primary or secondary hyperaldosteronism also may deplete whole-body potassium stores. In acidosis of any type, potassium ions may enter the blood stream as hydrogen ions enter the cells; administration of insulin produces the opposite effect, causing potassium to leave the plasma and go into the intracellular fluid.

Potassium loss can occur through the urinary or gastrointestinal tracts, due to renal tubular disorders, massive diuresis, hyperaldosteronism, diarrhea, intestinal fistulas, or vomiting. Loss of gastric contents causes massive loss of hydrogen ions, since the gastric juices are highly acidic. Severe vomiting and other conditions associated with alkalosis may be accompanied by hypopotassemia far more severe than the external loss would suggest.

WHOLE-BODY EXCESS

Hyperkalemia can result from decreased urinary output or from excessive intake. Whenever there is destruction of protein or body tissue, normally intracellular potassium is released into the blood stream. Thus severe accidental or operative trauma, burns, or wasting diseases impose a potassium load on the body. Usually these very conditions are associated with impaired renal function or impaired renal blood flow, or both, so that with the normal excretory route blocked, severe hyperkalemia may occur. High serum potassium levels may complicate adrenal insufficiency, acute renal failure, and the terminal stages of chronic renal disease.

ARTEFACTS

Artefactual elevation of the serum potassium levels can occur in improperly handled blood samples. Prolonged venous stasis during venipuncture can cause mild changes, and hemolysis of the specimen renders the potassium measurement worthless. Prompt separation of serum from cells is advisable so that intracellular potassium does not diffuse into the serum.

Chloride

Alteration of serum chloride is seldom a primary problem. Chlorides are excreted with cations during massive diuresis from any cause and are lost from the gastrointestinal tract in vomiting, diarrhea, or intestinal fistulas. Measurement of serum chloride usually is done for its inferential value. Serum chlorides are decreased (1) in conditions of acidosis when the anionic compartment is invaded by "unmeasured anions" from organic or other acids, (2) in conditions of gastrointestinal loss or obstruction, (3) in conditions of extracellular fluid excess such as edema and congestive heart failure, (4) in conditions of excessive urinary loss such as chronic renal failure or tubular acidosis, and (5) in certain abnormal states of the central nervous system. Hyperchloremia is rare, because sodium and chloride retention usually is accompanied by fluid retention as well. Severe dehydration, complete renal shut-down, and injudicious administration of ammonium chloride may elevate serum chloride concentrations.

REFERENCES

1. Astrup, P., Engle, K. Jorgensen, K., and Siggaard-Andersen, O.: *Definitions and terminology in blood acid-base chemistry.* Ann. N.Y. Acad. Sci. 133:59, 1966.
2. Alberti, K. G. M. M., and Nattrass, M.: *Lactic acidosis.* Lancet 2:25, 1977.
3. Bonnici, F., Smith, S., and Heese, H. deV.: *The anion gap.* Lancet 1:1304, 1977.
4. DeTroyer, A., Stolarczyk, A., deBeyl, D. Z., and Stryckmans, P.: *Value of anion-gap determination in multiple myeloma.* N. Engl. J. Med. 296:858, 1977.
5. Emmett, M., and Narins, R. G.: *Clinical use of the anion gap.* Medicine 56:38, 1977.
6. Gambino, S. R.: *pH and PCO_2,* in Meites, S. (ed.): *Standard Methods of Clinical Chemistry.* vol. 5. Academic Press, New York, 1965.
7. Hendry, E. B.: *Osmolality of human serum and of chemical solutions of biological importance.* Clin. Chem. 7:156, 1961.
8. Levinsky, N. G.: *Acidosis and alkalosis,* in Thorn, G. W., Adams, R. D., Braunwald, E., et al. (eds.): *Harrison's Principles of Internal Medicine.* ed. 8. McGraw-Hill, New York, 1977.
9. Levitin, H.: *Acid-base balance,* in Bondy, P. K., and Rosenberg, L. E. (eds.): *Duncan's Diseases of Metabolism.* ed. 7. W. B. Saunders, Philadelphia, 1974.
10. Narins, R. G., and Emmett, M.: *The anion gap.* Lancet 1:1304, 1977.
11. Nuttall, F. Q.: *Serum electrolytes and their relation to acid-base balance.* Arch. Intern. Med. 116:670, 1965.
12. Smithline, N., and Gardner, K. D.: *Gaps—anionic and osmolal.* J.A.M.A. 236:1594, 1976.
13. Winegrad, A. I., and Clements, R. S., Jr.: *Diabetic ketoacidosis.* Med. Clin. North Am. 55:899, 1971.

CHAPTER 11

SERUM ENZYMES OF DIAGNOSTIC IMPORTANCE

Enzymes are catalysts, enhancing the multiple reactions that collectively constitute body metabolism. Enzymes are highly specific in their activity, and all metabolizing cells contain some or many of these essential compounds. Certain tissues contain characteristic enzymes which enter the blood only when the cells to which they are confined are damaged or destroyed. The presence in the blood of significant quantities of these specific enzymes indicates the probable site of tissue damage. Small amounts circulate in the blood at all times. Because of differing analytic techniques and reporting units, there is great variation among laboratories in their normal values. The reader should note carefully the range of normal values reported for each enzyme by the specific laboratory he uses.

ALDOLASE

Aldolase, a glycolytic enzyme that splits fructose 1,6-diphosphate, is present most significantly in skeletal and heart muscle, although all cells contain a small amount, and the liver has a moderate concentration. Both colorimetric and spectrophotometric methods are used for measurement. The normal range in adult serum is 1.5 to 7.2 mM./min./L.,[40] using the method of Sibley and Lehninger.[38] Because aldolase is present within red blood cells, unhemolyzed serum must be used when enzyme activity is measured. Damage to skeletal muscle produces high serum levels of aldolase; this is particularly so in the case of progressive muscular dystrophy in which the level may be ten to fifteen times normal. There is no aldolase elevation in muscle diseases of neural origin such as neurogenic muscular atrophy, polio-myelitis, myasthenia gravis, and multiple sclerosis, but any of the inflammatory conditions involving muscle may cause moderately high values. In progressive muscular dystrophy, the aldolase level subsides as the disease progresses toward pronounced muscular wasting.

Despite the relatively low concentration in the liver, aldolase elevations to 17 to 80 international units (I.U.) per liter occur in early viral hepatitis. The sharp initial rise dissipates over the ensuing 2 or 3 weeks of the disease. Biliary obstruction and cirrhosis do not affect the aldolase level. Myocardial infarction may cause a slight rise, but aldolase determinations offer no advantage over transaminase determinations in diagnosing cardiac or hepatic disease. Serum aldolase also may rise with advanced prostatic carcinoma.

AMYLASE

Amylase splits starch into its component sugars. Its activity is extracellular, and salivary glands and the pancreas secrete the enzyme into the saliva and pancreatic fluid. Since a quantity of unsecreted enzyme exists within the secretory cells, damage to either the glandular cells or the secretory pathway may cause amylase to enter the blood stream. Amylase activity is measured by its effect upon a starch solution. This can be expressed either as the amount of sugar produced or as the amount of starch altered. In the Somogyi method, the resulting sugars are measured colorimetrically,[18] giving normal values of 40 to 140 units/dl.

In the dye method,[32] the enzyme acts upon a starch-dye substrate, and the amount of dye that the enzyme releases can be measured easily. This has good correlation with the saccharogenic method on serum, but values are much lower in urine, saliva, and pancreatic juice,[29] which do not have high protein concentration. Adding albumin to the specimen activates the enzyme and brings the results for this method into agreement with the saccharogenic technique.

Pancreatic Disease

Serum amylase elevations ordinarily indicate pancreatic disease. In acute pancreatitis, levels may rise to 600 Somogyi units within 4 hours of onset, reaching levels as high as 2000 units within a relatively short time.[40] The fall, like the rise, is rapid, and values may return to normal within 48 to 72 hours, even though active inflammation persists. Under these circumstances, elevated urinary amylase levels may be diagnostically revealing. In patients with severe abdominal pain, blood should be drawn for amylase levels before diagnostic or therapeutic measures are undertaken. Even without pancreatic disease, spasm of the sphincter of Oddi can elevate the serum amylase to as much as 600 units. Both morphine and certain radiopaque substances used in cholecystography induce significant spasm of the sphincter.

Other Diseases

Elevated serum amylase may accompany acute abdominal pain in certain cases of perforated peptic ulcer, empyema of the gallbladder, intestinal obstruction, ruptured ectopic pregnancy, or peritonitis from any cause.[27] In these cases, chemical irritation of the pancreas may cause transient pancreatitis, and the engorged permeable capillaries of the inflamed area readily absorb the enzyme from the biliary or intestinal fluid. Chronic pancreatitis produces less marked and rather variable elevations of serum amylase, and carcinoma of the pancreas characteristically does not affect the enzyme. Serum amylase levels as high as 700 to 900 units may follow disease of the parotid gland. Although enzyme determination is rarely needed for diagnosing disease of the salivary glands, it may be helpful in cases of mumps encephalitis or mumps orchitis with little overt salivary gland involvement. Separation of amylase activity into isoenzymes according to the gland of origin is feasible but presently not of diagnostic use.[27]

Amylase is excreted in the urine, and if the serum level has already decined, the urinary level may be useful diagnostically. Patients with severe renal disease may retain amylase in the serum, and elevation resulting from acute pancreatitis persists for an abnormally long time if the kidneys are diseased. Patients with the protein abnormality *macroamylasemia* have normal pancreatic function, but enzyme levels in the serum are high. Urine levels are normal, however, because the complex or polymerized molecule cannot cross the glomerular filter.[39]

CHOLINESTERASE

Two different cholinesterases have been identified, both of which hydrolyze acetylcholine and other cholinesters. One acts upon acetylcholine more rapidly than upon other cholinesters and is termed acetylcholinesterase, although formerly it was known as "true" cholinesterase. It is present in nearly all tissues, but especially in the gray matter of the central nervous system and in the conducting tissue, and is found in red blood cells but not in plasma. The less specific enzyme, formerly called pseudocholinesterase, acts indiscriminately upon a variety of cholinesters, including succinylcholine. This form, now known as cholinesterase, exists in plasma but not in red cells. Manufactured by the liver and present in a variety of organs, its physiologic role is imperfectly understood.

Acetylcholinesterase

Both cholinesterases are irreversibly inactivated by organophosphates, but it is acetylcholinesterase that is usually measured to document acute or chronic toxicity from this class of insecticides. The erythrocyte enzyme reflects toxicity more reliably than does the plasma activity,[11] and its regeneration after inhibition is much slower. Since, in a normal population, a rather wide range of activity exists, precise normal values are difficult to define, and a single value, measured during an episode of suspected organophosphate toxicity, may be difficult to interpret.

Knowledge of an individual's pre-exposure level can be extremely helpful; repeated surveillance of individuals known to be at risk for organophosphate exposure provides highly useful baseline data. Without comparison data for the individual, an activity level below 25 percent of the mean for the laboratory's normal population is considered diagnostically low.

Serum Cholinesterase

Serum, or plasma, cholinesterase exists in several genetically determined variants. The normal form, assayed by its activity on selected substrates in an appropriate buffer, can be measured as an index of liver function. Levels are decreased in parenchymatous liver disease, especially hepatitis and cirrhosis, and in such other conditions of disordered protein synthesis as malnutrition, carcinomatosis, and severe anemia. It is reported to be high in patients with nephrotic syndrome.[11] The enzyme is rarely measured for these conditions, since cholinesterase determination provides no information in addition to that supplied by the usual diagnostic tests for these diseases.

SUCCINYLCHOLINE SENSITIVITY

Although the intended physiologic role of cholinesterase is obscure, its absence can produce serious pharmacologic consequences. When patients lacking normal enzyme levels are exposed to suxamethonium (succinylcholine), protracted apnea and generalized muscle relaxation occurs, apparently due to failure to inactivate the ester. This condition constitutes a disease of medical progress, since succinylcholine enters the body only when given as a relaxant prior to anesthesia or electroconvulsive therapy. Individuals with the usual cholinesterase readily inactivate the drug; those with any of the variant enzymes appear unable to overcome the drug and sustain its exaggerated effects for several hours.

At least three variant genes have been identified, determining forms of cholinesterase described as dibucaine-resistant, fluoride-resistant, and "silent."[24] Dibucaine resistance has been known for many years, and the *dibucaine number* has long been used to classify heterozygotes and homozygotes for this atypical enzyme. Homozygotes, who comprise perhaps 0.1 to 0.5 percent of the white population,[25] are susceptible to succinylcholine apnea, but occasional heterozygotes also may show symptoms. The other forms are still less frequent. Symptomatically, the patients are similar, but the variants are fairly readily distinguished chemically.[16]

Accurate enzymatic determination is the only reliable way to identify patients at risk. A simple kit is available for screening, but its sensitivity appears insufficient to characterize those members of the general population for whom succinylcholine exposure may prove dangerous.[12]

CREATINE PHOSPHOKINASE

Creatine phosphokinase (CPK, also called creatine kinase or CK) catalyzes the reversible transfer of phosphate groups between creatine and phosphocreatine as well as between ADP and ATP. Most of the body's CPK resides in skeletal muscle, heart muscle, and the gastrointestinal tract; the brain is the only other major source. Lung, kidney, liver, and spleen contain tiny amounts, while red and white blood cells have virtually no CPK activity.

Total Serum Activity

CPK enters the blood stream rapidly following damage to muscle cells and slowly after brain tissue is damaged. Clearance is fairly rapid, occurring largely in the liver and, to a lesser extent, through renal excretion. Because of its limited tissue distribution and prompt appearance in the blood stream, CPK seemed at first to be an excellent marker for acute myocardial or skeletal muscle damage. It appeared to surpass transaminase and lactic dehydrogenase as a marker for myocardial infarction because it was not affected by the many noncardiac conditions that influence LDH and transaminase values. Serum CPK rises within 6 hours of damage to myocardial cells, reaching a peak at about 18 hours, and then falling to normal in 3 or 4 days.[33]

Unfortunately, total serum CPK proved unreliable as a specific indicator for acute myocardial damage because of its lability and sensitivity. Rather minor insults to skeletal muscle cause total serum levels to rise dramatically. Common occurrences such as vigorous exercise, a fall, or a deep intramuscular injection can elevate total CPK to significant levels. Surgical procedures that penetrate muscle layers invariably elevate the circulating enzyme. Since these events often coincide with clinical circumstances that point to myocardial infarction, total CPK determination has proved less useful than original workers predicted. Very high levels correlate well with myocardial necrosis, except in the first few days after cardiac surgery, when levels may rise to 200 I.U. or more, on the basis of operative trauma alone.[35] A moderately elevated level, however, could result from a small infarct, difficult to diagnose by other means, but also could represent a physiologic or false-positive rise. Because serum levels rise and fall so rapidly, the enzyme is particularly useful for diagnosing acute changes or extension of damage after a period of apparent healing.

MUSCLE DISEASES

Acute or ongoing damage to skeletal muscle causes serum CPK levels to skyrocket. The muscular dystrophies cause persisting elevations as high as 50 or 100 times the normal value. These changes reflect damage to functional muscle tissue and are seen early in the disease. As muscle mass declines, so does the amount of circulating CPK. In advanced disease, enzyme levels have little diagnostic or prognostic value. Serum CPK levels are higher than normal in most female carriers for Duchenne's muscular dystrophy, the common, X-linked type of muscular dystrophy. Because a wide range of enzyme values exists in women known to be carriers, the simple determination of serum CPK is insufficient for definitive diagnosis of the carrier state.

Polymyositis and early dermatomyositis are other conditions that cause serum CPK to rise dramatically. Severe hypothyroidism may cause a moderate rise in total CPK,[14] owing apparently to skeletal muscle deterioration.

Isoenzymes

The CPK molecule is a dimer composed of two subunits which may be of the same or different types. Two types have been identified: M, associated with muscle, and B, associated with brain. Skeletal muscle contains huge quantities of the MM dimer. Brain contains the BB dimer in modest amounts; GI tract also contains the BB form.[33] Heart muscle contains large amounts of MM but also has the hybrid dimer, MB. MB is not the predominant isoenzyme of heart muscle, but because it is present in no other tissue, it provides a unique marker for damage to myocardial cells.

The CPK isoenzymes can be separated by electrophoretic or ion-exchange techniques. Electrophoresis provides fairly rapid and quite distinct separation but requires some form of intensification so that low activity levels become apparent. The problem is that MM levels tend to overshadow MB activity. Since MB is not present in normal serum, mere demonstration of MB activity indicates damage to myocardial cells. Fluorescence intensification can be used to demonstrate qualitatively that an MB band is present on the electrophoretic strip. Quantitation of the separated isoenzymes is possible after elution from the electrophoretic strip or after ion-exchange separation.

MYOCARDIAL DAMAGE

Probably the most sensitive laboratory indication of myocardial necrosis is the presence in serum of CPK-MB. This occurs early, in the first day or two after damage,[15,41] and disappears fairly rapidly if no new necrosis follows. Patients hospitalized for actual or suspected infarction may continue to have high total CPK values if they receive intramuscular morphine injections, but decline in the MB level indicates that no additional myocardial cells are being destroyed.[33] Extremely important in differential diagnosis is the fact that CPK-MB does not rise after pulmonary embolism and congestive heart failure or during angina pectoris not accompanied by cellular necrosis.[33,41] All of these are conditions that may be difficult to distinguish from myocardial infarction in clinical and other laboratory findings.

Qualitative or semiquantitative demonstration of CPK-MB is unnecessary in clear-cut cases of myocardial infarction, but it provides invaluable information in diagnosis and management of early, small, or ambiguous episodes of myocardial damage and in distinguishing preinfarction angina from slowly evolving myocardial necrosis. With quantitative techniques, several workers have attempted to correlate serum CPK-MB levels with size of myocardial infarction.[33,42] The amount of measurable CPK-MB depends not only on the number of cells damaged, but also on the adequacy of circulation to the damaged area, the rate at which enzyme enters the blood stream, and the rate at which it is cleared or inactivated. Although preliminary results have shown good correlation between CPK-MB levels and infarct size, the degree of physiologic variation and technical difficulty make it unlikely that quantitative procedures will have widespread clinical applicability. Qualitative procedures, however, are assuming increasing importance in management of patients with cardiovascular diseases.

GAMMA-GLUTAMYL TRANSPEPTIDASE

Gamma-glutamyl transpeptidase (GGT) catalyzes transfer of glutamyl groups among different polypeptides and amino acids. Although fairly large quantities exist in the brush border of renal tubular cells, clinically significant enzyme found in the circulation derives from cells that line the smallest radicles of the biliary tract. Like alkaline phosphatase, it rises dramatically with obstructive diseases of the biliary tract and in hepatocarcinoma. In most hepatic parenchymal diseases, serum GGT levels rise early, and elevation persists as long as cellular derangement continues. The feature that distinguishes GGT from other enzymes used routinely in assessing liver function is its association with alcohol-induced liver disease.

Prolonged alcohol intake induces increased GGT content within cells. If just a few of these induced, enzyme-rich cells undergo necrosis, serum GGT levels rise perceptibly. Rosalski,[34] who has done most of the work with this enzyme, states that 75 percent of chronic alcoholics have mildly elevated GGT levels at all times, whether or not overt liver disease is seen. After heavy drinking, levels rise dramatically, beginning within 18 hours of intake at the level of six or more drinks per day. Measuring GGT levels may assist those who work with alcoholics in rehabilitation programs, since enzyme elevation provides objective evidence of recent drinking. Values return to normal 2 to 3 weeks after alcohol intake ceases.[34] There is not yet enough widespread experience with this enzyme to assess its pitfalls.

HYDROXYBUTYRATE DEHYDROGENASE

This enzyme catalyzes the interconversion between alpha-ketobutyric acid and hydroxybutyric acid. Its activity is entirely comparable to that of the fast-moving or cardiac component of lactic dehydrogenase, which has a high relative activity against the butyrate substrates, and discussion is deferred to the section on lactic dehydrogenase (see below).

LACTIC DEHYDROGENASE

This glycolytic enzyme catalyzes the reversible alteration between pyruvate and lactate. The spectrophotometric determination measures consumption of reduced DPN, and normal values are 200 to 450 units. Several colorimetric methods are available with entirely different units and normal values.

Isoenzymes

As an important part of the glycolytic process, LDH is present in nearly all metabolizing cells, but different tissues have enzyme of differing composition. The functioning LDH molecule is a tetramer, composed of four subunits. Two immunologically distinct subunits exist, called M (for voluntary muscle) and H (for heart). The tetramer can be all H, all M, or any combination of H and M. The all-H tetramer, called LDH_1, migrates rapidly toward the anode in an electrophoretic field. LDH_5, the all-M tetramer, migrates slowly in the opposite direction, toward the cathode. The other isoenzymes, LDH_2, LDH_3, and LDH_4, have intermediate patterns.

Serum LDH levels exist over a broad normal range. Males under age 50 have slightly higher mean normal values than do females of the same age. Values are highest in prepubertal children; after a sharp adolescent fall, they rise gradually with increasing age. When cell damage causes serum enzyme levels to rise, a rough proportion exists between number of cells damaged and magnitude of the enzyme elevation. If an individual with a low-normal serum LDH sustains a small amount of tissue damage, the resulting value may still fall within the overall normal range. Determining isoenzyme patterns can be especially helpful in these circumstances, since the proportion of circulating isoenzymes usually will undergo significant change.

TISSUE LOCATIONS

Heart muscle and red blood cells contain LDH_1. LDH_5 derives from liver and skeletal muscle, while LDH_3 is largely of pulmonary origin. The predominant isoenzyme in normal serum is LDH_2, which probably comes from cells of the reticuloendothelial system. Pancreas and placenta have LDH_4, and kidney has both LDH_4 and LDH_5. Renal cortex also may have moderate amounts of LDH_1.

When isoenzymes are distributed normally, LDH_2 is more prominent than LDH_1. Reversal of this two-greater-than-one ratio is significant evidence of myocardial or erythrocyte disease, whether or not total enzyme concentration increases.

Sample for Analysis

LDH determinations usually are done on serum, but they can be done on carefully drawn specimens of cerebrospinal fluid or cell-free fluids from other body cavities. When blood is drawn for LDH measurement, the serum should be separated promptly from cells and refrigerated if the test is not to be done immediately. The serum should not be frozen. Because red blood cells have such high LDH content, it is essential to avoid hemolysis.

Disease States

HEART DISEASE

Total LDH and LDH isoenzymes most often are measured to diagnose acute myocardial infarction. Total LDH levels rise rather slowly, beginning only 24 to 72 hours after infarction has occurred. The value remains high for 10 to 14 days afterward, making this an especially useful test for delayed diagnosis; for example, a patient may wait several days before seeking medical attention for his "indigestion." Isoenzyme proportions change long before the total LDH values rise. Within 4 hours of infarction, LDH_1 increases at the relative expense of LDH_2, and by 24 hours, there usually is a distinct reversal of the normal LDH_1/LDH_2 ratio. Similarly, the ratio of LDH_1 to LDH_2 remains elevated 3 or 4 days longer than does the level of total enzyme.

This reversal of LDH isoenzyme pattern is extremely valuable in distinguishing myocardial infarction from angina pectoris or other causes of chest pain and vascular instability. When infarction is extensive, total LDH rises, but other diseases may confound the interpretation unless isoenzymes are studied. Pulmonary disease without myocardial disease does not affect the ratio of LDH_1 and LDH_2. If circulatory collapse or severe congestive failure accompanies a heart attack, liver cells often undergo necrosis. This contributes to the total LDH level, and isoenzyme evaluation reveals a rise in LDH_5 and sometimes LDH_4 as well.

Inflammatory disease of the myocardium also elevates LDH_1. Active myocarditis produces an isoenzyme picture much like that of infarction, although total elevations are rarely as high. Operative trauma to the myocardium causes a relatively short-lived enzyme elevation. Abnormality of LDH_1 and LDH_2 that persists more than 5 or 6 days after an operation suggests that postoperative infarction has occurred.[28]

LIVER DISEASE

LDH_5 is the hepatic isoenzyme. Acute hepatitis causes total enzyme to rise enormously, all due to LDH_5. LDH levels do not correlate with the degree of jaundice, and LDH_5 usually rises several days before jaundice, if any, develops. Serum isoenzyme levels fall before the bilirubin does, and usually before the SGPT begins dropping. Drug-associated hepatitis also causes LDH_5 to rise impressively, but ascending cholangiitis causes only mild increase, and pure obstructive jaundice does not affect the LDH. The hepatitis of infectious mononucleosis affects LDH_5 only moderately, but total enzyme activity often is very high.

HEMATOLOGIC DISEASE

Pernicious anemia produces remarkably high total LDH values, mostly of LDH_1. Successful therapy with vitamin B_{12} reduces these levels extremely rapidly, even before reticulocytosis occurs. Hemolytic conditions of any kind elevate LDH_1 but may affect total enzyme only modestly. LDH_1 elevations provide the best evidence for the presence of hemolysis during an aplastic crisis.

Hematologic diseases cannot be distinguished with accuracy by means of isoenzyme patterns. In general, LDH_1 derives from red cells, LDH_2 from granulocytes, and LDH_3, LDH_4, and LDH_5 from damaged lymphocytes, but these rules are by no means invariable. Lymphomas, in particular, may cause impressive changes in LDH_2.

OTHER DISEASES

Lung tissue is rich in LDH₃, and destructive pulmonary processes cause LDH₃ to rise. Interpretation may be difficult, however, in pulmonary infarction because these infarcts, notoriously hemorrhagic, cause large-scale hemolysis of extravasated red cells. This causes LDH₁ to rise, confusing the desired distinction between pulmonary infarct and myocardial infarction.

For the most part, skeletal muscle contains LDH₅, together with some LDH₃ and LDH₄. LDH is less helpful in evaluating muscular disease than is creatine phosphokinase (CPK). In Duchenne's muscular dystrophy, the LDH pattern may be confusing because the rapidly migrating 1 and 2 isoenzymes predominate in both serum and the muscle itself, instead of the expected LHD₅. Following vigorous exercise, total LDH may rise several-fold, but the ratio between LDH₁ and LDH₂ remains normal. Increased LDH occurs sooner and drops more promptly after severe exercise than after acute myocardial damage.[21]

LEUCINE AMINOPEPTIDASE

Leucine aminopeptidase is a proteolytic enzyme that is present in pancreas, liver, and small intestine. Early observers[36] suggested its use in distinguishing carcinoma of the pancreas from other forms of obstructive biliary disease. Subsequent studies have shown that many types of hepatic and biliary diseases affect serum and urine levels of this enzyme, and its determination offers no advantages over the more easily obtained transaminase and alkaline phosphatase determinations.[23] When low-grade or confusing enzyme patterns occur, leucine aminopeptidase values may clarify the problem by pinpointing hepatobiliary tract disease, for which it is largely specific.

LIPASE

Lipase is a hydrolytic enzyme that is secreted by the pancreas into the duodenum where, aided by bile salts and calcium ions, it splits fatty acids from triglycerides. Like amylase, lipase exists within the secretory cells and appears in the blood stream following damage to the pancreas, the only organ known to produce it. Assay methods present certain technical difficulties, since the classic method requires 24 hours of incubation.[7] Subsequent modifications permit more rapid analysis, giving the test greater clinical applicability.

Normal values depend upon the method used, but serum levels are low in healthy states.

Acute pancreatitis is the most common cause of lipasemia. The lipase levels usually parallel serum amylase elevations early in the disease, but elevated lipase levels may persist up to a week after the acute episode. This makes lipase determinations helpful in the late diagnosis of acute pancreatitis. The enzyme is less useful in cases of chronic pancreatitis, chronic biliary tract disease, and pancreatic carcinoma. Diseases of the salivary gland do not affect lipase levels.

PHOSPHATASES

Phosphatases are hydrolytic enzymes that catalyze the cleavage of phosphate esters with little specificity as to preferred substrate. Two general types are recognized; that with a pH optimum of 4.5 to 5.5, called acid phosphatase, and that with a pH optimum between 9 and 10, called alkaline phosphatase. Although similar in catalytic effect, they are separated easily by altering the pH at which the test is run. Basically similar assays are used for both.

In the Bodansky method, β-glycerophosphate is the substrate, and the liberated inorganic phosphorus is measured. The original King-Armstrong method uses a phenylphosphate substrate and measures milligrams of phenol liberated. Various modifications are employed with each, and by varying the pH of the reaction mixture, each method can be used for either type of phosphatase. One Bodansky unit (B.U.) is equal to approximately 2.5 King-Armstrong (K.-A.) units. Normal serum levels for alkaline phosphatase are 1.5 to 4 B.U. or 3 to 13 K.-A. units. King and Wooten[22] give 1 to 3 K.-A. units as the normal range for acid phosphatase. For the Babson-Read method, using α-naphthyl phosphate as the substrate, normal acid phosphatase values are 0.5 to 5 Babson-Read units.[1]

Alkaline Phosphatase

Alkaline phosphatase activity derives from several different tissues. Serum alkaline phosphatase does not derive from alkaline phosphatase in white blood cells. The intracellular enzyme has completely different clinical significance from the circulating serum enzyme. Isoenzymes have been demonstrated as originating from liver, bone, placenta, and intestine, each with different properties which facilitate identification. That of bone origin is most readily inactivated by heat. Exposure to L-phenylalanine inhibits both the placental and intestinal forms. Electrophoresis, especially on polyacrylamide gel, probably gives the best separation, and immunologic specificity also can be demonstrated.

In normal adults, circulating alkaline phosphatase derives both from bone and liver[6] with children exhibiting significantly higher proportions of the osteoblastic form. The enzyme excreted in bile derives almost entirely from liver,[30] but biliary excretion probably is not the dominant metabolic pathway. Most of the enzyme produced appears to be degraded as part of the general protein pool, and is not excreted.[5] The phosphatase increase seen during pregnancy reflects placental manufacture. High serum levels of alkaline phosphatase have been reported following massive infusions of human albumin.[26] When the specifically placental isoenzyme was identified in these patients, the source was found to be the human placentas from which the albumin was prepared. Albumin preparations of non-placental origin do not produce this artefact.

BONE DISEASE

In conditions of pronounced osteoblastic activity, serum alkaline phosphatase activity is high. Prepubertal children have normal levels of 15 to 25 K.-A. units, and as bone growth ceases, the level declines to adult range. In conditions of retarded bone growth such as childhood hypothyroidism, alkaline phosphatase levels are low. Persistent elevation to childhood levels occurs in older patients whose skeletal growth continues abnormally, owing to disorders of skeletal maturation or excessive production of growth hormone.

The highest levels of alkaline phosphatase are found in Paget's disease and in hyperparathyroidism with skeletal involvement. In these conditions, values may reach 200 B.U., although more moderate elevations are the rule. Jaffe and Bodansky[19] noted that in Paget's disease a sudden rise from a stable and moderate elevation may signal the development of osteogenic sarcoma. Alkaline phosphatase is not elevated in hypervitaminosis D, which, like hyperparathyroidism, is associated with hypercalcemia and hypercalciuria. Vitamin D deficiency (rickets) in children may raise the serum level to 30 to 40 K.-A. units. Osteoblastic metastatic tumor may produce elevations to 20 to 30 B.U.,[40] while osteolytic metastases and foci of multiple myeloma do not affect the enzyme level.

HEPATOBILIARY DISEASE

Both hepatocellular disease and bile duct abnormalities affect the serum alkaline phosphatase level, which may rise to diagnostic levels in early obstructive disease before the serum bilirubin increases. Complete extrahepatic duct obstruction reliably causes elevations to 25 or 35 B.U. or higher, but much higher levels accompany inflammatory or proliferative changes affecting intrahepatic radicles. Biliary cirrhosis produces exceptionally high levels, but cholangiolitic hepatitis and infiltrative liver disease produce significant elevations. Infectious mononucleosis, even without overt signs of liver damage, may cause mildly elevated levels. Alkaline phosphatase levels may be more sensitive than transaminase levels in indicating infections, particularly granulomatous inflammation, or metastatic tumor infiltration.[5] Cirrhosis produces only mild changes in total alkaline phosphatase activity, but the intestinal isoenzyme may become apparent on electrophoresis, a finding associated almost exclusively with this form of liver disease.[6,8]

Acid Phosphatase

The function of acid phosphatase is not understood. It occurs primarily in the adult prostate gland and in erythrocytes, and the two organs contain rather different forms of the enzyme. Several methods are in use to separate the two forms. The Babson-Read method[1] uses a substrate specific for the prostatic enzyme, so that the erythrocyte portion does not interfere. Another fairly specific substrate is β-glycerophosphate, but with this method it is necessary to measure liberated inorganic phosphate which may be affected by pre-existing serum phosphate levels.[2] When phenylphosphate is used as the substrate, the two fractions can be partitioned by addition of L-tartrate. This inhibits the prostatic fraction, so that the difference between the total enzyme activity and the activity after inhibition represents the prostatic portion. The problem here is that the prostatic activity contributes only a small proportion to the total. Radioimmunoassay[13] is the most specific and most sensitive technique for detecting subtle changes in level of the prostatic enzyme.

Significantly elevated serum acid phosphatase nearly always points to metastatic carcinoma. Both total and prostatic fractions are elevated in approximately 80 percent of cases of prostatic carcinoma with metastasis to bone and in 10 to 25 percent of patients with prostatic tumor without metastases. If the tumor is successfully treated, enzyme levels decline within 3 to 4 days of surgical castration, or 3 to 4 weeks of estrogen therapy. Benign prostatic hyperplasia and prostatitis cause no change in the enzyme level as measured chemically. Radioimmunoassay results occasionally rise above normal in these conditions but not to the levels seen in prostatic cancer.[13]

Elevation of the nonprostatic fraction occurs in Gaucher's disease.[9] The best substrate for documenting this activity is p-nitrophenylphosphate (the Bessey-Lowry[3] technique) which is much less sensitive to the prostatic fraction than α-naphthyl phosphate or β-glycerophosphate.

TRANSAMINASES

Transaminases catalyze the reversible transfer of amino groups between various acids in the glycolytic cycle. In human tissues, two have been recognized, and both have glutamic acid as one of the substrates. Glutamic-oxalacetic transaminase (GOT) mediates between glutamic and oxalacetic acid, and glutamic-pyruvic transaminase (GPT) has pyruvic acid as the other substrate. The current formal practice is to refer to GOT as *aspartate aminotransferase* and to GPT as *alanine aminotransferase*. Acceptance of these terms has been gradual, and the older terms continue to be more widely understood. Very high concentrations of GOT occur in the heart and liver, and moderately large amounts are in skeletal muscle, kidney, and pancreas. Kidney, heart, and skeletal muscle, in decreasing order, have significant concentrations of GPT. Liver contains the highest concentrations of GPT, but even liver has three and a half times as much GOT as GPT. Both colorimetric and spectrophotometric methods of assay are used, and normal serum values vary from laboratory to laboratory, depending upon the technique.

Myocardial Infarction

Because intact myocardium contains abundant GOT, myocardial necrosis releases large quantities of the enzyme into the circulation. Within 6 to 10 hours after an acute infarction, significant elevation of the serum GOT occurs, reaching a maximum at 24 to 48 hours. In the absence of liver damage, recurrent elevation after the first peak has subsided indicates additional fresh necrosis. Numerous studies indicate correlation as high as 96 to 98 percent between myocardial infarction and elevated serum GOT.

Elevated serum GOT does not always indicate myocardial infarction, since severe arrhythmias and severe angina also have been reported to cause elevations. Uncomplicated congestive failure and uncomplicated pulmonary infarction probably cause little change, but secondary liver damage tends to complicate both clinical and enzyme diagnosis. Serum GPT levels rise less markedly and less consistently than GOT following myocardial infarction, owing perhaps to an initially lower concentration in the intact muscle.

Liver Disease

When hepatic cells are damaged, serum GOT and GPT levels rise. These enzyme changes occur early in the disease, whether damage is due to infectious or toxic hepatitis, central congestion, biliary obstruction, or active cirrhosis. The enzyme levels are especially useful in assessing subtle or early changes. In hepatitis, for example, transaminase levels rise several days before jaundice begins. The enzyme levels also fall rapidly and may return to normal while parenchymal changes are still active. A second rise tends to indicate a relapse. The serum GPT level returns to normal more slowly than does the GOT. In obstructive jaundice, there may be mild to moderate elevation, less striking than the change following hepatocellular disease. Mild elevation occurs in cases of active cirrhosis and metastatic tumor. While nonicteric cholecystitis does not alter the GOT and GPT levels, acute pancreatitis may cause some rise. Infectious mononucleosis often causes transaminase elevations, but the changes are less pronounced than the rise in LDH. Such muscle diseases as progressive muscular dystrophy and dermatomyositis may cause elevations in GOT with only minimal change in GPT, whereas myasthenia gravis and rheumatoid arthritis have no effect on either.

REFERENCES

1. Babson, A. L., and Read, P. A.: *A new assay for prostatic acid phosphatase in serum.* Am. J. Clin. Pathol. 32:88, 1959.
2. Babson, A. L., Read, P. A., and Phillips, G. E.: *The importance of the substrate in assays of acid phosphatase in serum.* Am. J. Clin. Pathol. 32:83, 1959.
3. Bessey, O. A., Lowry, O. H., and Brock, M. J.: *A method for the rapid determination of alkaline phosphatase with five cubic millimeters of serum.* J. Biol. Chem. 164:321, 1946.
4. Blythe, H., and Hughes, B. P.: *Pregnancy and serum-C.P.K. levels in potential carriers of "severe" X-linked muscular dystrophy.* Lancet 1:855, 1971.
5. Breen, K. J.: *Liver function tests.* Crit. Rev. Clin. Lab. Sci. 2:573, 1971.

6. Canapa-Anson, R., and Towe, J. F.: *Electrophoretic separation of tissue-specific serum alkaline phosphatases.* J. Clin. Pathol. 23:499, 1970.
7. Cherry, I. S., and Crandall, L. A.: *The specificity of pancreatic lipase: its appearance in the blood after pancreatic injury.* Am. J. Physiol. 100:266, 1932.
8. Connell, M. D., and Dinwoodie, A. J.: *Diagnostic use of serum alkaline phosphatase isoenzymes and 5-nucleotidase.* Clin. Chim. Acta 30:235, 1970.
9. Crocker, A. C., and Landing, B. H.: *Phosphatase studies in Gaucher's disease.* Metabolism 9:341, 1960.
10. Dawson, D. M., and Fine, I. H.: *Creatine kinase in human tissue.* Arch. Neurol. 16:175, 1967.
11. de la Huerga, J., Petrus, E. A., and Sherrick, J. C.: *Detection of cholinesterase inhibition,* in Sunderman, F. W., and Sunderman, F. W., Jr. (eds.): *Laboratory Diagnosis of Diseases Caused by Toxic Agents.* Warren H. Green, Inc., St. Louis, 1970.
12. Dietz, A. A., Rubinstein, H., and Lubrano, T.: *Detection of patients with low serum cholinesterase activity: inadequacy of "Acholest" method.* Clin. Chem. 18:565, 1972.
13. Foti, A. G., Cooper, J. F., Herschman, H., and Malvaez, R. R.: *Detection of prostatic cancer by solid-phase radioimmunoassay of serum prostatic acid phosphatase.* N. Engl. J. Med. 297:1357, 1977.
14. Gaede, J. T.: *Serum enzyme alterations in hypothyroidism before and after treatment.* J. Am. Geriatrics Soc. 25:199, 1977.
15. Galen, R. S., Reiffel, J. A., and Gambino, S. R.: *Diagnosis of acute myocardial infarction. Relative efficiency of serum enzyme and isoenzyme measurements.* J.A.M.A. 232:145, 1975.
16. Garry, P. J., Owen, G. M., and Lubin, A. H.: *Identification of serum cholinesterase fluoride variants by differential inhibition in tris and phosphate buffers.* Clin. Chem. 18:105, 1972.
17. Graig, F. A., and Ross, G.: *Serum creatine-phosphokinase in thyroid disease.* Metabolism 12:57, 1963.
18. Henry, R. J., and Chiamori, N.: *Study of the saccharogenic method for the determination of serum and urine amylase.* Clin. Chem. 6:434, 1960.
19. Jaffe, H. L., and Bodansky, A.: *Diagnostic significance of serum alkaline and acid phosphatase values in relation to bone disease.* Bull. N.Y. Acad. Med. 19:831, 1943.
20. Jennings, R. C., Brocklehurst, D., and Hirst, M.: *A rapid automated screening technique for the detection of placental-like phosphatase in malignant disease.* J. Clin. Pathol. 25:349, 1972.
21. Kamen, R. L., Goheen, B., Patton, R., and Raven, P.: *The effects of near maximum exercise on serum enzymes: the exercise profile versus the cardiac profile.* Clin. Chim. Acta 81:145, 1977.
22. King, E. J., and Wooten, I. D. P.: *Micro-Analysis in Medical Biochemistry.* ed. 3. Grune & Stratton, New York, 1956.
23. Kowlessar, O. D., Haeffner, L. J., Riley, E. M., and Sleisenger, M. H.: *Comparative study of serum leucine aminopeptidase, 5-nucleotidase, and nonspecific alkaline phosphatase in disease affecting the pancreas, hepatobiliary tree, and bone.* Am. J. Med. 31:231, 1961.
24. Lehmann, H., and Liddell, J.: *The cholinesterase variants,* in Stanbury,

J. B., Wyngaarden, J. B., and Frederickson, D. S. (eds.): *The Metabolic Basis of Inherited Diseases*. ed. 3. McGraw-Hill, New York, 1972.

25. Lubin, A. H., Garry, P. J., and Owen, G. M.: *Sex and population difference in the incidence of a plasma cholinesterase variant*. Science 173:161, 1971.

26. Mackie, J. A., Arvan, D. A., Mullen, J. L., and Rawnsley, H. M.: *Elevated serum alkaline phosphatase levels after the administration of certain preparations of human albumin*. Am. J. Surg. 121:57, 1971.

27. Meites, S.: *Amylase isoenzymes*. Crit. Rev. Clin. Lab. Sci. 2:103, 1971.

28. Mohiuddin, S. M., Raffetto, J., Sketch, M. H., et al.: *LDH isoenzymes and myocardial infarction in patients undergoing coronary bypass surgery: an excellent correlation*. Am. Heart J. 92:584, 1976.

29. O'Donnell, M. D., and McGeeney, K. F.: *Comparison of saccharagenic and "Phadebas" methods for amylase assay in biological fluids*. Enzyme 18:348, 1974.

30. Price, C. P., Hill, P. G., and Sammons, H. G.: *The nature of the alkaline phosphatase in bile*. J. Clin. Pathol. 25:149, 1972.

31. Ramdeo, I. N., and Joshi, K. C.: *Serum lactic dehydrogenase and its isoenzymes in hepatic disorders*. Am. J. Gastroenterol. 55:459, 1971.

32. Rinderkneckt, H., Wilding, P., and Haverback, B. J.: *A new method for the determination of α-amylase*. Experientia 23:805, 1967.

33. Roberts, P., and Sobel, B. E.: *CPK isoenzymes in evaluation of myocardial ischemic injury*. Hosp. Practice 11:55, 1976.

34. Rosalski, S. B.: *Gamma-glutamyl transpeptidase*. Adv. Clin. Chem. 17:53, 1975.

35. Rose, M. R., Glassman, E., Isom, O. W., and Spencer, F. C.: *Electrocardiographic and serum enzyme changes of myocardial infarction after coronary artery bypass surgery*. Am. J. Cardiol. 33:215, 1974.

36. Rutenberg, A. M., Goldbarg, J. A., and Pineda, E. P.: *Leucine aminopeptidase activity, observations in patients with cancer of the pancreas and other diseases*. N. Engl. J. Med. 259:469, 1958.

37. Shaw, R. F.: *Serum enzymes and prognosis in muscular dystrophy*. Lancet 1:856, 1971.

38. Sibley, J. A., and Lehninger, A. L.: *Determination of aldolase in animal tissues*. J. Biol. Chem. 177:859, 1949.

39. Snodgrass, P. J.: *Diseases of the pancreas*, in Thorn, G. W., Adams, R. D., Braunwald, E., et al. (eds.): *Harrison's Principles of Internal Medicine*. ed. 8. McGraw-Hill, New York, 1977.

40. Wilkinson, J. H.: *The Principles and Practice of Diagnostic Enzymology*. Year Book Medical Publishers, Chicago, 1976.

41. Wong, R., and Swallen, T. O.: *Cellulose acetate electrophoresis of creatine phosphokinase isoenzymes in the diagnosis of myocardial infarction*. Am. J. Clin. Pathol. 64:209, 1975.

42. Yasmineh, W. G., Pyle, R. B., and Nicoloff, D. M.: *The MB isoenzyme of creatine kinase in the quantitation of myocardial infarct size*. Am. J. Cardiol. 35:166, 1975.

43. Zavon, M. R.: *Treatment of organophosphorus and chlorinated hydrocarbon insecticide intoxications*. Mod. Treat. 8:503, 1971.

CHAPTER 12

LIVER FUNCTION TESTS

CLASSIFICATION OF LIVER DISEASE

It is useful to divide liver disease into three broad anatomic categories: disorders of circulation, disorders of the hepatobiliary system, and disorders of functioning liver cells. Each of these three systems can experience many types of disease, including inflammation, ischemia, infection, neoplasm, immune damage, acquired metabolic derangements, enzyme deficiencies, and chemical or physical toxicity.

Portal and Hepatic Circulation

Relatively few disorders affect only the circulatory system. By far the commonest is congestive heart failure, either acute or chronic. Congestive failure impairs return of blood from hepatic vein to right atrium. As venous pressure increases, liver cells are damaged by compression and by the hypoxia that accompanies slowed flow. Centrilobular cells are affected earlier and more severely than cells at the lobular periphery, because oxygenation is more precarious nearer the central veins.

Less common vascular problems are obstruction of the hepatic vein (Budd-Chiari syndrome) and thrombosis of the portal vein. Obstruction of the hepatic vein is more dangerous than congestive heart failure, because venous flow through the liver declines to exceedingly low levels. The clinical effects of portal vein obstruction usually reflect the underlying disease; circulatory effects, as such, are less prominent. Inflammation is the most common cause of portal vein obstruction, usually from amoebic infection, intraperitoneal infection, or pancreatitis. Obstruction occasionally results from cirrhosis or tumor.

Hepatobiliary Tract

The hepatobiliary tract can be divided into an *extrahepatic* portion, which includes the hepatic ducts, the gallbladder, the common bile duct, and the ampulla of Vater, where the common duct empties into the duodenum; and the *intrahepatic* portion, which begins with tiny collecting spaces between individual liver cells and gradually co-alesces into bile canaliculi, small bile duct radicles, and larger bile ducts located in the portal areas.

The extrahepatic bile ducts may sustain either obstructive or inflammatory damage. The earliest and most complete form of obstruction is congenital *biliary atresia*. In adult life, partial or progressive obstruction can occur with gallstones, ductal cysts, or pressure exerted by pancreatic or other adjacent neoplasms. Inflammation of gallbladder or bile ducts occurs fairly commonly. Cancer of the ducts or of the ampulla of Vater is much less frequent.

Inflammation is the usual cause of intrahepatic problems. *Cholestasis* refers to a slowing of the intrahepatic bile flow, often resulting from immune or toxic reactions to drugs, hormone therapy, or pregnancy. Inflammation often spreads upward from the larger extrahepatic ducts in a process called *ascending cholangiitis*. Most of this inflammation results from infection, from chemical irritation due to bile accumulation, or from immune-mediated processes. The proliferative, fibrosing process known as *biliary cirrhosis* quite probably has an immune origin. When there is severe hepatocellular disease, the intrahepatic bile ducts frequently suffer from secondary inflammation and scarring.

Hepatocellular Diseases

Innumerable processes affect the liver cells. It is useful to consider separately those with *focal* distribution and those which involve all lobules *diffusely*. Abscesses, primary or metastatic tumors, and the necrosis that follows portal vein obstruction are localized lesions. Granulomatous processes usually cause focal damage, especially tuberculosis and sarcoidosis. Leukemic or lymphomatous infiltration can either be generalized or cause focal loss of cellular activity. Focal processes usually cause recognizable defects on radioisotope scans and other radiologic investigations, but biopsy can be difficult, since a needle inserted transabdominally may miss the abnormal area.

CONGENITAL DISEASES

Diffuse parenchymal diseases may be congenital or acquired, acute or chronic. Congenital conditions include a variety of enzyme deficiencies that impair bilirubin excretion; enzyme defects in other systems often lead to gradual liver damage. Slowly developing cirrhosis is a long-term complication in α_1-antitrypsin deficiency, Wilson's disease (hepatolenticular degeneration), hemochromatosis, galactosemia, and glycogen storage disease.

ACQUIRED HEPATOCELLULAR DISEASES

Viral infections and drug or chemical toxins are the commonest causes of *acute* hepatocellular damage. Besides hepatitis A and hepatitis B (infectious and serum hepatitis respectively), numerous viruses can damage liver cells. Epstein-Barr virus and cytomegalovirus are well-recognized culprits, but there are many others. Acute hepatotoxins are easy to find: alcohol, anaesthetics (especially halothane), and organic solvents come immediately to mind, but antibiotics, anticonvulsants, psychoactive drugs, antihypertensive agents, and antimetabolites can be significantly hepatotoxic in significant numbers of people.[26] Less common and less well understood are the changes that occur in "acute fatty liver," a morphologic event that occurs in Reyes' disease,[7] some pregnancies, some cases of alcoholism, and sporadic other conditions.

  Chronic hepatocellular disease may follow acute damage or develop insidiously. The major categories are cirrhosis and chronic active hepatitis. *Cirrhosis* is a diffuse, chronic condition characterized by damage and regeneration of parenchymal cells, increase in connective tissue, and distortion of lobular architecture and blood flow patterns. The condition can be relentlessly progressive or can remain at a quiescent plateau. Any kind of liver damage can eventuate in cirrhosis, but the usual inciting causes are viral or toxic hepatitis, alcoholic liver damage, congestive heart failure, and disease of the biliary system. Except in acute, massive necrosis, liver disease severe enough to cause hepatic failure nearly always includes cirrhosis, which simply indicates progressive damage and attempts at repair.

  Chronic active hepatitis is a progressive process in which gradual damage to liver cells is accompanied by chronic inflammatory changes and variable evidence of immune dysfunction. Activity may wax and wane, and the course can range from a minimally significant chronic state to a rapidly progressive destructive process.[1]

Classification of Tests

The liver performs so many and such varied functions that no single laboratory procedure, or battery of laboratory tests, can evaluate them all. Tests, however, can be grouped according to the general functions they elucidate. These include tests of bilirubin metabolism and excretion; tests which indicate hepatocellular necrosis; tests that reflect decline or malfunction of specifically hepatic processes; tests with nonspecific findings that indicate generalized metabolic disorders; nonspecific tests of immune activity, which often become abnormal when liver disease exists; and tests for specific hepatotoxic agents, the virus of hepatitis B being the salient example.

BILIRUBIN METABOLISM AND EXCRETORY FUNCTION

The Origin and Fate of Bilirubin

Bilirubin originates from *heme*, the four-ringed, iron-containing, non-protein part of the hemoglobin molecule. Reticuloendothelial cells manufacture bilirubin as part of a degradation process directed largely at hemoglobin but also at heme components in myoglobin, peroxidase, and several of the electron receptors involved in ATP synthesis. Most hemoglobin—and hence most heme—is located in red cells, which have a normal life span of 120 days. Every day, 1/120th of a normal person's hemoglobin must be degraded into bilirubin. Other hemoproteins turn over more rapidly, contributing up to 10 to 15 percent of the total daily bilirubin load. Bilirubin levels increase if there is accelerated destruction of red cells or if red cell production is so flawed that some developing hemoglobin never circulates in mature red cells.

Bilirubin is produced wherever there are reticuloendothelial cells; the blood carries it to the liver, which processes it for excretion. When normal amounts are produced, circulating blood contains 0.1 to 0.3 mg./dl. of bilirubin en route to the liver. Prehepatic bilirubin is soluble in lipids but not in water; in plasma, most is bound to albumin, and plasma contains only minute amounts of unbound bilirubin. If albumin binding is impaired, unbound bilirubin enters the tissues. Most tissues suffer no damage other than pigmentation.

The exception is the lipid-rich developing central nervous system of the newborn. Newborns with excessive levels of unbound, prehepatic bilirubin may suffer irreversible neurologic damage from bilirubin deposition, a condition called *kernicterus*. Hypoxia, acidosis, and such drugs as salicylates interfere with albumin binding, but in adults, high bilirubin levels have little independent effect.

HEPATIC METABOLISM AND EXCRETION

Once bilirubin arrives at the liver, special mediators are needed to transfer the molecule across the cell membrane into the hepatocyte. . A single transfer system is used for transmembrane movement of bilirubin and other organic ions. Conjugating enzymes in the endoplasmic reticulum convert lipid-soluble bilirubin into water-soluble bilirubin glucuronide, a form that can be excreted into the bile. Small amounts normally are present in blood. Normal blood levels of conjugated, water-soluble bilirubin are approximately 0.3 to 1.3 mg./dl., three or four times the normal level of circulating unconjugated bilirubin.

Besides bilirubin, bile contains cholesterol, bile salts manufactured from cholesterol, and phospholipids. Bile enters the intestine, where the bile salts and phospholipids are instrumental in fat absorption. Intestinal bacteria convert bilirubin into *urobilinogen,* a colorless, water-soluble compound. Most urobilinogen travels through the intestine for fecal excretion, but a small amount is reabsorbed into the portal circulation. If bile flow is obstructed, either in the liver or in the extrahepatic bile ducts, neither bile salts nor bilirubin can reach the intestine, and excessive amounts enter the blood stream.

SIGNS OF JAUNDICE

The upper normal limit for serum bilirubin is 1.5 mg./dl., but within this total level, a rise in unconjugated, prehepatic bilirubin constitutes an abnormality. The unconjugated fraction increases with increased red cell destruction or hemoglobin turnover. The conjugated fraction rises in congestive heart failure, cirrhosis without active inflammation, and invasion of liver by metastatic tumor. Since conjugated bilirubin readily enters the urine, a minimal increase in posthepatic bilirubin may be apparent only by the presence of bilirubin in the urine. Bilirubin is never a normal urinary constituent; its presence signifies that excessive amounts of posthepatic bilirubin are in the circulation (see Table 16). Bilirubinuria

Table 16. Bilirubin Metabolism in Selected Liver Diseases

	Serum Bilirubin	Urine Bilirubin	Urine Urobilinogen	Fecal Urobilinogen	Comments
Vascular disorders:					
Congestive heart failure	↑ (both)	nl	nl	nl	
Hepatobiliary tract disorders:					
Extrahepatic obstruction	↑↑ or ↑↑↑ (direct)	↑	↓	↓	Serum bile acids rise.
Intrahepatic cholestasis	↑ (direct)	sl↑	nl	nl	
Cholecystitis	↑ (direct)	sl↑	nl	nl	
Biliary cirrhosis	↑ to ↑↑↑ (direct)	↑	nl	nl	Striking rise in serum bile acids; precedes jaundice.
Acute hepatocellular disease:					
Viral hepatitis	↑ or ↑↑	↑	sl↓	sl↓	Urine bilirubin may rise before serum levels.
Reye's syndrome	nl or sl↑	nl	nl	nl	
Alcoholic hepatitis	↑ or ↑↑	sl↑	nl	nl	
Drug-related liver damage	*	*	*	*	
Chronic hepatocellular disease:					
Fatty liver (alcoholic)	↑	nl	nl	nl	BSP retention becomes strikingly abnormal.
Chronic active hepatitis	↑	nl	nl	nl	
Cirrhosis	↑↑ (both)	nl or ↑	nl	nl	
Hyperbilirubinemia syndromes:					
Crigler-Najar	↑↑↑ (indirect)	nl	↓↓	↓↓	
Gilbert	↑ (indirect)	nl	nl	nl	
Dubin-Johnson	↑ or ↑↑ (both)	↑	nl or ↑	nl	
Red cell destruction (hemolysis)	↑ or ↑↑ (indirect)	nl	↑↑	↑↑	Evidence of shortened RBC survival; may have bilirubin gallstones

*Usually mimics either intrahepatic cholestasis or viral hepatitis.

may be the first indication of liver damage in viral hepatitis, occurring well before overt jaundice appears.

Chemical jaundice refers to a condition in which total serum bilirubin exceeds 1.5 mg./dl. Serum levels higher than 4.0 mg./dl. usually cause *clinical jaundice,* yellowing of sclerae or skin visible to the naked eye. Conjugated bilirubin can rise to extraordinary levels, but because normal liver cells have great reserve capacity for conjugating bilirubin, unconjugated bilirubin rarely rises above 5 mg./dl. unless hepatocellular damage exists.

TYPES OF JAUNDICE

Constitutional enzyme deficiencies cause lifelong mild elevation of unconjugated bilirubin levels.[3] *Gilbert's disease* is the commonest of these clinically innocuous conditions; *Dubin-Johnson* and *Rotor's syndromes* are due to less common enzyme deficiences. *Crigler-Najar's disease,* on the other hand, causes such severe unconjugated hyperbilirubinemia that kernicterus occurs early, and affected patients usually die in early childhood. Since cirrhosis and hepatitis of all kinds impair both conjugation and excretion of conjugated bilirubin, prehepatic and posthepatic fractions rise, sometimes to impressive levels. With biliary obstruction, biliary cirrhosis, and immune-mediated cholestasis, conjugated bilirubin dominates the jaundice, with little accumulation of the prehepatic form.

UROBILINOGEN

Unlike bilirubin, urobilinogen is a normal urinary component. It reflects the amount of bilirubin that enters the intestine, since urobilinogen originates in the gut and enters the blood stream only by enteric absorption. Increased urinary urobilinogen is an excellent indicator of hemolysis or inefficient erythropoiesis. If there is increased hemoglobin turnover, the liver processes and excretes increased amounts of bilirubin, and increased amounts of urobilinogen enter the blood. As long as hepatic function is normal, jaundice may be slight or nonexistent, and only the presence of increased urine urobilinogen testifies to the existence of hemolysis or inefficient erythropoiesis. Decreased urinary urobilinogen occurs with biliary obstruction, since no bile enters the intestine and there is no substrate from which colonic bacteria can make urobilinogen. Urine urobilinogen levels rarely are needed to diagnose obstruction, however, because the pale, grayish-white feces that occur with obstruction are virtually pathognomonic for the condition.

Tests of Bilirubin Transport Functions

Clinical jaundice, and even chemical jaundice, is easy to recognize. It is more difficult to document subtle distortion of hepatic function.[17] To demonstrate hepatic impairment so minimal that no bilirubin accumulates, dye excretion tests are extremely useful. Dye excretion tests are unnecessary in jaundiced patients, because increased serum bilirubin already is evidence of reduced excretory capacity. A possible exception might be the evaluation of enzyme functions in a patient with hemolysis and jaundice due to unconjugated bilirubin. Dye excretion tests are always abnormal in patients whose unconjugated hyperbilirubinemia results from genetically determined enzyme defects.

THE BSP TEST

Bromsulphalein (BSP, also called sodium sulfobromophthalein) is an anionic dye that the liver cell transports and excretes exactly as it does bilirubin. After intravenous infusion of BSP, the changing blood level reflects very sensitively the level of hepatocellular transport activity. In order to have normal clearance, there must be adequate blood flow to the liver; liver cells must clear the dye from the entering blood and must conjugate the dye before excreting the conjugated material into the bile.

Immediately after BSP is injected, the plasma level should be 10 mg./dl. The dose of BSP depends on body weight; 5 mg./kg. is the usual dose. Forty-five minutes after injection, the level of circulating dye is measured; a generally accepted normal result is to have less than 0.5 mg./dl. remaining in plasma. The result is expressed as "percent retention"; 0.5 mg./dl. is considered 5 percent of the injected dose.

ARTEFACTUAL RESULTS

Setting a normal threshold is difficult, however, because "percent retention" increases if the amount of body fat is high. Using body weight to calculate the injected dose assumes that plasma volume and body weight are directly proportional. This is not true, inasmuch as plasma volume in adipose tissue is less than in lean tissue. When an obese person is given a weight-adjusted dose, he probably receives more BSP than he should for his true plasma volume. This results in a higher plasma dye level 45 minutes after injection. Since the BSP test is useful precisely to demonstrate subtle departures from normal, this variable degree of inaccuracy makes the test suspect in obese patients.

The transport system used for BSP can be partially saturated by other materials. Dyes for radiographic visualization of the gallbladder interfere with BSP testing for several days, as may rifampin and other drugs. Patients whose plasma volume is excessively large will have spuriously low "retention" at 45 minutes. BSP, like bilirubin, is bound to albumin; when serum albumin levels are below 2.5 gm./dl., unbound BSP may filter directly into the urine and bypass the liver completely. This gives a falsely low plasma value at 45 minutes. Increased overall metabolism seems to impair excretion. When body temperature is over 103°F., abnormally high BSP values may occur without other evidence of hepatic dysfunction. High plasma levels of bilirubin or bile salts impair BSP excretion, but this should be no problem since the test is not done when jaundice exists.

INTERPRETING RESULTS

BSP results are genuinely abnormal in hepatocellular disease, in biliary tract obstruction, and in extrahepatic conditions that influence hepatic activity. The BSP test is helpful in indicating the beginning of viral or toxic hepatitis or the existence of continuing damage after the acute phase has passed.[18] Portal or nutritional cirrhosis nearly always causes abnormal BSP results, often to a degree that parallels disease activity. A liver with fatty metamorphosis but without inflammation or necrosis may clear BSP poorly, even when other liver function tests are normal. Cholelithiasis, cholecystitis, and partial obstruction of the biliary tract can affect BSP results before the occurrence of overt bilirubin retention.

Abnormalities of blood flow reduce the amount of BSP that the liver can clear. BSP results are abnormal in congestive heart failure, shock, or hepatic vein occlusion (Budd-Chiari syndrome); they also are abnormal when the liver is involved by metastatic tumor or by systemic diseases such as lymphoma, tuberculosis, sarcoidosis, or amyloidosis. The BSP test can be useful in the differential diagnosis of upper gastrointestinal tract bleeding; results are normal in peptic ulcer disease but abnormal in conditions secondary to cirrhosis-related portal hypertension.

The BSP test is not without hazards. Extravasation of dye, usually the result of poor injection techniques, can cause unpleasant damage to soft tissue. Systemic hypersensitivity or toxicity is rare and occurs predominantly if the dye is partially crystallized or incompletely dissolved before injection.

Bile Salts and Bile Acids

Levels of bile acids, which circulate largely as sodium salts, reflect both hepatocellular activity and biliary tract function. Bile salts are manufactured by liver cells and are concentrated in the bile. They serve as detergents in the intestine, where they enhance digestion and absorption of fats. With biliary tract obstruction, serum levels of bile acids rise, and intestinal levels decline. The itching that accompanies servere jaundice is due to circulation of bile salts. Their absence from the intestine causes steatorrhea and impaired absorption of fat-soluble vitamins. Excessive colonic levels produce watery diarrhea. Bile acids can be identified and measured by spectrophotometry and chromatography, procedures rarely applied to routine diagnosis of hepatobiliary disease but useful in special clinical circumstances.

It is possible to delineate subtle defects of hepatocellular function, ductal and intestinal motility, and mucosal activity by comparing bile salt levels in gallbladder bile, intestinal contents, and portal vein blood in such conditions as anicteric hepatitis, chronic active hepatitis, drug-related intrahepatic cholestasis, and neonatal cholestatic syndromes.[10]

HEPATOCELLULAR DAMAGE

When cells die, macromolecules normally confined within the cells escape into the interstitial fluid and thence to the blood stream. Different cell types contain unique combinations of enzymes; when these enzymes escape from dying cells into the blood stream, they provide valuable evidence about the cells that are affected. Although the nature of the enzymes is informative, it is not possible to calculate, from serum enzyme concentrations, the volume of tissue that has been damaged.

Relatively few enzymes are measured routinely for diagnostic purposes. In demonstrating liver damage, the principal enzymes are the transaminases, alkaline phosphatase, lactic dehydrogenase, leucine aminopeptidase, and gamma-glutamyl transpeptidase (see Table 17).

Table 17. Enzyme Changes in Selected Liver Diseases

	Alkaline Phosphatase	Transaminases	LDH*	Comments
Vascular disorders:				
Congestive heart failure	nl	↑ or ↑↑	↑ or ↑↑	
Hepatobiliary tract disorders:				
Extrahepatic obstruction	↑↑↑	nl to ↑↑	nl or sl ↑	Elevated lipids, especially nonesterified cholesterol. Vitamin K corrects prolonged prothrombin time. Autoantibodies are prominent.
Intrahepatic cholestasis	↑↑↑	nl to ↑↑	↑	
Biliary cirrhosis	↑↑	↑ or ↑↑	↑	
Cholecystitis	nl to ↑	nl or ↑	nl or ↑	Stones in common duct cause signs of extrahepatic obstruction.
Acute hepatocellular disease:				
Viral hepatitis	nl or ↑	↑↑↑	↑ or ↑↑	Tests for HB antigens and antibodies are important.
Reye's syndrome	nl	↑↑	↑↑	Prolonged prothrombin time, not corrected by vitamin K; low blood glucose, high ammonia
Alcoholic hepatitis	↑ or ↑↑	↑↑	↑	
Drug-induced liver damage	↑	↑	↑	
Infectious mononucleosis	nl or ↑	↑ or ↑↑	↑ or ↑↑	Some LDH is of hematopoietic origin.
Chronic hepatocellular disease:				
Fatty liver (alcoholic)	↑ or ↑↑	nl or sl ↑	nl or sl ↑	Hypergammaglobulinemia is common. Prolonged prothrombin time not corrected by vitamin K.
Chronic active hepatitis	↑	↑↑	↑	
Cirrhosis	nl or sl ↑	↑ or ↑↑	↑	

* Mostly LDH_4 and LDH_5.
† Resembles either intrahepatic cholestasis or viral hepatitis.

Transaminases

Transaminases catalyze the exchange of amino groups between an α-amino acid and an α-keto acid. Glutamic-oxalacetic transaminase (GOT) mediates the reaction: aspartic acid + oxoglutaric acid ⇌ oxalacetic acid + glutamic acid. Glutamic-pyruvic transaminase (GPT) mediates the reaction: pyruvic acid + glutamic acid ⇌ alanine + α-ketoglutaric acid. Analytic workers now prefer the term aminotransferase in place of transaminase, but the terminologic transition, in clinical settings, has been slow. The preferred term for GOT is *aspartate aminotransferase* and for GPT, *alanine aminotransferase*. We will continue to use the term transaminase in this edition, because it is more widely understood in general clinical parlance.

Neither GPT nor GOT is unique to the liver. Cardiac muscle has more GOT than any other tissue; liver is second, and parenchymal cells of skeletal muscle, kidney, brain, and other organs also contain substantial amounts. GPT is more specifically associated with the liver, but other tissues contain modest amounts. Enzyme levels rise very early in the course of most liver diseases, providing a more sensitive index of hepatic damage than do changes in bilirubin level. Circulating enzyme levels do not rise when cellular damage is merely functional; cells that permit enzymes to enter the circulation have been damaged irreversibly.

DIAGNOSTIC APPLICATIONS

Transaminase values rise much higher in parenchymal damage than in obstructive disease. Intrahepatic or extrahepatic obstruction may eventually injure liver cells, but jaundice usually precedes the enzyme rise, and serum transaminases rarely reach the levels seen in primary hepatocellular disease. Thus transaminase determinations are most useful as early indicators of hepatocellular disease and as a means of differentiating obstructive from hepatocellular jaundice. Several different methods, with different units, are used to measure transaminase activity. Values above 400 to 500 units are rare in obstructive disease but are common in viral hepatitis and chemical injury. Alcoholic hepatitis rarely causes more than modest elevation. Myocardial necrosis can elevate GOT levels to about 500 units, but if there is no liver damage, the GOT rise will be unaccompanied by rising GPT levels.

Some workers find the ratio of GOT to GPT a useful indicator of disease type.[18] At normally low baseline levels, GOT/GPT is less than unity (i.e., GPT levels are slightly higher). With severe hepatocellular damage of toxic or viral origin, both enzymes rise tremendously, but the GOT/GPT ratio remains less than one. GOT elevation that exceeds GPT (a ratio greater than one) nearly always occurs in cirrhosis and in hepatic involvement by metastatic tumor,[60] but total elevations are mild to moderate for both. After myocardial infarction, both GOT and GPT may rise, but GOT outstrips GPT to produce a ratio well above unity. Much of the GOT comes from the heart, while GPT elevation indicates liver damage that often accompanies circulatory embarrassment. Shock and circulatory collapse of any etiology may cause a fairly impressive rise in transaminase values, because centrilobular cells undergo ischemic necrosis.

Lactic Dehydrogenase

Lactic dehydrogenase (LDH) catalyzes the reversible conversion between lactic and pyruvic acids. This reaction is important in nearly all mammalian cells, and large quantities of LDH exist in many tissues. Red and white blood cells, skeletal muscle, cardiac muscle, and liver are especially rich sources of LDH, and serum LDH levels rise if damage occurs to any of these cell types. Different cell types contain the enzyme in subtly different forms, called *isoenzymes,* which can be exploited to pinpoint the cell of origin. Hepatic LDH moves slowly on electrophoresis and is readily inactivated by heat. When total serum LDH is high, it is important to determine which fractions are especially elevated (see p. 359).

Serum LDH rises in most types of hepatocellular injury, but this is not very useful in determining specific etiology. Mild to moderate elevation occurs in all forms of hepatitis, in obstructive jaundice, and in cirrhosis. Infectious mononucleosis, which usually includes some element of hepatitis, causes high total LDH levels, but part of this elevation derives from abnormally proliferating blood cells and not from liver. When carcinomas metastasize to the liver, serum LDH often rises impressively.

Alkaline Phosphatase

Alkaline phosphatase is not a single, well-characterized protein but rather a group of enzymes that catalyze, at an alkaline pH, the hydrolysis of organic phosphate esters. Other enzymes, with an acid pH optimum, are described as acid phosphatases (see pp. 362 to 365). The physiologic role of all the phosphatases is unclear. Three tissues contribute to the circulating enzyme level: bone, intestinal tract, and the hepatobiliary system. During pregnancy, a placental isoenzyme circulates as well. In a nonpregnant patient, elevation of total serum alkaline phosphatase usually reflects bone growth, conditions of abnormal bone turnover, or hepatobiliary disease. Alkaline phosphatase of bone origin can be distinguished from that of intestinal and/or hepatobiliary origin by using heat or a 2 M. urea solution to inactivate the bone-derived enzyme.

DIAGNOSTIC SIGNIFICANCE

Most hepatobiliary alkaline phosphatase comes from the biliary system. The enzyme is excreted through these ducts and is manufactured by epithelial cells that line the biliary system. Some phosphatase in the bile is manufactured by hepatic cells. Obstructive or inflammatory damage to the biliary tree causes a prompt increase in serum alkaline phosphatase levels. Hepatocellular damage that does not involve the biliary tract does not cause a systemic rise in alkaline phosphatase. The enzyme is most useful as a sensitive index of biliary tract disease, especially subtle degrees of intrahepatic or extrahepatic diseases, such as tuberculosis and sarcoidosis, probably because early involvement of portal areas irritates or stimulates biliary tract radicles.

When carcinoma metastasizes to liver, alkaline phosphatase often rises. Metastases to bone cause an increase in osseous alkaline phosphatase. Because some tumors appear to secrete alkaline phosphatase themselves, independent of hepatic or osseous metastases, alkaline phosphatase levels are not very helpful in the differential diagnosis of extensive carcinoma.

Other Enzymes

Numerous other enzymes are associated with the liver and biliary tract, but few have widespread diagnostic acceptance. An enzyme with specific phosphate-splitting activity is *5'-nucleotidase,* which has clinical significance comparable to nonspecific alkaline phosphatase. *Leucine aminopeptidase and gamma-glutamyl transpeptidase* are enzymes which, like the phosphatases, tend to rise with obstructive or inflammatory damage to the biliary system. Some workers believe that these offer advantages in distinguishing obstructive from hepatocellular jaundice; in diagnosing non-A, non-B hepatitis; or in detecting early damage or subtle signs of chronic or lingering disease.

Gamma-glutamyl transpeptidase, in particular, seems to be associated with alcoholic liver disease (see p. 357).

ABNORMALITIES OF HEPATOCELLULAR METABOLISM

Serum Protein Levels

Most serum proteins originate in the liver, except for the immunoglobulins. In addition to albumin and the coagulation proteins, the liver manufactures α and β globulins, notably ceruloplasmin, haptoglobin, and transferrin, as well as various lipoproteins. Manufacturing capacity is sufficiently great that serum levels drop significantly only when large numbers of liver cells have been damaged. The shorter the half-life in the circulation, the more rapidly a protein's serum concentration reflects changes in manufacturing level.[24]

ALBUMIN AND OTHER LIVER PROTEINS

As an index of fairly severe hepatocellular damage, serum albumin concentration is the simplest and most useful test. Prealbumin has the shortest half-life of all—only 2 days—thus it is the first to decline in acute liver disease, but it is more difficult to measure than albumin. Albumin, with a half-life of 21 days, declines only when liver dysfunction persists for some time. In acute hepatitis, for example, maintenance of near-normal albumin levels indicates that overall hepatic function is adequate, even if transaminase values go sky-high. A falling serum albumin level indicates more severe damage. Continuing low albumin levels accompanied by rising globulin values tend to indicate progression toward chronic damage, often with regeneration and an element of reactive immune activity. Ceruloplasmin levels drop with acute hepatocellular damage and rise with biliary tract disease. Obstructive disease also causes an increase in transferrin and the third component of complement, but measuring these proteins adds little to the diagnostic process in biliary tract disease.

GLOBULIN CONCENTRATION

Total globulins characteristically rise in chronic liver disease, an observation that cannot be explained adequately. Both total immunoglobulins and nonantibody proteins increase, but specific antibody levels show no consistent change. The generalized immunoglobulin rise seems to reflect an increase in overall immune activity, possibly resulting because the diseased liver fails to process, degrade, or in-activate antigenic material that normally enters the body. If this barrier function is absent, generalized immune stimulation causes increased production of immunoglobulins of all classes and specific-ities. It is not clear whether chronic hepatocellular damage actively stimulates autoimmune activity as well.

The most impressive globulin elevations accompany chronic active hepatitis and postnecrotic cirrhosis; these involve both IgG and IgM. Biliary cirrhosis characteristically causes an isolated rise in IgM. Alcoholic cirrhosis often causes a rise in serum IgA, as well as sub-stantial increases in IgG and IgM.

FLOCCULATION TESTS

In years past, flocculation tests were used to indicate the relative proportions of serum albumin and globulin. Albumin exerts a stabi-lizing effect on colloidal suspensions, while globulin causes colloi-dally suspended materials to precipitate. Zinc sulfate, ammonium sulfate, colloidal gold, and thymol can be used for this rough kind of estimation. Electrophoretic analysis of serum proteins has largely replaced these qualitative procedures.

ALPHA-1-ANTITRYPSIN

Alpha-1-antitrypsin, an α-globulin, has a unique but imperfectly under-stood relationship to liver disease. This protein inhibits several dif-ferent proteolytic enzymes, including trypsin. Its structure is gen-etically determined, and several abnormal variants have been found as autosomal-recessive traits. Persons with defective α_1-antitrypsin often have destructive and fibrotic changes in the lung (emphysema) and the liver (cirrhosis). Infants or young children with signs of ob-structive jaundice, cirrhosis, or portal hypertension should be ex-amined for this defect. Serum protein electrophoresis is an adequate screening test, since a significant decrease in the α-globulin band occurs if the defective enzyme is present.[22] In such cases, more specific analysis can be instituted to document the variety of defect in question.

Coagulation Proteins

Although the liver manufactures nearly all the coagulation factors, only a few change significantly when liver disease is present. The "liver factors," Factors II, VII, IX, and X, are the most responsive and the easiest to evaluate. In addition, Factor V may decline if liver damage is severe. Production of Factors II, VII, IX, and X depends on the presence of fat-soluble vitamin K and on adequate hepatocellular manufacturing capacity. Vitamin K may not reach the liver in cases of malabsorption or interference with bile acid activity. Vitamin K deficiency causes easily corrected depression of coagulation factors. Severe liver disease, on the other hand, causes coagulation abnormalities that cannot be reversed by administering vitamin K.

The prothrombin time (PT, see p. 74) is a sensitive reflection of changes in the vitamin K-dependent factors. Changes in Factor VII level affect the PT first, while changes in Factor X and Factor II become apparent later. Factor IX affects the partial thromboplastin time but not the PT. With hepatic dysfunction or vitamin K deficiency, the prothrombin time is prolonged. The two causes can be distinguished easily; injection of vitamin K corrects the PT within 48 hours (72 hours at the outside) in a patient with normal liver function but has little or no effect in liver disease.[4]

When liver disease exists, Factor V levels may show variable depression. Factor V influences the prothrombin time, but changing factor levels are difficult to quantitate. The changes of Factor V deficiency often coexist with documented failure to respond to vitamin K. Concentrates of the "liver complex" factors do not contain Factor V. Fresh-frozen plasma contains all the coagulation factors and usually is a better product for treating the hemostatic defects of chronic liver disease than are the more concentrated and more expensive commercially prepared products, which also carry a high hepatitis risk.

Cholesterol Metabolism

Much is unclear about the synthesis, transportation, and physiologic roles of cholesterol. The liver metabolizes preformed dietary cholesterol and also is important in de novo synthesis. Esterified cholesterol, and some nonesterified cholesterol, enters the blood stream from the liver. After conversion to bile acids and neutral steroids, cholesterol is excreted through the biliary system.

When there is biliary tract obstruction, serum cholesterol rises to double the normal levels. Serum phospholipid levels also double or triple when obstruction is extrahepatic. Intrahepatic cholestasis or biliary cirrhosis can elevate cholesterol levels to three or four times normal, with increase in both esterified and nonesterified forms.

Normally, 60 to 70 percent of total serum cholesterol is esterified; a fall in the ratio of esterified to nonesterified cholesterol accompanies diminished hepatocellular function, but with severe hepatocellular damage, both forms decline.[18]

Ammonia

The liver serves excretory as well as synthesizing functions. The liver takes carbon dioxide and ammonia and converts them to urea, the principal end product of protein metabolism. Some ammonia derives directly from metabolizing tissues and parenchymal organs, but most results from the interaction between intestinal bacteria and proteins in the luminal contents. This ammonia is absorbed into the portal venous system, which enters the liver. Normally, little ammonia circulates in the rest of the blood stream because the liver very efficiently extracts ammonia from portal blood and converts it to urea.

In severe liver disease, systemic ammonia levels rise. Except in really fulminant hepatic failure, rising serum ammonia does not result from failing hepatocellular function. The problem is largely one of circulation; portal blood flow is diverted, and metabolites are not exposed to adequate numbers of liver cells.[5] The load of ammonia and abnormal products is shunted directly from the portal system into the systemic blood. Although high levels of ammonia occur in incipient or established hepatic encephalopathy ("hepatic coma"), the ammonia itself probably does not cause the neurologic effects. Other materials, normally metabolized by hepatic cells but released by altered flow patterns into the systemic circulation, accompany the shunted ammonia and may well be the true effectors of CNS dysfunction.

IMMUNOLOGIC TESTS

Hepatic functions and immunologic activities often are interrelated. We have already described how serum immunoglobulin levels rise nonspecifically in many chronic liver diseases. Another disease in which immunology and hepatology interact is viral hepatitis, which is discussed in a later section. The remaining area we must consider is the ill-defined relationship between autoimmune phenomena and liver disease.

Despite intense investigation, the importance of cell-mediated autoimmunity in liver disease is not yet clear. The histologic appearance of several chronic inflammatory conditions strongly suggests immune activity, but experimental results are ambiguous or controversial, or both. No useful diagnostic tests have yet emerged from these investigations.

Autoantibodies

Three kinds of autoantibodies occur with moderate frequency in certain kinds of liver disease. The targets of these antibodies are smooth-muscle antigens, mitochondria, and such nuclear elements as soluble nuclear proteins and single-stranded DNA. When they occur, these antibodies have more diagnostic than etiologic significance. They do not appear to cause liver damage, but their presence makes some diagnoses more probable than others (see below). Fluorescein-labeled antiglobulin serum is used to demonstrate their presence after the patient's serum is incubated with frozen tissue sections. If the appropriate antibodies are present, they attach to the tissue and react with the antihuman globulin serum added afterward. All three antibodies are cross-reactive with tissues from various organs and from various host species.

SMOOTH-MUSCLE ANTIBODIES

Smooth-muscle antibodies react with the contractile protein *actin*, which seems to share some antigen with liver cells and probably with other cells. The IgG antibody against smooth muscle occurs in at least two-thirds of patients with chronic active hepatitis and in 30 to 40 percent of patients with primary biliary cirrhosis. It does occur sometimes in liver damage from infectious mononucleosis, acute viral hepatitis, or infiltrative tumors, suggesting that it develops as a response to damaged liver cells.

MITOCHONDRIAL ANTIBODIES

Mitochondrial antibodies react with those mitochondria engaged in the kind of high-energy transactions that occur in renal tubules or in secreting cells of the gastric mucosa. Meticulous technique is needed to avoid confusion with many other antibodies: those specific for the substrate organs, those that react with microsomal antigens, or those nonspecific immune reactants that occur in syphilis or SLE. Mitochondrial antibodies were originally associated with biliary cirrhosis, and in some series, up to 90 percent of patients with biliary cirrhosis have these antibodies.[23] Mitochondrial antibodies also occur in up to

25 percent of patients with chronic active hepatitis;[2] thus they cannot be considered specific for distinguishing biliary cirrhosis from other liver diseases.

ANTINUCLEAR ANTIBODIES

Antinuclear antibodies occur in many "collagen-vascular" diseases, some of which involve the liver. Anti-DNA is strongly correlated with active *systemic lupus erythematosus* (SLE). Ordinarily, patients with SLE do not have smooth muscle antibodies, even when liver damage exists. In contrast, the condition called *lupoid hepatitis* characteristically has both nuclear and smooth muscle antibodies. Lupoid hepatitis is a form of chronic active hepatitis that primarily affects young women; it is often accompanied by other autoimmune phenomena, such as organ-specific antibodies, rheumatoid factor, false-positive serologic tests for syphilis, and, sometimes, a weakly positive LE test. Gamma-globulin levels rise strikingly; transaminase and alkaline phosphatase levels are moderately elevated, but serum bilirubin usually remains low. Antinuclear antibodies also occur in primary biliary cirrhosis and after liver damage due to drugs or, occasionally, virus infection.

TESTS FOR VIRAL HEPATITIS

Many viral infections cause liver damage, but primary viral hepatitis classically has been divided into two types: *infectious hepatitis,* with a relatively short incubation period, fecal-oral transmission, and frequent association with common-source outbreaks; and *serum hepatitis,* with a long incubation period and transmission usually by parenteral inoculation, such as blood transfusion, injection of illicit drugs, or contaminated surgical, dental, or tattooing equipment. Today primary liver infections can be classified more accurately as immunologic identification of viral antigens and antibodies progresses.

Hepatitis A and Others

Hepatitis A is the disease previously called infectious hepatitis. Virus-like particles have been identified in the feces of acutely ill patients, and antibody to the viral antigen can be identified by immune electron microscopy.[8] At present, no routine tests are available for clinical diagnosis of hepatitis A antigen and antibody. *Hepatitis B,* formerly called serum hepatitis, results from infection with a DNA virus with multiple antigenic features. As these two forms of viral hepatitis are increasingly well understood, it has become obvious that much hepatitis is neither A nor B. Since it is unclear whether one or many viruses are responsible, this group of diseases has been cautiously christened *non-A, non-B hepatitis.* To qualify as non-A, non-B, the infection must be shown clearly not to have been due to Epstein-Barr virus (EBV) or to cytomegalovirus (CMV).[19]

Hepatitis B Antigens

The complete hepatitis B virion is called the *Dane particle.* It is 42 nm. in diameter and consists of a 28-nm. core containing DNA and protein and a surface envelope that contains protein, polysaccharide, and lipid.[20] The core antigen is called HB_cAg, while its identifying antibody is anti-HB_cAg. The surface material has several antigenic specificities, collectively characterized as HB_sAg; the antibody is anti-HB_sAg. Still another antigen, associated with hepatitis B but completely distinct from HB_sAg or HB_cAg, is called e. This may not be part of the virus, but instead may represent host proteins altered and rendered antigenic by viral activity.

During acute infection, HB_cAg is located in the nucleus of infected cells, while HB_sAg is found in the cytoplasm of infected liver cells and also in the patient's serum. HB_cAg, by itself, does not circulate. Dane particles contain HB_cAg completely enclosed in surface material; these circulate, along with isolated fragments of HB_sAg, in the blood of infected patients and of asymptomatic hepatitis carriers. HB_sAg often appears in the blood before the onset of clinical symptoms and may persist well after chemical signs of liver damage have disappeared. The e antigen circulates in about 10 percent of patients with HB_sAg antigenemia. Some workers believe that e-positive patients are more likely than e-negative patients to develop chronic liver disease or to become chronic carriers.[15]

HB_sAg can be demonstrated most sensitively, in serum or other body fluids, by radioimmunoassay or by reverse passive hemagglutination. Agar gel diffusion and counterimmunoelectrophoresis were used in early studies, but these are far less sensitive. Several antigenic subtypes exist, variously characterized as *adw, ayw, adr,* and *ayr.*[20] These are useful for epidemiologic and demographic studies but are unnecessary for routine diagnosis.

SIGNIFICANCE OF ANTIGEN TESTING

The presence of circulating surface antigen indicates that viable, multiplying viruses either are present or have been present. The test is useful in diagnosing active hepatitis B, chronic liver disease that follows hepatitis B infection, and the carrier state for the virus. Acute or chronic disease can be confirmed by abnormalities of other liver function tests, but there is no other reliable test for the carrier state. Blood or any body fluid that contains $HB_s Ag$ carries a high risk of HB transmission. True infectivity probably results only when the intact 42-nm. particle is present, but it is impossible to prove the absence of Dane particles if surface antigen fragments are present. Since 1970, increasingly sensitive $HB_s Ag$ tests have been applied to transfusion products; the incidence of post-transfusion hepatitis B has dropped significantly, although occasional cases of proven hepatitis B do follow transfusion of blood with negative $HB_s Ag$ tests, Although transfusion-related hepatitis B has declined, the overall incidence of the disease continues to rise steadily.[9]

The significance of the e antigen remains under study. The test is not widely available clinically; as a research tool, it is a promising indicator that chronic liver damage has occurred or is likely to occur.

Hepatitis B Antibodies

Anti-$HB_c Ag$, anti-$HB_s Ag$, and anti-e can be identified with suitable tests, but the procedures are more difficult to standardize and less widely available than tests for surface antigen. Seroconversion, the demonstration of antibody in a later serum when earlier specimens were antibody-free, indicates that infection has occurred. Since anti-$HB_c Ag$ does not persist very long after infection ceases, its presence indicates ongoing or very recent hepatocellular infection. The HB_c antigen is difficult to purify and concentrate, and tests for this antibody are not widely available. The presence of anti-$HB_c Ag$ in a patient currently or recently ill, or in one who has recently received blood, strongly suggests hepatitis B infection.

Antibody to the surface antigen (anti-$HB_s Ag$) can be detected for years after infection has been eradicated, but it also can coexist with circulating antigen. The antibody characteristically develops several weeks or months after antigen has circulated, but its development cannot be taken as evidence that infection has been overcome. An asymptomatic individual who has the antibody, but has no clinical history of hepatitis, can be presumed to have sustained subclinical or unrecognized infection at some previous time. It is not clear whether anti-HB$_s$Ag in donor blood makes hepatitis transmission more or less likely than after transfusion of blood with no detectible antibodies. Under intensive investigation is the role of anti-HB$_s$Ag as a hepatitis preventive. Both active and passive immunizations against hepatitis B are likely to become possible in the near future.

There is relatively little information on the development or significance of anti-e.

REFERENCES

1. *Acute and chronic hepatitis revisited. Review by an international group.* Lancet 2:914, 1977.
2. Archer, G. J., and Monie, R. D. H.: *Wilson's disease and chronic active hepatitis.* Lancet 1:486, 1977.
3. Berk, P. D., Wolkoff, A. W., and Berlin, N. I.: *Inborn errors of bilirubin metabolism.* Med. Clin. North Am. 59:803, 1975.
4. Black, M.: *Diagnostic methods in liver disease.* Med. Clin. North Am. 59:1015, 1975.
5. Cohn, J. N.: *Hepatocirculatory failure.* Med. Clin. North Am. 59:955, 1975.
6. Combes, B., and Schenker, S.: *Laboratory tests,* in Schiff, L., (ed.): *Diseases of the Liver.* ed. 4. J. B. Lippincott, Philadelphia, 1975.
7. De Vivo, D. C., and Keating, J. P.: *Reye's syndrome.* Adv. Pediatr. 22:175, 1976.
8. Feinstone, S. M., Kapikan, A. Z., and Purcell, R. H.: *Hepatitis A: detection by immune electron microscopy of a viruslike antigen associated with acute illness.* Science 182:1026, 1973.
9. *Hepatitis — United States, 1975–1976.* Morbid. Mortal. 26(22), June 3, 1977.
10. Javitt, N. B.: *Cholestatic jaundice.* Med. Clin. North Am. 59:817, 1975.
11. Klatskin, G.: *Toxic and drug-induced hepatitis,* in Schiff, L. (ed.): *Diseases of the Liver.* ed. 4. J. B. Lippincott, Philadelphia, 1975.
12. Koff, R. S.: *Postoperative jaundice.* Med. Clin. North Am. 59:823, 1975.
13. London, W. T.: *Hepatitis B virus and antigen-antibody complex diseases.* N. Engl. J. Med. 296:1528, 1977.
14. Maddrey, W. C., and Weber, F. L.: *Chronic hepatic encephalopathy.* Med. Clin. North Am. 59:937, 1975.
15. Magnius, L. O., Lindholm, A., Lundin, P., et al.: *A new antigen-antibody system: clinical significance in long-term carriers of hepatitis B surface antigen.* J.A.M.A. 231:356, 1975.
16. Melnick, J. L., Dreesman, G. R., and Hollinger, F. B.: *Approaching the control of viral hepatitis type B.* J. Infect. Dis. 133:210, 1976.
17. Mezey, E.: *Diagnosis of liver disease by laboratory methods,* in Halsted, J. A. (ed.): *The Laboratory in Clinical Medicine.* W. B. Saunders, Philadelphia, 1976.
18. Mezey, E.: *Specific liver diseases,* in Halsted, J. A. (ed.): *The Laboratory in Clinical Medicine.* W. B. Saunders, Philadelphia, 1976.
19. Mosley, J. W., Redeker, A. G., Feinstone, S. M., and Purcell, R. H.: *Multiple hepatitis viruses in multiple attacks of acute viral hepatitis.* N. Engl. J. Med. 296:75, 1977.

20. Robinson, W. S., and Lutwick, L. I.: *The virus of hepatitis, type B.* N. Engl. J. Med. 295:1168, 1232, 1976.
21. Scharschmidt, B. F.: *Approaches to the management of fulminant hepatic failure.* Med. Clin. North Am. 59:927, 1975.
22. Sharp, H. L.: *The current status of α-1-antitrypsin, a protease inhibitor, in gastrointestinal disease.* Gastroenterol. 70:611, 1976.
23. Sherlock, S., and Scheuer, P. J.: *The presentation and diagnosis of 100 patients with primary biliary cirrhosis.* N. Engl. J. Med. 289:674, 1973.
24. Skrede, S., Blomhoff, J. P., Elgjo, K., and Gjone, E.: *Serum proteins in diseases of the liver.* Scand. J. Clin. Lab. Invest. 35:399, 1975.
25. Solberg, H. E., Skrede, S., and Blomhoff, J. P.: *Diagnosis of liver diseases by laboratory results and discriminant analyses.* Scand. J. Clin. Lab. Invest. 35:713, 1975.
26. Zimmerman, H. J.: *Liver disease caused by medicinal agents.* Med. Clin. North Am. 59:897, 1975.

SECTION 4

MICROBIOLOGY

CHAPTER 13

MICROBIOLOGIC EXAMINATIONS

The exogenous invaders producing human disease are legion, ranging from viruses, the smallest known living entities, to worms and flukes of really substantial size. By convention, microbiology concerns itself with the plant kingdom, while animal parasitology occupies a separate niche. Most clinical microbiology laboratories isolate, identify, and cultivate bacteria and fungi, leaving to specialized laboratories the demanding techniques of virus and rickettsial cultivation.

BACTERIAL PROPERTIES

To some extent, certain pathologic processes can be correlated with the characteristics of the inciting organism. This kind of information is interesting, and useful to a point, but cannot fully explain the course of any one patient's disease. Nevertheless, we may profitably consider some elements determining the scope and nature of bacterial disease. The disease-producing organism must achieve an ecologic relationship with its hosts such that its continuation, as a species, is assured. This means that the agent must enter a host, multiply itself, leave the primary host, and then enter another host immediately or be able to survive independently. The cycle can be interrupted, in a single individual, by death of the host or cure of the disease, but (with the possible exception of the smallpox virus) it has not been possible to eradicate completely a disease-producing microorganism. Techniques of sanitation, asepsis, and sterilization attempt to prevent entry into hosts and transmission to other hosts, while therapeutic agents attempt to prevent multiplication of the organisms and prevent or correct deleterious effects of this multiplication.

Host-Invader Interactions

The body copes with bacterial invaders by cellular and humoral defenses. Both mononuclear and polymorphonuclear cells can attack invading organisms by engulfment or phagocytosis. Granulocytic leukocytes produce lytic substances which attack extracellular organisms as well as mediating intracellular destruction of the bacteria. Antibodies, both circulating and those on cell surfaces, may destroy the organism directly or alter its properties so that other cell-mediated defenses are more effective. The structure of certain tissues, such as the alveolar walls in the lungs, the fascial planes in muscle, and collagenous barriers in skin, contributes to mechanical confinement of the invader, thus concentrating and enhancing the body's other defenses. Bacteria, on the other hand, have various properties which protect them against the host's attacks, and the course of disease is the balance between these opposing forces.

SURFACE CHARACTERISTICS

The bacterial cell surface significantly affects the host-invader balance. Capsules or other surface characteristics may resist phagocytosis, thereby promoting bacterial multiplication. Pneumococcus, *H. influenzae*, and Klebsiella have capsules; the surface proteins of Group A streptococcus, although not a capsule, have antiphagocytic properties. This advantage to the bacteria is offset by the antigenic nature of capsular material and surface proteins (i.e., they stimulate the host to produce antibodies which inactivate or neutralize the antiphagocytic effect). The antigenic strength of these surface elements varies with different organisms and different strains of the same organism. The host's capacity to approach, engulf, and destroy the bacterial invader depends on individual factors as well. Immunologic competence, the numbers and functions of the leukocytes, the general state of protein metabolism, and the existence of adequate circulation and blood supply to the infected area all contribute to the outcome of the battle.

Immunologic stimulation and response are not the only determinants. Other bacterial products exert other effects. Many pathogenic staphylococci possess a coagulase which converts fibrinogen to fibrin. This deposits on the bacterial cell as an envelope which makes phagocytosis difficult. Although it is tempting to assign teleologic significance to this property, the role of coagulase in promoting staphylococcal infection is unproved. Hyaluronic acid, in the capsules of group A and C streptococci, is too similar to human polysaccharides to evoke antibodies, but it interferes nonetheless with phagocytosis.

BACTERIAL TOXINS

Bacteria produce a wide variety of extracellular substances with physiologic activity. Some of these produce disease directly, while others may enhance pathogenicity or be indifferent. For example, clostridial proteolytic enzymes and streptococcal hemolysins and proteases are not inherently pathogenic, but they assist bacterial multiplication or spread. Bacterial products which directly damage the host are called toxins. These are of two kinds. Exotoxins, produced by the cells, are secreted into the host's tissues or fluids and exert their effect independent of the presence or multiplication of the organism. Endotoxins are intrinsic to the organism, usually a lipopolysaccharide structural component, and these damage the host only when bacterial death or lysis liberates them into direct contact with host tissue.

EXOTOXINS. Exotoxins, not bacterial multiplication, mediate the harmful effects of such diseases as diphtheria, tetanus, botulism, and a variety of diarrheal syndromes ranging from "traveller's tummy" through staphylococcal food poisoning to cholera. Although the proteins are highly antigenic, they act so promptly that the patient usually dies or recovers before he can mount an antibody response. Exogenous antitoxins are used against the catastrophic effects of *C. tetani* and *C. botulinum* toxins. In cholera, diphtheria, and the gram-negative bacillary diseases, therapy aims more toward eradicating the organism than toward neutralizing the specific toxin.

ENDOTOXINS. The role of endotoxin depends partly on its quantity and mode of entry and partly on the biologic and immunologic condition of the patient. Endotoxins produce a generalized "toxic" state which may include fever, leukopenia, intravascular coagulation, and vascular and hemodynamic changes leading, in severe cases, to shock and death. On a weight-for-weight basis, exotoxins are far more potent than endotoxins, but a larger volume of morbidity and mortality derives from endotoxin effects, notably those of gram-negative bacilli. These multifarious systemic effects cannot be neutralized by specific antitoxins. The cell wall lipopolysaccharides mediate the antigenic identity of the organisms as the O (or somatic) antigens of the gram-negative rods, but diseases result from highly complex inter-actions of bacteria, host tissues, and immune response, rather than from chemical toxins alone.

ANTIBIOTICS

In the last 30 years, antimicrobial agents have altered radically the age-long battle between host and microbial invader. Bacterial growth can be altered by such factors as changes in pH, temperature, and nutrient environment, but antibacterial chemotherapy implies a dif-ferent attack. Antibiotics are chemical substances, produced by microorganisms, with the capacity to inhibit or destroy other micro-organisms in dilute solution. To be medically useful, the substance must selectively attack invading organisms without seriously impair-ing the host. Many bacteria, fungi, and actinomycetes produce anti-bacterial metabolites, but most are too toxic to human or other hosts or are too weakly active against other organisms to be therapeutically effective. Perhaps 50 or fewer have found medical employment, reflecting their ability selectively to damage or destroy the invader (usually a bacterial one) at reasonable pharmacologic dosage levels.

The ideal therapeutic agent should selectively interrupt some process vital to the invader, but absent or nonessential in the host's metabolism. The secondary results of such attack should not damage the host. Moreover, there should be no harmful secondary effects from the metabolic alteration, such as accumulation of toxic waste products or overgrowth by other invaders. No known drug or thera-peutic agent achieves this ideal completely.

Mechanisms of Action

Antibiotics can harm microorganisms in many ways, but some mech-anisms may prove as harmful to host as to invader. The major sites of antibiotic attack include cell wall synthesis, membrane function, protein synthesis, nucleic acid metabolism, and intermediary metab-olism. Most invading organisms have cell walls, but mammalian cells never do. Agents that interfere with cell wall synthesis are less likely to harm host cells than are drugs which inhibit or affect functions shared by all living cells, such as membrane function or protein and nucleic acid metabolism. Intermediary metabolism is another area where major differences exist, but it can be difficult to find specific exploitable metabolic pathways.

CELL WALLS

A rigid cell wall surrounds the bacterial cell, conferring on it shape, antigenic composition, and protection from mechanical and osmotic trauma. The essential components are peptidoglycans, consisting of polysaccharides and short-chain peptides which are manufactured in stages by the multiplying cell. Mature cells, their walls complete, are not affected by agents that interfere with peptidoglycan synthesis. If grown in special medium or under protected conditions, organisms can continue to multiply and mature without cell walls, growing into fragile, "naked" forms called *spheroplasts*. Antibiotics that inhibit cell wall synthesis induce the growth of spheroplasts under these artificial conditions.

Penicillin, penicillin derivatives, and the cephalosporins act on a late phase of cell wall synthesis, possibly by inhibiting enzyme activity or by substituting for some substrate to form a lethal or inhibitory intermediary. D-cycloserine acts by competitive inhibition; its structure allows it to substitute for D-alanine in cell wall synthesis. Organisms continue to grow if there is a high concentration of D-alanine or if they evolve alternate metabolic pathways that do not require D-alanine.

Bacitracin, effective predominantly against gram-positive organisms, inhibits a synthetic step earlier than that affected by penicillin. Vancomycin and ristocetin seem to act at still another site by means of mechanisms not at all clearly understood. Since these two drugs often remain effective against gram-positive organisms that have developed resistance to other agents, their mode of action must be quite different.

CELL MEMBRANES

Agents that affect the osmotic regulatory functions of cell membranes tend to be too toxic for clinical use. They act on resting as well as growing cells and must be selected carefully so as not to bind to host cells. Amphotericin B and nystatin are clinically useful because they bind selectively to sterol sites which are more numerous or more accessible in fungal membranes than in mammalian cells; nonetheless, amphotericin B carries substantial risk to the patient's kidneys. Also nephrotoxic are the polymyxins, used for their selective activity against gram-negative organisms but used with caution.

PROTEIN SYNTHESIS

Protein synthesis is such a complex process that it offers many sites for productive intervention. Since reactions occur entirely within cells, antimicrobial agents must penetrate the organisms and exert greater activity against bacterial processes than against pathways essential to mammalian cell function. The pathway from DNA to the finished protein includes transcription of RNA from the DNA template and translation of the RNA message through ribosomal interactions. It may be concluded that different antibiotics affect different phases.

Rifampin, a semisynthetic drug derived from Streptomyces strains, inhibits the DNA-dependent RNA polymerase that occurs in many bacteria but does not affect the mammalian form of the polymerase.[6] It has proved especially useful against M. *tuberculosis*, a slowly multiplying organism with unique chemical characteristics that render it impervious to many other antibiotics.

Interference with the smaller (30S) ribosomal subunit accounts for the activity of aminoglycosides and tetracyclines. Streptomycin, the first aminoglycoside to achieve clinical usefulness,[20] affects ribosomal action in many ways, causing outright inhibition of some synthetic steps and incorrect activity of others. Related agents, many of them less toxic, include neomycins, kanamycins, gentamycins, and spectinomycin. The aminoglycosides are lethal for many gram-negative organisms, but unfortunately, the bacteria can acquire unique ability to fight back. A single-step mutation produces high-grade resistance which can, moreover, be transmitted from one gram-negative organism to another (see below).

Tetracyclines are bacteriostatic agents ·that are most effective against the 30S ribosomal subunits of rapidly multiplying organisms. Many gram-negative and gram-positive organisms are initially sensitive but readily acquire resistance. Tetracyclines are particularly useful against rickettsiae, mycoplasmas, and chlamydiae.

The larger (50S) ribosomal subunit is the target for such varied agents as chloramphenicol, erythromycin, lincomycin, and clindamycin. All of these have potentially serious toxic effects on gastrointestinal tract, bone marrow, or liver cells, but they are invaluable for their breadth and efficiency of bactericidal action.

DNA SYNTHESIS

Considering the ubiquity and importance of DNA, it is hardly surprising that agents effective against DNA function or replication have little clinical application. An exception to this is griseofulvin, which inhibits specifically the mitosis of fungi whose walls contain chitin. This limits its clinical usefulness to superficial infections of hair, skin, and nails, but in this restricted sphere, it is effective and nontoxic.

INTERMEDIARY METABOLISM

The classic example of antimicrobial action through metabolic inhibition is the sulfonamide group. These are structural analogs of *para-aminobenzoic acid* (PABA) and act by substituting for PABA in bacterial metabolism. PABA is a precursor of folic acid, which is synthesized by many bacteria but not by man. Microorganisms which require preformed folic acid are not affected by the sulfonamides, and many initially sensitive organisms have developed pathways that bypass the PABA-requiring steps. At least for the present, organisms resistant to sulfonamides alone have proved largely susceptible to combination therapy in which the dehydrofolate reductase step of folate synthesis is inhibited at the same time that the PABA analog is given.

M. tuberculosis has been the target of several metabolic inhibitors not useful against other organisms. *Para-aminosalicylic acid* (PAS) acts as a competitive inhibitor of PABA, but only for this organism. Isoniazid, which resembles both niacin and pyridoxine, acts on the mycobacterium by means of an imperfectly understood mechanism. Giving PAS and isoniazid together reduces the likelihood that mutant organisms will develop that are resistant to either one.

Resistance to Antibiotics

The war between microorganisms and antibiotics continues unremittingly. "Wonder drugs" have not eradicated infectious disease; they have merely changed the conditions and natural history of many infections. Organisms display remarkable adaptive capacity, so that drugs effective today become ineffective against the same type of infection tomorrow. Effective adaptations that organisms can make include (1) membrane or cell wall changes so that drugs cannot enter; (2) adoption of metabolic pathways that bypass the step, substrate, or enzyme affected by the drug; and (3) elaboration of enzymes that inactivate the drug.[36] Alteration of microbial behavior requires alteration of genetic information. Once a resistant organism appears, its descendants also will display the properties that made the original cell resistant. Organisms change their genetic endowment either by mutation or by acquisition of new genetic material.

MUTATION

Mutation occurs spontaneously whenever cells divide. Whether or not a mutation survives to be perpetuated depends on its biologic effects and on the specific environment. Some genetic changes code for products that are directly lethal or, more often, that cause lethal dysfunction of some essential structure or activity. Other mutations give the organism altered metabolic properties which could be favorable, unfavorable, or neutral, depending on such environmental events as the availability of oxygen or CO_2 and the presence or absence of other organisms, other cells, or other chemicals.[32] The rate or the direction of mutation does not depend on environmental conditions, but these do influence survival of the mutant. In a population of organisms under attack by an antibiotic, a mutant capable of surviving the drug's effects will continue to multiply while other cells succumb. The fittest, in this setting, not only survives but becomes the predominant type.

A mutation that confers resistance to one antibiotic usually has no effect on response to other categories of drugs. If resistance develops to the simple, cheap, nontoxic agents first used for therapy, it is often possible to administer drugs with other actions. If emerging resistance seems especially likely or especially hazardous, it can be helpful to give two different drugs at once. Mutants capable of surviving against one have little chance of escaping the other. Chance, however, dictates that if many mutations continue, an organism will emerge eventually that resists both antibiotics.

GENETIC EXCHANGE

Chromosomal replication, with multiplication of genetically identical progeny, is not the only way that information passes from one organism to another. Bacteria possess extrachromosomal units that are genetically active. These autonomous molecules of DNA, called *plasmids*, are capable of directing protein synthesis and other actions independent of the chromosomal messages inherent in the cell. Plasmids can be exchanged between cells, either like members of a single species or dissimilar members of a larger family. Several transfer mechanisms exist. *Conjugation* involves structural mating between cells, and its occurrence depends upon the presence of genetic material that codes for this ability. *Transduction* is a passive process whereby viral infection carries material from one organism to another.

Extrachromosomal genetic units can code for ability to withstand antibiotic attack or to elaborate drug-inactivating enzymes. Chromosomal mutations usually confer resistance against a single action of a single drug, while extrachromosomal information tends to be more complex. The Enterobacteriaceae, highly pathogenic gram-negative bacilli that inhabit the gut, can develop resistance active simultaneously against chloramphenicol, tetracycline, streptomycin, and sulfonamides. This extrachromosomal *resistance factor,* called R, is transmitted among various organisms within the family in a manner quite independent of past or present exposure to the drugs. Not every organism that possesses this multidrug resistance can transmit it; the genetic information that allows conjugation to occur must be available as well. If both sets of information are present, however, the stage is set for the phenomenon called *infectious drug resistance.* Although many gram-negative organisms have acquired multiple resistance, potential plagues of resistant organisms sweeping through hospitals, populations, or continents have not materialized.

Ability to elaborate beta-lactamase, the enzyme that inactivates many forms of penicillin (penicillinase), also resides in plasmids. These occur in both gram-positive and gram-negative organisms and tend to develop in bacterial populations heavily exposed to penicillin. Other resistance properties may accompany penicillinase production. Transfer of penicillinase plasmids occurs by virus-mediated transduction. *Staphylococcus aureus* is the organism most notorious for possessing and exchanging this property, but *H. influenzae* and *N. gonorrhoeae* also have become involved.[31]

MICROBIOLOGIC TECHNIQUES

One vitally important function of diagnostic microbiology is the documentation of patterns of drug sensitivity and resistance in clinical pathogens. Before discussing these techniques, we must consider how pathogens are identified and implicated in clinical situations.

Bacteria are ubiquitous. They can be present in or on diseased tissue without causing the disease. Some bacteria cause disease in one site but grow harmlessly at some other one. Some bacteria cause disease but are difficult to culture. Identifying a significant pathogen requires that suitable clinical material be examined, that suitable microbiologic techniques be followed, and that resulting findings be interpreted in the light of general principles and individual circumstance.

Specimen Collection

Selection and handling of clinical material for examination seem to be simpler in theory than in practice. The principles are obvious. The specimen should be taken, when viable organisms are numerous, from a site where organisms are likely to be found. It should be collected before instituting antibacterial therapy and be handled without contaminating the specimen with outside organisms or spreading the patient's organisms to others. The specimen should be transported promptly to the laboratory and processed before relevant organisms have died or multiplied to levels which distort the true clinical picture. Any and all of these goals may fall short of achievement because of inadequate patient care, laboratory failure, poor cooperation from the patient himself, or plain bad luck.

TIME OF COLLECTION

The phase of the disease may be particularly critical and particularly difficult to control. Salmonella and Shigella are more easily cultured from stool specimens early in the illness, but the patient may not come for help until the process is well established. Brucella infections produce chronic, relapsing symptoms for months after cultures become negative. Recurrent bacteremias can produce persistent illness, but blood cultures taken between so-called showers may be negative. Tularemia and plague produce short-lived, early bacteremias, but once the organisms enter fixed tissue, they become extremely difficult to culture.

SITE OF COLLECTION

The site for culture is obvious when symptoms are localized, as with meningitis, abscesses, wound infections, or purulent pneumonias. More diffuse processes require greater selectivity, as, for example, in choosing among nasopharyngeal, throat, or sputum cultures for respiratory tract symptoms or in discriminating between the urinary tract and the genital tract as the origin of dysuria. When infection is deep-seated, culture material should come from deep in the tissue to avoid contamination with superficial organisms.

EFFECT OF MEDICATION

It may prove impossible to obtain a specimen before antibacterial therapy has begun. Ideally, therapy should await accurate diagnosis, or, when the need is acute, cultures should be taken just before medication is given. In practice, the patient may have been medicating himself and come to medical attention only when his own efforts have failed. The need for bacteriologic study may become urgent only after initial therapy has proved unsuccessful. Moreover, complications may occur which alter the initial diagnosis and require additional diagnostic study.

Antibiotic therapy does not always invalidate subsequent cultures. Sometimes penicillinase or some other anti-antibiotic is added to the culture medium; sometimes diluting the specimen will diminish the drug effect without suppressing the growth of significant organisms. If cultures must be taken after drugs have been given, laboratory personnel should be informed so that they can make suitable changes in culture techniques.

AVOIDING CONTAMINATION

Bacterial contamination may go in several directions. Organisms may spread from specimen to personnel, from personnel to specimen or from one specimen to another. Contamination of personnel usually results from carelessness or from inadequate containers. Sputum and feces containers tend to be the worst offenders, although urine collections, drainage tubes, and wound dressings are fertile sources of infection for the unwary. Spinal fluids and blood cultures are seldom handled sloppily, probably because the precautions necessary for obtaining the specimen are applied to the material throughout its processing.

Specimens should be collected with due concern for the desired results. This means meticulous cleansing of the skin before taking blood cultures or of the urethral meatus before taking urine samples. It also means excluding saliva from sputum specimens and avoiding admixture of urine with feces for stool culture. In these two latter instances, the cooperation of the patient is highly desirable; the extra time invested in instructing the patient may be rewarded by vastly improved specimen quality.

DELAY BEFORE CULTURING

A specimen may be examined immediately or transported down a corridor, or it may have to spend several days in the mail. Depending on the organism involved and the transport medium used, any of these can give excellent results. If delay must occur between collection and processing, the organisms must be protected from drying, pH change, and inimical temperatures. The bacterial population should be held near its original proportions without unduly encouraging or discouraging certain strains.

Because material on cotton swabs is particularly likely to dry, non-nutrient broth or holding medium is frequently used, even for short-term delays. Pathogens in urine, feces, and sputum specimens can survive refrigeration for a number of hours. Specimens with suspected shigellae, however, should be processed rapidly to avoid overgrowth by hardier, nonpathogenic organisms. Shigellae and salmonellae will survive for long periods if the fecal sample is smeared thinly on filter paper and air-dried. Such samples can be mailed, and the dried material later reconstituted in suitable medium.

Urine for cultures can be held at refrigerator temperatures for several days without affecting the validity of the results.[24] Spinal fluid, on the other hand, should be examined as soon as possible after lumbar puncture, partly because the clinical situation may be urgent, but also because such organisms as *H. influenzae* and meningococci are sensitive to environmental changes.

Direct Examination

Specimens are sent to the microbiology laboratory to answer several questions: Are any organisms present? If present, what are they? Are they causally related to the patient's disease? If they are pathogenic, what therapeutic agents can best be employed? Cultivating the organisms on culture medium gives the most accurate answers to these questions. Successful cultures require time for bacterial growth and depend upon the presence of viable organisms in the specimen as received. If time is short, or if the organisms may not be viable, direct microscopic examination of the material may be helpful.

WET MOUNTS

Most clinical specimens are stained and fixed for examination, but wet mounts are used to identify fungi and to demonstrate motile protozoa in, for example, trichomonal vaginitis or parastic diarrheas. A classic technique is the demonstration of Cryptococcus (formerly called Torula) in spinal fluids by adding India ink to the fluid. To find parasites or their ova, stool specimens can be emulsified, sometimes with added iodine, and examined in as fresh a condition as possible. Dark-field illumination enhances the visibility of motile organisms, notably spirochetes. All these techniques are excellent for immediate diagnosis, but their usefulness depends on the skill of the examiner, the presence of sufficient organisms to make detection feasible, and the morphologic features of these organisms which render them visible with relatively little processing.

STAINS

GRAM STAIN. Most bacteria are small and difficult to examine unstained. Their surface chemistry, however, permits combination with various stains to enhance visibility; differing chemical compositions permit differential staining reactions. The Gram stain and the acid-fast stain are the two most widely used. In the Gram stain, a purple-blue dye complex enters the organism when the smeared material is flooded with crystal violet and iodine. Once the dye complex has entered the cell, alcohol or acetone is added as a decolorizer. The alcohol dehydrates some bacterial walls, rendering them impermeable and preventing the escape of intracellular dye complex. In other organisms, presumably those with high lipid content, the organic solvent removes much of the cell-wall lipid, increasing permeability and permitting the dye complex to wash out of the interior. Bacteria which retain the blue-purple stain are called gram-positive, while those which alcohol decolorizes are called gram-negative. A contrasting counter stain (usually carbolfuchsin or safranin) is used to color the gram-negative organisms so that they can be seen and their morphology noted. Since retention of the dye complex depends on intact cell walls, organisms with absent or damaged walls will appear gram-negative, even if intact members of the species are gram-positive.

Besides differentiating organisms according to their cell wall composition, the Gram stain permits excellent visualization of bacteria, so that their morphology can be studied with some precision. Shape, relative size, and growth configuration all contribute to identification. Sputum, spinal fluid, urine, exudates, and other clinical specimens can be smeared, Gram-stained, and examined directly, in many cases permitting rapid presumptive diagnosis of bacterial infection. Centrifugation, with subsequent examination of the sediment, can be used to concentrate the organisms to readily detectible levels. The presence and nature of cells and the relation of organisms to the cells are additional diagnostic data available from properly made Gram-stained material. Gram stains also are used after organisms have been culti- vated to demonstrate the morphology of organisms comprising col- onies seen on culture. Modifications of the Gram stain are used to demonstrate bacteria in sections of fixed tissue, but morphologic detail may be altered by processing and sectioning.

ACID-FAST STAIN. The acid-fast stain also relies on cell wall proper- ties, especially the lipid content, but the principle is less well under- stood than that of the Gram stain. Again, the result is that intracellular dye resists decolorization, and acid-fast organisms are gram-positive as well. In the acid-fast procedure, carbolfuchsin is introduced into the cell with heat and acid. The cells accept the stain only with dif- ficulty, but once in, the stain remains despite further treatment. Or- ganisms which lack appropriate cell wall characteristics have no color after acid washing and can be seen only if counterstain is applied. The acid-fast technique, like Gram staining, can be used for direct examination of clinical material, for studying cultivated col- onies, and for documenting organisms in fixed tissue. Mycobacteria are most often sought with acid-fast staining procedures, but certain species of Nocardia are variably acid-fast, and Brucella sometimes can be identified in tissue sections by an appropriately modified acid-fast technique.

FLUORESCENCE TECHNIQUES

FLUORESCENT ANTIBODIES. A fairly new but increasingly useful technique for direct examination is fluorescence microscopy. The organisms are localized and identified by their reaction with a specific, fluorescein-labeled antibody. The theory is simple. If the appropriate organisms are present in the preparation, labeled antibody attaches to them, resulting in localized fluorescence. The antibody just rinses off if no bacteria are present or if the material contains bacteria of other specificities. The success of this technique depends on having a labeled, specific antiserum and on the presence of the specific organism. This cannot be used as an initial search tool for unknown bacteria. If the presence of a specific organism is suspected, for example in suspected diphtherial pharyngitis, gonorrheal urethritis, or H. influenzae meningitis, direct immunofluorescent examination can give a very rapid answer. The technique also can be used to identify strains and subspecies of organisms, if appropriate antibodies are available. Both the fluorescent dye and the antibody must be pure and of high quality, and the conjugation must be specific and firm.

INDIRECT IMMUNOFLUORESCENCE. Using indirect immunofluorescence is somewhat more flexible than using labeled specific antiserums. In the indirect technique, a battery of unlabeled specific antibodies can be used, and only a single serum, an anti-immunoglobulin or anti-antibody, need be labeled. Smears of clinical material are incubated with antibodies directed against the organisms suspected to be present. If the organism is present, the unlabeled antibody attaches to it, and subsequent addition of fluorescent antiglobulin serum produces fluorescence. If the antibody does not find its antigen, the subsequent fluorescent antiglobulin serum has nothing to attach to, and no fluorescence remains when the specimen is rinsed. In this way, a single conjugated serum can be used to demonstrate a variety of antigenic specificities, as long as all the specific, unlabeled antibodies react similarly with the conjugated antiglobulin serum. The antiglobulin serum must not react with the organisms or with any other material present on the slide.

Cultures

Ultimate diagnosis of infectious diseases depends on isolating, cultivating, and characterizing the organism. Most of clinical microbiology involves general and differential cultural techniques, exploiting the wide range of biochemical and morphologic characteristics of pathogenic flora. This chapter cannot detail the many media and techniques available, but we can consider profitably some of the general principles of culturing and show their clinical applications.

Different culture media may promote or discourage individual bacteria, and their use is dictated by the organisms likely to be found in a specimen. To some extent, the source of the specimen suggests the probable organisms and the manner in which the material should be handled. In anything but highly routine situations, however, the more information the microbiologist has about the clinical problem, the more directly he can achieve diagnostically significant results. Among the major considerations for the laboratory are whether or not to do anaerobic cultures, whether fast-growing contaminants or commensals are likely to be present and obscure the pathogen, and whether the suspected organism requires special culture media. The time devoted to a brief clinical note on microbiology requests can result in much faster and better culture interpretations.

BLOOD CULTURES

Blood is one of the few specimens routinely cultured in broth rather than on a solid medium. One major advantage of solid over liquid media is that they permit colonies to grow which are distinct from one another, so that mixed flora can be discriminated. Since most blood cultures reveal only a single organism, colony separation is rarely necessary, but up to 3 or 4 percent of blood cultures have two or more pathogens.[21] An advantage of broth culture is that dilution disperses the bactericidal effects of blood itself and of whatever drugs the patient may have received.

Routine cultures are placed in thioglycollate broth to permit growth of anaerobic or microaerophilic organisms, as well as in standard nutrient broths. Since growth may be slow, cultures appearing to be negative are kept for 15 days before the final verdict. Most growth occurs much earlier, and bacteria are encouraged to show themselves as early as possible. Initial broth cultures are subcultured quite early onto several aerobic and anaerobic media. Gram stain of the broth after overnight incubation may demonstrate early significant growth, but both Gram staining and subculturing must be done carefully to avoid contaminating the remaining material.

FINDINGS

Since blood stream invasion tends to be episodic, repeated blood cultures are desirable if bacteremia is suspected. Three to five cultures taken over a 24- to 48-hour period usually provide an adequate sampling, although if antibiotics are present, the number should be doubled. Drawing several samples also aids in evaluating contaminants. If the same organism is grown from several different cultures taken at several different times, then it probably has clinical significance. Septicemia carries a high mortality rate, but the nature of the patient population markedly affects these figures. In acute-care community hospitals, mortality runs in the 12 to 20 percent range, whereas mortality from septicemia in university hospitals runs much higher. Gram-negative sepsis is especially dangerous and occurs much more commonly in university and referral hospitals than in community hospitals.[30] The urinary tract is more often the primary infecting site than any other single system, but lung, hepatobiliary tract, endocardium, central nervous system, and peritoneal cavity often are the foci from which organisms enter the blood stream.

CONTAMINANTS

Contamination of blood cultures is by no means uncommon and usually occurs as the specimen is collected. The blood sample must be drawn through the skin, a fertile source of contaminants. Meticulous skin asepsis is essential; the detergents, alcohol sponges, or other cleansers used before most injections are not adequate. After superficial cleansing, the area should be treated with 3.5 percent tincture of iodine, unless severe iodine sensitivity is present. Although everyone knows that the cleansed area should not be touched, it is amazing how often the venipuncturist palpates the vein "just one last time, to be sure." When *Staphylococcus epidermidis* or diphtheroids are found in blood cultures, as happens frequently, the inclination is to consider them contaminants. *S. epidermidis*, however, may be a blood stream invader in patients with endocarditis or prosthetic heart valves; in debilitated or immunosuppressed patients, it may be rash to consider any organism nonpathogenic.

SPINAL FLUID

Cerebrospinal fluid normally contains no organisms and very few cells. Meningeal inflammation of any sort may increase the cell content and alter the chemical findings, but the demonstration of organisms signals particular clinical urgency. Because meningitis should be treated as promptly as possible, even the delay of primary culturing may be dangerous. Examining a Gram-stained spinal fluid smear may give a presumptive diagnosis, to be later confirmed after cultures have grown. Naked-eye examination can differentiate grossly purulent from clear fluid, but even a seemingly clear fluid can harbor organisms and increased numbers of mononuclear or neutrophilic leukocytes.

Immediate Examination

Spinal fluid specimens are ordinarily submitted to the laboratory in several aliquots. The cell count must be done on uncentrifuged material. Bacterial cultures must come from material handled under sterile conditions, and the centrifuged sediment may be preferable, since organisms and cells are concentrated into a small volume. The sediment is Gram-stained and examined after cultures have been taken. Because the shape and staining properties of several common organisms are fairly characteristic, presumptive diagnosis can be very rapid. *H. influenzae,* an increasingly frequent cause of meningitis in small children, may be difficult to find; its pleomorphic nature may be hard to distinguish from debris or nonviable organisms on the slide, since these, too, would be gram-negative. Another possible artefact is the presence of gram-positive or gram-negative rounded bodies resembling yeasts, which may be seen in spinal fluids shortly after performance of a myelogram.

BACTERIAL INFECTION

Aside from *H. influenzae,* the other common invaders, if present in large enough numbers, can be identified readily. *Neisseria meningitidis* (meningococcus) is a gram-negative diplococcus, while the pneumococcus is a gram-positive diplococcus. The clustered or chainlike patterns of staphylococcal and streptococcal growth are seldom appreciated in this kind of preparation. The distinction does not, however, affect the immediate therapy initiated. Coliform bacilli are gram-negative rods, while *Mycobacterium tuberculosis* is a gram-positive rod. Acid-fast stain of the smeared sediment should be done whenever clinically indicated, especially if the meningeal symptoms have been long-standing or vaguely defined or have not responded to therapy.

CRYPTOCOCCUS

Cryptococcus neoformans needs special treatment, since it may cause rather prolonged illness with very little cellular reaction. Being round, uniform cells the size of lymphocytes, cryptococci may be considered lymphocytes by the unwary examiner performing a cell count. Their diagnostic feature, however, is a large, clear capsule which stands in brilliant contrast to the carbon particles of added India ink. India ink examination is routine in many laboratories which examine spinal fluids, but the organisms may be sparse and difficult to demonstrate. A recently developed immunologic procedure can demonstrate cryptococcal antigen in spinal fluids even if direct examination and culture have been negative.[16]

Culture Media

Spinal fluid sediments are routinely cultured in several media. Since meningococci are sensitive to cold temperature, spinal fluid specimens should not be refrigerated if any delay occurs before culturing. Blood agar plates are useful for gram-positive cocci and gram-negative bacilli. Chocolate agar, in which prior heating renders the hemoglobin more accessible, is used for growing *H. influenzae* and meningococci. All these organisms are aerobes, but since 2 to 10 percent carbon dioxide enhances initial growth, these bacteria, like primary cultures from many other sources, are incubated in a CO_2-enriched atmosphere. Thioglycollate fluid medium permits isolation of bacteroides and other anaerobes. Individual laboratories have other media as part of their preferred protocol for spinal fluids. Special media for mycobacteria are inoculated if tuberculous meningitis is suspected, and the same applies to suspected fungal disease.

RESPIRATORY TRACT

The respiratory tract harbors a variety of organisms in the upper portion, but secretions from below the larynx normally contain few, if any, organisms. Lower respiratory secretions, however, must traverse the throat, tonsillar area, and mouth, and material from the posterior nasopharynx may drip down into the oropharynx or deeper.

Throat Cultures

The normal individual routinely carries in his throat substantial numbers of alpha-hemolytic streptococci and nonpathogenic species of Neisseria as well as varying populations of coagulase-negative staphylococci or even *Staphylococcus aureus*. Group A Streptococcus can be cultured from 11 to 24 percent of asymptomatic school children.[25] Other organisms which may inhabit the normal throat include *Hemophilus hemolyticus,* small numbers of pneumococci, gram-negative bacilli, yeasts, diphtheroids, occasional anaerobes, and gamma streptococci. Under suitable conditions many of these organisms can be pathogens or be difficult to distinguish from pathogenic species of the same genus. While nonpathogenic species of Neisseria may abound and must be distinguished from *N. meningitidis*, it must be remembered that healthy carriers may have *N. meningitidis* in the nasopharynx or carry pathogenic staphylococci without ill effect.

Obtaining and interpreting culture material from the respiratory tract requires both skill and judgment.

NASOPHARYNGEAL EXAMINATION

Personnel obtaining nasopharyngeal cultures should be careful to avoid contact between the tip of the swab and the proximal nasal mucosa. In adults, nasopharyngeal cultures are useful in detecting asymptomatic carriers of pathogenic flora. In small children, who frequently cannot produce sputum, nasopharyngeal culture is often used as an index of the bacteriologic condition of the bronchial tree. Pneumococcus, *H. influenzae,* and *N. meningitidis* frequently can be grown from nasopharyngeal specimens in children with meningitis from these organisms. Although cough plates are often recommended to isolate *Bordetella pertussis* from patients with whooping cough, nasopharyngeal cultures probably produce more positives. If Bordetella is suspected, Bordet-Gengou medium with added penicillin is used to inhibit the usual flora.

Classification of Streptococci

Throat cultures most often reveal acute streptococcal infections, but other forms of pharyngitis and tonsillitis must be considered. A word about classification of streptococci is in order here. Streptococci are gram-positive cocci which characteristically grow in chains. They thrive in animal and plant environments and are found in dust and water as well. Although several classifications are based on biologic or biochemical behavior, current practice leans toward serologic description. The antigenic characteristics of the polysaccharide C-substance are the basis for classification as groups A,B,C,D, and so on through O in the Lancefield system. Other antigenic classifications are available for distinctions within group A, of which M-precipitation and T-agglutination are examples. Most acute streptococcal diseases in humans result from group A organisms, although enterococci, which are group D, produce a spectrum of human disorders, and puerperal and neonatal infections have been caused by group B.

HEMOLYTIC PROPERTIES

Another diagnostic feature of streptococci is their capacity to hemolyze red blood cells in the culture medium. The type and amount of hemolysis varies not only with the organism, but also with the species of red cell. The following brief description relates to sheep blood agar. In alpha-hemolysis, a few cells immediately beneath the colony remain unhemolyzed, with the surrounding medium becoming "green" from partial hemolysis. Beta-hemolysis produces a clear, cell-free zone beneath and around the colony. The term *gamma* is applied to those streptococci which do not hemolyze at all.

DISTINGUISHING BETA-HEMOLYTIC ORGANISMS. Although nearly all Group A organisms are beta-hemolytic, organisms of other groups also may exhibit beta-hemolysis. Group A organisms can be distinguished from other beta-hemolytic colonies by their sensitivity to bacitracin, which does not inhibit growth of other groups. An error rate of 4 to 20 percent occurs with this approach, but with good technique, up to 90 percent accuracy usually can be achieved.[25] Group D organisms, only some of which produce beta-hemolysis, are distinctive in their ability to grow at 45° C. and to grow in the presence of sodium azide.

DISTINGUISHING STREPTOCOCCI FROM PNEUMOCOCCI. All streptococci resist dissolution by bile salts and grow on blood agar despite the presence of added ethylhydrocupreine (Optochin). These features do not help to discriminate among streptococcal groups but are useful in distinguishing streptococci from pneumococci in throat cultures and other sources where nonpathogenic streptococci and pneumococci may coexist.

NONSTREPTOCOCCAL PHARYNGITIS

Acute streptococcal pharyngitis lends itself to prompt bacteriologic diagnosis, since the organisms grow rapidly on agar plates and produce characteristic beta-hemolysis. Other causes of acute pharyngitis may be *S. aureus, H. influenzae,* various coliform bacilli, or pneumococci. To distinguish these as rapidly as possible on primary cultures, several different media are used to reveal differences in growth patterns, oxygen requirements, and colony morphology. If exudate is abundant or pseudomembranes are present, necrotizing streptococcal inflammation must be distinguished from diphtheria, candidiasis (thrush), or Vincent's angina, and examining stained smears may be most helpful. *C. diphtheriae* occasionally can be seen as gram-positive rods which often are somewhat pleomorphic, while Candida presents with budding yeast forms and occasional hyphal fragments. The organisms causing Vincent's angina are thought to be the gram-negative spirochete *Borrelia vincentii* and the pointed gram-negative rod *Fusobacterium fusiforme*. Cultivation of *C. diphtheriae* requires special media, usually Loeffler's agar (which includes coagulated serum) or Pai's culture (coagulated egg). Candida should be cultured on Sabouraud's medium. Morphologic examination of the smear or pseudomembrane gives better diagnostic results than do cultures for Vincent's angina, whereas direct smears tend to be less revealing than cultures in diagnosing diphtheria.

Sputum Culture

Lower respiratory tract disease is more complex than upper airway infection because the lungs can undergo such a variety of anatomic and physiologic changes, due to so many different invaders. The usual specimen subjected to microbiologic examination is sputum, but tracheal aspirates, bronchial washings, pleural fluid, and excised tissue all have a place in diagnosing intrathoracic disease. We will briefly consider tuberculosis and the fungus diseases in a later section and cannot give viral disease more than a passing nod.

Sputum remains the most frequent and most useful source for bacteriologic diagnosis. Sputum is, by definition, the secretion of the tracheobronchial tree. Admixture with saliva or nasopharyngeal material is unfortunately common, especially if the patient has been poorly instructed in coughing, and this severely impairs the diagnostic usefulness. Early morning is the best time to obtain a specimen, when overnight secretions are still in the tracheobronchial tree. The patient should be told to take several deep breaths—uncomfortably deep so as to provoke coughing. He should be encouraged to "hawk up" the deep material rather than to spit what first comes into his mouth. In general, acute bacterial pneumonias are associated with abundant sputum, as are bronchiectasis and certain phases of lung abscess, but scant production in no way rules out these diagnoses. Flecks of mucus, blood, or pus are especially likely to contain organisms and should be included in the material cultured.

COMMON ORGANISMS

The pneumococcus continues to be a common cause of acute pneumonia, and, despite advances in antibiotic therapy, carries severe morbidity and continuing high mortality, especially in older people and alcoholics. Antipneumococcal vaccine has recently been developed,[1] and prevention by vaccination may become a better way to reduce morbidity and mortality than treatment of established infection. *H. influenzae* is isolated from large numbers of adults,[33] as well as from the pediatric population. The gram-negative rods are increasingly associated with severe pneumonias, particularly in the elderly and debilitated, and in hospital-acquired infections. *E. coli,* Klebsiella, Proteus, and Pseudomonas are the prime offenders. *Staphylococcus aureus* often complicates the course of disease in children with mucoviscidosis or patients with bronchiectasis from any cause and may cause multiple abscesses as an opportunistic invader. Anaerobic organisms may be found in abscesses or empyema and always should be considered when sputum cultures are processed.

LEGIONNAIRES' DISEASE

Sputum culture is not effective in diagnosing Legionnaires' disease, the explosive epidemic pneumonia first identified in Philadelphia in 1976. All routine culture techniques were initially unsuccessful. Intensive microbiologic study has revealed the causative agent to be somewhat pleomorphic bacilli which sometimes can be grown from tissue sources on supplemented Mueller-Hinton agar. The most reliable culture technique is intraperitoneal inoculation of guinea pigs, with subculturing on the yolk sac of embryonated hen's eggs. This approach is hardly suitable for routine diagnostic laboratories. Numerous organisms can be demonstrated in sections of infected tissue stained with a silver impregnation technique,[7] but the technique is difficult to perform consistently and correctly.

Serologic diagnosis is currently the only reliable means of demonstrating that infection has occurred, and this, inevitably, means delayed or retrospective diagnosis. Suspect serum is incubated with a smear of organisms prepared from infected yolk sac, and fluorescent antiglobulin serum is used to indicate whether or not antibodies are present. Now that the Center for Disease Control can make the retrospective diagnosis fairly readily, it is clear that this organism causes both epidemic and sporadic cases of rapidly progressive, febrile pneumonia with nonproductive cough, pleuritic pain, and mild or modest leukocytosis. Mortality has been 16 to 20 percent.[14,15,22]

SPECIAL CONSIDERATIONS

Hospitalized patients, those receiving antibiotics, and those with altered physiologic responses are susceptible to innumerable insults.

The isolation, from sputum, of unusual organisms or of possible pathogens in small numbers only must be interpreted in the light of the patient's total condition. The existence and spread of nosocomial (hospital-induced) infection always should be an important consideration in evaluating sputum cultures.

URINARY TRACT

The urinary tract does not have a normal flora. The kidneys, ureters, and bladder are sterile, and the bacteria present at the urethral meatus ordinarily do not invade the deeper tissues. Urinary tract infection, however, is extremely common, and the range of recovered organisms is broad. The majority of urinary tract pathogens derive from the intestinal flora. Adequate understanding of urine cultures requires some understanding of the gram-negative bacilli, which include the enormously complex family Enterobacteriaceae and the families Bacteroidaceae and Pseudomonadaceae. The Brucellaceae, a family which includes Brucella, Hemophilus, Pasteurella, and Bordetella, also are gram-negative rods but rarely invade the urinary tract.

Classification of Enterobacteriaceae

The term *gram-negative enteric bacteria* refers by custom to the Enterobacteriaceae. One of the major large bowel inhabitants is Bacteroides, which are anaerobic gram-negative rods, but this group is not commonly considered in this context. The Enterobacteriaceae are gram-negative, nonspore-forming rods which grow well on a variety of artificial media. All ferment glucose and reduce nitrates to nitrites. Beyond these common attributes, they vary in motility, in carbohydrate and amino acid metabolism, in enzyme production, and in the antigenic characteristics of somatic (O) and flagellar (H) composition. Subdivision of the family into six tribes is based on both biochemical and antigenic features, and recent naming and classification of genera differs from older usage. Current taxonomy is based largely on the work of W. H. Ewing. The tribes and genera[39] are as follows:

Tribe	Genera
Eschericheae	Escherichia
	Shigella
Edwardsielleae	Edwardsiella
Salmonelleae	Salmonella
	Arizona
	Citrobacter
Klebsielleae	Klebsiella
	Enterobacter
	Serratia
Proteeae	Proteus
	Providencia
Erwinieae	Erwinia
	Pectobacterium

We cannot detail the distinctions among all the various species, serotypes, and bioserotypes subsumed in these genera. We must, however, consider some of the special purpose media used as initial diagnostic tests when enteric bacilli are isolated or suspected. Enteric bacilli grow well on most media, including blood agar, but gram-positive contaminants or nonpathogens often grow better, making isolation of the desired gram-negative organism more difficult.

PRIMARY CULTURES

Urine specimens often are inoculated onto an inhibitory medium, such as MacConkey's agar or eosin methylene blue (EMB), to encourage gram-negative isolates, and onto one or several general purpose or partially anaerobic media to demonstrate additional organisms. Both MacConkey's medium and EMB contain lactose in addition to other nutrients and a colored indicator. The coliform bacilli ferment lactose, thereby altering the indicator color, while Salmonella, Shigella, and Proteus do not. Thus the primary growth can supply prompt diagnostic clues.

Once primary cultures are available, each separate organism that is isolated should be subcultured on differential media. The critical step here is achieving pure cultures from the initial growth. Among the enormous range of possible biochemical distinctions, a few are

regularly used for preliminary screening. If more detailed differentiation is necessary, further cultures can be made later.

CARBOHYDRATE UTILIZATION

The most rapidly useful observations relate to carbohydrate utilization, motility, urea-splitting capacity, and some preliminary
metabolic characteristics. Inoculation of double or triple sugar
medium in a slanted tube permits rapid evaluation of carbohydrate
utilization. The slanted tube contains a low concentration of glucose
and a high concentration of lactose or sucrose or both. Fermentation
of small or large amounts of sugar produces pH changes which
impart characteristic color patterns. The pattern of growth and location of color changes reveal not only which sugars the organism
ferments, but also the speed of fermentation and the presence or
absence of gas production as a by-product. In general terms,
Escherichia, Klebsiella, Enterobacter, and some Proteus-Providence
groups rapidly ferment both lactose and glucose, with gas production. Glucose fermentation without lactose suggests the presence of
Salmonella, Shigella, some Proteus, some Citrobacter, and Serratia.
No color change occurs with Pseudomonas or Acinetobacter, because
these gram-negative rods are not Enterobacteriaceae and do not
ferment glucose.

UREASE PRODUCTION AND MOTILITY

Comparable pH-mediated color change is used to document urease
production. If the organisms split urea, incorporated into the
medium, the resulting alkaline pH converts the phenol red indicator
from yellow to red. Again, the speed with which the change occurs
has diagnostic implications. Proteus produces urease within a few
hours; Klebsiella, Enterobacter and Serratia split urea more slowly;
with the others, no color change occurs. The presence of motility
can be estimated in some cases by the degree of spreading growth
from a straight-line inoculation, while especially "stiff" media can be
used to measure the degree of motility. While Proteus is considered
the classic "spreader," nearly all the genera except Shigella and
Klebsiella exhibit some motility.

The series of four biochemical reactions referred to as IMViC
(indole, methyl red, Voges-Proskauer, and citrate) often helps
distinguish E. coli from Klebsiella and Enterobacter, which also
ferment lactose rapidly. The use of other diagnostic biochemical

tests depends on the magnitude of the clinical problem, and diagnostic charts and flow sheets are available for discriminating different species and variant behaviors.

Other Organisms

Not all urinary tract infections are due to gram-negative rods. Staphylococcus and enterococcus not uncommonly produce urinary tract disease. These often can be identified from their appearance in mixed cultures, or they may be isolated from cultures on media which partially inhibit gram-negative organisms. Contaminants, deriving from the periurethral tissues, tend to resemble skin flora— largely coagulase-negative staphylococci and diphtheroids, but organisms of fecal origin may appear in urine of noninfected individuals. Good technique in collecting the specimen reduces this problem, but the kind of perfunctory instructions given many patients makes a really "clean" voided specimen highly unlikely. If well-trained personnel perform the cleansing and the specimen is collected into a sterile container, results may be excellent.

Quantitation

The simple presence of bacteria need not imply clinical infection. It is generally agreed that 10^5 organisms per milliliter constitutes a clinically significant degree of bacteriuria. To some extent, this depends on the patient's physiologic condition. Urine that has remained in the bladder several hours will have a larger population, and very dilute urine will have a lower population, given the same degree of infection. It is preferable to collect and culture urine that has been in the bladder at least 2 hours; some laboratories recommend culturing the first morning specimen after overnight accumulation. Because bacteria multiply in the voided urine as well as in the bladder, prompt refrigeration is necessary if the specimen will not be processed immediately. At 4°C., multiplication is adequately inhibited for several days.

Quantitation is achieved by culturing a suitably measured or diluted volume of urine. Calibrated loops, delivering approximately 0.1 ml. of urine on a streak plate, permit rough estimation by counting the colonies that grow on the single plate. Greater accuracy results from making pour plates with serial dilutions. The colonies are evenly distributed, and the count can be made from that dilution giving the most legible plate. Although more accurate, this is far more time- and space-consuming than streaking a calibrated-loop specimen; thus each technique may be appropriate for different clinical situations.

QUICK QUANTITATION

A very quick, almost "bedside" screening procedure for significant bacteriuria is examination by Gram stain of uncentrifuged urine. If several bacteria can be seen on most of the oil-immersion fields, then the colony count will probably be 10^5 per ml. or more.[24]

CHEMICAL INDICATORS. Several screening techniques detect significant bacteriuria by the metabolic effect of large numbers of bacteria on an indicator. These vary in efficacy with the conditions of urine collection, the preservation of the reagents, the types of organisms present, and the need for rapid identification of the organism. When treating individual patients, quantitative or semi-quantitative culture methods probably provide more information in a shorter period of time than application of biochemical screening tests. Bacteriuria is demonstrated more effectively by specific tests for bacteria than by inference from urinalysis results since the presence of white cells or proteinuria correlates rather poorly with significant levels of bacterial invasion.

GASTROINTESTINAL TRACT

Microbiologic examination of the gastrointestinal tract is complicated by the normal presence of innumerable organisms of which more than 95 percent are anaerobes. The normal flora consists largely of Bacteroides species (gram-negative anaerobic rods); the enteric bacilli, mostly *E. coli* and Proteus species; intestinal streptococci (commonly called enterococci, Lancefield group D); and occasional yeasts and clostridia. All of these organisms can produce disease at sites other than their normal habitat, and pathogenic strains of usual commensals can produce significant gastrointestinal disease. Stool cultures in diarrhea or proctoscopic swabs in dysentery are the usual examinations requested, although gastric aspirate or duodenal or small intestinal specimens may be cultured under particular circumstances.[18]

Salmonella and Shigella

Salmonella and Shigella are the usual offenders in acute or chronic diarrheal disease in otherwise healthy adults.[17] While fairly numerous in acute infections, the organisms become difficult to find after several days of illness. The differential media described above may be useful for stool specimens, since gram-positive inhibition is desirable. More selective media, which suppress *E. coli* and Proteus on appropriately prepared plates, are used when Salmonella or Shigella are suspected. Another useful technique is to incubate a fecal sample in an enrichment broth, which permits Salmonella and Shigella to grow but temporarily suppresses *E. coli* and Proteus as well as gram-positive organisms. After 12 hours of incubation, the presumed pathogens would have a head start, and subcultures onto selective or differential media tend to yield maximal results. Shigella are rather fragile and may die if specimens are not processed promptly. They may be overwhelmed on occasion by the agents that suppress coliforms.

Characterization of Salmonella and Shigella, whether from stool, urine, blood, or other sources, is exceedingly complex. Following biochemical identification, serologic typing and subtyping can be done if suitable antisera are available. The techniques of serotyping are fairly simple, but the taxonomy and terminology are in a transitional state.

Pathogenic E. Coli

Although *E. coli* inhabits the normal colon, certain strains may cause disease, especially in infants. As serotyping of *E. coli* has been standardized, certain serotypes have been observed to cause disease, while others do not. Because morphology and biochemical reactions do not distinguish these, the diagnosis of enteropathogenic *E. coli* rests on accurate serotyping. The diagnosis may be suspected by the epidemic nature of the disease and failure to isolate any other pathogen. In these cases, the *E. coli* isolated from primary cultures can be serotyped directly. Some of the enteropathogenic *E. coli* produce exotoxins with activity similar to that of cholera organisms.[12] These toxigenic strains predominantly affect adults and are distinct from the strains which produce invasive, inflammatory changes and largely affect infants.

Vibrio Cholerae

In cholera cases, *Vibrio cholerae*, a species of small, motile, gram-negative rods, can be isolated readily from stool specimens. Since the vibrios are inhibited by most differential media and selective Salmonella-Shigella media, their cultivation depends upon prior suspicion and suitable plating. These organisms are bile-resistant. They grow best at a pH of 7.0, but their ability to grow at a pH as alkaline as 9.5 can be exploited for differential culturing.

Staphylococcal Disease

Staphylococci produce gastrointestinal disease in two ways. Hemolytic S. aureus and other staph organisms produce a highly potent exotoxin, which is heat stable, tasteless, and odorless. When bacteria multiply in prepared food, the resulting toxins may attain sufficient levels to produce the rapid onset of gastric and intestinal symptoms. Organisms cannot be grown from stool or vomitus in these cases, but culturing the contaminated foodstuffs permits rapid bacterial diagnosis.

Less dramatically acute, but clinically more worrisome, is the colitis produced by staphylococcal multiplication within the gut, often in patients whose normal flora has been altered by antibiotic therapy. Coagulase-positive staphylococci may be grown from normal stools on media that suppress enterococcal growth, but large numbers of these organisms on a nonselective medium have pathogenic significance. The staphylococci in these conditions often are resistant to the antibiotics previously given the patient.[17]

GENITAL TRACT

Suspected venereal disease usually provokes microbiologic examination of the male or female genital tract. The causative agent of gonorrhea, Neisseria gonorrhoeae, often can be isolated from the male urethra and from the female cervix uteri. In acute gonorrheal urethritis or cervicitis, Gram-stained smears of the exudate reveal intracellular gram-negative diplococci, a finding sufficiently pathognomonic that definitive treatment should be initiated without awaiting culture results. In chronic infections, the organisms may be sparse, but when there are systemic complications, prostatic secretions, joint fluid, or conjunctival exudate often contain readily visible organisms. Failure to culture gonococci, when clinical gonorrhea is suspected, may mean that the patient has been partially treated or has received antibiotics for some other condition.[29]

Gonococcus

N. gonorrhoeae, the gonococcus, is moderately fastidious and rather fragile. Specimens should be inoculated as soon as possible, since the organisms will not long survive at room temperature or warmer conditions without suitable nutrients. A transport medium may be used if delay is inevitable, and a few hours of refrigeration will not prevent subsequent growth. Since both urethral and cervical specimens may contain nonpathogenic contaminants, the material should be collected with care. Because lubricating jellies used to insert the vaginal speculum may damage gonococci, sterile saline or water should be used to moisten the instrument. Thayer-Martin medium, a chemically enriched blood or chocolate agar with added antibiotics, is the culture medium of choice. This is incubated in a high carbon dioxide atmosphere.

CHEMICAL TESTS

Growth from primary cultures can be identified as gonococcus by carbohydrate fermentation reactions on secondary media. The oxidase test, in which a colored indicator reveals the presence of the bacterial oxidizing enzyme, is characteristic of all species of Neisseria. Although it does not identify gonococcus specifically, in appropriate clinical conditions the results may be strongly suggestive. Fluorescent antibody tests offer the most rapid and accurate means of identification and can be used on colonies or directly on smears from the infected tissue.

Syphilis

Treponema pallidum, the causative agent of syphilis, cannot be cultivated on artificial media. Scrapings from primary, and especially secondary, lesions may be examined profitably under dark-field microscopy. When present, the treponemes are actively motile, spiral organisms. Dark-field examination often fails to reveal spirochetes, even when performed by experienced examiners; serologic diagnosis of syphilis is easier and more reliable.

Nonbacterial Infections

VAGINITIS

Two extremely common microbiologic agents involved in genital tract disease are *Trichomonas hominis* and *Candida albicans*. Trichomonas are protozoa. In saline-suspended material from vagina or urethra, they are swiftly moving, flagellated cells. Venereal transmission is common. The sexual partners of a woman with trichomonal vaginitis should also be examined and, if necessary, treated to prevent recurrent infestation. Monilial (candidal) vaginitis also is extremely common. It is diagnosed by observing characteristic budding or oval cells in KOH-suspended material from the vagina. When this organism invades the tissue, true hyphae can be identified, but vaginitis usually is a superficial infection.

URETHRITIS

In males, only 50 percent of acute urethritis is gonococcal. Syphilitic infection accounts for perhaps 10 percent of cases, and the organisms of lymphogranuloma for another 10 percent.[27] The remainder of cases result from agents that are difficult to culture or to diagnose, such as mycoplasmas and chlamydiae.

ANAEROBIC ORGANISMS

Anaerobes are organisms that grow only when oxygen pressure is low. Different bacteria have different requirements, ranging from intolerance of any oxygen at all to survival in modified room-air environments. To be classified as anaerobic, the organism must be unable to grow on agar surfaces exposed to room air augmented by up to 10 percent carbon dioxide.[28] Human commensals include far more anaerobes than aerobes. The normal flora of skin, mouth, and vagina includes many anaerobes, while in the intestinal tract, anaerobes outnumber aerobes by 1000 to 1.[19] Although many cause no problems for their human host, several groups of anaerobes cause severe infections when they reach normally sterile sites or find suitably anaerobic growth conditions in necrotic tissue.

Clinical Findings

Anaerobic organisms are frequent pathogens in deep abscesses, infected wounds, and closed infections in body cavities. Common predisposing events include aspiration of gastric contents, operations on the gut or biliary tract, deeply penetrating injuries, and abortions. Clinical suspicion should be high for abscesses at any site, but particularly in brain, female genital tract, and lung. Since anaerobes fail to grow under routine culture conditions, a "negative" culture report on obviously infected tissue should provoke search for anaerobes. The presence of gas in foul-smelling discharge provides another clue, as does the presence of septic thrombophlebitis, bacteremic jaundice, suppuration of necrotic tumors or operative sites, or a history of human bites.

Clostridia, which are spore-forming bacilli, have long been recognized as significant anaerobes, but in most clostridial infections, circulating toxins cause more clinical damage than do spreading organisms. With Bacteroides, Fusobacterium, Actinomyces, and Peptostreptococcus infections, local bacterial multiplication causes the clinical problems. The pathogenetic significance of other genera is less clear. Because multiple infecting organisms are the rule, not the exception, with anaerobes, it may be difficult to assign primary significance to any one agent.

Technical Considerations

Specimen collection and transportation are critical in culturing anaerobes. Unsuitable are specimens taken from surfaces normally colonized by anaerobes. Sputum, tracheal or bronchoscopic aspirates, feces, vaginal secretions, voided urine, and skin swabs cannot be evaluated for infecting anaerobes because a mixed flora of anaerobes normally is present. Appropriate specimens include carefully collected fluid from normally sterile sites, such as biliary tract, pleural spaces, or inside joints. Good for culture is material from the center of an abscess or deep in a wound, or tissue excised surgically. Once collected, the specimen must be transferred promptly to a transport vial filled with oxygen-free gas. Transport and culture equipment intended for anaerobic use should contain an indicator that documents continued absence of oxygen; often a reducing agent is added to neutralize any small quantities of oxygen inadvertently introduced. Methylene blue, which is colorless until exposed to oxygen, is a useful indicator.

To incubate anaerobic cultures, several methods are available. The simplest is the anaerobic jar. Oxygen can be evacuated mechanically, but the easiest technique makes clever use of the catalyst palladium to remove oxygen by combining it with hydrogen to form water. Another ingenious approach is the roll tube method, in which individual tubes of culture medium are surrounded by an oxygen-free environment that allows incubation in a standard incubator. The anaerobic glove box is a permanent installation in which all aspects of plating, incubation, and reading can be performed.

Since anaerobic cultures usually yield a mixed flora, a solid culture medium is preferable to broth. On a solid surface, different colonies can be distinguished, quantitated, and isolated for identification. In broth, however, the fastest-growing organism often monopolizes the picture. Since anaerobes tend to be fastidious in their growth requirements, supplemented media usually are necessary. Clostridium grows within 18 to 24 hours, but for most other anaerobes, as much as 5 to 7 days must pass before cultures can be called negative.

Anaerobes are identified by culture characteristics, Gram-stained morphology, motility, and analysis of metabolic behavior. Gas-liquid chromatography makes it possible to distinguish the acids and alcohols that different organisms produce. Fluorescent-labeled specific antiserums have proved useful for rapid identification of certain genera.

MYCOBACTERIA

Mycobacteria deserve separate discussion, even though these organisms can cause disease in all of the sites and tissues already mentioned. Tuberculosis is the infection caused by M. tuberculosis or by any of the other, less commonly encountered, "atypical" mycobacteria. Mycobacteria are nonmotile, nonspore-forming, aerobic or microaerophilic bacilli with a high lipid content. Although grampositive, they take the stain only with difficulty but are then exceedingly resistant to decolorizing. Their most salient staining characteristic is acid-fastness. Once a dye or staining agent enters the cell, it remains there despite vigorous treatment with acid-alcohol. The classic stains use carbolfuchsin with or without heating to encourage dye penetration.

Fluorescent Staining

The auramine-rhodamine technique[34] of fluorescent staining employs the same principle as does classic acid-fast staining. The fluorescent auramine-rhodamine solution, once attached to the mycobacteria, resists acid-alcohol decolorization. The end point, fluorescence as opposed to simple staining, is far easier to observe, so that lower-power objectives can be used for scanning. In this way, more material can be examined more thoroughly. The number of organisms found tends to be higher, so that the quantitation code of the National Tuberculosis Association (3 to 9 organisms per slide = rare; 10 or more per slide = few; more than 1 in each oil-immersion field = numerous) may need reinterpretation. In any laboratory which uses a consistent method and code, the clinical importance of the results is unchanged.

In both carbolfuchsin and fluorescent-stained smears, the finding of one or two stained bodies requires cautious interpretation, since artefacts and false positives are not infrequent. When one or two are found after 15 minutes of examination, additional material should be collected and examined.

Culture Techniques

Finding stained organisms offers rapid, presumptive evidence of mycobacterial infection but says nothing about the viability, the clinical significance, or even the identity of the organism. Accurate diagnosis requires meticulous technique, since the identity and drug susceptibility of infecting organisms have serious clinical implications. The mycobacteria are slow-growing, requiring complex media and freedom from more rapidly growing, competing organisms.

DANGER TO PERSONNEL

Prior to inoculation on media specially prepared for mycobacteria, most specimens are *decontaminated*. This does not mean rendering the specimen harmless to those who handle it. Mycobacteria constitute an ever-present threat to those who work with them. To avoid contagion, the conditions under which mycobacteria are processed, grown, and identified should be regulated carefully. Often less care is used in handling specimens from patients in whom tuberculous infection is not suspected, and these materials probably pose a greater danger than material in the specialized laboratory.

PROCESSING THE SPECIMEN

Decontamination attempts to kill off other organisms which might interfere with or overshadow mycobacterial growth. Sputum, bronchial secretions, and gastric washings are treated with strong alkali, which destroys other organisms but not the alkali-resistant mycobacteria.

This resistance is only relative, and mycobacteria almost certainly sustain some damage during the process.

Decontamination usually is combined with liquefaction to permit adequate mixing and sampling of tissue material. If shreds of tissue or purulent particles are visible, these should be separated and cultured directly, since they often harbor a high concentration of organisms. Specimens in which fewer organisms occur (e.g., urine, spinal fluid, or joint fluid) should not be subjected to harsh treatment. These materials often are concentrated, either by centrifugation or bacteria-trapping filtration.

Because other organisms so frequently are present, urine may pose a particular problem. An early-morning specimen should be collected under clean conditions. If urine volume and concentration are good, centrifuging the whole specimen may concentrate the mycobacteria sufficiently that the sediment can be decontaminated without completely losing the mycobacteria.

GROWTH CHARACTERISTICS

Mycobacteria can grow on simple media if the inoculum is really large, but cultivation from clinical material requires complex media and carefully regulated conditions. In differentiating mycobacteria, the rate of growth, colony characteristics, preferred temperature, and presence or absence of pigmentation provide important diagnostic clues. M. tuberculosis takes 2 or more weeks to grow at 37°C. and fails to grow at higher or lower temperatures. Although mature colonies appear cream-colored or buff, there is no distinct pigmentation; the warty, cauliflower-like appearance is quite characteristic. Because growth is so slow, cultures are kept for 6 weeks before "no growth" is reported.

A discussion of the biochemical tests and differential growth-promoting materials available for discriminating among mycobacteria is beyond the scope of this chapter. Culturing a mycobacterium does not always mean tuberculous disease. If M. tuberculosis is isolated or suspected, however, drug sensitivity studies should be initiated promptly. Drug resistance is increasingly prevalent, and patients may harbor more than one strain simultaneously, with various susceptibility patterns.

Antibiotic Resistance

Some strains of M. tuberculosis resistant to isoniazid have aberrant biochemical reactions; the catalase or peroxidase tests may serve as quick screening procedures for isoniazid resistance. Complete sensitivity testing is very time-consuming because the organisms are slow-growing to begin with. The primary culture must have sufficient growth to permit subculturing, and the subcultures must have enough growing time to reveal the drug effects. Cultures on drug-containing media must be compared with cultures plated onto drug-free medium of the same composition, and strains of known susceptibility should be included for comparison. Ordinarily, two different concentrations of the three commonly used drugs (isoniazid, p-aminosalicylic acid, and streptomycin) give sufficient information.

More extensive testing is necessary only with chronic, complicated, or highly resistant cases. Since the growth of partially resistant strains may be slow but highly significant, neither the microbiologist nor the clinician should lose patience after only 2 or 3 weeks. When many organisms are found on direct smears, sensitivity testing can be initiated simultaneously with primary cultures. If the presence of organisms is doubtful, the longer, indirect method is necessary. As a patient undergoes treatment, repeated cultures and repeated sensitivity trials are desirable, since changes in growth pattern and resistance are prognostically as well as therapeutically significant.

Tuberculin Testing

Tuberculin testing reveals whether or not an individual has cell-mediated immunity to M. tuberculosis or to other mycobacterial antigens. A positive test cannot be equated with ongoing disease. It indicates prior experience with the tubercle bacillus, but the disease may be dormant. When performed on a clinically ill patient, the tuberculin test helps rule tuberculosis in or out as the most likely diagnosis. In the early years of this century, most healthy adults had positive tuberculin tests. At present, about 10 percent of the population is positive on routine screening.[26] The tuberculin test has its greatest present usefulness in indicating recent exposure but not necessarily active infection. In a person known to have had a negative test, conversion to a positive reaction signals that potentially infective contact has occurred. When conversion occurs in children, adolescents, and populations at high risk, most workers begin antituberculous therapy without additional confirmation. In other cases, the clinician may elect to do more detailed diagnostic studies before deciding on treatment.

More than 90 percent of new active cases of tuberculosis occur in patients already tuberculin-positive;[26] this is strong evidence for reactivation of previously dormant disease. In those with documented conversion from negative to positive, the risk of developing active disease in the next year is 3.3 percent per year.[26] A similar risk exists for tuberculin-positive household contacts of a recently diagnosed case. Risks decline in various other categories. The lowest risk that active tuberculosis will develop in the following year occurs in healthy, tuberculin-negative persons, of whom only 1 in 50,000 will acquire the disease. Of persons without occupational exposure to the disease, about 4 per 1,000 convert from negative to positive each year.

False-positive tuberculin tests occur rarely, usually the result of misinterpreting hematoma or mechanical irritation as true hypersensitivity. The false-negative rate varies with the health of the population tested. In healthy individuals, fewer than 1 percent of those with active infection will give a negative reaction. False negatives become increasingly common with increasing age and general debility. Overwhelming tuberculous infection may inhibit the tuberculin reaction (anergy), and false negatives may occur in patients with sarcoidosis, disseminated cancer, or severe viral infections.

ANTIBIOTIC SENSITIVITY TESTING

Most bacteria grow much faster than mycobacteria, and sensitivity testing can be done rapidly and accurately. When optimum growth occurs in 12 to 18 hours, the effect of the drug on the organism becomes apparent as growth inhibition occurs around a central deposit of the drug. Because the process is brief, the zone of drug diffusion into the medium is finite and is easily measured and reproduced. When growth takes up to 6 weeks, diffusion would involve the entire culture medium but to an unstandardized, unreproducible degree. Incorporating a known concentration of drug into the medium avoids this problem but requires inoculating as many different plates (or segments of plates) as there are drug concentrations to be tested.

Single-Plate Tests

Many clinical microbiology laboratories use the Kirby-Bauer technique,[4] a reliable, single-plate method for measuring drug sensitivities of bacteria other than mycobacteria. In this method, paper disks impregnated with the desired drugs are placed on a standardized growth medium inoculated with a uniformly distributed bacterial suspension. The drugs diffuse out of the disks into the agar, at concentrations varying with the initial concentration in the disk and the drug's diffusability. When the disks and the growth conditions are properly standardized, the diameter of the zone of growth inhibition reflects reproducibly the organism's sensitivity to usual therapeutic serum levels of the drug.

This technique requires that the organism grow evenly and almost confluently on drug-free portions of the agar. In the original method, a broth suspension of culture was spread over the plate with a cotton swab, the density of suspension being adjusted to match the turbidity of a $BaSO_4$ standard. Variants of the technique employ different means for standardizing the suspension and spreading it uniformly on the plate.[2] The broth culture, of course, must be pure, for mixed cultures may give overlapping patterns of sensitivity and resistance, rendering the plate uninterpretable.

INTERPRETATION

Changes in incubation temperature, pH, and atmospheric composition will influence the results, and zone size must be measured accurately, especially with such drugs as polymyxin B and colistin, which diffuse rather slowly. Controls must be run frequently, using strains of known resistance, to insure that the disks remain potent and the medium is satisfactory.

Another problem relates to interpretation. Complete inhibition is easy to measure; so is complete drug resistance when the organism attains confluent growth up to and under the disk. In some cases, however, the results are equivocal and must be reported as such. The clinician also must remember that inhibition in vitro does not always insure clinical effectiveness. Among other determinants are the site and type of infection; the patient's cardiovascular, hepatic, and renal status; and the presence of steroids or other drugs.[37]

Drug Dilution Methods

Sometimes drug concentration is critical or the growth pattern is not adaptable to the plate and disk method. In such cases, sensitivity can be tested by drug dilution. One method is comparable to that described for mycobacteria in which various concentrations of drug are incorporated into agar plates. In another technique, broth tubes contain the drug dilutions, and the turbidity of the subsequent culture reflects the amount of bacterial multiplication. As with the single-plate disk methods, the pathogen should be in pure culture, although in the plate dilution test, the presence of more than one organism is more obvious than in broth tubes.

Primary Cultures

When speed is absolutely vital, antibiotic-containing disks are placed on the plates after primary inoculation. This is most effective after Gram stain or some other procedure has indicated bacteria to be present and has given some clue about their identity. After the primary culture has grown out and the organism or organisms have been identified, these tentative sensitivity results should be confirmed. In patients with persistent or mixed infections and in those who respond poorly to seemingly appropriate therapy, repeated isolations and a variety of susceptibility tests may be indicated.

MYCOTIC INFECTIONS

Laboratory diagnosis of mycotic infections follows the same theoretical approach as bacterial diagnosis. If clinical specimens contain the organisms in viable state, cultures on artificial media yield diagnostic growth. Problems arise, however, in distinguishing saprophytes in vivo or laboratory contaminants from significant pathogens. Pathogenic fungi coexist with bacteria, which may or may not also have pathogenic significance. Some fungi, ordinarily saprophytic, may become virulent in debilitated hosts. Systemic fungal infections may mimic bacterial disease, and unless special efforts are made, their presence may go undetected.

Superficial Infections

Fungal infections or mycoses are frequently categorized as superficial, cutaneous, subcutaneous, and systemic. Direct examination of skin scrapings or hair fragments often identifies superficial or cutaneous infections. Microscopic examination of NaOH- or KOH-suspended emulsions reveals morphologically characteristic hyphae or, occasionally, budding yeast forms. Cultural identification is made from growth on Sabouraud's dextrose agar, incubated at room temperature. Since the organisms tend to be slow-growing, cultures ordinarily are held for 30 days. Because skin and hair often harbor saprophytic bacteria and fungi in addition to pathogens, the culture medium may include antibiotics to suppress unwanted contaminants.

Subcutaneous Infections

Although they do not disseminate throughout the body, subcutaneous mycoses may be locally destructive and difficult to treat. *Sporotrichum schenckii* is one of the common agents in temperate climates, producing nodular or ulcerating lesions after superficial introduction of the spores. Most other infections are more frequent in, but not confined to, tropical or semitropical areas. Local introduction is through minor breaks in the skin, especially on bare feet, and a variety of fungal types may be involved. Nocardia, which are aerobic bacteria rather than fungi, may be isolated from lesions of this sort and grow in a fashion resembling fungi on Sabouraud's medium.

Direct examination of pus, scrapings, or fungous granules often permits rapid presumptive diagnosis, and most of the agents grow readily on Sabouraud's dextrose agar. Antibiotics inhibit cultivation of some pathogenic species. For this reason, two sets of Sabouraud's media often are inoculated, one with added antibiotics to prevent contaminating over-growth, and one unmodified, to give these sensitive organisms a chance to reveal themselves.

Systemic Infections

Systemic mycoses are becoming increasingly familiar to clinicians. These infections can be divided usefully into two groups: so-called primary disease and secondary, or opportunistic, invasion. In the first group are histoplasmosis, coccidioidomycosis, blastomycosis, paracoccidioidomycosis (South American blastomycosis), and systemic sporotrichosis. These illnesses, which afflict previously healthy individuals, must be recognized and treated on their own merits. The opportunistic infections attack patients with other diseases, who cannot mount effective defenses against agents which might not otherwise produce disease. This group includes systemic manifestations of infections with Candida, Aspergillus, Cryptococcus, and members of the class Phycomycetes, which produce mucormycosis.

PRIMARY INFECTION

Primary infections tend to present initially with pulmonary symptoms, although the respiratory tract cannot always be implicated as the portal of entry, and other organs sometimes are involved. Tissue sections and smears of pus contain yeast forms of the fungi. As with bacterial infections, definitive diagnosis requires cultivation for identification, although clinical data, skin testing, and the morphology of the tissue forms may suggest the diagnosis.

SECONDARY INFECTION

Opportunistic fungus infections occur when fungi normally present in the individual or his environment produce local or systemic damage. Aspergillus and the Phycomycetes are ubiquitous in the environment, and Candida is a normal commensal. These fungi grow frequently in cultured specimens, but without pathogenic significance. When large numbers of a single organism grow from repeated cultures of carefully obtained specimens, promptly processed, then pathogenic significance may be inferred. Since Cryptococcus is not a normal inhabitant of central nervous system, lung, or urinary tract, its presence in specimens, especially from debilitated or immunologically compromised patients, deserves prompt attention. Cryptococcal meningitis may develop as a primary disease, in which the organisms tend to be few and hard to demonstrate. The immunologic test for cryptococcal antigen sometimes helps in identifying these cases of seemingly aseptic, persisting meningitis.[16]

Candida is the most common fungal infection of compromised hosts. Immunosuppression, cancer, cancer therapy, and prior treatment with broad-spectrum antibiotics are common predisposing events. As surface invaders, fungi most often affect esophagus and bladder but may later spread to the lungs, nervous system, joints, and blood stream. The organisms sometimes can be cultured from urine or from esophageal brushings, but the most reliable technique is biopsy with subsequent culture and microscopic examination to evaluate depth of invasion. Aspergillus is the second commonest opportunist,[8] but it is often very difficult to diagnose. The lungs and the gastrointestinal tract are the usual sites of involvement, where symptoms are severe but nonspecific. Both Candida and Aspergillus may succumb to the cycloheximide placed in culture media to inhibit bacterial growth.[23] If these organisms are suspected, cycloheximide-free medium should be used in addition to routine fungus cultures. Cryptococcus enters through the lungs but spreads to the central nervous system. Histoplasmosis, in the compromised host, may take the usual pulmonary form, but also may spread to liver, spleen, or nervous system. Disseminated histoplasmosis can be documented more often by blood cultures than can any other fungus.[8] Mucormycosis, long thought to be exclusively the scourge of diabetics, is seen in leukemics and in patients receiving immunosuppressants.

The cultivation of viruses and mycoplasmas is a topic beyond our scope. Serologic approaches to these organisms are discussed in Chapter 14.

REFERENCES

1. Austrian, R.: *Pneumococcal infection and pneumococcal vaccine.* N. Engl. J. Med. 297:938, 1977.
2. Barry, A. L., Garcia, F., and Thrupp, L. D.: *An improved single-disk method for testing the antibiotic susceptibility of rapidly growing pathogens.* Am. J. Clin. Pathol. 53:149, 1970.
3. Bates, J. H.: *The changing scene in tuberculosis.* N. Engl. J. Med. 297:610, 1977.
4. Bauer, A. W., Kirby, W. M. M., Sherris, J. C., and Turck, M.: *Antibiotic susceptibility testing by a standardized single disk method.* Am. J. Clin. Pathol. 45:493, 1966.
5. Briggs, D. D., Jr.: *Pulmonary infections.* Med. Clin. North Am. 61:1163, 1977.
6. Carrizosa, I., and Kaye, D.: *Lincomycin, clindamycin, the tetracyclines, trimethoprim-sulfa methoxasole and rifampin,* in Hook, E. W., Mandell, G. L., Gwaltney, J. M., and Sande, M. A. (eds.): *Current Concepts of Infectious Diseases.* Wiley, New York, 1977.
7. Chandler, F. W., Hicklin, M. D., and Blackmon, J. A.: *Demonstration of the agent of Legionnaires' disease in tissue.* N. Engl. J. Med. 297:1218, 1977.
8. Codish, S. D., and Tobias, J. S.: *Managing systemic mycoses in the compromised host.* J.A.M.A. 235:2132, 1976.
9. Cohen, S.: *Cell mediated immunity and the inflammatory system.* Hum. Pathol. 7:249, 1976.
10. *Diagnostic Standards and Classification of Tuberculosis.* National Tuberculosis and Respiratory Disease Association, New York, 1969.
11. Eickhoff, T. C.: *Nosocomial infections,* in Hoeprich, P. D. (ed.): *Infectious Diseases.* ed. 2. Harper & Row, Hagerstown, Md., 1977.
12. Etkins, S., and Gorbach, S. L.: *Studies on enterotoxin from Escherichia coli associated with acute diarrhea in man.* J. Lab. Clin. Med. 78:81, 1971.
13. Ewing, W. H.: *Differentiation of Enterobacteriaceae by Biochemical Reactions.* rev. ed. DHEW Publication No. (CDC)74-8270, Atlanta, Georgia, 1973.
14. *Follow-up on sporadic cases of Legionnaires' disease—United States.* Morbid. Mortal. 26:408, 1977.
15. Fraser, D. W., Tsai, T. R., Orenstein, W., et al.: *Legionnaires' disease. Description of an epidemic of pneumonia.* N. Engl. J. Med. 297:1189, 1977.
16. Goodman, J. S., Kaufman, L., and Koenig, M. G.: *Diagnosis of cryptococcal meningitis: value of immunologic detection of cryptococcal antigen.* N. Engl. J. Med. 285:434, 1971.
17. Grady, G. F., and Keusch, G. T.: *Pathogenesis of bacterial diarrheas.* N. Engl. J. Med. 285:831, 1971.
18. Guerrant, R. L.: *The microbial diarrheas,* in Hook, E. W., Mandell, G. L., Gwaltney, J. M., and Sande, M. A. (eds.): *Current Concepts of Infectious Diseases.* Wiley, New York, 1977.
19. Hill, G. B.: *Introduction to the anaerobic bacteria: non-spore-forming anaerobes,* in Joklik, W. K., and Willett, H. P. (eds.): *Zinsser Microbiology.* ed. 16. Appleton-Century-Crofts, New York, 1976.
20. Hook, E. W.: *The aminoglycosides,* in Hook, E. W., Mandell, G. L., Gwalt-

ney, J. M., and Sonde, M. A. (eds.): *Current Concepts of Infectious Diseases.*
Wiley, New York, 1977.

21. McCarthy, L.: *Blood cultures.* Bull. Lab. Med. N.C. Mem. Hosp. 1, October
1975.

22. McDade, J. E., Shepard, C. C., Fraser, D. W., et al.: *Legionnaires' disease.
Isolation of a bacterium and demonstration of its role in other respiratory
disease.* N. Engl. J. Med. 297:1197, 1977.

23. McGinnis, M. R.: *Mycology of burns.* Bull. Lab. Med. N.C. Mem. Hosp. 13,
November 1976.

24. Mou, T. W., and Feldman, H. A.: *The enumeration and preservation of
bacteria in urine.* Am. J. Clin. Pathol. 35:572, 1961.

25. Peter, G., and Smith, A. L.: *Group A streptococcal infections of the skin
and pharynx.* N. Engl. J. Med. 297:311, 365, 1977.

26. Pitts, F. W.: *Tuberculosis, prevention and therapy,* in Hook, E. W., Mandell, G. L., Gwaltney, J. M., and Sande, M. A. (eds.): *Current Concepts of
Infectious Diseases.* Wiley, New York, 1977.

27. Rein, M. F.: *Management of gonorrhea, nongonococcal urethritis and
syphilis,* in Hook, E. W., Mandell, G. L. Gwaltney, J. M., and Sande, M. A.
(eds.): *Current Concepts of Infectious Diseases.* Wiley, New York, 1977.

28. Rosenblatt, J. E.: *Isolation and identification of anaerobic bacteria.* Hum.
Pathol. 7:177, 1976.

29. Rudolph, A. H.: *Control of gonorrhea.* J.A.M.A. 220:1587, 1972.

30. Scheckler, W. E.: *Septicemia in a community hospital—1970 through
1973.* J.A.M.A. 237:1938, 1977.

31. Slack, M. P. E., Wheldon, D. B., and Turk, D. C.: *A rapid test for beta-
lactamase production by* Haemophilus influenzae. Lancet 2:906, 1977.

32. Smith, H.: *Microbial surfaces in relation to pathogenicity.* Bacteriol. Rev.
41:475, 1977.

33. Tillotson, J. R., and Lerner, A. M.: Hemophilus influenzae *bronchopneumonia in adults.* Arch. Intern. Med. 121:428, 1968.

34. Truant, J. P., Brett, W. A., and Thomas, W., Jr.: *Fluorescence microscopy
of tubercle bacilli stained with auramine and rhodamine.* Henry Ford Hosp.
Med. J. 10:287, 1962.

35. Turck, M.: *New penicillins and cephalosporins,* in Hook, E. W., Mandell,
G. W., Gwaltney, J. M., and Sande, M. A. (eds.): *Current Concepts of Infectious Diseases.* Wiley, New York, 1977.

36. Weinstein, L., and Barza, M. J.: *Bacterial infections. An overview of the
development of basic and clinical knowledge.* Am. J. Med. Sci. 273:5,
1977.

37. Weinstein, L., and Dalton, A. C.: *Host determinants of response to antimicrobial agents.* N. Engl. J. Med. 279:467, 1968.

38. Young, L. S. (Moderator): *Gram-negative rod bacteremia: microbiologic,
immunologic and therapeutic considerations.* Ann. Intern. Med. 86:456,
1977.

39. Zwadyk P.: *Enterobacteriaceae: General Characteristics,* in Joklik, W. K.,
and Willett, H. P. (eds.): *Zinsser Microbiology.* ed. 16. Appleton-Century-
Crofts, New York, 1976.

CHAPTER 14

SEROLOGIC TESTS IN MICROBIOLOGY

ANTIBODIES TO SPECIFIC ORGANISMS

General Principles

In diagnostic microbiology, ongoing infection is documented by culturing organisms. Serologic diagnosis occurs after the fact, demonstrating that infection has occurred at some point in the past, allowing enough time for antibodies to develop. The requisite time lapse may be days, weeks, or months; the infection may be gone by the time demonstrable antibodies develop or organisms still may be present.

Most bacteria and viruses, as well as certain other microorganisms, characteristically provoke specific antibodies when introduced into an immunocompetent host. These antibodies may react with cell wall antigens or with products that the organism elaborates or secretes. For infections in which the invading organism can be cultured and identified readily, serologic diagnosis rarely is needed. When the infecting organism is evanescent or difficult to isolate, serologic diagnosis may be the only way to show that specific infection has occurred. Many viruses and rickettsiae cannot be cultured readily, whereas their antibodies are not hard to demonstrate. Bacterial diseases such as brucellosis and tularemia also are difficult to diagnose by direct culture.

SIGNIFICANCE OF ANTIBODIES

The fact that a patient's serum contains a particular antibody does not prove that his ongoing or recent illness was due to that organism.

Many antibodies persist for years; their presence merely indicates that the patient has experienced that organism at some time in the past. It is more useful diagnostically to demonstrate a rise in antibody level concomitant with, or shortly after, the illness. If serum has little or no antibody at the beginning of the illness, and if high levels are present in the "convalescent" sample drawn several weeks later, there is strong circumstantial evidence that the illness was due to that organism. This change from negative to positive for an antibody is called *seroconversion*. Antibody levels may not rise if effective antimicrobial therapy eradicates the infection before the immune system is fully activated.

TYPES OF RESPONSE

The rapidity of antibody rise depends partly on the size of the infecting dose, partly on the physiologic condition of the patient, and, most importantly, on whether the patient has been exposed pre-. viously to the organism. *Primary response*, in which the host has never before experienced the organism or its antigens, tends to take a minimum of several weeks; *secondary*, or *anamnestic*, responses occur within a few days. In the primary response, the antibody is usually IgM, best demonstrated in many cases by complement fixation or agglutination tests. IgG is the characteristic antibody in secondary responses.

Antibody activity is most easily measured semiquantitatively, using doubling dilutions for titration. The results of titration are never perfectly reproducible; on successive trials, a single sample can give results that vary as much as one doubling dilution above or below the original finding. For two samples to be considered significantly different, there must be a change of two or more doubling dilutions between them.

Antibacterial Antibodies

STREPTOCOCCUS

In acute streptococcal infections, culturing the organism usually is easy. Serologic testing becomes important primarily in the differential diagnosis of the poststreptococcal diseases: rheumatic fever, glomerulonephritis, and scarlet fever. These tests demonstrate antibodies against streptococcal enzymes, not against cell wall antigens. The antistreptolysin O (ASO) test is the most common of these. Streptolysin, the antigenic material, is secreted by group A streptococci and acts to hemolyze red cells, Less widely available, but useful in certain circumstances, is a test for antibodies against deoxyribonuclease B (the ADN-B test).

In the *ASO test*, antibodies, if present in the patient's serum, neutralize the hemolyzing capacity of commercially available reagent enzyme. Another version of the test uses particles coated with streptolysin; if antibody is present, the serum agglutinates the particles. For both procedures, serum is diluted 1:12, 1:50, 1:100, 1:125, 1:166, 1:250, 1:333, 1:500, 1:833, 1:1250, and 1:2500; the result is given as *Todd units*, the reciprocal of the dilution. ASO levels usually rise significantly 2 to 5 weeks after infection and begin falling about 4 to 6 weeks thereafter. Preinfection levels are re-established after 6 to 12 months.[16]

High serum ASO levels indicate recent prior infection by Streptococcus, a vital precondition for the diagnosis of rheumatic fever or poststreptococcal glomerulonephritis. It is difficult, however, to define "normal" levels, because they vary from group to group, depending on the extent of ongoing exposure to streptococci in the group. For healthy individuals not visibly recovering from recent infection, ASO levels tend to be higher in school-age children than in preschoolers or adults. In school-age children, finding levels above 250 Todd units indicates recent illness, whereas for adults, a lower figure of 125 or 166 would be significant.[17] ASO levels characteristically rise very little after streptococcal skin infections (pyoderma), although these infections can produce poststreptococcal diseases.

About 80 to 85 percent of patients with acute rheumatic fever have elevated ASO levels; the remaining 15 to 20 percent develop poststreptococcal complications without developing this specific poststreptococcal antibody.[29] Diagnostic confusion also can occur with patients whose illness is not rheumatic fever or glomerulonephritis but whose ASO levels are high because of unrelated recent streptococcal infection. Spuriously high results sometimes are seen in hyperglobulinemia due to liver disease. Artefacts also can cause problems. Oxidation of the reagent or contamination of the serum sample cause false positives. A hemolyzed serum sample is unsuitable for the hemolysis inhibition test, although the agglutination test still would be feasible.

The *ADN-B test* uses an indicator system of deoxyribonuclease and DNA to demonstrate the presence of antibodies. This enzyme depolymerizes DNA so that it cannot clot on exposure to alcohol or combine with certain colored compounds. [16] Following group A streptococcal infection, antibody to DNA-ase B develops later and persists longer than ASO antibodies. [9] ADN-B develops more reliably after streptococcal skin infections, and liver disease does not cause false positives. A false negative will occur, however, if the patient's serum contains DNA-ase of endogenous origin, which can occur in hemorrhagic pancreatitis. Fortunately, the population most susceptible to poststreptococcal disease and the population likely to have elevated endogenous DNA-ase overlap very little.

SALMONELLA (WIDAL TEST)

Up to 10 or 15 years ago, isolating and culturing enteric organisms was a difficult, chancy procedure; thus serodiagnosis was vital for clinical and epidemiologic study of diarrheal illness. Improved culture techniques and effective antimicrobial therapy have made agglutinin testing less important in distinguishing Salmonella infections from other diarrheal and febrile illnesses.

The flagellated organisms *Salmonella typhi* and *Salmonella enteritidis (paratyphi)* have both somatic (O) and flagellar (H) antigens, and the infected host usually forms antibodies against both. The Widal test is an agglutination procedure. Antibodies against H antigens form large, coarse, easily dispersed aggregates, while anti-O antibodies produce finely granular aggregates. [8]

The first week of illness affords the best chance of culturing organisms from stool samples, and antibodies have not had time to develop. Antibody titers rise to a peak in the following 4 weeks. H agglutinins often persist for years after the infection. Since O agglutinins persist only a few months, they are more reliable for diagnosing recent infection than are H antibodies. Many persons have continuing moderate levels of H or even of O agglutinins as a result of vaccination. [8] To diagnose recent Salmonella infection, one should document rising agglutinin titers between the acute and convalescent serum samples. A fourfold rise (two doubling dilutions) suggests ongoing infection with Salmonella.

The Widal test is not really specific for Salmonella. Patients with febrile or enteric illnesses from other causes [24] not infrequently have rising H and O agglutinins. Patients with liver disease and generalized increase in immunoglobulin levels have chronically high levels. It appears that either mucosal alteration or altered hepatic metabolism or both allow the patient's own colonic organisms increased exposure to the immune system. Illicit drug users characteristically have higher than normal Salmonella agglutinins;[8] this probably reflects poor hygienic practice and increased contact with enteric organisms of all sorts.

Some workers have reported that persisting antibodies to the Vi antigen of Salmonella indicate a chronic carrier state, because Vi agglutinins usually subside rapidly after infection clears. In recent years, this correlation has been somewhat discredited.[4]

TULAREMIA, BRUCELLOSIS, AND YERSINIA INFECTIONS

Some diseases are caused by infectious agents that are hazardous to handle even under laboratory conditions or are extremely difficult to culture. Serologic techniques are especially valuable in these cases. The organisms that cause plague (*Yersinia pestis*) and tularemia (*Franciscella tularensis*) are highly infective. Handling cultures may cause disease unless workers are experienced and isolation precautions are enforced. The organisms that cause brucellosis (*Brucella abortus*, *B. suis*, and *B. melitensis*) and some kinds of enteritis (*Yersinia enterocolitica*) can be cultured readily from lymph nodes but are extremely difficult to isolate from feces. Since lymph node biopsies are unsuitable for routine diagnosis, serologic tests are the easiest diagnostic approach. The agglutination procedure is the same as that used in Widal testing, and rising agglutinin titers correlate closely with clinical infection.[37]

In chronic or insidious diseases, the patient may not present himself for medical attention until the infection is well established. This makes it impossible to obtain an early serum sample against which later titers can be compared. It is important, therefore, to establish diagnostic significance in a single sample. Agglutinin titers above 1:256 have been found to indicate ongoing infection with *Y. pestis* or *Y. enterocolitica*. Antibody concentration of 1:80 or above is significant for *F. tularensis*, although in a single sample this could mean past, rather than present, infection. In tularemia, antibody levels take 4 to 6 weeks to reach their height; thus it is usually possible to draw several samples during the patient's illness.[37] Rising titers indicate ongoing infection.

Another name for brucellosis is *relapsing fever*; this name emphasizes the long, irregular clinical course of this disease. In a patient with brucellosis, the differential diagnosis will include many other febrile conditions; since Brucella organisms reliably evoke antibodies in an immunocompetent host, agglutination tests provide useful diagnostic information. A patient with recurrent fevers who does not have

Brucella antibodies almost certainly does not have brucellosis.[21] A patient with titers of 320 or above very likely does have brucellosis, unless he comes from a population endemically exposed to the pathogen. As many as 40 percent of healthy slaughterhouse workers have agglutinin levels up to 1:320.[21] This reflects the prevalence of Brucella organisms in their environment. Slaughterhouse workers also have a higher incidence of clinical brucellosis than any other group. For this reason, the agglutinin test cannot be considered uniformly applicable. Chronic exposure or previous vaccination make the agglutinin test almost useless. More complicated procedures for isolating and culturing the organism are necessary for diagnosis in such patients.

SEROLOGIC TESTS FOR SYPHILIS

Definitive microbiologic diagnosis of syphilis requires that *Treponema pallidum* be demonstrated in the involved tissues. *T. pallidum* cannot be cultured on artificial media. The organisms must be observed by dark-field microscopy, a difficult procedure under the best of circumstances. The motile organisms sometimes can be isolated by scraping the *chancre*, which is the inflammatory lesion that develops at the contact site during primary infection. Organisms are obtained more readily from the mucocutaneous lesions of the secondary phase, but often the patient fails to seek medical attention for the painless, self-limited lesions of either primary or secondary phase. The tertiary phase, which occurs years later, results from tissue hypersensitivity to treponemal antigens, not from the presence of viable organisms. It is very rare to find organisms during the tertiary phase. Serologic testing becomes extremely important in diagnosing this disease, the microbiologic diagnosis of which is so difficult. Infection with *T. pallidum* provokes both specific antitreponemal antibodies, which require sophisticated techniques for their demonstration, and nonspecific reaginic antibodies, which are easily demonstrated but can be diagnostically misleading.

Serologic tests for syphilis (STS) usually are performed on serum, but when the central nervous system is thought to be the site of tertiary syphilis, spinal fluid also can be tested. Serum reactivity sometimes disappears in the years between infection and the development of late CNS syphilis. In these cases, the presence in spinal fluid of nonspecific or specific antibodies may be the only indication that the neurologic disease is indeed syphilitic.

Reaginic Antibodies (Wasserman Reactivity)

Treponemal infection provokes development of IgM or IgG antibodies that react with a complex lipid-containing antigen called *cardiolipin*. Cardiolipin exists in many mammalian tissues, including fetal liver, which Wasserman used for the first serologic tests for syphilis. Bovine heart muscle is the source for commercial cardiolipin reagents. This anticardiolipin activity sometimes is called *reagin*; it is completely distinct from certain skin-sensitizing IgG antibodies which also are called reagin. Anticardiolipin reagin is not specific for treponemal infection or any other organism. It confers no protective benefits, and its presence in the circulation has no discernible immune effect, even though the antigen is present simultaneously in the host's tissues.

TEST PROCEDURE

The original Wasserman test was a complement fixation test. Descendants of this procedure currently in use include manual and automated variants of the Kolmer and the Kolmer-Reiter protein tests. The problems inherent in complement fixation procedures complicate these tests, but the results are sensitive, reproducible, and well adapted to laboratories experienced in complement fixation techniques.

More widely used are various flocculation procedures, of which the Venereal Disease Research Laboratory (VDRL) test is considered the present standard. VDRL testing requires heat-inactivated serum, carefully measured preparations of antigen and buffer, and well-controlled conditions of mechanical agitation, timing, and reading. A simpler and very effective variant is the rapid plasma reagin (RPR) test which uses unheated serum, less complicated antigen preparation, and less rigorous conditions of reading.[13] In both flocculation tests and complement fixation tests, serum reactivity is quantitated by dilution. Results are semiquantitative at best, and weakly positive results present especial problems in interpretation. Since technical problems may confuse the results, the first step in investigating any serum with a positive STS should be to repeat the test on a new serum sample.[33]

INTERPRETATION

Cardiolipin antibodies appear no sooner than 10 to 14 days after infection and often later than that. During the primary and highly infective phase, only 50 percent of patients will have positive reagin tests.[39] With the appearance of the secondary phase, 2 to 4 weeks after the chancre has disappeared, nearly all patients have a positive STS. The STS reverts to negative 6 to 8 months after successful treatment, if initiated during the primary phase. If treatment is begun after secondary manifestations have occurred, it takes a year or more for the STS to become negative. In patients treated 2 years or more after primary infection, the STS may never revert.[39]

Besides syphilis, many diseases induce Wasserman antibodies, but a positive STS from any cause other than *T. pallidum* infection is called a biologic false positive (BFP). The antibody apparently reflects altered immune reactivity to tissue constituents; thus it is not surprising that BFP's often accompany diseases of immune or uncertain etiology. The so-called collagen diseases, especially lupus erythematosus and rheumatoid arthritis, are notorious offenders.[18,22] Infectious mononucleosis, hepatitis, and leprosy, all conditions of aberrant reactivity to various organisms, frequently cause false positives.[38] Other conditions in which BFP should be considered include pregnancy, malaria, and the period that follows smallpox vaccination. To distinguish biologic false positives from the STS truly due to syphilis, one must search for specific antitreponemal antibodies.

Specific Treponemal Antibodies

TREPONEMA PALLIDUM IMMOBILIZATION

The first successful test for specific antibodies was the *Treponema pallidum* immobilization (TPI) test. The test requires viable, motile organisms, and *T. pallidum* cannot be cultured on synthetic media. Laboratory cultures must be grown in rabbit testes, an expensive and exacting procedure. To immobilize the organism, the antibody must have complement activity; since 25 to 30 percent of STS-positive serums are anticomplementary, almost a third of the tests will give ambiguous results. In addition, even trace amounts of penicillin immobilize the organisms spontaneously; this simulates a positive result whether antibody is present or not. Although highly sensitive and highly specific, the TPI test has so many technical and biologic pitfalls that it is now performed only occasionally and only at the Center for Disease Control in Atlanta, Georgia.[38]

FLUORESCENCE TESTING

A relatively simple, relatively specific test for treponemal antibodies uses the indirect fluorescence technique (see p. 220). Nonviable *T. pallidum* organisms can be applied to a glass slide, providing an antigen preparation that is stable and easily transported. The patient's serum is layered over the slide so that antibodies, if present, can attach to the fixed organisms. After incubation, the serum is washed away, and fluorescent antiglobulin serum is added. This is called the fluorescent treponemal antibody (FTA) test. Antibody present in the serum will attach to the organisms, and the fluorescent-labeled antiglobulin serum will attach to the antibody. If antibody is absent, the fluorescent antiserum has nothing to attach to.

Many patients have antibodies that react with treponemal cell walls but are not specific for *T. pallidum*. This reactivity for other treponemes can be removed by absorption with antigenic material prepared from nonpathogenic treponemes. Fluorescence testing of absorbed serum is called the absorbed fluorescent treponemal antibody test (FTA-ABS). The FTA-ABS is the best all-around procedure for distinguishing biologic false positives from true syphilitic positives and also for documenting syphilitic infection if clinical signs suggest the disease but cardiolipin tests are negative. It is not, however, suitable for use as a primary screening test; reagin tests perform this function more effectively and far more economically. [19]

FTA testing can be done on spinal fluid as well. Although spinal fluid need not be absorbed, several other modifications of the technique must be applied. Appropriately modified, the FTA test provides the most sensitive and specific test now available for syphilis of the central nervous system. [33, 38]

INTERPRETATION

The FTA-ABS usually becomes positive during the primary phase of syphilis. In the very earliest stages of spirochetemia and developing chancre, there has not been time for antibody of any kind to develop. Once seroconversion occurs, the FTA-ABS remains positive whether or not infection is treated. This makes it useful in investigating tertiary syphilis but not for determining whether past disease has been successfully treated. False-positive reactions due to globulin abnormalities, lupus erythematosus, and pregnancy are rare but do occur. [6] In these diseases, reactivity is weak and of an atypical morphologic pattern. [39] Lupus is the most common offender and occasionally gives a pattern of reactivity morphologically indistinguishable from a true positive. [31] The FTA-ABS will be positive in treponemal infections other than syphilis, such as yaws, pinta, and bejel. Because antigenic material from saprophytic or nonpathogenic organisms is used for absorption, antibodies to other pathogenic treponemes remain after the absorption process. A still more selective test, which weeds out nearly all false-positive FTA-ABS results, is the microhemagglutination assay for *T. pallidum* antibodies (MHA-TP). [25, 27]

VIRAL ANTIBODIES

Theoretical Considerations

Viral infections reliably induce antibody production in immunocompetent hosts. In principle, the range of viral serodiagnosis covers the entire spectrum of infectious viruses. For practical reasons, serologic techniques are used to diagnose relatively few viral diseases. Viral antigens are both numerous and changeable, even within a single strain of a single species. This makes it difficult to prepare effective antigenic reagents for widespread use. The reagent preparation must be reasonably stable on storage, with reliable biologic behavior and reproducible strength of activity. Specific infection should elicit antibodies of reproducible behavior so that a consistent test procedure can be used (e.g., complement fixation or neutralization of cytotoxicity). The antibodies must be directed against truly viral antigens, not against tissue elements altered by expsure to virus.

For serodiagnosis to be clinically and economically justifiable, its establishment should allow for useful therapeutic intervention, either to cure the patient himself or to prevent infection in others. So many viral illnesses are either self-limited or not amenable to treatment or prevention that it is difficult to justify expensive and time-consuming tests. Like viral isolation tests, viral serology has enormous importance in establishing etiology and transmission patterns for disease, but these are largely research or epidemiologic applications. Antibody testing has the most clinical use for infections due to rubella, hepatitis B, Epstein-Barr virus (EBV), and cytomegalovirus (CMV).

Rubella

Rubella (German measles) virus is clinically significant because it causes serious morphologic deformities of heart, ears, eyes, and other organs when it infects a first-trimester fetus. Except during these first months of intrauterine life, rubella infection is a benign, self-limited condition with few sequellae. Tests for rubella antibodies are useful in several different circumstances related to pregnancy. One consideration is to determine whether a woman of childbearing age is susceptible to rubella infection; another is to indicate whether an illness that complicates the first trimester of pregnancy really is rubella. Girls and nonpregnant young women found to lack antibodies should be vaccinated, after making sure that early pregnancy is not already in progress.

A woman already pregnant who is found to be susceptible to rubella should be followed at intervals to be sure that infection does not occur. Seroconversion during the first half of pregnancy is strong circumstantial evidence for infection, whether or not clinically apparent illness has occurred. The physician should discuss fully with the woman and her family the strong probability of fetal damage and consider the possibility of therapeutic abortion. Diagnostic problems are more difficult when a pregnant woman comes to medical attention only after recovering from illness or after known or possible exposure to the virus. In these circumstances, there is no chance to study a preinfection serum sample.

TYPES OF ANTIBODY

Hemagglutination-inhibiting (HI) antibodies occur earliest and last longest after rubella infection.[12] Antibody first becomes apparent as the rash fades and reaches peak levels about 2 weeks later. The hemagglutination inhibition test is sensitive, reliable, and relatively easy to perform.[32] HI antibody at concentrations of 1:8 or more indicates rubella infection at some time in the past. Levels below 1:8 indicate absence of past experience and a state of susceptibility. A fourfold rise in titer during illness is diagnostic of rubella infection.[28] If the only serum sample available is one drawn 2 or more weeks after the suspected illness, a high titer of HI antibody cannot distinguish between recent or long-past infection.

Complement-fixing (CF) rubella antibodies appear about a week after the rash disappears, somewhat later than HI antibodies. They achieve a peak level several weeks after HI levels peak and tend to decline after infection is past. If a pregnant woman is first seen several weeks after the illness, it still may be possible to demonstrate a rising titer of CF antibodies. If several samples show a stable, but elevated, level of CF antibody, it is quite probable that rubella infection occurred in the recent past, since CF titers rarely remain elevated for more than several months after the illness.[26]

Rubella antibodies also can be demonstrated by indirect immuno-fluorescence and by virus neutralization. These techniques have little clinical applicability. They are sometimes useful in evaluating apparent failures of rubella vaccination. Some individuals develop neutralizing antibodies and no other activities after viral exposure. Such a patient will appear to be seronegative, but the vaccinating dose does not elicit detectable antibody since the pre-existing neutralizing antibody suppresses the virus. Without special techniques to demonstrate prior rubella experience, it may appear that the patient is not only still rubella-susceptible, but also immunodeficient.[7]

Epstein-Barr Virus

The Epstein-Barr virus (EBV) is a herpesvirus which first was isolated from lymphoblasts in a culture prepared from Burkitt's lymphoma. Associations between EBV and human disease are rather confusing. Judging from antibody prevalence, one infers that EBV infection is extremely common but that recognizable disease is rare when infection occurs early. In developing nations and in socioeconomically deprived U.S. populations, at least 80 percent of 5-year-old children have antibodies; only 40 to 50 percent of economically privileged U.S. children have EBV antibodies.[1] In later life, seroconversion to EBV occurs after the patient experiences the clinical signs and symptoms of infectious mononucleosis. When EBV establishes a primary infection in an immunologically mature individual, it causes infectious mononucleosis. In the less mature individual, it causes no recognizable disease.

DNA characteristic of EBV can be identified in cells from Burkitt's lymphoma, a childhood neoplasm common in Africa and sporadically found elsewhere, and in nasopharyngeal carcinoma cells.[23] Viable virus particles do not occur spontaneously in these neoplastic cells, but explanted cells can be manipulated in cell culture so as to induce production of whole viruses. There is no evidence, however, that primary EBV infection is the cause of these or any other neo-plasms.[14] Normal human leukocytes exposed to EBV transform into lymphoblast-like cells which reproduce more generations, in cell cultures, than unexposed cells of the same original line.[1]

TYPES OF ANTIBODY

Numerous antibodies can be associated with the Epstein-Barr virus.

The most important, from the standpoint of the serology laboratory, are those directed against the capsid and against nuclear material. Acute infection elicits antibodies to viral capsid, which are demonstrated by indirect fluorescent techniques that employ virus-containing cultured lymphoid cells. Pre-illness serum from patients with infectious mononucleosis uniformly lacks these antibodies; serum drawn 1 or 2 weeks after onset of infectious mononucleosis almost always contains the antibody.[14] Within 3 to 4 weeks after illness begins, antibody to EB nuclear antigen becomes apparent.[11] Peak levels are established within 6 months, and high titers persist for life. The clinical course of the disease and the rate and intensity of antibody response are not correlated. Persons who once have had classical infectious mononucleosis retain lifelong protection against the disease. Other viruses may cause a somewhat similar syndrome, but heterophile-positive mononucleosis does not recur.

Patients with Burkitt's lymphoma or nasopharyngeal carcinoma uniformly have very potent anticapsid antibodies and also have antibodies against "early" antigen, an antigen produced in noninfected cultured cells by exposure to viral concentrates.[1] Antibody to "early" antigen indicates extensive or recent infection with EBV and also can be found in 80 percent of patients with active infectious mononucleosis.

Cytomegalovirus

Cytomegalovirus (CMV) is a herpesvirus which usually resides as a latent infection in cells of asymptomatic adults. It produces intensely damaging primary infection in the fetus or newborn and occasionally can cause symptomatic primary infection in adults. Immunologically mature patients produce both IgG and IgM anti-CMV antibodies, which can be demonstrated by complement fixation, indirect fluorescence technique, or neutralization of cytopathic viral effects on cultured cells.

Definitive diagnosis requires that the virus be cultured, usually from urine or saliva, and that viral antigens be demonstrable within infected cells.[35] This is especially important in evaluating sick infants. In adults, seroconversion alone is adequate presumptive evidence that CMV is the agent responsible for infectious mononucleosis-like illness or for hepatitis not associated with A or B activity, or for nonbacterial pneumonitis.

Infants acquire the virus transplacentally or during the birth process. The fetus suffering from intrauterine infection often produces

IgM antibodies detectible at birth or shortly thereafter. Intrapartum infection induces antibodies within weeks. IgM antibodies persist for some months after primary infection. IgM antibody present in an infant less than 2 years old indicates past infection but not necessarily ongoing or very recent infection. Half or more of all healthy adults have CMV antibodies at modest levels.[36] Reactivation of latent infection or primary infection by antigenically dissimilar strains can provoke a diagnostically significant fourfold rise in titer of complement-fixing antibodies.[35]

Hepatitis Virus

Hepatitis viruses are discussed in Chapter 12.

OTHER ORGANISMS

Rickettsiae

Rickettsiae are obligate intracellular parasites that enter human hosts after insect bites. Fever and headache characterize all the rickettsial diseases, and vasculitis and rash are prominent in all but Q fever. In the United States, Rocky Mountain spotted fever is by far the commonest rickettsial disease. Despite its name, the disease affects most heavily the southeastern part of the country, occurring largely in late spring and summer when exposure to ticks is greatest. Other rickettsial diseases of lesser incidence are Q fever; murine, scrub, and epidemic typhus; rickettsial pox; and Brill-Zinsser disease (recrudescent typhus).

Although rickettsiae have group and strain antigens capable of eliciting specific antibodies, laboratory procedures for demonstrating antirickettsial antibodies are not widely available. If prepared antigenic material is available, complement fixation tests are the best procedure. It is extremely difficult to isolate organisms from infected patients, partly because free organisms exist so very transiently in the blood stream and partly because culturing procedures are both exacting and hazardous. The *Weil-Felix test* is used for routine diagnosis of rickettsial infections. It is not specific for rickettsial antibodies and uses, as antigen, material from the bacterial genus Proteus.

THE WEIL-FELIX TEST

Rickettsial infection stimulates antibodies that cross-react with antigens found on certain strains of Proteus. As long as there is no concomitant Proteus infection, a rising titer of the appropriate anti-Proteus antibodies strongly suggests rickettsial disease (Table 18). Because rickettsial pox and Q fever do not produce these cross-reacting antibodies, the Weil-Felix test is noncontributory in these diseases.[30]

Testing each serum against the somatic (O) antigens of OX-19 and OX-2 of *Proteus vulgaris* and OX-K of *P. mirabilis* provides the most useful information, since different rickettsiae produce different patterns of reactivity. Antibody levels begin rising at the seventh to tenth day of illness unless successful antibiotic treatment aborts the immunologic response. Since Proteus is so widespread in the environment, most people have some level of Proteus antibodies at all times. If only one specimen is available for the Weil-Felix test, the antibody level must be 1:160 or above to be significant. If paired specimens are available, a fourfold rise in titer indicates ongoing rickettsial disease.[34]

Mycoplasma

Mycoplasma are small, free-living organisms which, unlike bacteria, exist without a cell wall. The cell membrane is in direct contact with the environment, and more than 50 different species have been identified from membrane antigens. Only *M. pneumoniae* is known to be pathogenic to man; it causes respiratory disease of gradual onset

Table 18. Weil-Felix Test Results in Rickettsial Diaseases

	OX-19	OX-2	OX-K
R. rickettsii (Rocky Mountain spotted fever)	+ to +++	+ to +++	neg.
R. prowazeki (Epidemic typhus)	+++	+	neg.
R. prowazeki (Recrudescent typhus or Brill-Zinsser disease)	+ or neg.	+ or neg.	neg.
R. typhi (Endemic, or murine, typhus)	+++	+	neg.
R. tsutsugamushi (Scrub typhus)	neg.	neg.	+++
R. akari (Rickettsialpox)	neg.	neg.	neg.
Coxiella burnetii (Q fever)	neg.	neg.	neg.

and several weeks' duration, characterized by fever and nonpurulent cough. In the past, this form of pneumonia was referred to as "primary atypical pneumonia," Eaton agent pneumonia, and "viral" pneumonia. Culture techniques for Mycoplasma and serologic techniques to identify mycoplasmal antibodies now make possible specific diagnosis of mycoplasmal pneumonia. Often, however, the time, expense, and technical requirements for specific diagnosis make it preferable to use nonspecific serologic findings for a presumptive diagnosis.

ANTIMYCOPLASMAL ANTIBODIES

Antibodies specific for mycoplasma develop a week to 10 days after illness begins. Various biologic reactivities exist, but the two most widely used diagnostic approaches are complement fixation and inhibition of metabolic activity. Viable cultures of Mycoplasma must be used for the metabolic inhibition test, and this limits its availability.

Complement-fixing antibodies at levels greater than 1:256[15] strongly suggest recent mycoplasmal infection. Levels less than this in a single specimen are not too helpful, because antibody often persists after infection has cleared. About 85 percent of patients with M. pneumoniae infection develop diagnostically significant elevations.[5] As with other serodiagnoses, a fourfold rise in titer between the onset of the disease and a sample drawn 2 or 3 weeks later provides the best evidence of infection. Some patients with pancreatitis develop mycoplasmal antibodies.[20] Conceivably, the lipid alterations resulting from liberation of pancreatic enzymes induce immunologic reactions similar to those against the lipid-rich mycoplasmal cell membranes.

Antibodies demonstrable by the metabolic inhibition test occur later and last longer than complement-fixing antibodies. False-positive inhibition results occur if the serum specimen contains antibiotics.[15]

COLD AGGLUTININS

In the first week of illness, many patients with M. pneumoniae pneumonia develop an antibody that reacts with the I antigen of human red blood cells. With the acute illness, the titer may reach 1:32 or more; it disappears after several weeks. This antibody precedes the appearance of antimycoplasmal antibodies and disappears much more rapidly.[15] The antibody agglutinates saline-suspended red blood cells at temperatures around 4°C., but agglutination is abolished by warming the cell-serum mixture to 37°C.

The laboratory test is a simple one, requiring only the incubation of serum with group O human cells. Positive results occur in one-half to two-thirds of patients with mycoplasmal pneumonia. About 20 percent of patients with adenovirus pneumonia also will have a positive cold agglutinin test, although, in general, titers are lower.[5] Rarely, a patient recovering from atypical pneumonia develops extremely high levels of cold agglutinins, with thermal properties that make clinically significant intravascular agglutination a real possibility. Very high cold agglutinin levels also can develop without apparent preceding infection. Idiopathic cold agglutinin disease of this sort sometimes precedes or accompanies the development of neoplasms of the lymphoreticular system. Mycoplasmal pneumonia, however, shows no association with lymphoreticular malignancies.

STREPTOCOCCUS MG ANTIBODY

Between 25 and 40 percent of patients with mycoplasmal pneumonia develop antibodies that react with the nonhemolytic streptococcal organism, Streptococcus MG. The nonspecific nature and unpredictable appearance of this antibody make it unsuitable as a present-day test for mycoplasmal pneumonia.

REFERENCES

1. Andiman, W. A., and Miller, G.: Epstein-Barr virus, in Rose, N. F., and Friedman, H. (eds.): Manual of Clinical Immunology. American Society for Microbiology, Washington, D.C., 1976.
2. Bergstrand, C. G., and Winblad, S.: Clinical manifestations of infection with Yersinia enterocolitica in children. Acta Paediatr. Scand. 63:875, 1974.
3. Blum, G., Ellner, P. D., McCarthy, L. R., and Papachristos, T.: Reliability of the treponemal hemagglutination test for the serodiagnosis of syphilis. J. Infect. Dis. 127:321, 1973.
4. Bokkenheuser, V., Suit, P., and Richardson, N.: A challenge to the validity of the Vi test for the detection of chronic typhoid carriers. Am. J. Public Health 54:1507, 1964.
5. Cate, T. R.: Mycoplasma, in Joklik, W. K., and Willett, H. P. (eds.): Zinsser Microbiology. Appleton-Century-Crofts, New York, 1976.
6. Cohen, P., Stout, G., and Ende, N.: Serologic reactivity in consecutive patients admitted to a general hospital: a comparison of the FTA-ABS, VDRL, and automated reagin tests. Arch. Intern. Med. 124:364, 1969.
7. Craddock-Watson, J. E.: Immunoglobulin responses after rubella infection. Ann. N.Y. Acad. Sci. 254:385, 1975.
8. Freter, R.: Agglutinin titration (Widal) for the diagnosis of enteric fever

and other enterobacterial infections, in Rose, N. R., and Friedman, H. (eds.): *Manual of Clinical Immunology.* American Society for Microbiology, Washington, D.C., 1976.

9. Goedvolk-DeGroot, L. E., Michel-Bensink, N., Van Es-Boon, M. M., et al: *Comparison of the titers of ASO, anti-DNase B, and antibodies against the group polysaccharide of group A streptococci in children with streptococcal infections.* J. Clin. Pathol. 27:891, 1974

10. Goldschneider, I.: *Bacterial allergy and immunity,* in Miescher, P. A., and Müller-Eberhard, H. J. (eds.): *Textbook of Immunopathology.* ed. 2. Grune & Stratton, New York, 1976.

11. Henle, G., Henle, W., and Horwitz, C. A.: *Antibodies to Epstein-Barr virus-associated nuclear antigen in infectious mononucleosis.* J. Infect. Dis. 130:231, 1974.

12 Herrmann, K. L., Halstead, S. B., Brandling-Bennett, A. D., et al.: *Rubella immunization. Persistence of antibody four years after a large-scale field trial.* J.A.M.A. 235:2201, 1976.

13. Jaffe, H. W.: *The laboratory diagnosis of syphilis. New concepts.* Ann. Intern. Med. 83:846, 1975.

14. Joncas, J. H.: *Clinical significance of the EB herpesvirus infection in man.* Prog. Med. Virol. 14:200, 1972.

15. Kenny, G. E.: *Serology of mycoplasmic infections,* in Rose, N. F., and Friedman, H. (eds.): *Manual of Clinical Immunology.* American Society for Microbiology, Washington, D.C., 1976.

16. Klein, G. C.: *Immune response to streptococcal infection,* in Rose, N. R., and Friedman, H. (eds.): *Manual of Clinical Immunology.* American Society for Microbiology, Washington, D.C., 1976.

17. Klein, G. C., Baker, C. N., and Jones, W. L.: *"Upper limits of normal" antistreptolysin O and antideoxyribonuclease B titers.* Appl. Microbiol. 21:999, 1971.

18. Kostant, G. H.: *Biologically false positive reaction to serologic tests for syphilis.* Bull. WHO 14:235, 1956.

19. Macfarlane, D. E., Hare, K., and Elias-Jones, T. F.: *Evaluation of automated large-scale screening tests for syphilis.* J. Clin. Pathol. 29:317, 1976.

20. Márdh, P.-A., and Ursing, B.: *The occurrence of acute pancreatitis in Mycoplasma pneumoniae infection.* Scand. J. Infect. Dis. 6:167, 1974.

21. McCullough, N. B.: *Immune response to Brucella,* in Rose, N. R., and Friedman, H. (eds.): *Manual of Clinical Immunology.* American Society for Microbiology, Washington, D.C., 1976.

22. Moore, J. E., and Lutz, W. B.: *The natural history of systemic lupus erythematosus: an approach to its study through biologic false positive reactions.* J. Chron. Dis. 1:297, 1955.

23. Nonoyama, M., Huang, C. H., Pagano, J. S., et al.: *DNA of Epstein-Barr virus selected in tissue of Burkitt's lymphoma and nasopharyngeal carcinoma.* Proc. Natl. Acad. Sci. U.S.A. 70:3265, 1973.

24. Olitzki, A.: *Enteric Fevers.* S. Karger, Basel, 1972.

25. Ovcinnikov, N. M., and Timcenko, G. F.: *The haemagglutination test (TPHA) in the serodiagnosis of syphilis.* WHO Document WHO/VDT/RES/74.394, 1974.

26. Person, D. A., and Herrman, E. C., Jr.: *Laboratory diagnosis of rubella*

virus infections and antibody determinations in routine medical practice. Mayo Clin. Proc. 46:477, 1971.

27. Rathler, T.: Hemagglutination test utilizing pathogenic Treponema pallidum for the sero-diagnosis of syphilis. Br. J. Vener. Dis. 43:181, 1967.

28. Rawls, W. E., and Chernesky, M. A.: Rubella virus, in Rose, N. F., and Friedman, H. (eds.): Manual of Clinical Immunology. American Society for Microbiology, Washington, D.C., 1976.

29. Read, S. E., and Zabriskie, J. B.: Immunological concepts in rheumatic fever pathogenesis, in Miescher, P. A., and Müller-Eberhard, H. J. (eds.): Textbook of immunopathology. ed. 2. Grune & Stratton, New York, 1976.

30. Sexton, D. J.: Rickettsiae, in Joklik, W. K., and Willett, H. P. (eds.): Zinsser Microbiology. Appleton-Century-Crofts, New York, 1976.

31. Shore, R. N., and Faricelli, J. A.: Borderline and reactive FTA-ABS results in lupus erythematosus. Arch. Dermatol. 113:37, 1977.

32. Smith, J. A.: Evaluation of a rubella hemagglutination inhibition test system. J. Clin. Microbiol. 3:5, 1976.

33. Sparling, P. F.: Diagnosis and treatment of syphilis. N. Engl. J. Med. 284:642, 1971.

34. Vinson, J. W.: Rickettsiae, in Rose, N. R., and Friedman, H. (eds.): Manual of Clinical Immunology. American Society for Microbiology, Washington, D.C., 1976.

35. Waner, J. L., Weller, T. H., and Kevy, S. V.: Patterns of cytomegaloviral complement-fixing antibody activity: a longitudinal study of blood donors. J. Infect. Dis. 127:538, 1973.

36. Waner, J. L., Weller, T. H., and Stewart, J. A.: Cytomegalovirus, in Rose, N. F., and Friedman, H. (eds.): Manual of Clinical Immunology. American Society for Microbiology, Washington, D. C., 1976.

37. Winblad, S.: Immune response to Yersinia and Pasteurella, in Rose, N. R., and Friedman, H. (eds.): Manual of Clinical Immunology. American Society for Microbiology, Washington, D.C., 1976.

38. Wood, R. M.: Tests for syphilis, in Rose, N. R., and Friedman, H. (eds.): Manual of Clinical Immunology. American Society for Microbiology, Washington, D.C., 1976.

39. Youmans, G. P., Paterson, P. Y., and Sommers, H. M.: The Biologic and Clinical Basis of Infectious Diseases. W. B. Saunders, Philadelphia, 1975.

SECTION 5

ENDOCRINE SYSTEM

CHAPTER 15

THE ENDOCRINE GLANDS

PITUITARY GLAND

Secretions of the pituitary gland control most of the other endocrine glands and directly affect various somatic tissues. The pituitary has two morphologically and embryologically distinct parts: the anterior glandular part, or adenohypophysis, and the posterior part, of neural origin, called the neurohypophysis. The two parts jointly occupy the sella turcica, but the functions and control of each part are separate.

Adenohypophysis

CELL TYPES AND HORMONES

The adenohypophysis secretes at least six hormones, several of which have more than one name. These are growth hormone (somatotropin); thyroid-stimulating hormone (TSH, thyrotropin); follicle-stimulating hormone (FSH); luteinizing hormone (LH, interstitial cell-stimulating hormone); luteotropic hormone (LTH, prolactin); and adrenal cortical-stimulating hormone (corticotropin, adrenal corticotropic hormone, ACTH).

Four major cell types, named for their affinity for tissue stains, comprise the anterior pituitary: acidophils, basophils, chromophobes, and amphophils. Although morphologic changes in various diseases suggest individual functions for individual cells, it is not certain which cells produce which hormones. Acidophils appear to be associated with growth hormone, and basophils with ACTH and thyrotropin.

461

Basophilic cells of slightly different appearance may secrete the gonadotropic hormones FSH and LH. The origin of prolactin is undetermined.

Other substances are associated with the pituitary, although their sites of origin and biologic nature are unclear. These are the melanocyte-stimulating hormone and the exophthalmos-producing factor, which is not the same as thyrotropin alone. Long-acting thyroid stimulator (LATS), a substance associated with hyperthyroidism, is probably not pituitary in origin. Present in the blood of hyperthyroid patients even after hypophysectomy,[1] it has many properties characteristic of gamma globulin, although an immune origin has not been demonstrated.

CORTICOTROPIN. Corticotropin (ACTH, adrenal cortical-stimulating hormone) has been intensively studied. Its primary action is upon the adrenal cortex, but it has extra-adrenal effects on fat, carbohydrate, and amino acid metabolism. Under its influence, glucocorticoids and adrenal estrogens and androgens enter the blood stream. Minimal aldosterone secretion may follow ACTH stimulation, but the pituitary does not exert primary control over the mineralocorticoids. ACTH secretion is, itself, controlled by hypothalamic response to the blood level of hydrocortisone. Hypothalamic secretions, elaborated in response to varying levels of circulating hormones, affect the production of other tropic hormones in addition to ACTH. Both bioassay and immunoassay procedures measure ACTH levels.

SOMATOTROPIN. Growth hormone exerts an imperfectly understood influence on the body as a whole. The results of somatotropic stimulation include increased amino acid transport and protein synthesis; mobilization of free fatty acids; and retention of calcium, phosphorus, sodium, potassium, and nitrogen. Approximately 4 to 10 mg. of growth hormone are found at all ages in the pituitary, which is believed to produce and store somatotropin. The very small amounts of circulating hormone are measured by immunoassay and radioimmunoassay procedures. Blood levels follow a diurnal pattern, and basal levels can be determined best early in the morning.[24]

THYROTROPIN. Thyroid-stimulating hormone promotes all synthesizing functions of the thyroid gland, resulting in increased gland weight and increased levels of circulating thyroid hormones. It is the change in these circulating levels that regulates TSH production, probably through hypothalamic mediation. Thyrotropin may independently affect connective tissue, but isolation of TSH from such associated proteins as exophthalmos-producing factor is so difficult that its extrathyroidal activity cannot be fully characterized. TSH is measured by bioassay and radioimmunoassay.

GONADOTROPINS. Production of the gonadotropins—follicle-stimulating hormone, luteinizing hormone, and luteotropic hormone—is apparently under hypothalamic control. In the female, follicle-stimulating hormone promotes maturation of the ovarian follicle. The maturing follicle produces estrogens, and as the level of circulating estrogen rises, luteinizing hormone is produced. Through combined LH and FSH activity, the ovum matures and the follicle ruptures. The secretory activity of the corpus luteum requires adequate levels of both luteinizing hormone and luteotropic hormone. The luteotropic hormone is also called prolactin because it initiates and sustains lactation, but successful milk secretion also requires the actions of estrogens, progesterone, growth hormone, and adrenal cortical hormones. In males, follicle-stimulating hormone promotes spermatogenesis, while luteinizing hormone stimulates the interstitial cells to secrete androgens. Both FSH and LH levels in the blood and urine can be measured by relatively uncomplicated bioassay and by immunoassay procedures.

DISEASES OF THE ANTERIOR PITUITARY

Pituitary abnormalities may be due to overproduction or underproduction of any or all of the adenohypophyseal hormones. Overproduction is almost always associated with gross or microscopic evidence of tumor. Underproduction usually follows hypophyseal destruction from disease or from operative procedures. In rare cases, there may be underproduction of isolated hormones, usually the gonadotropins, with no histologic or anatomic evidence of pituitary disease. Since the hypothalamus is so important to pituitary control, it is likely that isolated hormonal defects have their origin in individual loci of the hypothalamus.

SOMATOTROPIN DEFICIENCY. The most dramatic pituitary dysfunctions are disorders of growth hormone. Pituitary dwarfism occurs when postnatal supplies of somatotropin are inadequate; most such children have had normal intrauterine development. Craniopharyngioma causes approximately one-third of these cases, while the remainder are of unknown cause. Associated with retarded skeletal growth is retarded sexual maturation, although intelligence usually is normal. Despite reduced levels of thyroid and adrenal hormones, the patient generally is healthy, and there is no evidence of hypometabolism. Low fasting blood sugar is fairly common, but symptomatic hypoglycemia is unusual.

Differential Diagnosis. Pituitary dwarfism sometimes must be distinguished from so-called "primordial dwarfism," hypothyroidism, and gonadal aplasia. In primordial dwarfism, hormone production is normal, but the somatic tissues do not respond normally. Despite small stature, bone age and sexual development usually are normal, and thyroid and adrenal secretions are not diminished. In hypothyroidism, as in pituitary dwarfism, bone age and sexual development are retarded, but other clinical features point to childhood hypothyroidism, namely mental retardation, bradycardia, hypothermia, coarsening of skin and hair, and abnormal calcification of teeth and bones. Gonadal disorders, notably the XO chromosomal constitution, may be associated with short stature and failure of sexual maturation, but other physical abnormalities often are present, and the nuclear sex pattern is abnormal.

SOMATOTROPIN EXCESS. Overproduction of growth hormone occurs in eosinophilic or mixed adenomas. If overproduction precedes epiphyseal closure, striking long-bone enlargement produces gigantism. If the epiphyseal plates have fused, the facial and acral bones enlarge, producing the characteristic acromegalic appearance — enlarged facial features, protruding jaw, broad hands and feet, and enlargement of tongue and viscera. Advanced acromegaly is readily recognized, but frequently progression is gradual, and many years elapse before the diagnosis is made.

Laboratory Findings. Laboratory changes include altered carbohydrate metabolism, with diabetic glucose tolerance curve or frank diabetes mellitus; elevated BMR; increased glomerular and renal tubular function; elevated serum levels of alkaline phosphatase and inorganic phosphorus; and increased serum levels of growth hormone when assay is performed. Visual field defects are common if the pituitary tumor compresses the optic chiasm, and x-ray examination may show generalized osteoporosis as well as increased new bone formation.

CORTICOTROPIN EXCESS. The pituitary basophilic cells apparently produce ACTH, and increased levels of ACTH are frequently associated with basophilic adenomas. Autopsy series on patients with adrenal hyperfunction reveal that approximately one-fourth have pituitary tumors. Patients who have undergone bilateral adrenalectomy for treatment of Cushing's disease subsequently may develop basophil or chromophobe adenomas, but Addison's disease, in which ACTH production also is high, is not often associated with pituitary tumors.

Serum ACTH is measured by bioassay and immunoassay. Existence of an ACTH-producing tumor may be suggested if administration of a potent glucocorticoid, such as dexamethasone, fails to suppress ACTH production or if corticosteroid excretion does not fall after the suppressor drug is given. Since excessive steroid production, unresponsive to suppressor drugs, can occur with either pituitary or adrenal gland tumors, both glands must be evaluated. X-ray examination of both areas may be helpful in the differential diagnosis. Certain nonpituitary tumors, notably those of the lung and pancreas, may secrete an ACTH-like substance and produce hyperadrenalism.

OTHER HORMONES. Other pituitary hormones may be present in excess, but ACTH and somatotropin are by far the most common. Excess prolactin has been invoked to explain lactorrhea in women with acromegaly, and lactorrhea associated with amenorrhea may be the presenting symptom of pituitary tumor. Thyrotropin disorders are extremely rare. Most hyperthyroidism appears to arise from intrathyroid abnormalities.

PANHYPOPITUITARISM. Generalized hypopituitarism may occur when more than three-quarters of the gland is destroyed by surgical ablation, tumor, or non-neoplastic destruction. The first deficiency to appear clinically is of gonadotropin, followed by somatotropin (noticeable only in children), thyrotropin, and lastly corticotropin. Non-neoplastic destruction nearly always is due to infarction, often following hemorrhagic shock, as in Sheehan's syndrome in which hypopituitarism follows obstetric bleeding. Such infections as tuberculosis and syphilis formerly caused pituitary destruction, but are now very rare. Very rarely, hemochromatosis, Hand-Schüller-Christian disease, or noninfectious giant cell granuloma may destroy the gland, while some patients with hypopituitarism are found at autopsy to have diffuse fibrosis of unknown cause.

Differential Diagnosis. Hypopituitarism must be distinguished from other conditions of hypometabolism, loss of gonadal function, and anemia. When pituitary infarction follows obstetric shock, lactation does not occur, the menses do not resume, and there is gradually progressive disability. In long-standing hypopituitarism, there is genital atrophy, generalized depigmentation, sparsity of body hair, and evidence of thyroid and adrenal hypofunction. Cachexia is uncommon, distinguishing hypopituitarism from anorexia nervosa. The skin is waxy with fine wrinkles and diminished sweating.

Diagnosis rests on evaluation of hormonal levels. Urinary gonadotropins are low, a finding especially significant in older individuals, since normal young adults may have variably low gonadotropin excretion. Urinary excretion of 17-ketosteroids and 17-OH steroids is low, but the levels rise following 3 or 4 days of ACTH stimulation. After adrenal function has been established, pituitary failure is documented by administering the adrenal blocking agent metyrapone, which normally causes ACTH stimulation and marked increase in urinary steroids. All the tests of thyroid function are low, including BMR, ^{131}I uptake, circulating thyroxine, and the like, but after several days of TSH stimulation, thyroid function returns to normal.

End-Organ Failure. Pituitary failure results in endocrine hypofunction, but the target organs can be stimulated to normal function by exogenous tropic hormones. It may be difficult to distinguish between severe primary hypothyroidism and long-standing hypopituitarism since, in both cases, hypometabolism and decreased adrenal and genital function are observed. The thyroid gland, after prolonged absence of TSH stimulation, may atrophy so severely that the TSH stimulation test remains negative. In such cases, the thyroid gland usually is extremely small, while primary causes of hypothyroidism frequently produce a normal-sized or enlarged gland. Unfortunately, this difference in size is not of universal occurrence. Anorexia nervosa may present another difficult diagnostic problem, since amenorrhea and loss of thyroid and adrenal function can occur with this as well as other types of chronic malnutrition. Hypopituitarism, however, usually is characterized by a better nutritional state, loss of body hair, and loss of pigmentation. In chronic malnutrition, urinary steroid excretion tends to be higher than in hypopituitarism.

Indirect Tests. As specific hormonal tests become available, indirect tests of pituitary function are less important. Hypoglycemia, insulin hyper-reactivity, anemia, hyponatremia, and increased water retention are nonspecific findings of inconstant occurrence and should not be considered diagnostic. Such tests as insulin tolerance and water tolerance may be dangerous for the patient, and they provide less information than direct hormonal evaluation.

Neurohypophysis

The posterior, neural portion of the pituitary is a storehouse rather than a producer of hormones. The neurohypophyseal hormones originate in the hypothalamus and travel down the neurohypophyseal tract to the pituitary pars nervosa. Two hormones are involved: vasopressin, also called antidiuretic hormone (ADH), and oxytocin. Their structures are remarkably similar, but the difference of one amino acid confers different properties on each.

FUNCTIONS OF ADH

The two names of one hormone—vasopressin and antidiuretic hormone—signal its two actions. It stimulates vascular smooth muscle contraction, and it affects renal fluid excretion. The pressor effect occurs to a mild degree in anesthetized patients, but it is probably of little physiologic significance. Highly significant, however, is the antidiuretic effect. Diabetes insipidus, the clinical condition caused by neurohypophyseal insufficiency, is a dramatic example of physiologic derangement.

Antidiuretic hormone directly affects the distal convoluted tubule of the nephron. Emerging from the loop of Henle, urine is markedly hypotonic relative to the plasma in adjacent capillaries. ADH permits water to diffuse through the distal tubular epithelium, going from the dilute fluid in the tubule to the relatively concentrated medium of plasma. Without ADH, water cannot traverse the epithelium, so that large quantities of dilute urine are excreted. Changes in plasma osmolality appear to regulate ADH production, although changes in blood volume also may play a part. Nicotine, morphine, and ether promote ADH secretion, while alcohol produces diuresis by inhibiting ADH production.

FUNCTION OF OXYTOCIN

Oxytocin also has two effects: it promotes uterine contraction and stimulates milk ejection. Neither the mechanism of oxytocic effects nor the interrelationship between ADH secretion and oxytocin release is clearly understood. Patients with diabetes insipidus have normal labor and successful lactation. Isolated deficiency or excess of oxytocin has not been reported, but oxytocin deficiency occurs in patients with panhypopituitarism, especially with postpartum pituitary necrosis.

DIABETES INSIPIDUS

Diabetes insipidus may follow neoplastic and, occasionally, traumatic or granulomatous destruction of the fibers connecting the hypothalamus with the neurohypophysis. Hypothalamic disease, with or without apparent histologic change, may cause ADH deficiency. The presenting symptom is enormous urine output, characteristically 7 to 11 L. daily, but even more in many cases. The urine is pale and dilute with a specific gravity of less than 1.005. If patients with diabetes insipidus do not consume enormous amounts of water, they become dehydrated rapidly, since urine output continues despite diminished fluid intake. The basal metabolic rate sometimes is elevated. In some cases of pituitary destruction, x-ray examination, electroencephalogram, chemical or bacteriologic studies, or visual field determination may reveal abnormalities diagnostic of the primary disease.

DIFFERENTIAL DIAGNOSIS. Before diabetes insipidus is proved conclusively, two points must be confirmed. The kidneys must be capable of response to ADH, and the patient must be incapable of producing ADH after appropriate stimulation. To be excluded are psychogenic polydipsia, nephrogenic diabetes insipidus, and acquired renal damage. In hyperparathyroidism or vitamin D intoxication, hypercalcemia may cause ADH-resistant polyuria, but this is diagnosed readily by serum electrolyte studies. Administration of exogenous ADH has no effect on patients with nephrogenic (vasopressin-resistant) diabetes insipidus. Exogenous ADH causes a marked but short-lived increase in urine osmolality, both in true diabetes insipidus and in psychogenic polydipsia. The differential diagnosis is made by demonstrating secretory response, or lack of it, to changes in plasma osmolality.

WATER DEPRIVATION TEST. In the water deprivation test, water is withheld until 2 to 5 percent of the body weight is lost. This usually requires 6 to 12 hours, during which time the patient must be watched constantly, for patients with psychogenic polydipsia may display extreme cunning in obtaining illicit fluids, while patients with diabetes insipidus may collapse from dehydration. Carefully monitored stimulation by hypertonic sodium chloride or nicotine also may be used to alter plasma osmolality. However the change is produced, increased plasma osmolality causes decreased urine volume and increased urine concentration in a patient with an intact neurohypophyseal system and responsive kidneys. The patient with diabetes insipidus continues massive urine excretion, although the specific gravity may rise slightly.

INAPPROPRIATE ADH SECRETION

The observation that certain patients have expanded total body water and continuing low serum osmolality has suggested that ADH can be secreted independent of any volumetric or osmometric stimulus.[3] Bronchogenic carcinoma has been shown to elaborate a material indistinguishable from ADH, and many other intrathoracic lesions and intracranial abnormalities produce similar clinical findings. Excessive ADH activity leads to water retention with dilutional hyponatremia. This stimulates increased glomerular filtration and sodium excretion, resulting in net sodium loss and a urine significantly hyperosmolar to the serum.

ADRENAL CORTEX

The adrenal gland, like the pituitary, consists of two functionally and embryologically distinct portions. The cortex is of mesodermal origin and secretes hormones essential to maintain life. The medulla derives from the ectoderm, and its secretions, though important for normal existence, are not vital.

Steroids and Their Structures

The cortical hormones have as their basic structure the cyclopentanoperhydrophenanthrene ring, a 17-carbon structure. Specific hormones derive their functions and characteristic chemical and physical properties from additional groups present on several of the carbon atoms. Although innumerable active and intermediate compounds are known, the major adrenocortical products can be grouped fairly simply (Fig. 19).

STEROID STRUCTURE
AND NOMENCLATURE

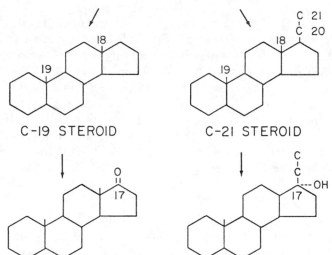

BASIC STEROID NUCLEUS

C-19 STEROID   C-21 STEROID

17-KETOSTEROID   17-HYDROXYCORTICOSTEROID

Figure 19. Structure and nomenclature of principal steroids in the adrenal cortex. (Redrawn with permission from Williams, G. H., Dluhy, R. G., and Thorn, G. W., in Thorn, G. W., et al. (eds.): *Harrison's Principles of Internal Medicine.* ed. 8. McGraw-Hill, 1977.)

ZONES OF PRODUCTION

The outer and middle zones of the adrenal cortex produce hormones with 21 carbon atoms. Those with a hydroxyl group at position 17 are called 17-hydroxycorticosteroids or glucocorticoids, since one of their significant effects is on glucose metabolism. Twenty-one carbon corticoids without the OH group at C-17 principally affect mineral metabolism and are called mineralocorticoids. The inner zone of the cortex produces steroids with 19 carbon atoms and a ketone group at C-17. These have androgenic activity and are produced in both males and females. All adrenocortical hormones derive from cholesterol and acetate through a multitude of enzymatic reactions.

MEASUREMENT OF STEROIDS

In research work and detailed diagnostic procedures, bioassays can yield highly reproducible results; however, in clinical endocrinology, chemical determinations and immunoassay and competitive protein-binding techniques are useful and much more readily available. Screening chemical procedures are done on urinary excretion products, although serum levels sometimes are measured. Urinary steroids can be divided conveniently into three major groups: 17-ketosteroids (17-KS), 17-ketogenic steroids (17-KGS), and 17-hydroxy-corticosteroids (17-OH corticosteroids, 17-OHCS). It is unfortunate that the terms are so similar, because the substances measured are quite different. These differences are presented in Figure 20.

17-KETOSTEROIDS. Steroids with 19 carbon atoms and a ketone group at C-17 are called 17-ketosteroids and usually are measured by the Zimmerman reaction. Not all 17-ketosteroids derive from adrenal hormones. Among the excreted 17-ketosteroids in the mature male are metabolites of testicular androgens, and the normal 17-ketosteroid levels for men are significantly higher than for women. In normal adult males, the 24-hour excretion of 17-ketosteroids is 7 to 25 mg. with a mean of 15 mg. Normal adult females excrete 5 to 15 mg. of 17-ketosteroids daily with a mean of 10 mg. Prior to puberty, this sex difference is absent.

17-KETOGENIC STEROIDS. A rather similar term describes a completely different group of compounds. The term 17-ketogenic steroid refers to compounds having 21 carbon atoms and a hydroxyl group at C-17. This hydroxyl group can be converted to a ketone group by oxidation, which also removes the side chain of C-20 and C-21 regardless of its nature. The group of compounds capable of oxidation to 17-KS includes several glucocorticoid derivatives as well as pregnanetriol. These compounds sometimes are called *Norymberski steroids,* after the method used for their determination. In both men and women, normal excretion of 17-ketogenic steroids is 5 to 20 mg. in 24 hours. The original urinary 17-ketosteroids either must be inactivated or measured separately before the 17-ketogenic steroids are studied.

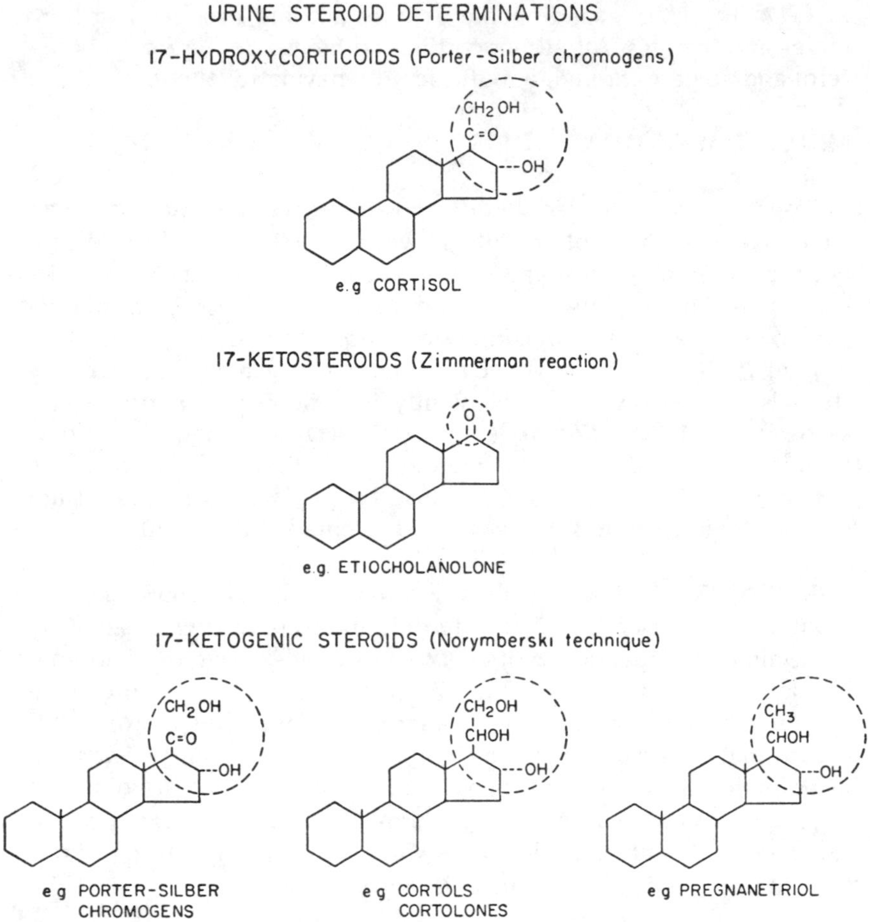
URINE STEROID DETERMINATIONS
17-HYDROXYCORTICOIDS (Porter-Silber chromogens)
CH2 OH
C=O
OH
e.g CORTISOL
17-KETOSTEROIDS (Zimmerman reaction)
O
e.g. ETIOCHOLANOLONE
17-KETOGENIC STEROIDS (Norymberski technique)
CH2 OH
C=O
OH
e g PORTER-SILBER CHROMOGENS
CH2OH
CHOH
OH
e g CORTOLS CORTOLONES
CH3
CHOH
OH
e g PREGNANETRIOL

Figure 20. Reactive groups that participate in the tests used for measuring urinary steroids. (Redrawn with permission from Dluhy, R. G., and Thorn, G. W., in Thorn, G. W., et al. (eds.): *Harrison's Principles of Internal Medicine.* ed. 8. McGraw-Hill, New York, 1977.)

17-HYDROXYCORTICOSTEROIDS. A third group of urinary compounds is called the 17-hydroxycorticosteroids, a misleading term since not every 21-carbon compound with a 17-hydroxyl group is included. The steroids included are those with 21 carbons and a dihydroxyacetone side chain. This combination of hydroxyl groups at C-17 and C-21 and a ketone group at C-20 reacts with phenylhydrazine to form a yellow compound. This is the Porter-Silber reaction, and these steroids often are called *Porter-Silber* *chromogens.* Included in this group are aldosterone and several metabolites of glucocorticoids. Owing to its high potency, aldosterone contributes little to the total quantity of urinary 17-OH corticosteroids, even in conditions of excess. The normal 24-hour excretion of Porter-Silber chromogens is 1 to 10 mg. with slight variation depending on the method used to extract the compounds.

Two slightly different methods are used for extracting the Porter-Silber chromogens, and results usually are expressed in terms of the method used. The Glenn-Nelson method gives slightly higher normal values than the Reddy method.

It is worth noting that 17-OH corticosteroids and 17-ketogenic steroids are related. The Porter-Silber chromogens are, in fact, 17-ketogenic steroids, since their 17-hydroxyl group can be oxidized to a ketone. The compounds commonly designated 17-hydroxycorticosteroids normally contribute approximately 40 percent of the total 17-ketogenic steroids.

ALDOSTERONE. Circulating aldosterone is measured by radioimmunoassay. Levels exhibit circadian variation, with peak concentration occurring in the morning and lower levels in the evening. Potassium loading or sodium restriction will increase circulating aldosterone, and change from supine to upright position causes increased secretion. Normal plasma levels, drawn from a supine patient, are 1 to 5 ng./dl. plasma.[37]

OTHER PRODUCTS. In addition to the groups of compounds described, a multitude of other products can be extracted from blood, urine, or the adrenal gland itself. Because of the exacting requirements for determination, these products are not used in routine clinical diagnosis.

Indirect Tests of Adrenal Function

Clinicians evaluated adrenocortical function long before steroids were isolated and purified. Adrenal hormones produce so many effects that many different derangements could be studied and manipulated. More specific information now can be obtained through steroid determinations, especially in tests using purified ACTH and other hormone preparations.

The classical indirect studies of adrenal function relate to glucose metabolism, fluid balance, and hematologic findings. These procedures have little diagnostic significance now that hormonal measurements are readily available. The Thorn test, in which circulating eosinophils decline to less than 50 percent of their baseline level after ACTH administration, may be combined with other procedures employing ACTH. No indirect tests of androgenic function are needed, since history and physical examination testify to sexual changes, and determination of urinary 17-ketosteroids now can confirm the clinical impression.

Direct Tests of Steroid Production

ACTH STIMULATION

The Thorn test was the first of the more specific tests of adrenal function, but it remains an inferential procedure. Direct measurement of steroid output following ACTH stimulation is more reliable. To provide maximum information, this test should include four or five daily doses of 50 units of ACTH with measurement, every 24 hours, of 17-ketosteroid and 17-hydroxycorticosteroid excretion. Of critical importance is the accurate collection and measurement of urinary output, and it may be advisable to monitor the adequacy of collection by measuring creatinine content of each 24-hour sample.

NORMAL RISE IN 17-OHCS. Once complete collection is assured, changes in ketosteroid and hydroxysteroid excretion mirror adrenal response. In the patient with potentially normal adrenal glands and inadequate pituitary function, steroid output rises progressively over the 5 days of the test. On the last day, the 17-hydroxycorticosteroids should be five to ten times the starting level, while ketosteroids increase twofold to threefold. Patients with partial adrenal function respond to intensive stimulation with a mild rise in hydroxycorticoids but no significant change in the ketosteroids. If the 17-OHCS rise less than 2 mg. in 24 hours, marked adrenal insufficiency can be inferred.

TESTS OF PITUITARY-ADRENAL AXIS

Both the pituitary and the adrenal glands are important in regulating corticosteroid production. Glucocorticoid levels are controlled by ACTH secretion, and ACTH secretion depends, in turn, on the amount of adrenal hormones in the circulation. Two tests are available to measure the integrity of this "feedback" mechanism. In the dexamethasone suppression test, the pituitary perceives high levels of circulating hormones, and it should respond by curtailing ACTH production, causing subsequent diminished excretion of steroid metabolites. In the metyrapone test, hormone synthesis is blocked, and the pituitary tries to increase the level of active hormones by producing more and more ACTH, thus provoking more and more synthesis of the inactive precursors.

DEXAMETHASONE SUPPRESSION TEST. Both dexamethasone and 9-alpha-fluorohydrocortisone are potent glucocorticoids causing marked metabolic effect and pituitary suppression with little quantitative change in steroid excretion. Either drug could be used for this test, but 9-alpha-fluorohydrocortisone produces sodium retention, an undesirable side effect. Following baseline determination of 24-hour 17-hydroxycorticosteroid excretion, 0.5 mg. of dexamethasone is given every 6 hours for 2 days. In patients with a normally responsive pituitary-adrenal axis, steroid production drops in response to decreased ACTH stimulation, usually to 2.5 mg. or less per 24 hours, on the second day of medication.

Increased Dexamethasone Dosage. Patients with Cushing's disease from any cause fail to show a drop in steroid excretion after the total dose of 4 mg. Often it is possible to distinguish bilateral hyperplasia from adrenal tumor as the cause of adrenal hyperfunction by repeating the dexamethasone test with higher dosage. In patients with bilateral hyperplasia, administration of 2 mg. of dexamethasone every 6 hours for eight doses usually produces a fall in 17-OH corticosteroid excretion to 50 percent or less of the basal value, while patients with adenomas are unaffected by the total dose of 16 mg. Patients with Cushing's disease associated with pituitary gland tumors may have suppressed steroid excretion after the larger, but not the smaller, dose of dexamethasone.[37]

Rapid Dexamethasone Test. To avoid the disadvantages of prolonged medication and the pitfalls of repeated 24-hour urine collections, a rapid screening test of dexamethasone suppression has been introduced. In this simplified version, 1 mg. of oral dexamethasone is given at midnight, and in the morning a 5-hour urine sample is collected. The total 17-OH corticosteroids and the creatinine content in the 5-hour sample are determined, and the ratio of steroid to creatinine excretion is calculated as

$$\frac{mg.\ 17\text{-}OHCS}{mg.\ creatinine} \times 1000.$$

Good separation can be obtained between normal individuals and patients with Cushing's disease. The mean normal excretion of 17-OHCS after the single suppressing dose is 0.1 mg. with a mean steroid-creatinine ratio of 0.6. The mean values for patients with Cushing's disease are 3.2 mg. of 17-OHCS total and a steroid-creatinine ratio of 20.4.[37]

METYRAPONE TEST. This test measures the ability of the pituitary gland to correct declining levels of circulating cortisol. Metyrapone (SU 4885) inhibits certain enzymes required to convert 17-OH precursors into cortisol. When the drug is given, cortisol levels decline, while precursor products accumulate. If the pituitary is normally responsive, increasing ACTH levels cause acceleration of efforts at synthesis and further accumulation of the 17-OH precursors. Urine is collected in 24-hour aliquots during and for 1 day after oral administration of 500 or 750 mg. of metyrapone every 4 hours for 24 hours. The 24-hour excretion of 17-hydroxycorticosteroids on the last day of collection should be at least double the baseline excretion. Since the result will be abnormal if the adrenals cannot respond to stimulation, this test should be done only if the ACTH stimulation test gives normal results. Chlorpromazine interferes with the normal response to metyrapone and should not be given during the testing period.

Evaluation of Adrenal Disorders

Tests of adrenocortical function are used to evaluate the four major groups of adrenal dysfunction: Cushing's syndrome (excess of glucocorticoids), hyperaldosteronism, adrenal virilism, and Addison's disease (adrenal hypofunction).

CUSHING'S SYNDROME

The commonest cause of glucocorticoid excess is adrenal hyperplasia, with adenoma and carcinoma together accounting for approximately one-fourth of the total number of cases. Bilateral hyperplasia apparently results from increased ACTH stimulation or possibly from inherent end-organ hypersensitivity. In some cases, pituitary tumors are found; in others the defect is ascribed to hypothalamic dysfunction without anatomic changes. Certain nonendocrine tumors, notably small cell carcinomas of the lung, secrete substances with ACTH-like activity.

USUAL FINDINGS. Cushing's syndrome, of whatever origin, is characterized by elevated urine and plasma levels of 17-OH corticosteroids and usually by increased 17-ketosteroids as well. The normal diurnal cycle, with lower steroid production at night, usually is diminished or absent. Patients have eosinopenia of less than 100 per cubic millimeter, mild neutrophilia, and a variable degree of lymphopenia. Serum uric acid levels are low, and increased uric acid is excreted in the urine. The glucose tolerance curve is abnormal, and overt diabetes is a fairly common related finding. Abnormalities of serum electrolytes are not always present, although potassium and chloride levels may be low.

RESPONSE TO MEDICATIONS. Hyperplasia is characterized by hyperreactivity to exogenous ACTH with double or triple the normal rise in urinary 17-OH corticosteroids and 17-ketosteroids. When hyperplasia is due to hypothalamic dysfunction or pituitary tumor, dexamethasone suppression is sluggish, and doses of 2 mg. every 6 hours may be needed to produce even moderate suppression. Apparently the 0.5 mg. dose is too small to contrast with the already high levels of circulating hormone. ACTH-producing carcinomas of nonpituitary origin secrete ACTH independent of circulating hormone level, and the resultant steroid overproduction is not altered by dexamethasone or metyrapone. Patients with hypothalamic dysfunction, on the other hand, respond dramatically to metyrapone; when cortisol production is blocked, ACTH is produced in still greater amounts, and the hyperplastic gland responds enthusiastically with accelerated hydroxysteroid production.

DIFFERENTIAL FINDINGS. Adenomas may be difficult to evaluate. Some remain amenable to ACTH, while others, although not carcinomas, nevertheless behave autonomously. Adenomas responsive to changes in ACTH frequently react to exogenous ACTH by increasing 17-OH steroid production much more than 17-ketosteroid production. ACTH-sensitive, or partially autonomous, adenomas respond to dexamethasone suppression as do hyperplastic glands: high doses are needed to induce suppression. The pituitary-adrenal axis is, however, distorted; metyrapone produces relatively little effect in these patients. This could be due, perhaps, to reduced pituitary ACTH-producing capacity following prolonged steroid elevation, but patients with bilateral hyperplasia have a striking response to metyrapone. The highest combined levels of 17-hydroxycorticosteroids and 17-ketosteroids occur in adrenal carcinoma.

Neither ACTH stimulation nor dexamethasone suppression alters steroid excretion, and the remaining potentially responsive glandular tissue frequently atrophies. Autonomous benign adenomas cannot be distinguished from carcinomas by laboratory tests.

HYPERALDOSTERONISM

The syndrome of hyperaldosteronism is a relative newcomer to lists of adrenal malfunctions. Primary hyperaldosteronism usually is due to a relatively small and usually benign adenoma producing only the mineralocorticoid, so that 17-hydroxycorticosteroid and 17-ketosteroid levels are normal. In some cases of cortical hyperplasia, there is increased secretion of all the cortical steroids, with the mineral effect of the glucocorticoids enhancing the effect of aldosterone. Secondary hyperaldosteronism results when continuing stimulation promotes adrenal secretion, producing excessive potassium loss and other physiologic concomitants of hormonal effect, without altering the underlying problem. Accelerated hypertension and states of persistent edema may produce this picture.

PHYSIOLOGY. Aldosterone is potent in promoting the exchange of sodium for potassium in the distal convoluted tubule, resulting in sodium retention and potassium excretion. Sodium retention increases extracellular fluid (ECF) volume through passive transfer of water. ECF volume changes regulate aldosterone secretion through the renin-angiotensin system, whereby a perceived drop in ECF causes the kidney to secrete renin, which activates angiotensin, which directly stimulates the adrenal to secrete aldosterone. The cycle normally is completed when aldosterone-induced sodium retention repletes the ECF, causing renin production to cease. Very subtle volume changes alter renin activity levels. The stimulus of upright posture produces sufficient shifts in fluid compartments to serve as a renin-inducer; renin measurments before and after posture change, combined with serial determinations of blood and urinary electrolytes, permit excellent assessment of this complicated interrelationship.

In primary hyperaldosteronism, autonomous hormone production permanently depresses renin activity. Most patients have persistent diastolic hypertension, for reasons which are not fully clear, but do not manifest edema. Since early or mild hyperaldosteronism need not manifest pronounced hypokalemia,[7] it has been suggested that much "essential" hypertension actually may be due to excessive aldosterone secretion. Studies of renin activity and potassium metabolism have not been conclusive.[38]

In secondary hyperaldosteronism, the adrenal responds appropriately to renin stimulation, but the renin levels remain inappropriately high. Accelerated hypertension is a common cause, and persistent edema, as from cirrhosis or nephrotic syndrome, also increases aldosterone production. The stimulus to excess renin production in these conditions presumably arises from alterations in renal arterial dynamics, causing a physiologically perceived hypovolemia, regardless of the actual whole-body state of fluid volume.

LABORATORY FINDINGS. Low serum potassium characterizes both primary and secondary hyperaldosteronism. Serum sodium tends to be high in the primary form, and in severe cases increased bicarbonate levels and metabolic alkalosis compound the problem. In addition to excessive urinary potassium, there is usually impaired urinary concentrating ability and neutral or alkaline urine. Patients with primary aldosteronism have low levels of renin activity, which fails to increase in the upright position. Persistently high renin activity occurs in secondary aldosteronism, and serum sodium levels tend to be lower than in the primary form.

ELECTROLYTE RESPONSES. Although aldosterone is not easily measured, its physiologic effects on urinary sodium and potassium are readily observed. In a patient with suspected hyperaldosteronism, dietary manipulation can give valuable information. After measurement of sodium and potassium excreted while the patient eats a relatively normal diet of 80 to 100 mEq. sodium and 100 mEq. potassium daily, the sodium intake can be reduced to 10 mEq. per day, while the potassium intake remains unchanged. The normal individual will respond to sodium depletion by increasing aldosterone production, resulting in increased potassium excretion over a 5-day period. Sodium excretion falls with sodium restriction. In the patient with autonomous overproduction of aldosterone, there may be little change in hormone secretion. Indeed, potassium excretion tends to fall during sodium restriction, for the tubular urine contains less sodium to be exchanged for potassium.

Salt Loading. After a period of restricted sodium intake, a high sodium regimen (200 mEq. per day) can be instituted, again with constant potassium intake. The normal individual promptly suppresses aldosterone secretion, and urinary potassium falls significantly during 5 days of salt loading. In the patient with primary hyperaldosteronism, the excess sodium is excreted adequately, so that an increased sodium load traverses the distal tubule. This accentuates the tendency toward potassium exchange, and potassium excretion increases over the baseline level. Patients with secondary hyperaldosteronism also react abnormally to a salt load administered after sodium deprivation. These patients reabsorb the excess sodium, resulting in accentuated hypernatremia and edema and in diminished sodium excretion. Because the sodium is reabsorbed in the proximal tubule, the sodium load in the distal tubule is too small to affect potassium excretion to a significant degree; therefore, in secondary hyperaldosteronism, increased potassium excretion does not occur, and urinary sodium excretion is abnormally low.

Serum levels of sodium and potassium should be monitored throughout the test, especially since symptoms of severe hypokalemia may complicate the salt-loading portion of the procedure. Whenever urinary electrolytes are measured, the values should be checked against the serum values to avoid misinterpretation of abnormal results.

ADRENAL VIRILISM

The clinical signs of adrenal virilism vary with age and sex. Among these are the inappropriate appearance of masculine traits in prepubertal children of either sex, virilization in mature females, and less easily recognized accentuation of the male secondary sex characteristics in mature men. There are two forms of adrenal virilism with two different etiologies.

DEFECTIVE SYNTHESIS. Congenital adrenal virilism results from any of several inborn enzymatic defects in cortisol synthesis. As glucocorticoids are normally synthesized, many preliminary products are 19-carbon steroids with androgenic properties. If normal cortisol production is blocked by enzyme deficiencies, ACTH secretion continues at a high level, producing glandular hyperplasia which results in continuing high levels of the precursor substances. A number of different genetically determined defects have been implicated.

Despite the inborn nature of the disease, symptoms may become manifest at any time, although most cases are recognized at birth or in early childhood. The effect of massive doses of androgenically active steroids in utero is masculinization of the female infant, who may appear to be a pseudohermaphrodite, or production, in the male infant, of macrogenitosomia. If aldosterone production is impaired along with cortisol synthesis, there may be sodium loss and potassium retention in the so-called salt-losing type of adrenal virilism.

Laboratory Findings. Primary laboratory findings in adrenal virilism include increased levels of plasma and urine 17-ketosteroids, decreased 17-hydroxysteroids, and high levels of circulating ACTH. The most common defect, that of inadequate 21-hydroxylation, produces high levels of pregnanetriol, a 21-carbon steroid. Because this compound is measured in the 17-ketogenic steroids, in these cases there will be high levels of 17-ketogenic steroids but low 17-hydroxysteroids.

In most patients with congenital adrenal hyperplasia, the gland remains sensitive to ACTH stimulation. Exogenous ACTH further elevates the already high levels of 17-ketosteroids, but 17-hydroxycorticosteroids do not rise. A rare form of the syndrome arises from a defect of 11β-hydroxylation, and 17-OH precursors of cortisol accumulate, analogous to the situation when normal individuals receive metyrapone. In this form, 17-hydroxycorticosteroids are elevated, and increased mineralocorticoid activity and hypertension are present.

TUMORS. Occasional cases of adrenal virilism in adults are due to late manifestations of congenital enzyme defects. More often, however, they are due to hyperplasia or tumor. Benign androgenic hyperplasia, in which 17-ketosteroids are elevated but 17-hydroxycorticosteroids are normal, is rarely seen. Adrenal virilization usually is due to carcinoma, and generally there are increased 17-hydroxycorticosteroids in addition to the high levels of 17-ketosteroids.

ADDISON'S DISEASE

The clinical findings of chronic adrenal hypofunction are the reverse of those in Cushing's syndrome. The former include weight loss, hypotension, nausea and vomiting, and hyponatremia with elevated serum potassium. Weakness is a constant finding, hypoglycemia may occur, and there is increased sensitivity to insulin. Characteristically, the basal metabolic rate is low in patients with Addison's disease, but other tests of thyroid function are normal if the pituitary gland is intact.

LABORATORY FINDINGS. When chronic adrenal hypofunction is suspected, the initial test will be determination of 24-hour 17-ketosteroid and 17-hydroxycorticosteroid excretion rates. These may be in the low-normal range or frankly low: 3 to 6 mg./24 hours and 0 to 2 mg./24 hours, respectively. The diagnosis of primary adrenal insufficiency is confirmed by failure of the adrenal glands to respond to ACTH stimulation. In some cases of partial insufficiency, an initial small rise in steroid excretion is followed by falling levels, despite continuing ACTH stimulation. This may represent exhaustion of the maximally stimulated gland. High plasma levels of ACTH are found with primary adrenal deficiency.

Secondary adrenal hypofunction occurs when ACTH production is deficient. When ACTH deficiency has been of short duration, the adrenals maintain their responsiveness to exogenous stimulation, and by the fourth or fifth day of ACTH administration, urine 17-hydroxy-corticosteroid levels may rise by as much as tenfold. The rise in 17-ketosteroids is also prompt.

SECONDARY ADRENAL ATROPHY. Prolonged ACTH deficiency causes severe adrenal atrophy and is ordinarily iatrogenic, due to prolonged steroid medication. Following prolonged steroid medication, the glands may take from several weeks to several months to recover their function and reactivity. Prolonged stimulation causes gradual rise in steroid excretion, 17-hydroxycortico-steroids generally rising first. Once adrenal reactivity has been established, pituitary response can be tested. Pituitary responsiveness to changes in circulating cortisol returns later than adrenal sensitivity, once exogenous therapy is discontinued.

ADRENAL MEDULLA

The adrenal medulla, although entirely surrounded by cortex, has no functional or histologic resemblance to the cortex. The principal cell type is the chromaffin cell, which bears within its cytoplasmic granules the two hormones of the adrenal medulla. These are the two catecholamines, epinephrine and norepinephrine, both mediating the "fight or flight" reflexes, but producing slightly different physiologic effects. Chemically, their only difference is that epinephrine has a methyl group that norepinephrine lacks.

Hormone Synthesis and Degradation

Epinephrine is the major medullary hormone. Of total secreted and stored hormone, approximately 80 percent is epinephrine. Norepinephrine, however, predominates in the urine, much of it deriving from postganglionic synapses of the autonomic nervous system. The synthesis and degradation of the two compounds are similar, and most clinical laboratories do not distinguish between the two hormones. Catecholamine synthesis starts with the amino acid phenylalanine, which is oxidized to tyrosine. Subsequent oxidative and other reactions produce norepinephrine, to which a methyl group is added in epinephrine synthesis. For both substances, the degradative end products are acids, usually studied in terms of 3-methoxy-4-hydroxymandelic acid, also called vanillylmandelic acid (VMA). The enzyme monoamine oxidase is required for VMA production.

EPINEPHRINE AND NOREPINEPHRINE

Catecholamine secretion is stimulated by cholinergic nerve impulses and by such stimuli as physiologic or psychologic stress, hypoxia, hemorrhage, and a number of drugs, among them reserpine, histamine, and nicotine. The two hormones have disparate cardiovascular effects: norepinephrine constricts vascular smooth muscle, slows the heart rate, and raises both systolic and diastolic blood pressure, while epinephrine increases heart rate and cardiac output and produces only systolic hypertension. Both increase the metabolic rate, raise the blood sugar, and cause elevated plasma fatty-acid levels. Despite their widespread and dramatic physiologic effects, the medullary catecholamines are not essential for life. Bilateral adrenalectomy, in fact, may alter urinary catecholamine excretion very little, since urinary levels derive largely from norepinephrine synthesized at sympathetic nerve endings.

Pheochromocytoma

The adrenal medulla is much simpler to discuss than the adrenal cortex. Only one condition is clinically significant—the tumor pheochromocytoma. This may be either benign or malignant; distinction, difficult even after histologic examination, is impossible by laboratory testing. Characteristically, pheochromocytoma is seen with intermittent or sustained hypertension, although the generalized symptoms of nervousness, weight loss, palpitations, headache, and paroxysmal sweating may first bring the patient to medical attention. Since many other conditions may cause hypertension, with or without the additional symptoms, the diagnosis of pheochromocytoma rests on demonstrating increased adrenomedullary secretion. Urinary and plasma catecholamines are measured fluorometrically after careful absorption, elution, and oxidation. The normal quantities in plasma are small, less than $1\mu g./L.$[2] Urinary catecholamine excretion is less than 100 $\mu g.$ per 24 hours, although the metabolites metanephrine and normetanephrine are excreted in larger quantities and constitute a fairly accurate index of physiologically active amines.[2] The quantities are so small and the procedure so exacting that catecholamines ordinarily are measured only in reference laboratories.

VMA EXCRETION

Urinary vanillylmandelic acid (VMA) frequently is measured to indicate catecholamine production. Both VMA and catecholamine measurement require a 24-hour urine specimen kept at a pH of 3.0 or below by collection in 6N hydrochloric acid. Normal values for 24-hour VMA excretion depend somewhat upon the method used, one method giving a range of 1.8 to 10.8 mg.; another widely used method has a range of 0.7 to 6.8 mg. The findings in pheochromocytoma do not overlap either normal range, ranging from 15 to 90 mg. in 24 hours in one series.[35] Elevated VMA levels occur occasionally in retinoblastoma, carotid body tumor, malignant carcinoid, and acrodynia. Urinary VMA frequently is high in the presence of neuroblastoma and ganglioneuroma, which secrete dopa, an oxidation product of tyrosine. Mild elevations may occur with childbirth, surgical or traumatic stress, and burns.

ARTEFACTS. Certain chemicals distort the tests for both catecholamines and VMA, and it is customary to forbid dietary intake of potential interfering substances such as coffee, tea, bananas, and anything containing vanilla. Sunderman[35] states, however, that the VMA elevation induced by ingestion of four bananas does not exceed the upper limits of normal, and newer methods of VMA measurement are not affected by dietary intake. Insulin may increase catecholamine excretion, but therapeutic doses do not affect VMA levels. Insulin shock therapy, however, is followed by rising VMA excretion. Monoamine oxidase inhibitors naturally depress VMA excretion, since that enzyme is necessary to degrade catecholamines. Oral chlorpromazine may cause a moderately low level, and slight decrease may follow morphine or Pentothal administration. Intramuscular reserpine causes a moderate rise in VMA levels.

PRESSOR TESTS

Classical diagnostic procedures for pheochromocytoma employ manipulation of blood pressure. In patients with initial pressure below 170/110 mm. Hg, the histamine test is used. Intravenous injection of 0.01 to 0.025 mg. histamine causes a prompt, dramatic rise in blood pressure if pheochromocytoma is present. Often this is preceded by a cold pressor test, since general vasomotor instability may mimic a positive result. The diastolic pressure rise after histamine injection should be at least 50 mm. Hg higher than the elevation provoked by immersion of one hand in cold water. To reverse a possibly disastrous hypertensive response, antihypertensive agents should be immediately available. Urine collected after the test should contain increased catecholamines or their metabolites.

Phentolamine (Regitine) promptly antagonizes the hypertension induced by excess catecholamine. This drug is an antidote for untoward responses to the histamine test, and it can be used diagnostically in patients with baseline blood pressure above 170/110 mm. Hg. In hypertensive patients with pheochromocytoma, intravenous phentolamine provokes a systolic drop of at least 35 mm. and a diastolic drop of 25 mm. or more.

THYROID GLAND

Introductory Physiology

The thyroid gland synthesizes its hormones from iodine and the essential amino acid tyrosine. Most of the body's iodine enters through the alimentary tract as iodide (I^-), but under certain circumstances, the lungs and skin may be portals of entry. Of the iodine that enters the body, approximately one-third enters the thyroid gland and the remaining two-thirds leaves the body in urine.

SYNTHESIS OF THYROID HORMONES

In the thyroid gland, enzymes oxidize iodide to organic iodine, which is incorporated into monoiodotyrosine and diiodotyrosine. These one- and two-iodine-containing compounds are building blocks for the active thyroid hormones thyroxine (T_4), which has four iodine molecules, and triiodothyronine (T_3), which has three. These synthesizing steps occur in the intrafollicular colloid, mediated by enzymes from epithelial cells which line the follicle. A single complex molecule, thyroglobulin, is the principal constituent of follicular colloid, and hormonal synthesis occurs within the thyroglobulin molecule.

Once formed, the thyroid hormones are loosely bound to thyroglobulin and can be cleaved enzymatically and liberated into the blood stream. In the blood, the hormones are bound fairly tightly to thyroid-binding globulin and other serum proteins. Thyroxine has a far higher affinity for thyroid-binding globulin than has triiodothyronine.

The pituitary hormone thyrotropin (thyroid-stimulating hormone, TSH) stimulates all stages of hormonal synthesis including uptake of circulating iodide, synthesis of new hormone, and release of formed hormone. The level of circulating hormone regulates the level of thyrotropic activity by a feedback mechanism, although the metabolic activity of adrenal and gonadal hormones exerts some influence on TSH production.

EFFECTS OF THYROID HORMONES

Control of oxygen consumption is the most conspicuous biologic effect of the thyroid hormones, a physiologic variable measured in simplest fashion by the basal metabolic rate. Thyroid hormones also influence carbohydrate and protein metabolism, the mobilization of electrolytes, and the conversion of carotene to vitamin A. Although the mechanism is not known, thyroid hormones are essential for development of the central nervous system, and the thyroid-deficient infant suffers irreversible mental damage. The thyroid-deficient adult may have slowed deep-tendon reflexes and diffuse psychomotor retardation, but these changes are reversible with hormone replacement therapy.

FACTORS THAT DECREASE THYROID ACTIVITY

Genetically determined enzyme deficiencies may interfere with iodine metabolism at any step, causing congenital goiter. Much more frequently, depressed thyroid function results from external causes. Exogenous thyroid hormone suppresses hormone production by depressing TSH levels. Drugs of the thiocyanate and perchlorate groups interfere with iodide concentration, while thiourea and thiouracil prevent incorporation of thyroidal iodine into organic compounds. The antithyroid effects of iodine are not fully understood but probably include inhibition both of iodine binding and of hormonal release, while radioactive iodine selectively irradiates hormonally active tissue, owing to its concentration in the actively functioning gland.

Tests of Thyroid Function

THE BASAL METABOLIC RATE

The oldest and least specific test of thyroid function is the basal metabolic rate (BMR). This measurement of oxygen consumption is expressed as kilocalories expended per square meter of body surface per hour, with the fasted patient in a condition of mental and physical repose. In clinical use, the results are expressed as a percentage of the expected normal, with suitable corrections made for the individual patient's height, weight, age, and sex. As more specific tests have become available, the BMR, a general test subject to many artefactual alterations, has lost its usefulness.

NONHORMONAL TESTS

Thyroid hormones affect the synthesis, degradation, and intermediate metabolism of adipose tissue and circulating lipids, and abnormalities of endocrine function are reflected in altered lipid levels. In hyperthyroidism, degradation and excretion increase more than synthesis, resulting in low circulating levels of cholesterol, phospholipids, and triglycerides; hypothyroidism slows catabolism more than it affects synthesis, and hypercholesterolemia and hypertriglyceridemia reliably accompany myxedema. This produces a predominantly pre-beta lipoprotein pattern when lipids are partitioned,[10] and increased cholesterol levels may be the earliest indicator of impending hypothyroidism. Hypothyroidism secondary to pituitary failure, however, does not cause lipids to rise.[16] In an obviously hypothyroid patient, a normal serum cholesterol level should direct attention to the pituitary. Cholesterol levels drop to normal within 2 or 3 weeks after successful therapy for hypothyroidism has been initiated.

In severe hypothyroidism, serum levels of muscle-associated enzymes tend to rise. Total creatine phosphokinase (CPK) and lactic dehydrogenase (LDH) values rise moderately, and isoenzyme partition reveals skeletal muscle to be the source.[12]

Hormone Concentration in the Blood

Thyroxine (T_4) concentration is normally 25 to 50 times greater than that of triiodothyronine (T_3 levels). Most tests for thyroid hormone levels measure primarily thyroxine, and ordinarily this information is clinically sufficient. Only in unusual circumstances is it necessary to determine T_3 and T_4 separately. Older tests for hormone levels measured serum iodine content, from which the levels were extrapolated. Accurate, specific measurements of T_4 and T_3 are now possible and have largely superseded tests of iodine content. It is important, however, to understand the differences between these procedures.

IODINE MEASUREMENTS

The oldest test for circulating thyroid hormone is the *protein-bound iodine (PBI) test.* This measures the iodine present in a precipitate of serum proteins. Because most thyroxine is bound to carrier protein, the PBI includes nearly all the hormonal iodine. It also includes T_3 iodine and a group of loosely defined compounds called *iodoproteins.* Normal serum rarely contains many iodoproteins, which are largely precursors of T_3 and T_4 and other molecules usually confined to the thyroid gland. Normal PBI values are 3.5 to 8.0 μg./dl., expressed as iodine. The problem with the PBI test is that exogenous organic and inorganic iodine-containing compounds artefactually elevate the results. Notable offenders are cough medicines, vaginal suppositories, skin preparations, multivitamin preparations, and radiographic contrast media.

The *butanol-extractible iodine (BEI) test* uses a solvent rather than precipitation to remove iodine-containing material from serum. Inorganic iodides do not contaminate BEI results, and one- and two-iodine hormonal precursors are excluded. Normal values range between 3.2 and 6.5 μg./dl. Radiographic contrast media, some of which remain in the body as detectible iodides for many years, distort BEI values as much as PBI values.

It is possible to separate thyroxine and T_3 from the binding protein and measure iodinated material separately from the associated proteins. Passing serum through a column of anion-exchange resin causes T_4 and T_3 to remain in the column and proteins, including iodoproteins, to pass through for discard. With this "T_4 by column" technique, inorganic iodides are not a problem, but results can be thrown off by high concentrations of iodinated radiographic media. Normal values are 3.0 to 7.0 μg./dl. of iodine or 4.4 to 9.8 μg./dl. expressed as thyroxine. Iodine contributes 65 percent of the weight of thyroxine.

THYROXINE MEASUREMENT

Direct measurement of thyroxine bypasses the issue of iodine contamination. The best current test for thyroxine concentrations uses the technique of competitive protein binding. This procedure, developed by Murphy and Pattee, is sometimes called thyroxine by displacement (T_4D), thyroxine by Murphy-Pattee (T_4MP), or thyroxine by competitive protein binding (T_4CPB). The first step is to extract all T_4 from the serum specimen. The patient's T_4 is then incubated with a known quantity of thyroid-binding globulin fully saturated with radiolabeled T_4. The proportion of labeled T_4 displaced from the reagent globulin directly reflects the level of nonlabeled T_4 present in the test specimen. Although T_3 accompanies T_4 in the extraction process, it has such low affinity for thyroid-binding globulin that it does not affect the results.

Normal values for T_4 by displacement are 4 to 11 μg./dl., expressed as thyroxine. Because the numbers involved in reporting total thyroxine are substantially higher than the numbers many clinicians are accustomed to seeing when iodine is reported, some laboratories multiply the thyroxine results by 0.65 to give a value for thyroxine iodine. This practice has little to recommend it for routine use but can be useful in the specific setting of directly comparing to T_4D iodine levels with PBI.

When there has been physical disruption of thyroid tissue, iodoproteins normally confined to the gland may enter the blood stream. This occurs especially in Hashimoto's thyroiditis and subacute thyroiditis and may sometimes occur with thyroid neoplasms. Under these conditions, PBI values are significantly higher than the iodine content present in thyroxine alone. It is, of course, essential that contamination by exogenous iodides be ruled out as a cause of high PBI.

Thyroxine levels measured by this method are not affected by iodine artefacts but do rise and fall with anything that affects the amount of thyroid-binding globulin or the affinity of T_4 for its carrier. Increased TBG levels occur in pregnancy, after administration of exogenous estrogen or oral contraceptives, in viral hepatitis, and in genetically determined peculiarities of protein manufacture. Under these conditions, the T_4 values will be high, but the patient is euthyroid. Conversely, a low T_4, due to decreased TBG levels, occurs when androgenic steroids are given, when there is acromegaly or excessive glucocorticoids, when there is excessive renal or intestinal protein wastage, in starvation or illness severe enough to cause prolonged protein degradation, or in genetically determined defects of TBG synthesis.

Radioimmunoassay can be used to measure serum thyroxine. The results, and the conditions that affect the results, are entirely similar to those for T_4D determination.

TRIIODOTHYRONINE MEASUREMENT

Triiodothyronine (T_3) can be measured effectively only by radioimmunoassay. It is present at far lower concentrations than T_4 but is biologically more active and has a much shorter serum half-life. Some T_4 undergoes conversion to T_3 at the site of peripheral activity, and some workers believe that all T_4 is physiologically effective only through conversion to T_3. The relationships between unbound T_4, T_3 and the patient's metabolic status remain under intense investigation. In laboratory testing, it is important to avoid nonphysiologic conversion of T_4 to T_3. Radioimmunoassay escapes this pitfall, which had produced serious problems with efforts to measure T_3 by competitive protein-binding techniques. Normal T_3 values are about 120 ng./dl.[16]

RADIOACTIVE IODINE WITHIN THE BODY

The body metabolizes all the isotopes of iodine in identical fashion, so that introduction of radioactive isotopes provides a convenient marker for studying iodine physiology. The isotope most frequently used is ^{131}I, which has a half-life of 8 days and is considered adequately safe for all patients except pregnant women.

Since radioactive iodine is absorbed and metabolized exactly as is stable iodine, the rate of its metabolism accurately reflects the state of iodine kinetics. Direct proportionality can be assumed, however, only if the total iodine pool is of normal size for the individual being tested. If the iodine pool is expanded, as following ingestion of iodinated medications or contrast media, then the administered dose of radioactive iodine occupies an abnormally small proportion of the total body iodine, and only a small percentage will appear to be metabolized. Similarly, the radioactive iodine will appear to be metabolized very rapidly if the total iodine pool is small, since the administered dose occupies an excessively large proportion of the total supply.

EPITHYROID UPTAKE. In this test, a known dose of radioactive iodine is given either by mouth or intravenously. The rate at which radioactivity increases over the thyroid gland reflects the speed with which the gland traps iodine. The remainder of the administered dose is excreted in the urine.

There are several variants of this procedure, depending upon the timing of the subsequent counts. Radioactivity over the thyroid can be measured as soon as 10 minutes after intravenous administration of a tracer dose. Following oral administration, significant uptake occurs within 1 hour. This follows a rather characteristic curve over the subsequent 24 hours.

Perhaps the most commonly used test of thyroidal radioactive iodine uptake employs an epithyroid count 1 hour and then 24 hours after oral ingestion of a tracer dose. In hyperthyroid patients, the whole process of uptake, hormonal synthesis, and subsequent release of formed hormone may be so rapid that in 24 hours much of the labeled iodine has already left the gland. If the 1-hour count is high, it may be desirable to do a 6-hour count to catch peak activity before thyroidal radioactivity declines. In normal individuals, the epithyroid count made 24 hours after an oral dose of ^{131}I ranges between 5 and 30 percent of the administered radioactivity.

Artefacts That Lower [131]I Uptake. The most common factitious cause of depressed radioactive iodine uptake is intake of exogenous iodine, which enlarges the body's total iodine pool. In addition to the obvious sources of exogenous iodine, such as cough preparations and x-ray media, there may be absorption of iodine through the skin from suntan lotions or nail polish. Enriched breakfast cereals, amebicides, vaginal and anal suppositories, and some vitamin-mineral preparations may be unsuspected offenders in enlarging the iodine pool.

If the administered iodine dose is not absorbed, as in severe diarrhea or intestinal malabsorption syndromes, the thyroidal uptake may appear low even though the gland is functioning normally. Rapid diuresis during the test period may deplete the supply of available iodine, causing an apparently low percentage of iodine uptake. Drugs that depress thyroid function will, of course, depress the radioactive iodine uptake, and ACTH and corticosteroids may have this effect, as may phenylbutazone, arsenicals, and cobalt and other heavy metals. Administration of thiouracils may cause a high 6-hour uptake, but the overall uptake at 24 hours is lower than normal.

Artefacts That Elevate [131]I Uptake. The converse of the above conditions may cause a seemingly high uptake in euthyroid individuals. Hypoiodinism, with resultant failure to dilute the tracer dose, causes a large percentage of the administered dose to appear in the thyroid. Renal failure, with decreased excretion of the administered dose over the 24 hours of the test, may permit excessive amounts of the tracer radioactivity to enter the gland. Because different artefacts have different effects, more than one test of thyroid function usually is advisable.

THYROID STIMULATION TEST. The thyroid gland may have impaired ^{131}I uptake because of intrinsic disease or because it is insufficiently stimulated by the pituitary. Thyroidal responsiveness can be measured following administration of thyroid-stimulating hormone (TSH) which is available commercially. In normal individuals, ^{131}I uptake increases within 8 to 10 hours after TSH is given. Subsequently, the serum level of protein-bound iodine rises, and the thyroid gland itself increases in weight.[9] This latter change is not easily measured, but the increase in iodine uptake and serum hormone level constitutes a valuable diagnostic test. Different workers suggest different dose schedules for this test. Although 5 to 10 USP units of thyrotropin usually provoke increased activity, some workers prefer to stimulate the gland maximally, giving injections of TSH for 3 to 5 days before measuring the stimulated uptake.[9] If the initially low uptake is due to inadequate pituitary stimulation of an intrinsically normal thyroid, TSH administration should increase ^{131}I uptake by at least 10 percent, and the PBI should rise 1.5 μg./dl. or more. The rise in ^{131}I uptake is measured in absolute units, that is, a rise from 15 percent uptake in 24 hours to 25 percent uptake in 24 hours constitutes a 10 percent increase. The rise is not measured as a 10 percent increment of the baseline value. Failure of TSH to increase ^{131}I uptake indicates primary end-organ failure.

Clinical Applications. TSH stimulation of thyroid function is more dramatic in patients with low-normal ^{131}I uptake—in the range of 15 percent. Individuals with considerably higher 24-hour uptakes have a relatively small increment following stimulation, but these patients ordinarily would not need the test. The thyroid stimulation test can be used even if a patient is receiving thyroid replacement therapy, but inorganic iodine not only invalidates ^{131}I uptake results, but may antagonize TSH stimulation as well.

Besides distinguishing primary from secondary hypothyroidism, the TSH test can suggest the level of glandular activity. Patients with a decreased volume of functioning thyroid following subtotal thyroidectomy, irradiation therapy, or thyroiditis may have normal or low-normal ^{131}I uptake but fail to respond to thyrotropin stimulation. Such patients, with low "thyroid reserve," need prolonged observation in order that incipient myxedema may be forestalled.

THYROID SUPPRESSION TEST. The interrelationship of thyroid and pituitary is used in investigating high thyroidal iodine uptake. In normal individuals, administration of thyroid hormone causes lessened ^{131}I uptake, since the increased level of circulating hormone depresses TSH production. If the thyroid-pituitary axis functions normally, ^{131}I uptake after thyroid medication should be less than 20 percent in 24 hours. Patients with Graves' disease have little or no suppression, owing, perhaps in part, to the effect of the long-acting thyroid stimulator. Unfortunately, some patients with nontoxic goiters have inadequate thyroid suppression, and some euthyroid patients have suppression failure for as long as 5 years after successful therapy for Graves' disease.

RESIN T_3 UPTAKE

In the circulating blood, thyroid hormone exists principally as thyroxine, which is bound to thyroid-binding globulin (TBG). Because the amount of circulating TBG is independent of the amount of thyroid hormone it is carrying, the degree to which thyroid-binding globulin is saturated indirectly indicates the level of circulating hormone.

In the T_3 uptake test (Fig. 21), a known amount of ^{131}I-labeled triiodothyronine (T_3) is added to a sample of blood. Unoccupied sites on the thyroid-binding globulin will combine with the added labeled hormone. The leftover labeled hormone remains free and unbound in the plasma. Variations of the test use different methods to measure the unbound labeled T_3. As the test was originally performed, labeled T_3 was added to fluid whole blood. Whatever hormone was left, after the TBG sites were filled, then attached itself to the red cells. The amount of leftover radioactive hormone could be measured by separating plasma from cells and determining red cell radioactivity. A later modification employs plasma alone, avoiding the problem of variable hematocrits. In this technique, labeled T_3 is added to plasma in the presence of finely divided resin particles or a sponge. The resin or sponge adsorbs the leftover hormone, and the radioactivity of the separated material reflects the amount of hormone that could not attach to binding sites.

INTERPRETATION. Both tests are interpreted in the same way. If large quantities of endogenous hormone are present, nearly all the

Principle of T₃ Uptake Test

EUTHYROID

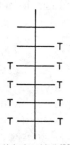

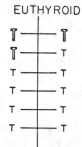

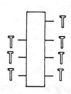

Thyroid-binding globulin(TBG), with 12 available binding sites, 9 of which are occupied by endogenous thyroxine (T)

When 10 units of radioactive thyroxine (T̄) are added, 3 attach to the TBG and 7 are left over

Indicator substance picks up the left-over radioactive hormone, which can easily be measured

HYPOTHYROID

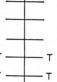

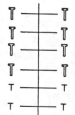

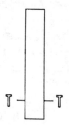

Thyroid-binding globulin with 12 available binding sites, only 4 of which are carrying endogenous hormone

When 10 units of radioactive thyroxine are added, 8 attach to the TBG and only 2 are left over

Indicator substance picks up the 2 left-over radioactive units. The radioactivity of the indicator in hypothyroidism is much less than if normal amounts of thyroid hormone were present.

HYPERTHYROID

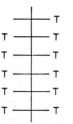

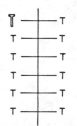

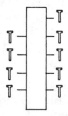

Thyroid binding globulin with 12 available binding sites, 11 of which are occupied by endogenous hormone

When 10 units of radioactive thyroxine are added, only one can attach to the TBG, and 9 are left over

Indicator substance picks up the 9 left-over radioactive units. The radioactivity of the indicator in hyperthyroidism is much greater than if normal amounts of thyroid hormone were present.

Figure 21. Schematic depiction of the principle of the T₃ uptake test. This is an example of competitive binding (see also p. 200, Fig. 13).

available thyroid-binding sites are occupied, and few sites will be free to bind the test dose of labeled hormone. Therefore, a large amount will attach to the secondary binding substance, be this resin or red cells. If there is only a small amount of circulating hormone, many binding sites will be available to combine with the labeled hormone, and relatively little will remain for the secondary binding substance. Thus, in hyperthyroid conditions, the red cell or resin uptake is high; that is, a large amount of administered hormone is left over from the nearly saturated TBG. In hypothyroidism, the red cell or resin uptake is low because the nearly empty TBG attaches most of the labeled dose, and little radioactivity attaches to the secondary site.

This test is useful for patients on iodine-containing medications, since iodine-containing material does not affect the results. The patient is spared exposure to radioisotopes since the radioactive material is added to the blood sample. Unfortunately, the quantity of thyroid-binding globulin varies from individual to individual, and this may affect the results. For example, normal T_3 uptake could occur in a hyperthyroid patient if his TBG level were sufficiently high to accommodate the added tracer dose as well as his own hormone.

ARTEFACTS AFFECTING T_3 UPTAKE. The T_3 uptake does not always correlate well with abnormal results of other tests, possibly because the level of thyroid-binding globulin is somewhat variable. Certain conditions are known to alter the level of TBG and introduce arte-facts into the test's usefulness. Thyroid-binding globulin is elevated in pregnancy, in patients taking estrogens and contraceptive hor-mone combinations, and in patients with estrogen-secreting tumors. In these conditions, resin T_3 uptake is correspondingly lowered to seemingly hypothyroid levels, despite normal thyroid function. Con-versely, androgen administration may decrease the amount of thyroid-binding protein. Conditions that depress the plasma proteins are associated with high T_3 uptakes because the amount of TBG is re-duced. Thus high values are found in nephrotic syndrome and severe liver disease. Dilantin and salicylate, which compete with thyroxine for TBG sites, may cause a seemingly high T_3 uptake.

THYROID ANTIBODIES

Antibodies to three types of thyroid antigens have been noted in patients with various thyroid diseases. Of these, two are essentially research tools, while tests for the third are clinically useful and readily available. Most patients with Hashimoto's thyroiditis (Hashimoto's struma, struma lymphomatosa, chronic lymphocytic thyroiditis) and some with primary myxedema have antibodies to human thyroglobulin, and it is highly probable that these diseases have an autoimmune basis. Thyroglobulin antibodies can be demonstrated quite simply, since they cause agglutination. Tanned red cells or latex particles can be coated with thyroglobulin. When these coated particles are mixed with a serum that contains the antibody, readily visible agglutination occurs. The tanned cell technique is the more sensitive, while the latex particle test is suitable as a screening technique.

The other two antibodies react with the epithelium of thyroid follicles and with an unidentified component of colloid. These may acquire greater clinical significance as they are studied more fully.

CLINICAL APPLICATION. Antibody tests are useful in the differential diagnosis of thyroid enlargement, with antibody usually present in Hashimoto's thyroiditis and absent in cases of nodular colloid goiter or carcinoma. The distinctions are by no means clear-cut, since up to 8 percent of normal individuals may possess thyroglobulin antibodies, and up to 20 percent of patients with "simple" hypothyroidism also may have detectible antibody.[16] It may be that in some thyrotoxic patients, high antibody titers are associated with widespread, progressive thyroiditis which subsequently terminates in hypothyroidism.

Diagnosis of Thyroidal Abnormalities

Thyroid disease can be divided profitably into five clinical categories: simple goiter, hypothyroidism, hyperthyroidism, thyroiditis, and neoplasms. These categories are not mutually exclusive, since transitions occur from any one to any of several others.

SIMPLE GOITER

Simple, or nontoxic, goiter implies an enlarged gland whose function may be normal or depressed. In most cases, enlargement is due to persistent or intermittent TSH stimulation, resulting from persistent or intermittent deficiency of circulating thyroxine. The end result of hypothyroidism or euthyroidism depends on how successfully the gland responds to stimulation.

A euthyroid patient with a so-called simple goiter should have a normal BMR, normal thyroxine, and normal T_3 uptake. The thyroidal ^{131}I uptake may be normal or, if the gland is especially large, increased. TSH stimulation frequently causes relatively little response since the gland is already functioning at or near capacity. Simple goiter is not associated with circulating thyroid antibodies. Some patients with simple goiter gradually become hypothyroid; a few become hyperthyroid after a long course of multinodular goiter.

HYPOTHYROIDISM

Hypothyroidism can occur at any stage of life, from fetus to late adulthood, and may be due to primary thyroidal dysfunction, inadequate pituitary function, or such exogenous factors as drugs or thyroidectomy. In hypothyroidism, the BMR, PBI, or T_4 and epithyroid ^{131}I uptake are depressed, as is red cell or resin T_3 uptake. If the hypothyroidism is due to defective hormonal synthesis, as in severe iodine deficiency or certain congenital disorders, high TSH levels may cause a normal or high epithyroid iodine uptake. Occasionally, thyroid antibody titers are elevated in this condition, suggesting the possibility of autoimmune origin.

Certain tests have particular areas of usefulness. The thyroid stimulation test may differentiate primary thyroidal dysfunction from pituitary insufficiency as the cause of hypothyroidism. Patients with hypothyroidism occasionally resemble patients with nephrosis who also have edema, blunted sensorium, high cholesterol, and a low PBI. The epithyroid ^{131}I uptake may help to make this distinction, being normal in nephrosis. Serum creatine kinase and LDH levels may be increased in hypothyroidism, apparently reflecting skeletal muscle alterations, since it is the muscle LDH isoenzyme that increases.[12]

HYPERTHYROIDISM

Hyperthyroidism may manifest itself in symptoms referable to many organs or systems, notably the cardiovascular system and gastrointestinal tract. The full-blown picture of Graves' disease is not difficult to diagnose, but in many patients, one or several symptoms may throw the classical syndrome out of balance. When hyperthyroidism is a possible diagnosis, elevation of the PBI or T_4, high thyroidal iodine uptake, and high red cell or resin T_3 uptake are reliable indicators. Thyrotropin stimulation alters very little the thyroidal iodine uptake, because hyperthyroidism, like toxic adenoma, may be associated with autonomous activity of the target gland. This autonomy remains unaltered by administration of exogenous thyroid hormones which normally depress TSH levels and reduce the ^{131}I uptake. Thyroid antibodies may occur, but their diagnostic significance is limited. Additional findings in hyperthyroid patients may include low serum cholesterol and creatinuria.

THYROIDITIS

Thyroiditis of the lymphocytic type (Hashimoto's struma) causes the highest thyroglobulin antibody titers. A characteristic finding early in the disease is a low or normal PBI associated with an elevated ^{131}I uptake. This occurs when iodinated protein escapes from the gland into the blood where it affects the PBI test but does not elevate T_4 results. Because it is not hormonally active, however, the pituitary responds with increased TSH production, which results in a high iodine uptake. Ultimately, however, the gland becomes unable to respond, and ^{131}I uptake diminishes to hypothyroid levels if the disease progresses. In some patients, the ^{131}I uptake is higher than normal at 6 hours but declines to normal or even subnormal levels by the 24-hour reading. The abnormal iodinated protein is not butanol-extractable so that in the early stage of Hashimoto's thyroiditis, the BEI or column-T_4 determination will be abnormally lower than the PBI.

TUMORS

Neoplasms of the thyroid gland include adenomas and carcinoma of varying histologic types. Characteristically, adenomas secrete hormones and may cause hyperthyroidism. Hyperfunctioning, or toxic, adenomas are diagnosed most readily by isotopic scanning procedures, in which the adenomas appear as localized areas of increased radioactivity, sometimes surrounded by areas of depressed function. Thyroid carcinomas, on the other hand, usually cause no endocrine disorder, although many well-differentiated tumors concentrate iodine and secrete hormone. History and physical examination may suggest the diagnosis, especially if there is a history of radiation to the neck in childhood. Nodular goiter and Hashimoto's thyroiditis are part of the differential diagnosis, and antibody determinations may be helpful in these cases. In cancer of the thyroid, the BMR, T_4, and tests employing radioactive iodine usually are normal. A localized area of decreased isotope concentration in a scan may suggest an area of malignant change, but it is hardly diagnostic. The diagnosis of thyroid carcinoma cannot be made or excluded by laboratory examination alone.

PARATHYROID GLANDS

The parathyroid glands, which may vary in number from two to ten, produce only one hormone. Parathyroid hormone, or parathormone, regulates calcium and phosphorus metabolism, but its specific activity has been the topic of endless debate and experimentation. Through its effect on plasma calcium concentration, parathormone influences neuromuscular function in all organs and affects a wide spectrum of body functions.

Parathormone Effects

Present concepts suggest that parathormone has at least two specific effects, and it is probably fruitless to argue over which is primary. The hormone mobilizes calcium directly from bone into the blood; it also suppresses renal tubular resorption of phosphate, promoting active urinary excretion of phosphate. Because the serum levels of calcium and inorganic phosphorus are inversely proportional, the two effects are interrelated. The end result is elevation of serum calcium and depression of serum inorganic phosphorus. Parathormone production appears to be regulated by the level of serum calcium, with no influence from tropic hormones.

SERUM CALCIUM AND PHOSPHORUS

The normal concentration of serum calcium is 9 to 11 mg./dl., also expressed as 4.5 to 5.5 mEq./L. Since approximately half is bound to the serum proteins, abnormal protein levels may distort the results of a calcium determination, despite normal ion concentration. The proportion of ionized and bound calcium can be calculated when the total calcium and total protein are known. The normal value for serum inorganic phosphorus is 2.5 to 4 mg./dl. in adults, and 4 to 5 mg./dl. in children.

Hypoparathyroidism

The commonest cause of parathyroid insufficiency is removal of the parathyroid glands by operation, either intentionally in parathyroidectomy or inadvertently in thyroidectomy. Inflammation, trauma, or other destructive processes are less likely to disrupt endocrine function because the glands are widely separated in the neck, and the undisturbed glands can compensate for loss of one or several others. Idiopathic hypofunction can occur in childhood or maturity, causing destruction, scarring, and atrophy which may have an autoimmune basis. Because the symptoms are prompt and dramatic and because physicians are alert to the possibility, acute hypoparathyroidism is readily diagnosed after operations on the neck. Chronic hypoparathyroidism presents a more difficult diagnostic problem. Symptoms in either form arise from low serum concentration of ionized calcium. Nonparathyroid causes of persistently low serum calcium include rickets, osteomalacia, severe steatorrhea, and renal failure.

TETANY

Tetany, a condition of increased neuromuscular irritability, may occur when the serum calcium drops to 7.5 mg./dl. or lower. Tetany sometimes occurs in patients with alkalosis or hyperventilation, but in these conditions the normal total calcium level in the serum eliminates hypoparathyroidism as a possible cause. Neuro-muscular irritability may be manifest as cramps of the skeletal muscles or as laryngospasm, hypermotility of the gastrointestinal tract, or convulsive disorders. Chronic hypoparathyroidism also may present with central nervous system disorders, lenticular cataracts, and growth disorders of the hair, nails, and skin.

LABORATORY FINDINGS

The diagnosis of hypoparathyroidism depends upon demonstrating consistent depression of serum calcium below 7.5 mg./dl., with elevation of serum phosphate to 4 to 6 mg./dl. The serum magnesium level may be reduced from the normal of 2.0 or 2.5 mg./dl. to 1.5 to 1.8 mg./dl. Urinary calcium usually is absent, and addition of Sulkowitch reagent to the urine sample produces no turbidity. Phosphaturia is difficult to evaluate because it varies with dietary intake; even without parathormone activity, increased intake of phosphate results in increased excretion.

EXCRETION TESTS. The Ellsworth-Howard test provides a fairly reliable index of parathyroid function, comparing unmodified phosphate excretion against excretion stimulated by exogenous parathormone. A standard dose of parathyroid extract is given, and phosphate excretion is measured at hourly intervals for 3 to 5 hours. In normal individuals, phosphate excretion rises five- or sixfold; in patients with hypoparathyroidism, the elevation may be tenfold or greater. Certain patients whose symptoms suggest hypoparathyroidism have a rise no greater than twofold. This condition is known as pseudohypoparathyroidism, due probably to faulty renal response to parathormone rather than to hormonal insufficiency.

Other tests of calcium or phosphorus balance require the strict supervision and standardization of a metabolic ward. Nonparathyroid causes of hypocalcemia include excessive fecal calcium loss in intestinal malabsorption syndromes and also phosphate retention due to renal disease. Distinction from hypoparathyroidism usually causes no difficulty. Vitamin D deficiency or rickets of renal origin also causes hypocalcemia along with more obvious signs of the primary disease.

Hyperparathyroidism

Excessive parathormone activity may be due to hyperplastic enlargement of all the glands or to adenomatous enlargement of only one or two. Sometimes hyperplasia is idiopathic, but frequently diseases of other organs cause changes in mineral metabolism that induce increased parathormone secretion. Since primary hyperparathyroidism damages kidneys, bones, lungs, and stomach, and diseases of each of these organs can induce secondary hyperparathyroidism, it may be difficult to distinguish the cart from the horse.

CLINICAL SYMPTOMS

The symptoms of primary hyperparathyroidism develop insidiously, usually in adults and more often in females than in males. Increased calcium is mobilized from bone, and increased phosphorus is lost in the urine, leading to a variety of symptoms due to hypercalcemia, skeletal changes, and renal disease. The clinical symptoms almost always include weakness, anorexia, and vague aches and pains. Other nonspecific findings may include hyperextensibility of the joints, bradycardia, constipation, and anemia. The increased urinary solute load often produces polyuria, which is followed by polydipsia. Renal parenchymal damage and nephrolithiasis may impair the ability to concentrate urine above a specific gravity of 1.022. In advanced hyperparathyroidism, widespread bone cysts may occur, often associated with osteoporosis, pathologic fractures, incomplete healing, and bizarre skeletal deformities. Some of the excessive circulating calcium may be deposited as ectopic calcification of kidneys, lungs, stomach, blood vessels, or myocardium. Less readily explained is the frequent occurrence of intractable peptic ulcer, pancreatitis, or deposition of corneal opacities (band keratitis).

LABORATORY FINDINGS

The laboratory findings in uncomplicated hyperparathyroidism are characteristic. The serum calcium is elevated above 12 mg./dl. and often much higher. The serum inorganic phosphorus is decreased below 2.5 mg./dl. The urine contains large quantities of calcium and phosphorus, even if the diet is relatively low in phosphates. The serum alkaline phosphatase rises only with extensive skeletal involvement fairly late in the disease.

When hypercalcemia suggests hyperparathyroidism, several tests of mineral metabolism may provide moderate assistance. Intravenous infusion of calcium, which normally suppresses parathormone secretion and thus decreases urinary phosphate excretion, does not alter urinary phosphate levels in primary hyperparathyroidism. Unfortunately, other causes of hypercalcemia may produce similar results and, even in normal individuals, diurnal variation of phosphate excretion may be great enough to distort the test results.

PHOSPHATE REABSORPTION. Tubular reabsorption of phosphate can be measured directly, but the results are valid only if other urinary functions are demonstrated to be normal. The test itself is simple enough, requiring only collection of a timed urine specimen and a blood sample taken during the collecting period. The calculation compares relative serum and urine levels of creatinine and phosphorus, using the formula

$$TRP = \left[1 - \frac{UP \times SC}{UC \times SP} \right] \times 100$$

where TRP is the tubular reabsorption of phosphorus expressed as a percentage, U refers to urine concentration, S to serum concentration, C to creatinine, and P to phosphorus. The normal TRP is 90 percent or greater; in hyperparathyroidism, values are less than 85 percent.

DIFFERENTIAL DIAGNOSIS

The difficulty in diagnosing hyperparathyroidism is in distinguishing it from other causes of hypercalcemia. The most common nonparathyroid etiologies for hypercalcemia are malignant tumors, with or without apparent skeletal involvement; multiple myeloma; sarcoidosis; therapy with thiazide drugs; vitamin D intoxication; and milk-alkali syndrome. Moreover, calcium mobilization accompanying enforced inactivity (acute bone atrophy[14]) may raise serum calcium to disturbing levels. A 10-day course of cortisone may assist in differential diagnosis, since serum calcium levels decline in patients with sarcoidosis, myeloma, and vitamin D overload and are unresponsive when hyperparathyroidism exists. The hypercalcemia accompanying malignant tumors responds unpredictably.[14] Thiazide-induced hypercalcemia usually is mild and recedes within a month after cessation of therapy. Increased serum protein levels elevate total circulating calcium at a rate of approximately 0.8 mg./dl. calcium for each 1 gm./dl. of elevated albumin or globulin,[32] and serum protein studies should be a part of every hypercalcemia workup. Parathormone can be measured directly by radioimmunoassay, but this may not be diagnostic when hypercalcemia results from the secretion of parathormone-like substance from solid malignant tumors. Table 19 outlines characteristic serum and urine alterations in many conditions affecting calcium and phosphorus metabolism.

SECONDARY HYPERPARATHYROIDISM

Secondary hyperparathyroidism is more common than primary hyperplasia or adenoma. The usual cause is advanced renal disease, in which phosphate retention causes reciprocal reduction of serum calcium. The low calcium level stimulates the parathyroids, which may overrespond and become hyperplastic. In such cases, both serum calcium and serum phosphate are elevated, and the skeletal, neuromuscular, and gastrointestinal complications of hyperparathyroidism are superimposed on the clinical picture of severe renal disease. The renal disease usually is well documented, and elevations of serum phosphates, urea, and creatinine are diagnostic. In the presence of demonstrated renal disease and elevated serum phosphate, an elevated or even high-normal calcium level indicates secondary hyperparathyroidism. Hyperparathyroidism may complicate renal disease without overt hypercalcemia, and skeletal changes may be the first sign of its presence.

PANCREAS

Pancreatic endocrine function resides in the islets of Langerhans, which produce two different, major hormones. The beta cells pro-

Table 19. Summary of Chemical Features of Diseases with Disturbed Plasma Calcium and Phosphate*

Disease	Serum			Urine	
	Calcium	Phosphate	Alkaline Phosphatase	Calcium	Phosphate
Hyperpara-thyroidism	Increased	Decreased	Normal or increased	Increased	Increased
Paget's disease	Normal	Normal	Increased	Normal	Normal
Hypopara-thyroidism	Decreased	Increased	Normal	Decreased	Decreased
Renal insufficiency	Decreased	Increased	Normal or increased	Decreased	Decreased
Osteomalacia	Decreased or normal	Decreased	Increased	Decreased	Decreased
Senile osteoporosis	Normal	Normal	Normal	Normal	Normal
Multiple myeloma	Normal to increased	Normal	Normal	Normal to increased	Normal to decreased
Milk-alkali syndrome	Increased	Normal to increased	Normal	Normal to decreased	Normal to decreased
Vitamin D intoxication	Increased	Increased	Normal	Increased	Decreased
Metastatic carcinoma	Normal to increased	Normal	Normal to increased	Increased	Normal
Sarcoidosis	Increased	Normal to increased	Normal to increased	Increased	Decreased
Hyper-ventilation (alkalosis)	Normal	Normal	Normal	Normal	Normal

*From Bernstein, D. S., and Thorn, G. W., in Wintrobe, M. M., et al. (eds.): *Harrison's Principles of Internal Medicine.* ed. 6. McGraw-Hill, New York, 1970.

duce insulin, the body's hypoglycemic agent, while the alpha cells produce glucagon, a hyperglycemic agent that promotes glycogenolysis.

Diabetes Mellitus

The term *diabetes mellitus* denotes merely the presence of large volumes of sugar-containing urine. Many different sugars can be abnormal constituents of urine, but glucose is the relevant sugar in diabetes. Many events can provoke a positive test for urinary glucose (see p. 569); in diabetes, the urine contains glucose because high blood glucose levels impose so much glucose on the glomerular filtrate that tubular reabsorptive capacity is exceeded. Many circumstances can induce elevations, either acute or long-standing, of blood glucose levels. Diabetes mellitus refers to a defect of carbohydrate metabolism due, at least in part, to genetic factors and characterized by a relative or absolute lack of insulin activity, often associated with abnormalities of nerves and blood vessel walls.

OTHER EFFECTS ON CARBOHYDRATE METABOLISM

Glucose metabolism is affected by several hormones other than insulin, which is the product of beta cells of the islets of Langerhans, the endocrine portion of the pancreas. *Glucagon,* produced by the alpha cells in the pancreatic islets, promotes release of glucose from stored glycogen, thereby inducing short-lived hyperglycemia. Glucagon is under increasing scrutiny as a significant factor in diabetic ketoacidosis, and there is evidence that effective glucagon regulation is faulty in diabetics,[26] but its role remains highly speculative. *Epinephrine* and *norepinephrine,* products of the adrenal medulla, stimulate glycogenolysis and gluconeogenesis, the manufacture of glucose from fatty acid or amino acid precursors. Moreover, they decrease the rate at which muscle cells utilize glucose and inhibit insulin secretion. *Hormones of the adrenal cortex* markedly enhance gluconeogenesis and also antagonize the effects of insulin. *Growth hormone* stimulates protein synthesis from amino acid precursors, thereby reducing gluconeogenesis. Its overall effect is to increase blood sugar levels by reducing peripheral utilization of carbohydrate and antagonizing the effects of insulin. In *pregnancy,* insulin activity is lessened by an increase in plasma free fatty acids and probably by placental degradation of insulin. Pregnancy also stimulates secretion of adrenal corticosteroids and of *placental lactogen* (see p. 530), the effects of which mimic those of growth hormone.

DISEASES WITH SECONDARY EFFECTS. Hyperglycemia, often transient but sometimes prolonged, commonly accompanies acute illness severe enough to constitute systemic stress. Infections, burns, and acute liver disease are especially likely to cause a diabetes-like syndrome that disappears upon recovery. The complicated, prolonged metabolic and hormonal burden of pregnancy provokes many changes in carbohydrate metabolism (see p. 534). Adrenal gland hyperfunction, either cortical or medullary, alters carbohydrate metabolism; exogenous administration of adrenal hormones complicates interpretation of most tests of carbohydrate metabolism. Severe liver disease and chronic hepatic failure impair many mechanisms of glucose homeostasis, leading to conditions of hyperglycemia or hypoglycemia. Estrogen administration interferes with glucose regulation, as does prolonged over- or underconsumption of carbohydrates.

PANCREATIC DAMAGE. Although the pancreas has impressive reserve capacity, loss of more than 80 percent of functioning gland tissue can cause insulin deficiency. Experimentally, several drugs can induce diabetes on this basis, but in human patients, tumors and severe inflammatory destruction are the agents of tissue loss. The massive deposition of hemosiderin that occurs in hemochromatosis sometimes damages enough pancreatic cells that diabetes ensues. Hemosiderin is a colored compound, and tissues in which there are large quantities often have a rusty or golden appearance; the diabetes that occurs after long-standing pigment deposition is sometimes called *bronze diabetes.*

DIAGNOSING DIABETES MELLITUS

PREVALENCE. Since precise diagnostic standards for diabetes do not exist, it is difficult to state exactly when diabetes is present and when it is not. Many patients with established disease are sufficiently asymptomatic that they do not seek medical attention and hence remain undiagnosed. Some patients with obvious genetic predisposition exhibit overt diabetes under certain conditions of weight, diet, or hormonal status but not under others. All these factors make it difficult to state the frequency of diabetes in the population.

Diabetes becomes increasingly prevalent as age increases. It is more common in women than in men and in obese populations as compared to groups of lean people. One overall estimate is that diabetes affects between 1 and 5 percent of the entire U.S. population, achieving a peak frequency, in one study, of 18 percent in women at age 70.[25]

Although genetic influences are clearly important, no distinct inheritance pattern is obvious. Most workers believe that several genes are involved and that somatic influences are also important. Concordance in identical twins is only 70 percent and in fraternal twins is 10 percent.[8,29] In the general population, diabetes in a close family member imposes a two- to fourfold risk that an individual will develop diabetes. Association with HLA-D phenotype has been established for juvenile-onset diabetes but not for maturity-onset disease.[28] Genetic transmission, related at least in part to what seems to be a dominant gene, can be discerned for maturity-onset diabetes but less clearly for that of juvenile onset.

PRESENTATION. Diabetes can present in two fashions sufficiently distinct from each other that many workers consider them to be two different diseases. In *juvenile-onset diabetes,* the patient is usually younger than 25 (often a child or adolescent) and slender. Onset is sudden and symptomatic, and control is difficult. Circulating insulin levels are virtually zero, and oral antidiabetic agents that work by stimulating insulin synthesis have no therapeutic effect. *Maturity-onset* diabetes tends to affect fat people over 40. The disease may be asymptomatic and usually responds predictably to relatively simple treatment regimens. Weight loss alone may correct the carbohydrate abnormality, and insulin dosage, if needed, remains fairly constant. Oral diabetic agents may be extremely useful in this group.

Another set of diagnostic categories relates to the stage to which this constitutionally determined disease has progressed. *Overt diabetes* is the active disease, accompanied by glycosuria and fasting hyperglycemia. *Chemical diabetes* is the condition in which the patient's fasting blood sugar is normal but carbohydrate loads are handled poorly. Postprandial blood glucose levels are high, and the glucose tolerance curve has a diabetic shape. In *suspected diabetes,* both fasting glucose and the glucose tolerance curve are normal under normal conditions, but abnormal glucose tolerance can be elicited by such stresses as pregnancy, systemic illness, or administration of corticosteroids. Hardest of all to conceptualize and almost impossible to diagnose except in the identical twin of a known diabetic is *pre-diabetes.* This refers to the metabolic state of an individual who possesses the one or several genes that predispose to the disease but who has not yet developed any defect in carbohydrate metabolism.

SCREENING FOR DIABETES. For a disease as widespread and as protractedly degenerative as diabetes, it is important to have simple, inexpensive techniques to single out those who deserve more detailed diagnostic consideration. Index of suspicion is important. Persons with a family history of diabetes or a personal history of obstetrical complications, premature onset of vascular disease, obesity, or hypoglycemic episodes should be kept under closer surveillance than otherwise normal persons in the same age groups.

The simplest procedure is *screening urine for glucose*. Paper strips impregnated with glucose oxidase are both sensitive and specific for glycosuria, and the technique is simplicity itself. A patient, hitherto unsuspected of metabolic abnormality, with a positive glucose dip strip test for urinary glucose should be subjected to further testing. A negative test is satisfactory evidence that glycosuria is absent. This does not mean that glucose metabolism is perfectly normal; it simply means the patient is not spilling glucose at that time and probably does not have florid diabetes mellitus.

The *fasting blood sugar* test is slightly more difficult to perform than urine testing, since it requires venipuncture and laboratory analysis of the sample. In an adequately nourished patient, a fasting blood sugar within normal limits (below 90 to 110 mg./dl., depending on method) effectively rules out overt diabetes. A fasting blood glucose, drawn and analyzed under appropriate conditions, above 120 mg./dl. is fairly strong evidence that diabetes is present. Further testing is hardly required in patients with significantly elevated fasting glucose levels.

An elevated *postprandial blood glucose level* indicates some abnormality in glucose metabolism but cannot be considered adequate for diagnosing diabetes. Blood glucose should return to fasting levels 3 hours after eating, but if the patient is in an unknown metabolic condition and the meal has not been standardized for carbohydrate content or speed of absorption, the results may be difficult to interpret. Post-breakfast sampling is usually more informative than samples drawn after lunch.[6]

ORAL GLUCOSE TOLERANCE TEST. Either inadequate nutritional state or excess carbohydrate can impair glucose metabolism. The patient should consume a diet adequate in protein and calories, containing 150 to 300 gm. of carbohydrate daily for at least 3 days before the test. Patients on a weight-reduction diet should discontinue it for 5 days before the test; medications should be discontinued for 3 days before the test; and oral contraceptives should be discontinued for a full cycle before testing.

Several different protocols are used for glucose tolerance testing.

Glucose loads vary from a standard dose of 100 gm. to levels based on actual weight, "ideal" weight, or calculated surface area. Mild disagreement also exists about the levels at which an unequivocal diagnosis of diabetes can be made. Most protocols stop after 2 or 3 hours, but in patients with early or equivocal disease, it may be useful to continue the test for 5 hours. Values at 4 and 5 hours which are significantly below the fasting level signify inability to mobilize stored glucose appropriately and may be the first signs of inadequate carbohydrate homeostasis. Deficient renal function and hyperglycemia impair glucose utilization; the hypermetabolism of hyperthyroidism causes a prompt, elevated peak followed by a decline that is more rapid than normal. Liver disease or heavy alcohol intake may also affect the results. Glucose tolerance patterns may vary considerably for the same individual at different times, even under well-standardized conditions. When results are borderline or seemingly normal in a patient whose clinical story is highly suspicious, it is worthwhile to repeat the study a month or two later.

Patients with a normal fasting blood glucose and abnormal glucose tolerance curves may present a problem in management. Treatment with insulin or oral hypoglycemic agents is usually not indicated, but if the patient is overweight, weight reduction should be strongly promoted. Such patients have substantially increased likelihood of developing symptomatic diabetes in the next several years. Weight reduction improves blood pressure levels as well as carbohydrate metabolism and can be expected to reduce the likelihood of severely progressive vascular disease. Unfortunately, the relationships among blood glucose levels, consistency of diabetic "control," and development of vascular complications are by no means clear-cut.

COMPLICATIONS OF DIABETES

CHRONIC CHANGES. Once diabetes has been diagnosed, treatment is usually monitored by repeated urinalysis for glucose and by periodic examination of blood glucose levels and levels of glycosylated hemoglobins.[40] Systemic changes due to microangiopathies, arteriosclerosis, and neuropathy cannot be monitored by laboratory examinations, but there is much interest in observing the correlation between degenerative changes and increased levels of glycosylated "minor" hemoglobins.[41] Another indication for repeated urinalysis is the increased incidence of urinary tract infections in diabetics. If pyelonephritis occurs, urinalysis reveals proteinuria, pyuria, and bacteriuria, along with increased glycosuria and ketonuria. Progressive kidney damage due to diffuse glomerulosclerosis may cause progressive functional change, terminating in excretion of protein and casts, but nodular glomerulosclerosis (Kimmelstiehl-Wilson lesion) does not have a characteristic urinary profile.

Another chronic complication of diabetes is nerve root damage, which may increase spinal fluid protein levels to 50 to 100 mg./dl. but does not cause pleocytosis.

ACUTE KETOACIDOSIS. Of the acute complications of diabetes, ketoacidosis is the one in which laboratory findings change most rapidly and most critically. At the beginning, blood glucose is elevated and there are ketones in the serum. When the body cannot meet its caloric requirements from circulating glucose, it mobilizes fat as an energy source, and the ketone bodies—acetoacetic acid, acetone, and beta-hydroxybutyric acid—are end products of this inefficient metabolic expedient. The normal serum ketone level is zero. Changes in the ketone level can be monitored by testing suitably diluted serum or plasma with Acetest powder. Large quantities of glucose and ketones appear in the urine, requiring excretion of cations to balance ketotic acids. Ketone bodies in the blood cause acidosis, and as the blood pH falls, respiration is increased. At a pH of 7.2, Kussmaul respiration may become obvious; this reduces the body's CO_2 supply but does not get rid of excess hydrogen ions.

LABORATORY FINDINGS. The results of diuresis, cation loss, and massive respiratory effort include depletion of sodium, potassium, calcium, and other cations; pronounced drop in CO_2 combining power; progressive dehydration with consequent fall in renal plasma flow and glomerular filtration rate; accentuated hyperglycemia because of diminishing renal clearance; temperature elevation due to dehydration; and leukocytosis of 15,000 to 30,000/mm.[3] due simply to these physiologic derangements. If infection was the precipitating event, fever and leukocytosis will be even greater.

Potassium metabolism is especially sensitive to these changes. When hydrogen ions become more numerous in the blood, they enter the fixed cells in exchange for intracellular potassium which comes out into the plasma. The serum potassium level changes with influx of intracellular potassium and irretrievable loss through the kidneys, and the blood value at any given moment cannot reflect the massive depletion of whole-body supplies.[1] Serum sodium determinations are affected by the same complex problems.

DIFFERENTIAL DIAGNOSIS. The differential diagnosis of diabetic ketoacidosis frequently must include hypoglycemic coma and salicylate intoxication. Blood glucose levels easily distinguish diabetic coma from insulin coma, and a still more rapid distinction may be obtained in doubtful cases by treating the patient with intravenous injection of 100 ml. of a 50 percent solution of glucose. If the problem is diabetic ketoacidosis, an additional 50 gm. of glucose will not aggravate the problem, but if the problem is hypoglycemia, dramatic improvement occurs. Further differentiating points are that hypoglycemia is usually of rapid onset and is characterized by shallow respiration rather than the deep Kussmaul respiration of diabetic coma. Salicylate intoxication may superficially resemble diabetic coma, since acidosis and Kussmaul respiration frequently are observed, and reducing substances are present in urine. Salicylate metabolites can be distinguished readily from urinary glucose by means of glucose oxidase testing, and the blood glucose, of course, is not elevated in salicylism.

Hypoglycemia

Symptomatic hypoglycemia usually results from functioning islet cell tumors, either benign or malignant, but sometimes occurs with early diabetes or with "functional" hyperinsulinism in which no histologic lesion is present. More rarely still, severe liver disease, pituitary or adrenal insufficiency, inborn enzymatic defects, or nonpancreatic tumors may cause spontaneous hypoglycemia. The diagnosis of hypoglycemia is made when low blood glucose levels accompany objective or subjective symptoms. Whipple's triad, originally applied to the diagnosis of islet cell tumors, documents hypoglycemia due to any cause: symptomatic attack, with blood glucose level less than 50 mg./dl. and relief of symptoms by glucose administration.

TOLBUTAMIDE TEST

Insulin-producing tumors occur most frequently in middle life and usually are benign. The distinction between benign and malignant may be difficult even after microscopic examination, and multiple tumors are common in either form. Characteristic findings in insulin-producing tumors are increasingly severe symptoms during prolonged fast, aggravation by exercise, and a positive tolbutamide test. In the tolbutamide test, blood samples drawn 15, 30, 45, 60, 90, 120, 150,

and 180 minutes after intravenous administration of 1 gm. of tolbutamide are compared with the fasting glucose level. In normal individuals or in those with functional hyperinsulinism, blood glucose returns to at least 70 percent of fasting level within 3 hours. Patients
with insulinomas have continued, marked hypoglycemia, sometimes
with neurologic symptoms that force the physician to administer
glucose and terminate the test. If insulin assays are available, elevated plasma insulin activity can be shown to follow this stimulus.
The tolbutamide test cannot be used if fasting glucose levels are
below 50 mg./dl., and false-positive results may occur in cases of
severe liver disease, alcoholism, starvation, and occasional nonpancreatic tumors.

EFFECT OF FASTING

Induction of a 24- to 72-hour fast may be helpful for diagnosis because, in functional hyperinsulinism, fasting produces little alteration
in the glucose level, and exercise after a period of fasting causes
blood glucose to rise. In patients with insulin-producing tumors, the
blood glucose level falls progressively during the fast, and exercise
may induce hypoglycemia if the fast itself has not produced symptoms.

REACTIVE HYPOGLYCEMIA

In reactive functional hyperinsulinism, rising blood sugar levels
appear to stimulate excessive insulin secretion. Thus, after large
amounts of carbohydrate are consumed, a normal mild hyperglycemia may be followed in 2 to 4 hours by signs and symptoms of
hypoglycemia. An oral glucose tolerance test reveals the same pattern;
glucose levels rise no higher than normal, but decline is excessive
and hypoglycemia occurs in 2 to 4 hours. A type of reactive hypoglycemia may occur in mild diabetes; in these cases, insulin secretion
appears to be delayed. Blood sugar levels rise to diabetic levels, and
then a delayed, overenthusiastic insulin response causes subsequent
hypoglycemia.

Noninsulin-Producing Islet Cell Adenomas

Hormonal products of nonbeta islet cell tumors produce the Zollinger-
Ellison (Z-E) syndrome of refractory, often atypically located gastric
ulcers; intense gastric hyperacidity; and, often, watery diarrhea and

malabsorption. These tumors, which may be single or multiple, produce enormous quantities of gastrin, which stimulates enormous gastric acid production, which in turn produces mucosal ulceration, impaired fat metabolism, and sometimes impaired vitamin B_{12} absorption,[34] each of which can lead to further symptoms. Surgical extirpation of the tumors may be difficult or impossible, but total gastrectomy prevents acid production and usually provides the best cure. After successful gastrectomy, extrapancreatic tumor nodules may disappear.

ACID SECRETION

Zollinger-Ellison syndrome should be considered when medical management fails to control peptic ulcer symptoms. Measurement of gastric acidity is the best diagnostic tool but is not infallible. The diagnosis is suggested when overnight free acid secretion is 100 mEq. or more, if 1-hour basal output exceeds 15 mEq., or if basal secretion is 60 percent or more of maximally stimulated secretion. Serum gastrin can be measured by radioimmunoassay, with Z-E patients having tenfold or greater elevations over normal range. This is not foolproof either, since gastrin secretion may be intermittent, and a single specimen may be unrevealing.

OTHER SYNDROMES

A histologically different nonbeta cell tumor produces a different clinical picture, characterized by massive watery diarrhea (up to 8 L. in 24 hours), hypokalemic alkalosis, and sometimes a diabetic glucose tolerance curve but without gastric hyperacidity. The hormonal product of this tumor has not been characterized. While complete tumor resection promptly relieves the symptoms, recurrences are not uncommon.

Pancreatic islet cell tumors frequently are part of the syndrome of polyendocrine adenomatosis, with peptic ulceration present in more than half the cases. Demonstration of nonbeta cell adenomas should prompt careful examination for evidence of parathyroid, pituitary, adrenal, or thyroid adenomas as well.

OVARIES

The ovaries contain three types of cells: germ cells, somatic cells of the cortex, and medullary cells which share a common origin with the adrenal cortex. The germ cells have no endocrine function. Rather, they are influenced by pituitary and other hormones and propelled toward ovulation or involution. The cortical cells differentiate into the granulosa and theca cells of the ovarian follicle which produce estrogens and progestins, respectively. Medullary cells, usually scattered sparsely at the hilus, retain the capacity to produce androgens, usually in very small amounts.

Hormones and Their Effects

The ovaries and the pituitary are linked in a reciprocal relationship. Critical levels of estrogen induce secretion of follicle-stimulating hormone (FSH) which in turn promotes estrogen production. Follicle-stimulating hormone and luteinizing hormone (LH) together induce ovulation, after which FSH and estrogen levels decline, while LH and progesterone secretion increase. Under the influence of LH, the ruptured follicle becomes the corpus luteum, and luteotropic hormone promotes continued elaboration of progesterone. Shortly before menstruation, progesterone secretion declines, and there is a second, but lower, peak of estrogen production.

Progesterone and the estrogens are steroids, evolving by way of cholesterol from acetate fractions. The pathway is such that progesterone is a precursor of testosterone, which is a precursor of the estrogens. Many estrogen metabolites have been isolated, but the three principal substances, in order of diminishing potency, are estradiol, estrone, and estriol. In the maturing child, estrogens induce the secondary sex characteristics and closure of the epiphyses. Estrogen, in the female adult, thickens and cornifies the vaginal mucosa and produces uterine enlargement, salt and water retention, and mammary stimulation. Estrogen renders the endometrium sensitive to subsequent stimulation by progesterone. Progesterone has its major effect on the endometrium, which enters the secretory phase and becomes ready for implantation of the blastocyst if fertilization has occurred.

Measuring Ovarian Secretion

Measurement of the ovarian hormones is difficult. Both bioassay and chemical methods are available, but the chemical methods are difficult and expensive, while the bioassay methods are time-consuming and, like all bioassays, rather difficult to standardize. Radioimmunoassay gives the most sensitive and reproducible results. Progesterone usually is measured as its principal excreted metabolite, pregnanediol. Estrogen and pregnanediol determinations involve enzymic hydrolysis and chromatographic separation followed by spectrophotometry.

A NOTE ON PREGNANETRIOL. Pregnanediol should not be confused with pregnanetriol, despite the similarity of names. Pregnanetriol arises, not from progesterone, but from 17-hydroxyprogesterone, a precursor in adrenal corticoid synthesis, and elevated pregnanetriol levels occur in congenital adrenal cortical hyperplasia.

PROGESTERONE EFFECTS

Because direct hormonal measurement is somewhat difficult, ovarian function is commonly evaluated indirectly. In the adult, estrogenic function can be inferred from the degree of cornification of vaginal epithelial cells. Progesterone activity is evaluated by the presence or absence of secretory changes in an endometrial biopsy taken at the appropriate phase of the menstrual cycle. Body temperature change also indicates progesterone activity; a sustained rise of 1°F. in the basal temperature implies that ovulation has occurred.

Hypofunction

Ovarian hypofunction usually means estrogen deficiency, since an isolated deficiency of progesterone is rare. Combined deficiency of estrogen and progesterone results in menstrual irregularities and difficulty in conceiving. Estrogen deficiency may be due to primary ovarian insufficiency; or normal ovaries may be stimulated inadequately if pituitary gonadotropins are deficient. In the prepubertal child, primary or secondary ovarian hypofunction causes failure of sexual maturation and eunuchoid skeletal growth. Loss of ovarian function in a previously normal mature woman causes amenorrhea or oligomenorrhea, and this may be followed by regression of certain secondary sex characteristics. Actual masculinization does not occur unless androgen excess accompanies estrogen deficiency.

INSUFFICIENCY DUE TO PITUITARY PROBLEMS

Secondary ovarian insufficiency is diagnosed by demonstration of persistently low levels of pituitary gonadotropins. Since this may be due to tumor, infarction, infiltration, or idiopathic glandular failure, evaluation should include measurement of other pituitary functions, as well as evaluation of radiographic changes, visual fields, and other tests relating to potential disorders of the pituitary.

INSUFFICIENCY DUE TO OVARIAN PROBLEMS

Primary ovarian insufficiency nearly always is associated with high levels of pituitary gonadotropins, once the age of normal puberty is attained. Primary insufficiency may be due to congenital hypoplasia or dysgenesis of the ovaries, scarring from infections, or changes from irradiation or surgery. In the normal menopause, pituitary gonadotropins reach high levels, and in the condition described as *premature climacteric,* there is a similar elevation of gonadotropin associated with diminished numbers of germinal follicles and diminished ovarian responsiveness.

CHROMOSOMAL ABNORMALITY. In *gonadal dysgenesis* (Turner's syndrome), gonadotropin levels are high because there is no ovarian tissue to respond. In this condition, the individual has only 45 chromosomes instead of the normal complement of 46. The missing chromosome is the second sex chromosome—the patient has neither a Y chromosome, which induces testicular development, nor the second X chromosome of the female genotype. This condition can be recognized by the absence, from epithelial cells, of the Barr body, a tiny mass of chromatin material thought to represent the involuted, inactive second X chromosome.

SYSTEMIC DISEASES

Ovarian hypofunction may be caused by certain systemic diseases such as chronic renal disease, advanced malignant disease, severe hypothyroidism, anorexia nervosa, or other conditions of generalized hypometabolism. In some cases, psychogenic factors appear to cause amenorrhea by depressing gonadotropin secretion. Depression of gonadotropin secretion also may occur in patients with androgenic adrenal hyperfunction. Apparently, the high levels of androgen inhibit gonadotropin secretion.

Hyperfunction

PRECOCIOUS MATURATION

If the prepubertal ovary produces any hormones, it is hyperfunctioning. This leads to early appearance of female secondary sex characteristics and the occurrence of uterine bleeding. If hypothalamic disease is the cause of early maturation, cyclical gonadotropin and ovarian hormone production may lead to ovulation and fertility at a very early age. Such children demonstrate all the cyclic changes in hormone excretion, vaginal cornification, and endometrial morphology that occur in mature women. In many cases, no morphologic lesion is found in the hypothalamus and, except for early maturation (i.e., menarche before age 10) and short stature, the children prove to be normal. The children are short because the adult levels of estrogen cause the epiphyses to close very early.

In a few cases, precocious puberty is due to granulosa-theca cell tumors of the ovary. These children have high urinary levels of estrogen, low levels of gonadotropin, and ordinarily a palpable ovarian mass.

Another cause for early feminization and estrogen excretion is ingestion of exogenous estrogens. This may occur when children swallow estrogen-containing pills or cosmetics belonging to adults, or it may be due to the presence of contaminating estrogenic compounds in other drugs.

OVARIAN TUMORS

Relatively few ovarian tumors produce hormones. The most common hormonally active ovarian neoplasms are granulosa-theca cell tumors, which account for approximately 10 percent of the solid ovarian tumors. These secrete estrogens which appear in the urine at very high levels. Frequently noted are other changes related to excessive estrogen production, such as irregular uterine bleeding, uterine and breast enlargement, and salt and water retention. Certain rare ovarian tumors, notably the arrhenoblastomas, produce androgens. Virilizing signs generally include hirsutism, acne, deepening of the voice, clitoral enlargement, involution of the breasts, and cessation of menses. Despite rather marked clinical virilization, urinary 17-ketosteroids may not be markedly elevated. Adrenal disease is a more common cause of significant 17-ketosteroid excess, especially congenital hyperplasia in children and virilizing adrenal carcinoma at all ages.

Uterine Bleeding

Functional uterine bleeding, an extremely common complaint, might be considered evidence of ovarian hyperfunction in the sense that excessive estrogen stimulates an endometrium insufficiently counter-balanced by progesterone. The precise defect may be difficult to pinpoint, since rather subtle upsets of the pituitary-ovary relationship can result in irregular uterine bleeding. Once coagulation disorders, pregnancy, and infection have been eliminated as causes, laboratory procedures offer little for diagnosis. Endometrial biopsy or curettage usually shows only changes due to estrogen stimulation, but cu-rettage is advisable, especially in older women, to rule out endo-metrial carcinoma.

Female Infertility

Diagnostic regimens for involuntary infertility are beyond the scope of this discussion, but a few points should be considered. In addition to evaluation of the general health of each partner, certain specific laboratory procedures are indicated. Patency of the cervix, uterus, and fallopian tubes should be determined by insufflation or dye instillation.

LABORATORY FINDINGS

Evidence that ovulation and progesterone secretion have occurred is usually indirect. If the endometrium, at the onset of the menses, has a secretory pattern or if there has been sustained rise in basal body temperature, it may be inferred that the hormonal cycle is normal. At the time of expected ovulation, it may be helpful to examine the cervical mucus for normally occurring changes in clarity, increased glucose content, tensile strength (ability to form a thread). and presence of crystalline, fernlike pattern where the mucus dries on a glass slide. In some women, inadequate progesterone secretion is inferred from low urinary levels of pregnanediol and the demon-stration of atypical secretory patterns in the postovulation endo-metrium. If ovulation has not occurred but gonadotropin levels are normal, suitable hormonal therapy sometimes induces ovulatory cycles. Repeated demonstration of low gonadotropin levels points to hypothalamic or pituitary disease, while excessively high levels of gonadotropin indicate failure of ovarian response. In patients with primary amenorrhea, cytologic examination for sex chromatin pattern is indicated despite outward evidence of feminine habitus.

STEIN-LEVENTHAL SYNDROME

Many young women are first seen with secondary amenorrhea, mild hirsutism, and infertility problems. Certain such women have bilaterally enlarged cystic ovaries surrounded by a tough grayish-white capsule, a condition known as the Stein-Leventhal syndrome. These women have anovulatory cycles, normal or low levels of FSH, and LH levels which tend to be quite high but fluctuate widely.[11] Suggested causes include the production of abnormal adrenocortical hormones, production of increased quantities of testosterone by the ovarian stromal cells, inhibition of FSH production by prolonged estrogen production, and alterations in hypothalamic mechanisms. Ordinarily estrogen production is normal or high, and urinary 17-ketosteroids are within normal limits. Some women with the Stein-Leventhal syndrome, and certain others with idiopathic hirsutism, have been shown to excrete excessive 17-ketosteroids, and 17-hydroxy-corticosteroids after ACTH administration. Additional support for adrenal hyperreactivity and possible hyperfunction as the etiology is the finding that certain such women succeed in conception when intrinsic ACTH production is partially suppressed by administration of small doses of glucocorticoids.

TESTES

The testes perform two functions: elaboration of the male hormones, predominantly testosterone, and the production of spermatozoa, the male gametes. The Leydig, or interstitial, cells secrete testosterone under the influence of the interstitial cell-stimulating hormone (ICSH, which is apparently the same as luteinizing hormone in females). Testosterone is a 19-carbon hormone but not a 17-ketosteroid. Its excreted metabolites, however, can be measured as 17-ketosteroids and constitute approximately one-third of the total 17-ketosteroid excretion in adult males. The remaining two-thirds derive from the adrenal and are present in both males and females. Testosterone stimulates the seminiferous tubules, but actual spermatogenesis is largely regulated by the pituitary gonadotropin called, in the female, follicle-stimulating hormone (FSH).

Hormones and Their Functions

Interstitial cells are active during fetal development, secreting products that direct genital development toward the masculine habitus, but testicular function is largely dormant in the male from birth to puberty. An upsurge of pituitary gonadotropins heralds the onset of puberty and promotes secretion of testosterone, which initiates male secondary sex characteristics. Following puberty, abnormally diminished testosterone production is associated with high levels of pituitary gonadotropin, but the relationship between testes and pituitary is somewhat unclear. Some men with diminished spermatogenesis have elevated gonadotropin levels, despite normal excretion of testosterone metabolites.

Laboratory evaluation of testicular function rests upon measurement of androgen secretion and examination of the seminal fluid. Testosterone is measured when hypogonadism is suspected, and spermatogenesis is evaluated when a couple desire children but have difficulty conceiving.

Hypogonadism

Hypogonadism cannot be suspected in an outwardly normal male child until after the age of expected puberty. Individuals vary so markedly that delayed maturation and hypogonadism are difficult to differentiate until after the patient is 19 or 20 years old. As with other endocrine defects, testosterone deficiency may be due to primary testicular failure or may be secondary to inadequate pituitary stimulation. The clinical findings of primary and secondary hypogonadism are the same. When first seen, the individual displays eunuchoid features of excessive growth of long bones, high-pitched voice, absence of male pattern of hair distribution, poor muscular development, and infantile external genitalia. These physical findings are not present in the mature male whose testes were damaged after puberty.

PRIMARY GONADAL INSUFFICIENCY

In patients with primary testicular disorders, urinary gonadotropin levels are high after the age of expected puberty. One of the commoner causes of primary dysfunction is *Klinefelter's syndrome,* in which there is a supernumerary X chromosome. These patients have a positive sex-chromatin pattern, despite male habitus. Primary testicular disorders in men with normal chromosomal complement usually are due to anatomic or developmental abnormalities demonstrable by testicular biopsy.

SECONDARY GONADAL INSUFFICIENCY

Patients with low gonadotropin levels may have complete or incomplete pituitary hypofunction. The gonadotropins suffer first when the pituitary is damaged, so that what appears to be an isolated defect in gonadotropin production is sometimes the first sign of progressive pituitary destruction. Demonstration of gonadotropin deficiency should prompt a careful search for the cause of pituitary disease: x-rays of the sella turcica and examination of visual fields to demonstrate tumor; serologic tests for syphilis; x-ray examination and immunologic evaluation for tuberculosis; and hematologic examination to rule out multiple myeloma. Gynecomastia cannot be associated reliably with estrogen levels or with changes in testosterone production and appears to require the presence of gonadotropins. Patients with pituitary failure do not develop gynecomastia despite the absence of testosterone.

Hypergonadism

Hypergonadism becomes apparent most readily in young boys in whom secondary sex characteristics appear unexpectedly early. Gonadotropin levels usually are increased above preadolescent levels, sometimes due to demonstrable tumor in the region of the hypothalamus. In some boys, early maturation appears to be a hereditary constitutional syndrome without anatomic abnormalities. Since testosterone is a potent androgen, there may be minimal change in 17-ketosteroid excretion in the early phases of precocious puberty. Subsequently, an adult pattern of 17-ketosteroid excretion develops, consistent with the developmental rather than chronologic age.

17-KETOSTEROIDS

Early maturation with high levels of urinary 17-ketosteroids may be due to testicular tumors or, more commonly, to adrenal cortical hyperplasia. The 17-ketosteroid levels are especially high with congenital adrenal hyperplasia (adrenogenital syndrome) or tumors. In contrast to the full maturation produced by pituitary or constitutional precocious puberty, androgen overproduction does not stimulate spermatogenesis, and the testes remain preadolescent in size. Urinary gonadotropins are virtually absent, presumably due to high levels of functioning hormones.

TUMORS

Hormonally active testicular tumors are relatively rare even in adults. Choriocarcinoma and those teratomas that contain chorionic elements may produce chorionic gonadotropin, which gives a positive reaction in a "pregnancy test." Patients with such tumors also have elevated levels of urinary estrogens. Tumors of the interstitial cells may produce androgen or estrogen or both. In prepubertal boys, interstitial cell tumors cause precocious development of male secondary sex characteristics, but androgen excess causes little clinical change in mature men. The rare estrogen-producing tumors are associated with gynecomastia and decrease of libido and testicular size.

Semen Examination

Evaluation of an infertile couple should include examination of the seminal fluid within 1 or 2 hours of ejaculation. Because rubber condoms may damage the spermatic morphology and motility and because coitus interruptus may cause the first portion of the ejaculate to be lost, masturbation is probably the best means of obtaining the specimen.

The ejaculate should be evaluated for quantity, viscosity, sperm count, and morphology and motility of the sperm. Normal volume is 3 to 5 ml.; both smaller volumes (1 to 2 ml.) and larger volumes (6 to 10 ml.) are associated with lessened fertility for reasons not presently clear. The normal sperm count is approximately 60 to 250 million/ml., but documented impregnation has occurred with lower counts, and several authorities[20,39] mention 6 to 10 million/ml. as the lowest possible limits at which conception is possible.

Motility and morphology must be evaluated subjectively. The combined effects of motility, morphology, and total sperm count influence fertility, and a high percentage of inactive or bizarre sperm is associated with decreased fertility. The viscosity of the seminal fluid may vary. The presence of a coagulum is very common shortly after ejaculation, but as this normally liquifies within a few minutes, failure to liquify should be considered abnormal.

Testicular biopsy may be indicated if the ejaculate contains no sperm at all, since there is always the possibility that an abnormality of the epididymis or vas deferens is preventing emission of normally produced sperm. Male infertility is difficult to evaluate and highly uncertain to treat. In primary spermatogenic arrest, FSH levels are persistently high, indicating that successful spermatogenesis exerts a negative feedback on FSH production. The levels of LH cannot be correlated reliably with sperm production, and hormonal manipulation has not been successful in correcting abnormalities of spermatogenesis.

REFERENCES

1. Alberti, K. G. M. M., and Hockaday, T. D. R.: *Diabetic coma: a reappraisal after five years.* Clin. Endocrinol. Metabol. 6:421, 1977.
2. Axelrod, J., and Weinshilboum, R.: *Catecholamines.* N. Engl. J. Med. 287:237, 1972.
3. Bartter, F. C., and Schwartz, W. B.: *The syndrome of inappropriate secretion of antidiuretic hormone.* Am. J. Med. 42:790, 1967.
4. Beierwaltes, W. H.: *Thyroiditis.* Ann. N.Y. Acad. Sci. 124:586, 1965.
5. Bondy, P. K.: *The adrenal cortex,* in Bondy, P. K., and Rosenberg, L. E. (eds.): *Duncan's Diseases of Metabolism.* ed. 7. W. B. Saunders, Philadelphia, 1974.
6. Bowen, A. J., and Reeves, R. L.: *Diurnal variation in glucose tolerance.* Arch. Intern. Med. 119:261, 1967.
7. Conn, J. W., Cohen, E. L., Rovner, D. R., and Nesbit, R. M.: *Normokalemic primary aldosteronism.* J.A.M.A. 193:200, 1965.
8. Felig, P.: *New insights and old concepts.* Arch. Inte   Med. 137:569, 1977.
9. Fore, W., and Wynn, J.: *The thyrotropin stimulation test.* Am. J. Med. 40:90, 1966.
10. Fowler, P. B. S., Swale, J., and Andrews, H.: *Hypercholesterolemia in borderline hypothyroidism: stage of premyxoedema.* Lancet 2:488, 1970.
11. Franchimont, P.: *Human gonadotrophin secretion.* J. R. Coll. Physicians Lond. 6:283, 1972.
12. Gaede, J. T.: *Serum enzyme alterations in hypothyroidism before and after treatment.* J. Am. Geriatr. Soc. 25:199, 1977.
13. Genuth, S. M., Houser, H. B., Carter, J. R., Jr., et al.: *Community screening for diabetes by blood glucose measurement. Results of a five-year experience.* Diabetes 25:1110, 1976.
14. Goldsmith, R. S.: *Treatment of hypercalcemia.* Med. Clin. North Am. 56:951, 1972.
15. Hays, R. M.: *Antidiuretic hormone.* N. Engl. Med. 295:659, 1976.
16. Ingbar, S. H., and Woeber, K. A.: *The thyroid gland,* in Williams, R. H. (ed.): *Textbook of Endocrinology.* ed. 5. W. B. Saunders, Philadelphia, 1974.
17. Jaspan, J. B., and Rubenstein, A. H.: *Circulating glucagon: plasma profiles and metabolism in health and disease.* Diabetes 26:887, 1977.
18. Kumar, M. S., Safa, A. M., Deodhar, S. D., and Schumacher, O. P.: *Evaluation of T_4 radioimmunoassay as a screening test for thyroid function.* Cleve. Clin Q. 44:1, 1977.
19. Lauler, D. P.: *Pre-operative diagnosis of primary aldosteronism.* Am. J. Med. 41:855, 1966.
20. MacLeod, J.: *The semen examination.* Clin. Obstet. Gynecol. 8:115, 1965.
21. McGarry, J. D., and Foster, D. W.: *Ketogenesis and its regulation.* Am. J. Med. 61:9, 1976.

22. Mulrow, P. J.: *The adrenal cortex.* Annu. Rev. Physiol. 34:409, 1972.
23. Murphy, B. E. P., Pattee, C. J. and Gold, A.: *Clinical evaluation of a new method for the determination of serum thyroxine.* J. Clin. Endocrinol. Metab. 26:247, 1966.
24. Ontjes, D. A., and Ney, R. L.: *Tests of anterior pituitary function.* Metabolism 21:159, 1972.
25. O'Sullivan, J. B., and Mahan, C. M.: *Prospective study of 352 young patients with chemical diabetes.* N. Engl. J. Med. 278:1038, 1968.
26. Pek, S.: *Glucagon and diabetes.* Clin. Endocrinol. Metabol. 6:333, 1977.
27. Permutt, M. A.: *Postprandial hypoglycemia.* Diabetes 25:719, 1976.
28. Potts, J. T., Jr., and Deftos, L. J.: *Parathyroid hormone, calcitonin, vitamin D, bone and bone mineral metabolism,* in Bondy, P. K., and Rosenberg, L. E. (eds.): *Duncan's Diseases of Metabolism.* ed. 7. W. B. Saunders, Philadelphia, 1974.
29. Pyke, D. A.: *Genetics of diabetes.* Clin. Endocrinol. Metabol. 6:285, 1977.
30. Robbins, J., Rall, J. E., and Gorden, P.: *The thyroid and iodine metabolism,* in Bondy, P. K., and Rosenberg, L. E. (eds.): *Duncan's Diseases of Metabolism.* ed. 7. W. B. Saunders, Philadelphia, 1974.
31. Rubinstein, P., Suciu-Foca, N., and Nicholson, J. F.: *Genetics of juvenile diabetes mellitus. A recessive gene closely linked to HLA-D and with 50 percent penetrance.* N. Engl. Med. 297:1036, 1977.
32. Scholz, D. A., Purnell, D. C., Goldsmith, R. S., et al: *Diagnostic considerations in hypercalcemic syndromes.* Med. Clin. North Am. 56:941, 1972.
33. Schwartz, N. B., and McCormack, C. E.: *Reproduction: gonadal function and its regulation.* Annu. Rev. Physiol. 34:425, 1972.
34. Shimoda, S. S., Saunders, D. R., and Rubin, C. E.: *The Zollinger-Ellison syndrome with steatorrhea. II. The mechanism of fat and vitamin B_{12} malabsorption.* Gastroenterology 55:705, 1968.
35. Sunderman, F. W., Jr.: *Measurements of vanillylmandelic acid for the diagnosis of pheocromocytoma and neuroblastoma.* Am. J. Clin. Pathol. 42:481, 1964.
36. Unger, R. H., and Ocri, L.: *The essential role of glucagon in the pathogenesis of diabetes mellitus.* Lancet 1:14, 1975.
37. Williams, G. H., Dluhy, R. G., and Thorn, G. W.: *Diseases of the adrenal cortex,* in Thorn, G. W., Adams, R. D., Braunwald, E., et al.: *Harrison's Principles of Internal Medicine.* ed. 8. McGraw-Hill, New York, 1977.
38. Wisenbaugh, P. E., Garst, J. B., Hull, C., et al.: *Renin, aldosterone, sodium and hypertension.* Am. J. Med. 52:175, 1972.
39. Zorgniotti, A. W., and Hotchkiss, R. S.: *Male infertility.* Clin. Obstet. Gynecol. 8:128, 1965.
40. *Glycosylated hemoglobins.* Lancet 2:22, 1977.
41. Peterson, C. M., and Jones, R. L.: *Minor hemoglobins, diabetic "control," and diseases of postsynthetic protein modification.* Ann. Intern. Med. 87:489, 1977.

CHAPTER 16

PREGNANCY

Pregnancy deserves a chapter to itself since the condition is neither a disease nor a normal state. Although the etiology is straightforward, the physiologic changes are complex.

TESTS FOR THE EXISTENCE OF PREGNANCY

Fertilization occurs within several days of ovulation at the midpoint of the menstrual cycle. The fertilized ovum floats down the fallopian tube into the uterus, where it implants on the welcoming secretory endometrium. Shortly after implantation, on the twenty-first to twenty-third day of the cycle, chorionic gonadotropin production begins.[39] Virtually all laboratory tests for the diagnosis of pregnancy measure the presence of chorionic gonadotropin, a hormone unique to the trophoblast.

Until the 1960s, pregnancy tests were bioassays in which the presence of human chorionic gonadotropin (HCG) in serum or urine was demonstrated by its effect on animals. The earliest tests used mice and rabbits; subsequent tests used female rats or male frogs. These biologic tests now have been largely supplanted by immunologic tests which are more accurate, easier to perform, and do not require the laboratory to maintain animal facilities. In addition, the results are less subject to artefactual distortion by drugs the patient may be taking.

Principle of Immunologic Tests

The immunologic tests rely upon commercially available antihuman chorionic gonadotropin antibody (anti-HCG). The presence of HCG in serum or urine is documented by alteration in antibody activity, as shown by an indicator system. Red cells or latex particles are coated with human chorionic gonadotropin in such a concentration that unmistakable agglutination occurs upon contact with the antibody. When the test is performed, the patient's serum or urine is incubated with the antibody; HCG, if present, reacts with and thereby inactivates the antibody. The incubated mixture of antibody and sample is then added to the indicator. If HG was present in the sample, the antibody is inactivated, and the red cells or particles remain unagglutinated. If the sample does not contain HCG, the antibody remains active, and agglutination occurs (Fig. 22). Commercial testing kits include positive and negative control samples along with the vial of anti-HCG.

RESULTS OF IMMUNOLOGIC TESTING

Immunologic tests have an accuracy rate of 95 to 99 percent as compared with a range of 65 to 97 percent accuracy with the rat ovarian hyperemia test.[15,31] Because the immunologic tests are sensitive to lower concentrations of HCG than the bioassays, the test becomes positive earlier in the pregnancy. Positives have been reported as early as 16 days after ovulation (2 days after the first missed period), and most tests are reliable at 3 weeks after the first missed period. The tests with red cell indicators tend to be more sensitive than those which use latex particles. Since chorionic gonadotropin has some immunologic resemblance to the luteinizing hormone (LH) of the pituitary, some cross-reactivity occurs, and excessively sensitive tests would be subject to false positives from high levels of LH. Immunologic tests can be quantitated by diluting the urine or serum sample and comparing it with control dilutions of known potency.

Pregnancy tests should be performed on the first voided morning specimen, since this is the most concentrated urine. Although quantitative study of 24-hour samples is necessary to measure total hormonal excretion, the level in the first morning specimen parallels fairly closely the range of total excretion.

VALUE OF ASSAY PROCEDURES

Since immunologic assay is so much easier to perform than bioassay, serial determinations of HCG levels are simple and practical for studying women suspected of abnormal pregnancy or malignant

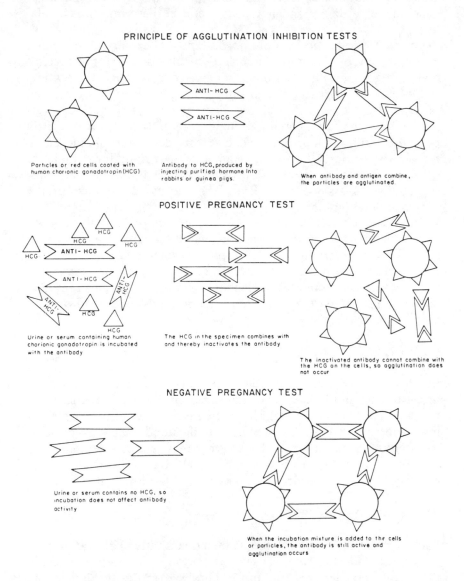

PRINCIPLE OF AGGLUTINATION INHIBITION TESTS

Particles or red cells coated with human chorionic gonadotropin (HCG)

Antibody to HCG, produced by injecting purified hormone into rabbits or guinea pigs.

When antibody and antigen combine, the particles are agglutinated.

POSITIVE PREGNANCY TEST

Urine or serum containing human chorionic gonadotropin is incubated with the antibody

The HCG in the specimen combines with and thereby inactivates the antibody

The inactivated antibody cannot combine with the HCG on the cells, so agglutination does not occur

NEGATIVE PREGNANCY TEST

Urine or serum contains no HCG, so incubation does not affect antibody activity

When the incubation mixture is added to the cells or particles, the antibody is still active and agglutination occurs

Figure 22. Immunologic tests for demonstration of pregnancy use an antibody against chorionic gonadotropin in an agglutination inhibition technique (see also Figure 11, p. 195).

trophoblastic disease. As a rule, less HCG is excreted in ectopic than in normal pregnancies. Only two-thirds of women with ectopic pregnancy have positive pregnancy tests,[12] and in these, the titer is relatively low.

Abortion is followed by a prompt fall in HCG excretion. In women with a history of abortion, serial determinations during the first trimester are especially useful during episodes of vaginal spotting. If the HCG level remains high during an episode of spotting, the pregnancy is likely to continue.[40] Since the range of values varies from one woman to another, a single determination provides little prognostic information, but repeated tests can establish the curve for any particular woman. In women with hydatidiform mole or choriocarcinoma, or in men with trophoblastic tumors of the testis, repeated HCG assays can indicate the success of therapy or the presence of recurrence.

Chorionic gonadotropin excretion reaches its peak at the twelfth to fourteenth week of gestation, and thereafter falls to a fairly constant level. By secreting gonadotropin, the placenta stimulates the corpus luteum to produce the steroids necessary to maintain pregnancy. As gonadotropin levels decline, the placenta begins secreting its own steroids, and the pregnancy becomes independent of ovarian protection.

PLACENTAL HORMONES

Besides chorionic gonadotropin, the placenta secretes estrogens, progesterone, and human placental lactogen (HPL). All of these can be measured in the maternal blood stream or urine, but their physiologic functions are so incompletely understood that it is difficult to interpret quantitative findings. Pregnancy-related hormones are measured as a means to assess fetal well-being and to evaluate the effects of therapy intended to improve fetal development.

Relationships to Pregnancy

Each of these hormones follows its own quantitative curve at various stages of pregnancy. Total estrogen excretion increases progressively throughout pregnancy, rising most sharply after the thirtieth week. Pregnanediol, the excretory product of progesterone, rises steadily until 30 to 34 weeks, and then remains level or falls slightly. Human placental lactogen rises steadily throughout much of pregnancy, maintaining a high plateau during the last trimester. The range of normal values is wide for all the hormones and, even for a single individual, pronounced variation occurs from day to day.

Since we do not know how these hormones or their metabolites influence fetal development, or which aspects of fetoplacental function they represent, it is difficult to know which tests are useful for prenatal medical care. It is still more difficult to interpret a single result obtained by testing an apparently normal pregnant woman who suddenly develops bleeding, fever, toxemia, or other worrisome signs. Given the range of normal variation, it is almost essential that each woman serve as her own control.[18] In following a high-risk pregnancy, sequential values should be obtained to construct a curve for that individual pregnancy; marked departure from that established norm indicates a change in fetal or placental development. When a previously normal woman unexpectedly has clinical problems, it may be necessary to extrapolate from only a few results and hope for the best.

Estriol

Maternal estriol derives partly from the placenta and partly from the fetal adrenal glands. Estriol levels in maternal urine are additionally influenced by the woman's excretory function and urine volume. Urinary estriol correlates fairly well with fetal growth rate; anencephalic pregnancies have consistently low levels because pituitary aplasia causes adrenal gland hypofunction.[1] When serial estriol levels are available, a sharp downward trend indicates probable fetal difficulty. This can be defined as a drop of 30 to 40 percent below previous levels, observed on 2 consecutive days,[1] or a fall of 35 percent or more, on a single day, from the average of the preceding 3 days' values.[33] Frequent sampling is especially useful in women with hypertension or impending toxemia. Diabetic women often show such wide swings in value that a valid downward trend is hard to document until it is too late to help the fetus; nevertheless, these women should be followed as closely as possible.

Progesterone

Pregnanediol is the most easily measured metabolite of progesterone, but there is only modest correlation between pregnanediol levels in urine and circulating plasma progesterone.[18] Urinary pregnanediol levels drop with severe placental dysfunction, but this occurs too late to allow detection or correlation of impending problems. Pro-

gesterone derives entirely from the placenta with no fetal contribu-
tion. Urinary pregnanediol levels may remain unchanged despite
severe fetal distress or·even death.

Human Placental Lactogen

Although produced by the placenta, human placental lactogen (HPL)
exerts its entire known effects on the mother. Like growth hormone,
it causes relative insulin resistance and an increased level of circulating free fatty acids. Plasma and urine HPL levels reflect placental
size and tend to be high in diabetic mothers. Despite good statistical
correlation between HPL levels and placental weight, urinary HPL
levels have little predictive value for any individual pregnancy.
Plasma HPL levels below 4 μg./ml. frequently indicate retarded
growth, especially if total estrogen also is low.[17] HPL levels fall in
toxemia, and declining values sometimes can help in distinguishing
incomplete abortion from threatened abortion.[18]

PHYSIOLOGIC CHANGES IN PREGNANCY

Pregnancy causes plasma volume to increase enormously, peaking at
about 34 weeks.[21] Complex changes in hormonal relationships and
sodium regulation produce this volume expansion, which in turn
demands increased cardiac and renal workload and leads to dilution
of many blood constituents. Measurements made on whole blood,
plasma, or serum must be interpreted with this volume increase in
mind.

Hematologic System

RED BLOOD CELLS

Red cell production increases during pregnancy but not as much as
plasma volume. If iron stores are adequate, red cell mass increases
by 400 to 450 ml.,[9] but hemogloblin concentration and hematocrit
decline. Hemoglobin concentration below 10.5 gm./dl. should be
considered abnormally low, even when hemodilution is greatest.
Reticulocyte counts rise, especially in the middle trimester; reticulocyte counts of 2.0 to 5.0 percent may result from pregnancy alone
without indicating additional hematopoietic stress.

 Anemia occurs very commonly during pregnancy, with iron deficiency the most common etiology. Red cells are small, hypochromic,

and irregularly shaped; serum iron levels are low, with low transferrin saturation; and bone marrow iron is absent.

Megaloblastic anemia also is common. The conceptus drains off substantial amounts of folic acid and modest amounts of vitamin B_{12}. In addition, the mother's tissues absorb more folate and B_{12} than usual, and there is increased excretion of the dialyzable fraction of folic acid.[9] Serum folate levels decline from the nonpregnant normal in all pregnancies, but red cell folate levels remain unchanged unless deficiency exists. Both serum and red cell levels of vitamin B_{12} decline in normal pregnancies, a phenomenon also seen in women taking oral contraceptives.

WHITE BLOOD CELLS

In the last half of pregnancy, granulocyte levels rise, but lymphocyte levels remain unchanged, resulting in increases in total white count to as much as 15,000/mm.[3] with a relative granulocytosis. Up to 25 percent of pregnant women have occasional metamyelocytes or myelocytes in the peripheral blood.[9] The hematologic picture often resembles that seen in infection or other tissue stress. There is an increase in the number of neutrophils giving a positive nitroblue tetrazolium test; leukocyte alkaline phosphatase values rise; and Döhle bodies are seen not infrequently. These findings must be interpreted with caution. While it is undesirable to initiate too quickly an intensive, expensive search for infection, it is even worse to overlook acute infection on the grounds that the laboratory findings represent physiologic variation. History, physical findings, and the results of sputum and urine examination usually clarify doubtful cases.

THE COAGULATION SYSTEM

Fibrinogen levels rise throughout pregnancy, reaching levels of 400 to 600 mg./dl. in the third trimester. Plasminogen levels also increase, but total fibrinolytic activity declines, owing possibly to a fall in circulating plasminogen activator or to the presence of placental inhibitors.[3] Venous thrombosis occurs more often in pregnant than in nonpregnant women of comparable age and health. It is not clear how this increase in fibrinogen and decrease in relative fibrinolytic activity relate to the incidence of thrombosis, if in fact they relate at all. Assayed activity of Factors VII, VIII, and X increases somewhat, but this does not consistently affect the prothrombin time or partial thromboplastin time.

In normal pregnancy, circulating fibrinogen degradation products (FDPs) do not increase. If FDPs are detected in a pregnant woman without obvious coagulopathy, the cause is probably liver disease or toxemia. The liver normally clears the circulating blood of activated coagulation factors and fibrinogen degradation products. In pregnancy, despite the increase in blood volume and total cardiac output, blood flow to the liver does not increase. The result is a relative decline in hepatic blood flow which accentuates minor degrees of hepatic failure.

Serum Proteins

Many proteins increase during pregnancy. This is especially striking for thyroid- and cortisol-binding proteins and causes total circulating hormone levels to increase significantly during pregnancy. Serum concentrations also rise during pregnancy for β-lipoproteins, transferrin, ceruloplasmin, α_1-antitrypsin, several complement components, and a pregnancy-associated protein that migrates as an α_2-macroglobulin.[37] A twofold rise in fibrinogen levels causes the erythrocyte sedimentation rate to increase. Levels of IgG and IgA decline, but IgM concentrations remain unchanged. Serum albumin concentration falls by as much as 0.5 to 0.8 gm./dl. Hemodilution causes part of this drop, but there is also a failure to increase manufacture despite acceleration of albumin degradation.[37]

The Endocrine System

THYROID GLAND

Plasma concentration of thyroxine-binding globulin (TBG) increases markedly with pregnancy. The rise begins shortly after fertilization, and continues until it reaches an elevated plateau at 12 weeks. Failure to initiate this rise after fertilization suggests hypothyroidism or estrogen deficiency, conditions which severely reduce the likelihood of successful pregnancy.[38] Plasma thyroxine levels rise along with the TBG, but TBG increases more than the hormone does. This means that the level of TBG saturation declines. In vitro tests of T_3 uptake (see p. 493) fall into the nonpregnant hypothyroid range during normal pregnancy. The increase in circulating thyroxine affects only the bound fraction; the active, unbound fraction does not increase. Values for total thyroxine, and for PBI or BEI, fall into the hyperthyroid range during normal pregnancy. Effective thyroxine ratio and levels of thyroid stimulating hormone (TSH) remain normal in euthyroid pregnant women.[4]

Pregnant women can become hyperthyroid, and hyperthyroid women can become pregnant. Laboratory values can be elevated moderately without causing concern, but T_4 values above 13 μg./dl. or resin T_3 uptake in the euthyroid range suggest true thyroid hyperactivity. Hypothyroidism and pregnancy coexist less frequently. With severe hypothyroidism, conception rarely occurs, and suboptimal thyroid activity makes it difficult to maintain a pregnancy.

ADRENAL GLANDS

Both cortisol and cortisol-binding protein increase with pregnancy, but the relation between bound and free hormone is less clear-cut than with bound and free thyroid hormone. Cortisol values remain elevated throughout the day, and there is flattening of the usual diurnal curve.[29] Women taking oral contraceptives have an elevated morning peak for free cortisol but not elevated round-the-clock levels. The rate of cortisol production actually declines slightly, but the plasma half-life is increased during pregnancy, and there is exaggerated response to ACTH stimulation. It may be difficult to diagnose adrenal hyperfunction during pregnancy, but suppression of steroid secretion following dexamethasone administration persists in normal pregnancy. Cortisol levels in the "normal" range and failure of ACTH response indicate diminished adrenal function during pregnancy.

Aldosterone, the sodium-conserving, potassium-depleting hormone of the outermost part of the adrenal cortex, is increased throughout pregnancy. Pregnancy produces a cumulative total sodium retention of about 500 to 900 mEq.,[21] but plasma volume increases beyond this level, and there is a decline in effective osmolality due to sodium. Since the increases in plasma volume, cardiac output, and glomerular filtration rate combine to impose a huge sodium load on the pregnant kidney, adequate sodium retention is essential. During pregnancy, the flexibility of aldosterone production declines. Urinary sodium loss rises if excessive sodium is present, but when sodium deprivation occurs, there is inappropriate sodium loss before sodium retention readjusts.[21] The increased aldosterone activity does not cause potassium wastage. Aldosterone secretion declines with advancing toxemia. In pre-eclampsia, the level of above-normal production drops; in established toxemia, levels fall below nonpregnant states.[26]

HORMONES AFFECTING CARBOHYDRATE METABOLISM

During pregnancy, insulin production increases, but the need for insulin increases simultaneously. The combined effects of increased cortisol, increased estrogen, increased progesterone, and circulating placental lactogen reduce the entry of glucose into cells and increase the circulation of free fatty acids.[20] In normal pregnancies, compensatory insulin production counteracts these tendencies, and fasting blood glucose levels remain in the normal range or even drop slightly.[36] Glucose absorption diminishes somewhat; oral glucose tolerance curves are essentially normal, but there is slight, progressive increase in the time required for serum glucose levels to peak.

The metabolic stress of pregnancy may push the pancreas beyond its ability to respond, unmasking a latent diabetic state. *Gestational diabetes* is abnormal insulin metabolism that occurs only during pregnancy and reverts to normal when pregnancy terminates. Many women with gestational diabetes have abnormal glucose tolerance curves between pregnancies but do not have glycosuria or fasting hyperglycemia unless some other stress supervenes. Most such women eventually become overtly diabetic.

Glycosuria during pregnancy does not necessarily indicate gestational diabetes. Pregnancy imposes such a glucose load on the tubular reabsorptive capacity that glycosuria is a common event and need not, on a single random specimen, set off a major search for diabetes. More significant is consistent glycosuria or glycosuria in older women, in obese women, in women with a family history of diabetes, or in those with a history of bearing deformed babies or babies weighing over 9½ pounds.

Renal Function

Both absolute blood volume and the relative renal blood flow increase in pregnancy. The glomerular filtration rate increases by as much as 50 percent, and response to altered posture or to sodium load becomes exaggerated. Because of increased filtration, increased amounts of electrolytes, proteins, vitamins, and nitrogenous products pass through the tubules. Urinary loss of sodium, calcium, protein, and urea increases, causing a small but consistent drop in serum levels of these constituents. A woman in the last half of pregnancy whose serum calcium or urea is in the "high normal" range should be considered abnormal.

Throughout pregnancy, the calyces, renal pelves, and ureters are widened and slack. Urine flow slows, and complete emptying becomes more difficult. These are among the factors causing increased susceptibility to urinary tract infections during pregnancy.

Liver Function

The most conspicuous pregnancy-associated change in standard "liver function tests" is a two- to fourfold rise in alkaline phosphatase. The placenta manufactures a specific alkaline phosphatase isoenzyme whose physiologic function is unknown. The hepatobiliary form of the enzyme does not increase, and circulating transaminase levels do not change in normal pregnancy.

The liver is largely responsible for the increased production of proteins during pregnancy. The binding proteins are most conspicuous in this regard. Cortisol- and thyroxine-binding proteins increase significantly; testosterone-binding protein, ceruloplasmin, and transferrin also increase. Fibrinogen rises to double the prepregnancy levels. Albumin manufacture, however, does not seem to increase. Since albumin degradation increases and plasma volume expands, failure to increase synthesis causes circulatory levels to drop by as much as 500 to 750 mg./dl. or even more.

Pregnancy also affects lipid metabolism; concentrations of all the major lipid classes increase. Cholesterol and the low-density lipoproteins increase about twofold, while triglycerides increase even more markedly. Heparin-stimulated lipase and esterase activities decline.

LIVER DISEASE

Perhaps the most dangerous liver disease in pregnancy is *acute fatty liver*, a disease of unknown etiology that carries a very high mortality. Laboratory findings are unpredictable, but often there is a significant fall in albumin levels as well as a moderate prolongation of prothrombin time. Regulatory activity also is impaired, commonly accompanied by falling blood glucose and rising ammonia levels. The transaminases rarely rise past the 300 to 500 unit range, and there is moderate jaundice to about 10 mg./dl. Alkaline phosphatase, however, rises very little.

Cholestasis of pregnancy affects the values associated with biliary function. Alkaline phosphatase, all of it hepatobiliary, increases markedly, and serum bile acids rise astronomically. Serum bilirubin does not increase as much, rarely going above 5 mg./dl. Hepato-cellular function is not affected significantly, and transaminases, prothrombin time, and albumin levels change very little.

PRENATAL EXAMINATION OF THE FETUS

Amniocentesis has revolutionized prenatal diagnosis. The fluid itself can be subjected to biochemical and spectrophotometric analysis, and the suspended cells can be observed, cultured, and analyzed. Amniocentesis is done for a variety of reasons: estimation of fetal maturity and fetal response to environmental problems; establishment of fetal chromosome complement; documentation of enzyme deficiencies or other biochemical abnormalities; and diagnosis of structural malformations.

Evaluating Fetal Condition

When there is a question of terminating pregnancy early, either by cesarean section or induced labor, the obstetrician needs some indication of fetal maturity and well-being. This allows realistic assessment of relative risk between allowing the fetus to remain in an adverse uterine environment or bringing too immature an infant into a hostile world. Several biochemical measurements on amniotic fluid give good, but not absolute, prognostic information.

BILE PIGMENTS

Hemolytic disease of the newborn causes severe intrauterine hemolysis, which discolors the amniotic fluid. Standard chemical techniques are unsuitable for measuring amniotic fluid bilirubin, but the various bilirubin-related pigments can be quantitated spectrophotometrically. The informative wavelength is 450 mμ. If bile pigments are present, optical density increases in that range, forming a "hump" whose magnitude reflects the pigment concentration.

The earlier in pregnancy the hump occurs, the greater the danger of intrauterine damage or death. It has been possible, by compiling data on many at-risk pregnancies, to correlate the level of pigment accumulation with fetal danger at different gestational ages. It is necessary first to establish that maternal antibody is the cause of intrauterine hemolysis. This is done by screening the mother's serum for an isoimmune red cell antibody capable of crossing the placenta.

Most often the antibody is anti-Rh$_o$(D). Nearly all the rest react with other antigens of the Rh system, but innumerable different antibodies have caused isolated examples of severe hemolytic disease.

A woman with a potent antibody should have amniocentesis at 24 to 28 weeks or even earlier if previous pregnancies have been severely affected. The frequency of subsequent tests depends on the initial findings. Values are compared against a chart that estimates the danger of different pigment levels at different gestational ages. Accurate estimation of gestational age is important; this requires a reliable menstrual history and, often, ultrasonographic determination of fetal size. When there is clear evidence of danger to the fetus, the obstetrician must decide whether to attempt intrauterine therapy or to induce labor. The crucial factor in determining survival of premature infants tends to be maturity of the fetal lung, which can be estimated in part by biochemical analysis of amniotic fluid.

LECITHIN/SPHINGOMYELIN RATIO

The leading killer of premature infants is *respiratory distress syndrome*, also called *hyaline membrane disease*. Immature lungs become atelectatic shortly after birth because respiratory movements cannot overcome the surface forces that make alveolar membranes adhere to one another. If sufficient surfactant material lubricates the alveolar surfaces, the alveoli do not collapse and respiration occurs normally. Surfactant activity depends on physical interactions between complex lipid molecules. The lipid concentration in amniotic fluid reflects the lipids present in intrapulmonary secretions; this makes it possible to estimate pulmonary surfactant levels by analyzing the amniotic fluid. The two lipids that give the most information are *lecithin* (L) and *sphingomyelin* (S).

Sphingomyelin in the amniotic fluid remains fairly constant throughout pregnancy, in the range of 4 to 6 mg./dl. Lecithin rises slowly during the first two trimesters and sharply at about 35 weeks. At 30 to 34 weeks, lecithin concentration usually is about 6 to 9 mg./dl.; after 35 weeks, this increases rapidly to 15 to 20 mg./dl. The absolute values for lecithin and sphingomyelin are less important than the ratio between them. Mature lung function correlates strongly with L/S ratios of 2.0 or above. Infants born with amniotic fluid L/S ratios below 1.5 have a 70 percent risk of respiratory distress syndrome.[14] With an L/S ratio between 1.5 and 2.0, the risk is 40 percent; at 2.0 or above, the risk of respiratory distress syndrome is 1 to 2 percent.

PROBLEMS WITH THE L/S RATIO. Measuring lecithin and sphingo-myelin is exacting, requiring rapid processing, careful centrifugation, and numerous steps for extraction and isolation. Fetal blood, maternal blood, and meconium can cause technical interference. There is a bedside technique for estimating L/S ratio which bypasses the need for tedious chemical quantitation but is highly liable to false-negative results.[32] In the "shake test," a carefully measured aliquot of amniotic fluid is added to 95 percent ethyl alcohol and saline. After the tube has been shaken vigorously, persistence of bubbles 15 minutes later indicates an L/S ratio of 2.0 or above. Poor technique, dirty glass-ware, or contamination of specimen frequently causes false nega-tives. If bubbles persist, it is safe to assume that adequate lecithin is present. If the "shake test" is negative, complete analysis is necessary.

There is disagreement about how maternal or fetal disease affects pulmonary maturation and lecithin development. Many workers believe that the L/S ratio has less predictive value in diabetic than in normal pregnancies.[32] Others disagree, citing comparable incidence of respiratory distress at comparable L/S ratios for children born to diabetic or nondiabetic mothers.[10] An extensive study of high-risk pregnancies[25] attempted to correlate L/S ratio, gestational age as estimated clinically at birth, and incidence of respiratory distress. It was found that in pregnancies complicated by severe pre-eclampsia, severe diabetes, major hemoglobinopathies, chronic bleeding, pla-cental insufficiency, or prolonged rupture of membranes, an L/S ratio of 2.0 or more occurred at an earlier gestational age than would normally occur. The mature L/S ratio was attained later than expected in pregnancies complicated by less severe diabetes, collagen dis-eases, hepatitis, renal disease, and hemolytic disease of the newborn. Altogether there was a 20 percent discrepancy rate between matura-tion estimated by prenatal L/S ratio and findings on clinical evalua-tion after birth. In these complicated pregnancies, 5 percent of infants with an L/S ratio of 2.0 or greater had respiratory distress; of the 423 infants with an L/S ratio of 2.0 or more, however, respiratory distress was classified as severe in only three.

CREATININE

Amniotic fluid accumulates creatinine from fetal urine; the quan-tity reflects maturity of the fetal kidney. Amniotic fluid creatinine concentration begins to rise sharply at about 34 gestational weeks. Between 30 and 34 weeks, levels run about 1.3 to 1.7 mg./dl.; by 37 weeks, 94 percent of pregnancies have creatinine concentrations at or above 2.0 mg./dl.[30] The problem with measuring creatinine is that renal function and pulmonary function do not always mature in parallel. If the L/S level is low and creatinine indicates good renal development, the pulmonary findings tend to carry more weight in the decision-making process.

Establishing Fetal Chromosome Complement

The fetal karyotype can be established by culturing cells harvested from the amniotic fluid. Karyotyping reveals the sex of the fetus, the number of chromosomes present, and severe abnormalities of chromosomal structure. For most X-linked diseases, precise prenatal diagnosis is not possible. In a pregnancy at risk for such serious X-linked conditions as hemophilia or Duchenne's muscular dystrophy, knowledge of fetal sex may be sufficient information.

Chromosomal abnormalities are rather common, occurring in some series in as many as 50 to 60 percent of first trimester pregnancies that abort spontaneously.[23,35] Of stillborn infants, 5 percent have been found to have abnormal karyotypes, and 0.5 percent of liveborn infants have some demonstrable chromosomal defect. Additional X chromosomes and trisomy of chromosome 21 are the commonest events.

WHICH PREGNANCIES SHOULD BE EXAMINED?

Amniocentesis during the second trimester carries rather slight risk,[28] but the possibilities of bleeding or infection exist, and the expense and anxiety are considerable. Families in which there has been one child or fetus with a chromosomal abnormality have much more than a chance risk of another abnormal pregnancy. After one pregnancy complicated by trisomy, the risk of further children with excessive chromosome number is 2 to 5 percent.[24] Women with one or more previous abnormal infants are a high-risk group whose later pregnancies should be monitored with amniocentesis.

The risk of chromosomal abnormality rises with advancing age. One estimate is that one in 70 mothers between ages 35 and 40 will have an aneuploid infant; between ages 40 and 45, at least one in 62 will be abnormal.[35] Most clinicians believe that all pregnancies in women over age 40 should be monitored; many would lower the age threshold to 35.

If either parent is known to be a carrier for chromosomal translocation, there is a high risk that the infant will have a translocation defect, notably Down's syndrome. If it is the mother who carries the translocation, the observed incidence is about 10 percent in offspring. If the father is the carrier, the risk drops to 2 or 3 percent but remains substantial.[35] Any pregnancy in which either parent is known to have a structurally abnormal chromosome should be monitored.

WHAT CAN BE LEARNED?

Abnormality of chromosome number (aneuploidy) is the easiest kind of prenatal diagnosis. With chromosomes, more is not better. Autosomal trisomies always cause mental deficiency and physical deformities. Trisomy 21 causes Down's syndrome; trisomies of 18 or 13 are less common and cause more severe mental and physical abnormalities.

Either X or Y chromosome can be present in excess. The XXY karyotype occurs once in every 600 female births; XYY occurs once in each 1000 male births.[11] Aneuploidy of the sex chromosomes causes reduced fertility and, usually, some degree of physical change. Mental retardation is not invariable, but slightly subnormal intelligence occurs very commonly in this category. The existence of an unpaired X chromosome (Turner's syndrome, with an incidence of 1 in 3000 female births) causes much reduced fertility, but reproductive failure is not absolute. Body habitus is slightly abnormal, and intelligence often is borderline or reduced. The presence of an unpaired Y chromosome seems to be incompatible with fetal development.

With sophisticated techniques of chromosome identification, it is possible to identify translocations, inversions, and other structural defects. The significance of these abnormalities is less clear than for the more easily identified numerical aberrations.

WHAT CAN GO WRONG?

Culturing cells and preparing the karyotype take 4 to 6 weeks. If the cells fail to grow or if the cultured cells prove to be maternal in origin, it may be too late in the pregnancy to begin the process again. Artefacts in the culture flasks occasionally induce abnormalities not present in the original cells. For this reason, several duplicate cultures usually are prepared. This makes it easier to evaluate the significance of different findings in different flasks or of an isolated abnormality present in one flask but not in others. If one or several cultures yield results suggesting genetic mosaicism, it is extremely difficult to interpret subsequent observations in which only one cell type is found.

Enzyme or Biochemical Abnormalities

To diagnose a biochemical problem before birth, the informative cells, tissue, or fluid must be available. The cells in amniotic fluid derive from the fetal membranes and from skin, oral and vaginal epithelium, urogenital tract, and umbilical cord. If a disease is due to enzymes found only in some internal organ, this deficiency cannot be demonstrated directly on cultured cells. Sometimes the absence of an enzyme in an inaccessible site creates abnormalities of amniotic fluid composition, but if not, intrauterine diagnosis becomes difficult or impossible.

It is also very difficult to identify conditions that become apparent only late in pregnancy. Defects in synthesis of the hemoglobin beta chain are an example of this problem, since hemoglobin A is not produced in large quantity until the third trimester.

Despite these problems, the list of genetically determined diseases susceptible to prenatal diagnosis is truly impressive.[22,24] Prominent among these are the carbohydrate and lipid storage diseases, in which diagnostically abnormal products often can be found in amniotic fluid itself or in uncultured cells. Disorders of amino acid metabolism often cause abnormality of amniotic fluid composition; in other amino acid disorders, the enzyme deficiency can be noted in cultured cells. Less well established are techniques for measuring hormone levels in amniotic fluid or for observing abnormal nucleic acid metabolism in cell culture lines.

SELECTION OF CASES

It is both difficult and expensive to diagnose most metabolic diseases, and there must be a high index of suspicion before the procedure is undertaken. Usually the birth of one abnormal infant is the first indication that the family is at risk. Precise diagnosis of the first abnormal child is essential in order to know what tests to perform in subsequent pregnancies. For some autosomal-recessive disorders, notably Tay-Sachs disease and sickle cell anemia, it is reasonably simple to identify carriers. If two known carriers mate, it is desirable to monitor all pregnancies without waiting for a first-affected infant.

A serious pitfall in diagnosing autosomal-recessive disorders is the necessity to distinguish a homozygous fetus from a heterozygote. For many biochemical disorders, specific abnormalities occur only in the homozygote, but in some enzyme deficiencies, the distinction may be difficult or impossible.

Another problem is to establish normal values. One must have enough data about normal pregnancies to know what level of abnormality is significant. It is obviously impossible to run normal controls along with every at-risk case, and it is difficult to accumulate an adequate series of normal results for every enzyme and every metabolite that needs to be studied.

Structural Abnormalities

Most congenital malformations are multifactorial. No single gene or chromosome lies at the root of the problem. Often both genetic peculiarities and intrauterine circumstances have etiologic importance, and the defect results from the additive effects of several genes or of genes plus environment. Common multifactorial conditions include defects of the atrial septum; cleft lip and palate; closure defects of the neural tube, ranging from anencephaly to all degrees of meningomyelocoele; hypospadias; and pyloric stenosis.

Risks for these multifactorial defects vary, reflecting to some extent the distribution of a gene or genes in the population.[16] Common in the white population are hypospadias (6 per 1000 live births) and neural tube defects (4 per 1000). Atrial septal defect and clubfoot have an incidence of 1 per 1000, while the risk of cleft palate is 5 per 10,000. The risk is much greater in pregnancies that follow the birth of an affected infant. Risk increases enormously with the number of previously affected children and the severity of their malformations.

Relatively few multifactorial defects can be diagnosed before birth. Ultrasound techniques now allow detection of limb defects and abnormalities of head size. With increasingly sophisticated ultrasonic techniques, it is becoming possible to visualize gross structural distortions of heart, alimentary tract, and excretory system.[22] Still highly experimental is direct visual examination by fetoscopy, sometimes combined with biopsy of fetal tissues.

ALPHA-FETOPROTEIN

One common malformation, closure defects of the neural tube, can be diagnosed with 90 to 95 percent certainty by analyzing amniotic fluid levels of α-fetoprotein (AFP).[5] AFP is manufactured by the fetal liver, beginning at the sixth week and rising to a maximum during the second trimester. Brisk fetal production continues to about the thirty-second week, but amniotic fluid concentration declines as the volume of amniotic fluid increases. AFP concentration in fetal serum is several hundred times that in amniotic fluid throughout the entire pregnancy.

If the neural tube fails to close properly, enormous amounts of AFP enter the amniotic fluid. The reasons for this are not clear but appear to be related to increased exudation of fetal protein across the exposed chorionic plexus. Except for the confounding conditions mentioned below, the difference between normal and abnormal amniotic fluid AFP levels is dramatic. Although actual values vary from laboratory to laboratory, diagnostic accuracy is 90 percent or better in most experimental settings. AFP levels in maternal serum have proved more difficult to standardize. Some centers report excellent results with this noninvasive technique for screening mothers at risk,[22] while others have been less successful.

The most common cause of artificially high amniotic fluid levels is contamination by fetal blood. Since fetal blood contains so much AFP, a very small puncture or hemorrhage can confuse the results. Sometimes this artefact can be detected by noting fetal hemoglobin in the fluid, but this may not be helpful if the bleeding occurred in the past. Another problem is incorrect dating of the pregnancy. Normal AFP values change markedly with gestational age. Ultrasound is an extremely useful adjunct to AFP measurement because it helps in estimating fetal size and also in establishing the presence of severe structural malformations. Other conditions characterized by high amniotic fluid AFP are severe omphalocoele and congenital nephrosis. Omphalocoele often can be detected with ultrasonic visualization, but congenital nephrosis is an internal defect of renal tubular function, and no structural changes can be seen.

SCREENING NEWBORNS

Screening refers to the process of testing unselected populations to uncover asymptomatic, unsuspected, or untreated disease. Screening is useful if the diseases uncovered can be treated or controlled, so that the patient and society in general derive benefit from learning the diagnosis. Early discovery of an untreatable condition has questionable value. The usefulness of screening programs depends on the frequency with which the disease occurs in the population; the incidence of false-positive and false-negative results; the cost and feasibility of confirming suggestive positives; the cost of the screening technique; and the probable outcome of treating the disease once diagnosis has been established.

Enzyme Deficiencies

Several genetically determined diseases can be detected effectively in the newborn period and treatment instituted before irreversible damage occurs. Most are relatively rare deficiencies of enzymes in intermediary metabolism; treatment requires years or a lifetime of stringent adherence to a dietary regimen. Phenylketonuria, galactosemia, homocystinuria, and maple syrup urine disease are the metabolic conditions most easily and most beneficially sought. The consequences of failure to diagnose the condition or to maintain treatment once the diagnosis is established are progressive mental and physical deterioration, a tragedy to the patient and his family, and a lifelong burden to society.

Congenital hypothyroidism, which occurs in about 1 of every 5000 live births,[2] can be diagnosed by radioimmunoassay for circulating thyroxine. Hormone replacement therapy prevents the catastrophic intellectual deterioration that occurs if cretinism remains untreated for just a few months. Screening techniques are relatively cheap, accurate, and effective. Although these endocrine and metabolic conditions are relatively rare, the logistics and economics of diagnosis and the effectiveness of therapy combine to make screening worthwhile.

Cystic Fibrosis

For one of the commonest and most disabling congenital diseases, there is no truly effective screening procedure. Cystic fibrosis affects as many as 1 in 2000 white children, causing severe disability and early death if not vigorously and unremittingly treated. The most reliable diagnostic procedure is measurement of sweat electrolytes, a test that is difficult, time-consuming, and expensive but thoroughly justified if even the suspicion of disease exists. It is not, however, a screening technique. Tests suitable for application to every newborn on every obstetrical service still carry unacceptably high false-negative rates. Most are based on "dip-stick" procedures to measure proteins in meconium. More promising are simple techniques to measure enzyme activity in early stool samples,[6] but none has achieved widespread adoption.

Hemoglobinopathies

The commonest genetic disease that affects black infants is sickle cell anemia, an abnormality of adult hemoglobin. It is easy to screen adults for the presence of sickle hemoglobin because large amounts are present. Newborns have such a high proportion of fetal hemoglobin that simple screening techniques cannot be applied. Modified electrophoretic techniques can be used to identify infants with abnormal hemoglobins, but this type of screening is not routinely done, in part because of the expense and the technical difficulties involved, but in large measure because there is no curative or palliative therapy available. The major advantage of diagnosing hemoglobinopathies before symptoms occur is the opportunity to maintain surveillance over these children for whom there is high risk of severe infections and retarded growth.

REFERENCES

1. Beling, C.: *Estrogens,* in Fuchs, F., and Klopper, A., (eds.): *Endocrinology of Pregnancy.* ed. 2. Harper & Row, Hagerstown, Md., 1977.
2. Bennett, A. J. E.: *New England regional newborn screening program.* N. Engl. J. Med. 297:1178, 1977.
3. Bonnar, J.: *The blood coagulation and fibrinolytic systems during pregnancy.* Clinics Obstet. Gynaecol. 2:321, 1975.
4. Burrow, G. N.: *Thyroid and parathyroid function in pregnancy,* in Fuchs, F., and Klopper, A. (eds.): *Endocrinology of Pregnancy.* ed. 2. Harper & Row, Hagerstown, Md., 1977.
5. Cowchock, F. S.: *Use of alpha-fetoprotein in prenatal diagnosis.* Clin. Obstet. Gynecol. 19:871, 1976.
6. Crossley, J. R., Berryman, C. C., and Elliott, R. B.: *Cystic-fibrosis screening in the newborn.* Lancet 2:1093, 1977.
7. Erbe, R. W.: *Current concepts in genetics: principles of medical genetics.* N. Engl. J. Med. 294:381, 480, 1976.
8. Farrell, P. M., and Kotas, R. V.: *The prevention of hyaline membrane disease: new concepts and approaches to therapy.* Adv. Pediatr. 23:213, 1976.
9. Fleming, A. F.: *Haematological changes in pregnancy.* Clin. Obstet. Gynaecol. 2:269, 1975.
10. Gabbe, S. G., Lowensohn, R. J., Mestman, J. H., et al.: *Lecithin/sphingomyelin ratio in pregnancies complicated by diabetes mellitus.* Am. J. Obstet. Gynecol. 128:757, 1977.
11. Gerald, P. S.: *Current concepts in genetics: sex chromosome disorders.* N. Engl. J. Med. 294:706, 1976.

12. Glass, R. H., and Jesurn, H. M.: *Immunologic pregnancy tests in ectopic pregnancy.* Obstet. Gynecol. 27:66, 1966.
13. Gluck, L., Kulovich, M. V., Borer, R. C., Jr., et al.: *Diagnosis of the respiratory distress syndrome by amniocentesis.* Am. J. Obstet. Gynecol. 109:440, 1971.
14. Harvey, D., Parkinson, C. E., and Campbell, S.: *Risk of respiratory distress syndrome.* Lancet 1:42, 1975.
15. Henry, J. B., Little, W. A., and Christian, C. D.: *Modified immunologic test for pregnancy.* Am. J. Clin. Pathol. 42:109, 1964.
16. Holmes, L. B.: *Current concepts in genetics: congenital malformations.* N. Engl. J. Med. 295:204, 1976.
17. Josimovich, J. B.: *Human placental lactogen,* in Fuchs, F., and Klopper, A. (eds.): *Endocrinology of Pregnancy.* ed. 2. Harper & Row, Hagerstown, Md., 1977.
18. Klopper, A.: *Choice of hormone assay in the assessment of fetoplacental function,* in Fuchs, F., and Klopper, A. (eds.): *Endocrinology of Pregnancy.* ed. 2. Harper & Row, Hagerstown, Md., 1977.
19. Klopper, A., and Fuchs, F.: *Prostaglandins,* in Fuchs, F., and Klopper, A., (eds.): *Endocrinology of Pregnancy.* ed. 2. Harper & Row, Hagerstown, Md., 1977.
20. Lind, T.: *Changes in carbohydrate metabolism during pregnancy.* Clin. Obstet. Gynaecol. 2:395, 1975.
21. Lindheimer, M. D., and Katz, A. I.: *Renal changes during pregnancy. Their relevance to volume homeostasis.* Clin. Obstet. Gynaecol. 2:345, 1975.
22. Mennuti, M. T.: *Prenatal diagnosis: current status.* N. Engl. J. Med. 297:1004, 1977.
23. Miller, O. J., and Breg, W. R.: *Current concepts in genetics: autosomal chromosome disorders and variations.* N. Engl. J. Med. 294:596, 1976.
24. Milunsky, A.: *Current concepts in genetics: prenatal diagnosis of genetic disorders.* N. Engl. J. Med. 295:377, 1976.
25. Morrison, J. C., Whybrow, W. D., Bucovaz, E. T., et al.: *The lecithin/sphingomyelin ratio in cases associated with fetomaternal disease.* Am. J. Obstet. Gynecol. 127:363, 1977.
26. Mulrow, P. J.: *Renin aldosterone system in pregnancy,* in Fuchs, F., and Klopper, A. (eds.): *Endocrinology of Pregnancy.* ed. 2. Harper & Row, Hagerstown, Md., 1977.
27. Nadler, H. L.: *Prenatal detection of genetic defects.* Adv. Pediatr. 22:1, 1976.
28. NICHD National Registry for Amniocentesis Study Group: *Midtrimester amniocentesis for prenatal diagnosis.* J.A.M.A. 236:1471, 1976.
29. Peterson, R. E.: *Cortisol,* in Fuchs, F., and Klopper, A., (eds.): *Endocrinology of Pregnancy.* ed. 2. Harper & Row, Hagerstown, Md., 1977.
30. Pitkin, R. M., and Zwirek, S. J.: *Amniotic fluid creatinine.* Am. J. Obstet. Gynecol. 98:1135, 1967.
31. Powell, J., Stevens, V. C., Dickey, R. P., and Ullery, J. C.: *Immunologic pregnancy testing in urine and serum.* Am. J. Obstet. Gynecol. 96:844, 1966.
32. Pritchard, J. A., and Macdonald, P. C.: *Williams' Obstetrics.* ed. 15. Appleton-Century-Crofts, New York, 1976.
33. Quilligan, E. J., and Collea, J. V.: *Fetal monitoring in pregnancy.* Adv. Pediatr. 22:83, 1976.

34. Rhine, S. A.: *Prenatal genetic diagnosis and metabolic disorders.* Clin. Obstet. Gynecol. 19:855, 1976.
35. Simpson, J. L., and Martin, A. O.: *Prenatal diagnosis of cytogenetic disorders.* Clin. Obstet. Gynecol. 19:841, 1976.
36. Spellacy, W. N.: *Insulin, glucagon and growth hormone in pregnancy,* in Fuchs, F., and Klopper, A. (eds.): *Endocrinology of Pregnancy.* ed. 2. Harper & Row, Hagerstown, Md., 1977.
37. Studd, J.: *The plasma proteins in pregnancy.* Clin. Obstet. Gynecol. 2:285, 1975.
38. Tunbridge, W. M. G., and Hall, R.: *Thyroid function in pregnancy.* Clin. Obstet. Gynaecol. 2:381, 1975.
39. Vaitukaitis, J. L.: *Human chorionic gonadotropin,* in Fuchs, F., and Klopper, A. (eds.): *Endocrinology of Pregnancy.* ed. 2. Harper & Row, Hagerstown, Md., 1977.
40. Whitelaw, M. J., and Nola, V. F.: *Accuracy of the immunologic pregnancy test in early pregnancy and abortion.* Obstet. Gynecol. 27:69, 1966.

SECTION 6

OTHER TESTS

CHAPTER 17

URINE

PHYSIOLOGY

The Nephron

The kidneys, which together constitute 0.5 percent of total body
weight, receive 20 percent of cardiac output, a testimonial to the
complexity and importance of renal function. Approximately 1500 L.
of blood pass through the kidneys each day; approximately 150 L. of
fluid per day enter the proximal convoluted tubules as potential
urine; approximately 1.5 L. per day is the usual output for a metabolically stable adult. The magnitude of renal activity is obvious.
The functional unit of renal activity is the nephron, of which each
kidney contains approximately 1.5 million. Comprising the nephron
are the glomerular capillary loop, the proximal convoluted tubule,
the loop of Henle, the distal convoluted tubule, and the collecting
duct, which unites with other ducts to connect, ultimately, with the
renal pelvis.

GLOMERULAR FUNCTION

Glomerular blood flow is regulated by the afferent (preglomerular)
and efferent (postglomerular) arterioles. The principal function of
the glomerular capillary loop is filtration, whereby fluid and associated solutes leave the blood stream for processing into urine. Filtration pressure, the push that expels fluid from the capillary lumen,
is the net sum of outward-directed hydrostatic pressure and in-pulling

551

colloid osmotic pressure. Serum protein levels principally determine osmotic pressure, while changes in arteriolar constriction regulate the intracapillary hydrostatic pressure.

After leaving the capillary lumen, the filtrate traverses a maze of cellular and acellular elements which permit plasma solutes to pass but restrict larger molecules, notably proteins. Small amounts of the smallest plasma proteins normally enter the filtrate. Hemoglobin, a compact, spherical molecule, can readily pass the filter, but its presence in plasma is highly abnormal. Abnormal quantities of protein may enter the filtrate if hydrostatic pressure is exceptionally high, if there is damage to the endothelial basement membrane or epithelial structures comprising the physical barrier, or if exceptionally small protein molecules are present in plasma for any reason.

THE PROXIMAL TUBULE

The 150 L. of filtrate that enter the convoluted tubule contain more than a kilogram of sodium chloride and innumerable other constituents. While traversing the proximal convoluted tubule, the urine-to-be loses 80 to 85 percent of its water and salt and virtually all its sugar, amino acids, and proteins. The epithelial cells lining this segment expend energy in the reabsorption of sodium; water and chloride passively accompany the reabsorbed sodium back into the general circulation. This portion of salt and water regulation does not respond to changing physiologic stimuli, and final regulation occurs more distally.

SECRETION AND ABSORPTION. The proximal tubular cells transport a multitude of other substances, most of them from the tubular lumen into capillary blood, but some are secreted in the reverse direction, so that urinary concentration exceeds the filtered level. These transport mechanisms depend upon the coupling of transported substance with an intracellular carrier, and their capacity is finite. The exact nature of these carriers is unknown, although certain common reabsorptive pathways are known to exist. Glucose, fructose, xylose, and galactose share one system; different classes of amino acids share several different systems. Secretion, which is net transport from blood or interstitial fluid into tubular urine, employs comparable carrier systems. One well-defined common secretory pathway is shared by such organic ions as penicillin, *para*-aminohippuric acid (PAH), and phenolsulfonphthalein (PSP). The tubules can clear a small amount of protein from the filtrate by a carrier system involving lipoprotein complexes, but the maximum capacity is quite low.

Measurement of absorptive or secretory capacity for a given substance provides a functional estimate of tubular epithelial capacity; the descriptive term for maximum rate of tubular transport is T_m, the substance being specified by a subscript, as $T_{m(PAH)}$ or $T_{m(glucose)}$. If the tubular fluid contains more glucose, for example, than the reabsorptive mechanism can handle, the T_m is exceeded, and the excess material remains in the urine.

THE LOOP OF HENLE

Fluid and electrolyte recovery in the proximal tubule reduces the minute volume of tubular content from 120 ml. to 20 ml., but excretion at this rate would still produce 29 L. of urine per day. Entering the loop of Henle, the tubular fluid is isosmotic with plasma (i.e., approximately 300 mOsm./L). The loop descends into the renal medulla, where the interstitial fluid is highly hypertonic. Water and electrolytes move between tubular lumen and interstitial fluid in a complex series of relationships known as *countercurrent multiplication of concentration*. Following its passage through Henle's loop, the fluid entering the distal convoluted tubule is hypotonic to the concentrated interstitial fluid just outside the tubule.

THE DISTAL TUBULE

In the distal convoluted tubule and collecting ducts, the day-to-day, minute-to-minute adjustments of volume and electrolyte composition occur. Antidiuretic hormone (ADH) controls volume excretion by varying the interaction between dilute tubular contents and concentrated interstitial fluid. When ADH is present, the wall of these segments becomes permeable to solute-free water. From the interstitial fluid, this water returns to the circulation, thus conserving body water and leaving urine fairly concentrated. Without ADH, the walls resist water movement, the tubular fluid remains hypotonic, and large volumes of dilute urine are excreted.

Both proximal and distal convoluted tubules participate in acid-base and potassium ion regulation. In the proximal tubule, potassium and bicarbonate are removed from the filtrate, while hydrogen ion content of the tubular fluid increases. The proximal tubular epithelium regenerates bicarbonate ions and restores them to the circulation along with sodium ions. In the distal tubule, the epithelium adjusts the excretion of hydrogen and potassium ions; as long as the organism maintains approximate metabolic equilibrium, these ions are excreted in a roughly reciprocal fashion. Excess hydrogen ions are excreted by combination with ammonia (to form ammonium ions) or with filtered buffers such as $HPO_3^=$. When H^+ excretion is increased, urinary K^+ concentration diminishes. If whole-body potassium stores are low, K^+ will be conserved and H^+ excreted. This may occur even if the stimulus to K^+ depletion is one which leads to overall alkalosis; thus the urine may be paradoxically acid in the face of whole-body alkalosis.

Physiologic Derangements

Renal function is so intimately dependent upon the interrelations of blood vessels and epithelial elements that distinct separation of disease states is very difficult. It is useful to consider vascular disease, glomerular disease, and tubular disorders in separate categories, but the glomerulus is, after all, a tuft of blood vessels, and tubular function at all levels in the nephron requires interchange with interstitial fluid and the capillaries of the interstitium.

Acute drop in renal perfusion reduces urine flow because of decreased filtration and, if severe, because of hypoxic damage to the metabolically active and highly vulnerable tubular epithelial cells. Marked increase in arterial or arteriolar pressure leads to structural changes in the blood vessels, originally to protect against damage but leading to irreversible changes if prolonged.

SITES OF DAMAGE

If the glomerulus sustains damage either from inflammatory conditions or vascular disease, its filtration functions suffer, and large molecules such as serum proteins or even intact erythrocytes or leukocytes can enter the tubular contents. Damage to the tubular cells impairs their secretory and reabsorptive capacities and interferes with the regulatory mechanisms for electrolyte and acid-base control, as well as control of volume and concentration. If the interstitium of cortex or medulla is altered by inflammation, scarring, or deposition of abnormal elements, then concentrating power and metabolic exchange will be affected.

ABNORMAL URINARY CONSTITUENTS

Red or white blood cells may enter the urine from any level in the urinary tract. If these cellular elements or other constituents originate in the kidney and spend sufficient time in the tubules, they may become packed together and assume the shape of the tubular lumen. These are called casts and, when seen in the urine, are incontrovertible evidence of intrarenal disease. Red or white cells of renal origin sometimes may appear loose in the urine, and desquamated tubular epithelial cells sometimes are found in urinary sediment. More often, however, the inciting abnormality sets up conditions conducive to cast formation.

CAST FORMATION. Casts consist of inspissated tubular contents passed directly into urine and therefore reflect fairly accurately the presence of renal parenchymal disease. Hyaline casts, composed largely of the Tamm-Horsfall mucoprotein which is a product of the normal nephron, are present in small numbers in normal urine, but increase when urinary protein is increased and urine is highly concentrated. Increased acidity and electrolyte concentration enhance precipitation of Tamm-Horsfall mucoprotein.[28] The sticky protein casts attract white cells or tubular cells to their surface, and cellular inclusions in hyaline casts are fairly common. Bilirubin or hemoglobin, if present in the urine, may lend color to these normally colorless cylinders. Mucous threads, fibers, and other artefacts occasionally may be mistaken for hyaline casts, which are difficult to see against a brightly lighted background. Other kinds of casts include cellular elements or debris from blood or epithelial cells and appear granular or overtly cellular. These are more obvious on microscopic examination and often accompany more destructive renal processes.

CHEMICAL ABNORMALITIES. The chemical composition of urine depends on the nature of the material which enters the tubular filtrate, that is, the composition of blood as it reflects systemic metabolism and the activity of the nephron in modifying the filtrate. For some substances, comparison of blood and urine levels provides some idea of the site of abnormality. For others, urinary composition may be an important clue to systemic disease. The urinary levels of sodium, potassium, calcium, phosphates, and bicarbonate reflect both renal and systemic problems and must be evaluated with many variables in mind. Routine urinalysis ordinarily includes a qualitative search for such common pathologically significant elements as glucose, ketone bodies, protein, blood, and bile pigments. When specific diseases are under consideration, a host of other qualitative or quantitative procedures may be indicated. Table 20 shows values of the constituents of normal urine.

RENAL FUNCTION TESTS

Glomerular Blood Flow

Urine constitutes an end point of renal function, but a single specimen, or even a timed collection, often cannot provide information about the dynamics of the functioning kidney. Several well-established procedures are available to investigate glomerular flow rate and tubular excretory capacity. The volume of blood going through the glomerulus cannot, of course, be partitioned and measured separately from the total renal blood flow. Instead, the glomerular flow is inferred from the rate at which certain materials leave the circulation and enter the filtrate, resulting in a figure called the glomerular filtration rate.

INULIN CLEARANCE

Glomerular filtration rate (GFR) usually is expressed in terms of clearance, a figure representing the amount of plasma from which some substance is totally cleared in 1 minute. Such clearing does not actually occur, nor could it be measured precisely if it did. Clearance is calculated by comparing the amount of substance excreted with the concentration of that substance in the plasma, that is, the amount available to the kidney for excretion. The amount excreted is measured readily; it is the concentration of the substance in the urine (U) multiplied by the volume of urine excreted in the selected time (V). Dividing the amount excreted by the concentration in plasma (P) tells how many milliliters of plasma yielded that amount of material, assuming that each milliliter of plasma flowing through the glomerulus released all its substance into the urine. The clearance formula, then, is

$$\frac{U \times V}{P} \ .$$

Table 20. Normal Values for Urine

Test	Normal Values	Remarks
Addis count	WBC 1,800,000; RBC 500,000; casts (hyaline) 0–5000	Rinse bottle with 10% neutral formalin and discard excess 12-hr. specimen.
Albumin		
Qualitative	Negative	Single specimen
Quantitative	10–100 mg./24 hr.	24-hr. specimen
Aldosterone	2–23 μg./24 hr.	24-hr. specimen; keep refrigerated.
Amino acid nitrogen	100–290 mg./24 hr.	24-hr. specimen; collect in thymol; refrigerate
Ammonia	700 mg./24 hr.	24-hr. specimen
Amylase	2–50 Wohlgemuth u./ml.	Single specimen
Amylase, total in 24-hr.	6–30 Wohlgemuth u./ml. Up to 5000 Somogyi u./24 hr.	24-hr. specimen
Bence-Jones protein	Negative	First morning specimen
Bilirubin	Negative	Single specimen
Blood, occult	Negative	Single specimen
Calcium		
Sulkowitch	Positive 1 +	Single specimen
Quantitative	30–150 mg./24 hr.	Average diet
	100–250 mg./24 hr.	High-calcium diet; 24-hr. specimen
Catecholamines	Less than 230 μg. in 24 hr.	24-hr. specimen; use 1 ml. conc. H_2SO_4 for preservative
Chloride	110–250 mEq./24 hr.	24-hr. specimen
Coproporphyrin	50–200 μg./24 hr. Children: 0–80 μg./24 hr.	24-hr. specimen in 5 gm. of Na_2CO_3
Creatine	Less then 100 mg. in 24 hr., or less than 6% of creatinine. Pregnancy: up to 12% of creatinine. Children under 1 yr.: may equal creatinine. Children over 1 yr.: up to 30% creatinine	24-hr. specimen
Creatinine	Females: 0.8–1.7 gm./24 hr. Males: 1–1.9 gm./24 hr.	24-hr. specimen
Estrogens	Females: 4–60 μg./24 hr. Males: 4–25 μg./24 hr.	24-hr. specimen; refrigerate

Table 20. Continued

Test	Normal Values	Remarks
Fishberg concentration test	Specific gravity: 1.022 to 1.032	Collect specimens at 7, 8, and 10 a.m.
Fishberg dilution test	Volume of 40 ml. in first hour with specific gravity 1.000 to 1.003	Collect 4 hourly specimens after patient drinks 1200 ml. of water.
Glucose		
Qualitative	Negative	Single specimen
Quantitative	50–500 mg./24 hr.	24-hr. specimen
Gonadotropic hormone, pituitary	10 to 15 mouse uterine u./24 hr.	24-hr. specimen; collect with toluene
17-Hydroxycorticosteroids	Females: 2-8 mg./24 hr. Males: 3-10 mg./24 hr.	24-hr. specimen; tranquilizers interfere
5-Hydroxyindole-acetic acid	2–9 mg./24 hr.	24-hr. specimen; tranquilizers interfere
Indican	4–20 mg./24 hr.	24-hr. specimen
17-Ketosteriods	24-hr. excretion:	24-hr. specimen

Age	Females	Males
10	1–4 mg.	1–4 mg.
20–30	4-16 mg.	6-26 mg.
50	3-9 mg.	5-18 mg.
70	1–7 mg.	2–10 mg.

Test	Normal Values	Remarks
Lead	0.021–0.038 mg./L.	24-hr. specimen
pH	4.8 to 7.8	Single specimen
Phenylpyruvic acid	Negative	Single specimen
Phosphorus	0.9–1.3 gm./24 hr.	24-hr. specimen
Porphobilinogen	Negative	Single specimen
Potassium	25–100 mEq./24 hr.	24-hr. specimen
Pregnanediol	Children: negative. Females: 1-8 mg./24 hr. Males: 0–1 mg./24 hr.	24-hr. specimen; refrigerate
Pregnanetriol	Children: Less than 0.5 mg./24 hr. Females: 0.5–2 mg./24 hr. Males: 1.0–2.0 mg./24 hr.	24-hr. specimen; refrigerate
Protein		
Bence-Jones	Negative	First morning specimen
Qualitative	Negative	Single specimen
Quantitative	10–100 mg./24 hr.	24-hr. specimen
Serotonin	See 5-Hydroxyindoleacetic acid	
Sodium	About 110 mEq./24 hr.	24-hr. specimen
Specific gravity	1.002–1.030	Single specimen
	1.015–1.025	24-hr. specimen

Table 20. Continued

Test	Normal Values	Remarks
Sugars	Negative	Single specimen
Urea clearance	Maximum: 75 ml. Standard: 54 ml.	Serum and urine
Uric acid	0.5-1.0 gm./24 hr.	24-hr. specimen
Urobilinogen		
Semiquantitative	Up to 1 Ehrlich u./2 hr.	2-hr. specimen; collect between 1 and 3 p.m.
Quantitative	1.0–4.0 mg./24 hr.	24-hr. specimen; collect in dark container with 5 gm. of Na_2CO_3
Vanillylmandelic acid	0.7–6.8 mg./24 hr.	24-hr. specimen in 3 ml. 25% H_2SO_4; omit fruit and coffee 2 days before test
Volume	Adults: 1000–1500 ml./24 hr. (about 15–21 ml./kg. body wt.) Children: 3 to 4 times as much as adults per kg. of body wt.	

MEASUREMENT. Accurate measurement of clearance requires that the substance be one that can be measured accurately at both plasma and urine levels. It also requires that the proportion of urinary concentration to plasma concentration [U]/[P] be constant over a wide range of plasma levels and that the substance not be secreted, absorbed, or metabolized. The substance that fulfills these requirements best is inulin, a metabolically inert polysaccharide of fructose.

The rate of plasma flow through the glomerulus can be measured very accurately if inulin is infused at such a rate that a constant plasma level is maintained and complete, meticulous urine collection is achieved. The glomerular filtration rate, as so determined, is 124 ± 15 ml. of plasma/min./1.73 m.^{2} of body surface in healthy young men and 110 ± 15 ml./1.73 m.^{2} for healthy young women.[22] These values diminish slightly with aging, even when no demonstrable renal disease coexists.

ABNORMALITIES. Diseases that affect the glomerular tuft and renal vascular disease have the most immediate effect on GFR, but any significant degree of renal disease can diminish the filtration rate. Nonrenal conditions which impair small vessel circulation also may decrease glomerular plasma flow; these include congestive heart failure, cirrhosis with ascitic accumulation, shock from any cause, and dehydration.

ENDOGENOUS CLEARANCE TESTS

Inulin clearance is not suitable for routine laboratory use because the plasma levels must be monitored by frequent and very accurate measurement, and urine collection must be extremely careful. From research studies using inulin clearance, however, has come knowledge of the relative accuracies and shortcomings of other clearance techniques. In clinical situations, glomerular filtration rate usually is estimated from values for urea clearance or creatinine clearance. Both procedures have shortcomings, but creatinine clearance is perhaps more widely used. Both are endogenous clearance tests, meaning that the substance measured is already present in the circulation. This makes it unnecessary to achieve and maintain a constant plasma level of the material during the test period, since the assumption is made that the plasma level remains stable for this period. A highly unstable metabolite, such as glucose, could not be used.

CREATININE CLEARANCE. One problem affecting both creatinine and urea is that excretory levels reflect more than just filtration. The tubules normally secrete a small amount of creatinine into the urine and reabsorb a moderate amount of urea. When plasma creatinine is high, secretion is enhanced. Since patients with impaired renal function have increased plasma creatinine, the degree of inaccuracy is cumulative. For this reason, creatinine clearance rates in seriously ill patients cannot be referred usefully to absolute normal values. A better approach is to follow sequential values in an individual patient who then serves as his own control.

For creatinine clearance, a 12- or 24-hour urine specimen is collected. The sample for plasma determination should be drawn sometime during this period. Plasma levels are normally so low (0.7 to 1.5 mg./dl.) that strictly accurate determinations are difficult. In addition, plasma contains noncreatinine reactants which are chromogenic in the alkaline picrate procedure usually employed. This small degree of error probably is balanced in calculation, however, by the inaccuracy that results from tubular secretion.

UREA CLEARANCE. Tubular reabsorption of urea presents a more serious problem, because the rate of absorption varies with the rate of urine flow. When flow is slow, quite a lot of filtered urea is removed. For reasonably reliable results, urine flow must be 2 ml./min. or greater. The fact that plasma urea concentrations are somewhat more variable than creatinine levels is one reason for using a shorter collection period for urea than for creatinine clearance. If urea clearance is measured during two consecutive 1-hour collections, sufficient hydration can be achieved that urine flow remains above 2 ml./min., and plasma fluctuations are unlikely to be serious. The short collection periods, however, may introduce serious artefacts if bladder emptying is incomplete.

NORMAL VALUES. The values for creatinine clearance, properly done, bear a close relationship to those measured by inulin clearance. Normal creatinine clearance values are approximately 125 ml./min. for men and 110 ml./min. for women. Urea clearance often is expressed in terms of percentage of normal function instead of in absolute terms. The normal or 100 percent level is taken as 75 ml./min. if urine flow has been 2 ml./min. or greater and 54 ml./min. (calculated with the square root of the urine volume) if flow was less than 2 ml./min. Values between 75 and 125 percent of normal indicate adequate filtration function.

Tubular Transport Mechanisms

Inulin does not undergo tubular transport, but certain other materials enter the urine both by glomerular filtration and tubular secretion. Comparing this excretion against purely glomerular excretion permits estimation of tubular transport capacity. A single transport path is known to secrete phenolsulfonphthalein (PSP) and *para*-aminohippuric acid (PAH) into the urine and also to transport penicillin, glucuronides, and such x-ray contrast media as Diodrast. That portion of PSP or PAH which is bound to plasma proteins does not pass the glomerular filter but reaches the tubules from the postglomerular interstitial circulation. At fairly low plasma levels, virtually all the PAH in a volume of blood can be removed by one passage through the kidney; one passage removes about 50 percent of the PSP. The excretory rate of these substances varies with the renal blood flow and the degree of tubular function.

PAH EXCRETION

Since PAH is excreted both by tubular secretion and glomerular filtration, tubular transport capacity (T_m) can be measured by comparing PAH excretion with the values for glomerular filtration rate obtained by inulin clearance. The increment of PAH over inulin values
represents the tubular capacity. Both technical and clinical problems
limit widespread employment of this approach.

PSP EXCRETION

Simpler than measuring PAH excretion but still a useful measure of
tubular transport is measuring PSP excretion. In this test, urinary
content of PSP is measured at 15, 30, 60, and 120 minutes after intravenous injection. With normal renal blood flow, normal tubular
function, and unobstructed urine flow, at least 25 percent of the total
dose should appear in urine at 15 minutes, and 60 to 70 percent
should have been excreted within an hour.

Since the plasma PSP level achieved with the usual dose does not
reach the maximum capacity of normally functioning tubules, the
amount of dye excreted relates more closely to the amount of blood
coming in contact with the tubules than to the functional capacity
of the tubular epithelium. If obstruction and oliguria are ruled out,
reduced early (15-minute) PSP excretion is more likely to indicate impaired renal perfusion than diminished tubular function. Congestive
heart failure or isolated renal vascular disease can produce abnormal
PSP results before the degree of circulatory impairment reduces
tubular function. Depressed tubular function rarely occurs without
impaired perfusion. Markedly abnormal PSP results indicate extensive
damage, and the 1-hour total excretion will be reduced.

PROBLEMS IN INTERPRETATION. Since injected contrast media,
chlorothiazide, penicillin G, and PSP all share a common tubular
mechanism, the test should not be performed if these drugs are in
use. Patients with severe hypoproteinemia may excrete unexpectedly
large amounts of PSP because more dye is unbound and filterable,
thus bypassing tubular transport. It is essential that the accurately
measured dose be completely injected, and, because the collecting
periods are so short, the patient must be thoroughly hydrated.

CONCENTRATING ABILITY

Regulation of urine concentration occurs primarily in the medulla, where the interstitial fluid is intensely hyperosmolar relative to the tubular fluid. Sodium and chloride reabsorption occur across the wall of the ascending limb of the loop of Henle.[16] Water is removed in the inner medulla, where antidiuretic hormone (ADH, vasopressin) alters tubular permeability to allow more or less water to return to the circulation.[10] Impaired concentrating ability may be the first indication of systemic conditions such as hypercalcemia or amyloidosis, which affect the kidney by altering the countercurrent multiplier mechanism of the medulla. It is often the first sign that infection or other inflammatory conditions have damaged renal parenchyma.

SPECIFIC GRAVITY

Several different means are available to measure urine concentration, that is, the relative amounts of solute and water. The oldest is measurement of specific gravity, using a float or urinometer which has been calibrated against distilled water. The specific gravity of urine from normal individuals can vary between 1.000 and 1.035. The procedure requires a large volume of urine and careful technique to avoid contaminating the specimen or misusing or misreading the urinometer. Other technical problems include the need to correct for temperature changes and the necessity for frequent instrument calibration. Simpler, but employing the same basic principles, is measurement of urinary solute load by its refractive effect on transmitted light. This can be measured easily on a few drops of urine without temperature interference. Urine refractometers are calibrated to translate refractive index directly to specific gravity.

SIGNIFICANT ALTERATIONS.   Specific gravity and refraction are influenced by the number and the nature of the solute particles. Large molecules in the urine, particularly proteins, glucose, and radiopaque dyes, exert a disproportionate effect on specific gravity. Artefact introduced by these substances may obscure small but significant changes in true concentration. The specific gravity of plasma, which contains proteins, glucose, lipids, and other macromolecules, is approximately 1.010. When the kidneys lose their ability to concentrate or dilute, excreted urine cannot reflect responses to physiologic stimuli, and urine specific gravity becomes fixed at 1.010, the plasma level.

OSMOLALITY

An index of renal function more sensitive than specific gravity is urine osmolality. Osmolality reflects only the number of solute particles in a fluid, regardless of their size or composition. Osmolality is measured by the effect of solute particles on the freezing point of a fluid. Pure water freezes at 0°C. A single osmole, which is 1 gram-molecular weight of an undissociated solute dissolved in 1 kg. of water, depresses the freezing point to −1.86°C. Osmolality is expressed as osmoles (Osm.) or milliosmoles (mOsm.) per kilogram of water.

Normal plasma has a mean osmolality of 285 mOsm./kg. with a range of 280 to 300. Sodium, chloride, and bicarbonate contribute more than 90 percent of this value. Urine osmolality can vary between 50 and 1400 mOsm./kg.,[16] depending on the burden of fluid and solutes presented to the kidney and the ability of the kidney to fulfill physiologic needs. Urea contributes a major portion of urinary osmotic activity.

Osmolality and specific gravity correlate roughly. A specific gravity of 1.022 corresponds to an osmolality of 800 mOsm./kg. Since osmolality can be measured accurately over a far greater range and to far finer grades of distinction, it offers a more flexible diagnostic instrument than measurement of specific gravity. In addition, the substances that disproportionately alter specific gravity, notably high sugar concentrations, x-ray contrast media, and abnormal proteins, do not greatly affect osmolality. Changes in osmolality reflect systemic physiologic conditions and renal concentrating ability more accurately than does changing specific gravity.

SIGNIFICANT ALTERATIONS. Serum osmolality rises with hyperglycemia, uremia, hemoconcentration from most causes, and the presence of circulating abnormal solutes, as in certain kinds of acidosis and shock. Under these conditions, urine osmolality also should be elevated. One effect of antidiuretic hormone (ADH) is to lower serum osmolality, producing relative urinary hyperosmolality until physiologic or pharmacologic measures achieve metabolic stabilization. Persistently high urine osmolality in the face of serum hyposmolality and hyponatremia suggests "inappropriate" ADH secretion. Urine is hyposmolar to serum in most types of physiologic or induced diuresis. Osmotic diuresis, which can occur with uremia and hyperglycemia as well as after infusion of mannitol or other substances, leads to urine which is isosmolar with serum.

VALUE OF RANDOM SPECIMENS. Determining the specific gravity or osmolality of a random urine specimen provides a spot check of renal concentrating ability but in an uncontrolled fashion. A standard of adequate concentrating ability is achievement, under appropriate stimulus, of urinary specific gravity of 1.025, or osmolality of 900 mOsm./kg. If a random specimen, often the first or second voided morning specimen, attains these or higher levels, than adequate concentrating function can be inferred, and further testing is unnecessary. Care must be taken that none of the above-mentioned artefacts has spuriously raised the specific gravity. If concentrating ability requires further study, the patient can be subjected to controlled water deprivation, and subsequent concentrating ability observed.

CONCENTRATION TESTS

THE MOSENTHAL TEST. The classical concentration test is that of Mosenthal, requiring a 24-hour period of water deprivation, although relatively normal food intake is permitted. Following a day and a night of fluid restriction, the patient saves the first voided morning specimen but remains recumbent. After 1 hour of recumbency, he voids again, and then after 1 hour of upright activity, he saves the third specimen voided. Of these three specimens, at least one should have a specific gravity of 1.025. The first specimen is usually the most concentrated, but patients with congestive heart failure or mobilizing edema fluid for any reason may have a relatively dilute overnight specimen; thus the second or third specimen would become more concentrated. Comparing the second and third specimen also permits detection of orthostatic proteinuria.

FOURTEEN-HOUR DEPRIVATION. A shorter period of fluid restriction is easier to control and gives similarly useful results. If the patient eats his evening meal before 6 p.m. and takes no fluids thereafter, the morning specimens will reflect 14 hours without intake. The first voided morning specimen should be discarded, since the overnight accumulation may include dilute urine from the early evening. Sampling the second voided specimen measures concentrating ability during a short period of known fluid restriction. The second morning sample should achieve either a minimum osmolality of 850 mOsm./kg. or a specific gravity of 1.026. If this concentration is not achieved, additional samples can be measured by prolonging the fluid restriction for another 6 hours. In some physiologically normal individuals, water deprivation for 22 hours may be necessary before maximum concentrating ability is induced.[24]

SIGNIFICANCE. Failure to concentrate normally indicates renal damage which may be localized to the medulla or may involve the entire nephron. Impaired concentrating ability may be the first sign of subtle damage or an early indicator of unsuspected infection. Needless to say, patient cooperation is essential. Before diagnosing impaired concentrating ability, the physician must be sure that the patient has not taken nocturnal fluids, either accidentally or deliberately. Diminished concentrating ability usually means damaged kidneys, but rare etiologies may include pituitary dysfunction with reduced antidiuretic hormone (ADH) production or renal insensitivity to ADH. Both these possibilities can be investigated by noting the response to exogenous ADH.

Concentration tests are meaningless in patients taking diuretic drugs. Metabolically induced conditions of osmotic diuresis or increased solute load also invalidate the results, since renal concentrating ability is inversely proportional to the solute load. The patient should be in a state of adequate diet and normal hydration. Protein deficiency impairs renal concentrating ability, and patients who have been markedly overhydrated for several days may have impaired concentration if dehydration is then imposed.[24]

Renal damage also can impair diluting ability, but this is less readily demonstrated than impairment of maximum concentration and gives no more information than concentration testing.

ROUTINE URINALYSIS

Routine urinalysis includes the observation of color, concentration, and pH of the urine, along with microscopic examination of formed elements and a search for pathologically significant elements not normally present, such as glucose, protein, blood, ketones, and bile pigments. The technology of routine urinalysis has changed from manual tests for individual constituents to use of chemical-impregnated paper strips and reagent tablets. The results offer equal or greater accuracy, as long as the limitations are appreciated, and much greater speed and convenience. The strips should be protected from moisture or volatile fumes and should not be used if discolored. Personnel using the strips should avoid touching the test areas with their fingers. In reading the results, recommended time intervals are important, and a good light is indispensable.

Urine pH

Urinary pH is measured only roughly. The normal pH is slightly acid, approximately 6 when the usual acid-residue diet is consumed. The limits of pH variation are from 4.5 to nearly 9. The combination of bromthymol blue and methyl red used in the testing strips permits discrimination to approximately one-half pH unit within this range.

Urine acidification requires metabolic work by the kidney, including reabsorption and reconstitution of bicarbonate ion, ammonium ion excretion, and excretion of free hydrogen ions. With good renal function, urine pH tends to reflect plasma pH, permitting compensation when acid-base derangements are present, but there are several notable exceptions.

SIGNIFICANT ALTERATIONS

If tubular function is deficient, the kidney may be unable to produce an appropriate gradient between urine and plasma pH. This syndrome of renal tubular acidosis may be primary, due to congenital or acquired renal disease and resulting in subsequent metabolic abnormalities if uncorrected, or it may be secondary to other conditions which produce acidosis and also impair renal activity. Urine may be inappropriately acid during metabolic alkalosis, because of obligatory hydrogen ion excretion if potassium is severely depleted. With the kind of severe dehydration and salt loss that tends to produce this picture, ketones and organic acids frequently accumulate, enhancing urinary acidity and ultimately producing a picture of mixed alkalosis and acidosis.

ALKALINITY. Significantly, alkaline urines are relatively rare. They may result from a diet disproportionately high in fruits and vegetables and low in meat protein or from alkalinizing drugs given to prevent precipitation of urate or other stones. Since ammonia-splitting bacteria convert urine from acid to alkaline, a strongly alkaline reaction may mean that the specimen has been sitting around too long. If a freshly voided specimen is alkaline, urinary tract infection should be investigated.

ACIDITY. Strongly acid reactions accompany nearly all forms of acidosis except, as mentioned above, when there is intrinsic or acquired renal damage. A test of acidifying capacity is the administration of large doses of ammonium chloride (12 gm. daily for 3 days), which should result in urine acidification to pH 4.5 to 5.5. In renal tubular failure, pH fails to go below 6 or 6.5. High meat diets and acidifying drugs produce persistently acid urine.

Color

Normal urine ranges in color from pale yellow to deep gold, depending on the concentration of solutes. Although usually clear, urine may turn cloudy on standing if urates precipitate in acid urine or phosphates precipitate at alkaline pH. The most common pathologically significant color changes result from the presence of blood, hemoglobin degradation products, or bilirubin and its metabolites. Fresh blood imparts a cloudy reddish-pink or reddish-brown appearance; deeper brown or brownish-gray shades develop if urinary acidity converts hemoglobin to acid hematin or methemoglobin. Myoglobin also produces a reddish-brown appearance. Closely related chemically to hemoglobin, myoglobin may enter urine after severe destruction of muscle, the only tissue that contains myoglobin.

HEMOGLOBIN TESTING

Virtually all tests for hemoglobin, in urine, feces, and other materials, exploit the peroxidase properties of the molecule, whereby oxygen catalytically released from hydrogen peroxide affects an indicator color. For urine, orthotoluidine is used as indicator, and it is sensitive to hemoglobin in extremely low concentrations. Myoglobin, when present, also produces a positive test. Since the test detects hemoglobin free in solution, it sometimes fails to reveal that intact red cells are present. Microscopic examination of the centrifuged sediment is the best way to demonstrate red blood cells in the urine, while orthotoluidine testing is valuable if hemoglobinuria is of other origin or if red cells originally present have lysed. Both chemical and microscopic examinations should be applied to all specimens, since neither test will reliably detect all significant abnormalities.

Blood can enter the urine from trauma, hemorrhage, infarction, or infection at any level in the urinary system. Cell-free hemoglobinuria, if not the result of red cell lysis after the urine is voided, indicates intravascular hemolysis, usually due to acquired hemolytic anemia of the cold agglutinin type, paroxysmal nocturnal hemoglobinuria, drug-induced hemolysis, or transfusion reactions.

FREE HEMOGLOBIN. Extracellular hemoglobin enters urine only after the hemoglobin-binding capacity of plasma haptoglobin is exceeded. Normal haptoglobin levels can bind as much as 3 gm. of hemoglobin, the amount released from approximately 20 ml. of blood. Hemoglobinuria begins within 1 or 2 hours of an acute hemolytic event and usually does not persist beyond 24 hours, although hemosiderin may be excreted for 3 to 5 days thereafter. In paroxysmal nocturnal hemoglobinuria, as in other states of persistent or repeated hemolysis, the sediment may contain hemosiderin granules in casts or in the cytoplasm of epithelial cells. Its presence is detected by treating the sediment with ammonium sulfide, which highlights the hemosiderin as distinct black granules.

OTHER SIGNIFICANT COLORS

Bilirubin and related pigments produce shades ranging from orange through yellow to greenish-brown. Chemical tests for these products are described later in the chapter. Uncommon but diagnostically significant causes for peculiar coloration include the following: clear urine which turns dark red on standing suggests porphobilinogen excretion, found in acute intermittent porphyria; clear urine which turns brown or black on standing suggests homogentisic acid, excreted in the amino acid disorder alkaptonuria, or melanogen, excreted in disseminated malignant melanoma.

ARTEFACTUAL CHANGES

A number of drugs or dietary items affect urine color but in themselves have little pathologic importance. Pyridium, used to relieve the pain of bladder and other urinary tract diseases, imparts a lurid orange hue. The vitamin riboflavin, in large doses, turns urine bright orange. Certain dyestuffs in candies or drugs may sometimes produce red or yellow urine. Alkaline urine turns red in the presence of several related substances including excreted phenolphthalein, sometimes used as a laxative, phenolsulfonphthalein (PSP) which has laxative effect but usually is administered for a renal function test, and Bromsulphalein (BSP) which is used in liver function testing. Large quantities of phenacetin, used in innumerable proprietary pain-relieving preparations, may turn urine brownish-gray or black.[20] The anticonvulsant drug Dilantin and psychoactive drugs of the phenothiazine group may cause pink, red, or reddish-brown urine.

Sugar

Normal urine contains virtually no sugar. Although approximately 250 gm. of glucose passes through the kidneys daily, no more than

100 mg. are excreted in 24 hours. Glucose may occur in urine (gly-cosuria) if high blood glucose levels produce a glucose load in the filtrate which exceeds the kidneys' reabsorptive capacity or if the proximal tubules perform this reabsorptive function imperfectly. Sugar in urine was known by the ancients to be abnormal, and perhaps the earliest form of urinalysis was tasting the urine; the term diabetes mellitus means "flow of sweet urine."

COPPER REDUCTION TESTS

The classic present-day test for glucose is Benedict's test, in which the sugar reduces blue alkaline cupric sulfate to red cuprous oxide. This measures reducing activity, not glucose or even carbohydrates specifically. In addition to such sugars as fructose and galactose, other urinary constituents which may reduce copper sulfate are creatinine, uric acid, salicylates, and homogentisic acid. In addition, drugs or contaminants such as ascorbic acid or some antibiotics may cause spurious positives.

Benedict's test is sensitive to concentrations of 50 to 80 mg. glucose per 100 ml. urine and can be quantitated roughly according to the color and quantity of the precipitate. The single-tablet copper reduction test (Clinitest) employs the same reagents and is slightly less sensitive but far easier than Benedict's test, which requires boiling.

GLUCOSE OXIDASE TESTS

Reagent-impregnated paper strips and several automated procedures employ a different, highly sensitive and highly specific test for glucose. The strips contain glucose oxidase which reacts with glucose to produce gluconic acid and hydrogen peroxide. The hydrogen peroxide induces color change in orthotoluidine or some other colored indicator, to a degree proportional to the glucose concentration. Adventitious hydrogen peroxide or bleach in the urine container will, of course, produce a false positive, while large quantities of ascorbic acid in the urine delay or abolish the color development. Other reducing substances have no effect on the glucose oxidase methods.

NONGLUCOSE SUGARS

Under some conditions, demonstration of sugars other than glucose is highly significant, and the specificity of glucose oxidase is a liability, not an advantage. This is especially true in the urine of young

infants, when galactosuria is a more significant finding than glycosuria. Galactose in urine may signal the presence of the potentially
disastrous hereditary condition galactosemia; infants' urines should
be screened with a copper-reduction, not a glucose-oxidase, technique. Since galactose will be excreted only if the child is ingesting
milk in moderate quantities, galactosemia cannot be diagnosed by
urine testing during the immediate newborn period.

Other sugars which reduce copper and may be found in urine
include lactose, fructose, and five-carbon sugars. Their presence may
signify dietary peculiarities or congenital metabolic abnormalities
which usually are fairly benign except for galactosemia. Pregnant
and lactating women may excrete lactose; since glycosuria is very
common in pregnancy, the presence of lactose or other sugars will
not be noted unless specific tests are done. Both chemical and
chromatographic tests are used to identify specific sugars.

Ketones

If tissue needs outstrip the body's available glucose supplies, fat
combustion substitutes as an energy supply. Since fat metabolism is
less efficient, metabolic end products accumulate, and these ketone
bodies are excreted in the urine. The three ketone bodies found in
urine are betahydroxybutyric acid, which accounts for nearly 80
percent of the ketones present; acetoacetic acid (just under 20
percent); and acetone, which comprises no more than a very small
percentage.[12] The nitroprusside test generally used for screening
ketonuria identifies only acetoacetic acid and acetone, but all three
are excreted in parallel proportions, and there is no particular virtue
in partitioning the ketones present.

SIGNIFICANCE

Any condition of acute metabolic demand with reduced intake, often
exacerbated by fluid and nutrient loss through diarrhea or vomiting
or both, can produce ketonuria. In children, stress which might not
outstrip an adult's glucose metabolism will produce ketonuria. In
adults, significant ketonuria most frequently accompanies uncontrolled episodes of diabetes when glucose is present but not functionally available for metabolism. The degree of ketonuria roughly
reflects the severity of metabolic stress, but accurate quantitation is
unnecessary. Reporting excretion as trace, slight, moderate, and
severe ketonuria usually is sufficient.

Reagent strips impregnated with nitroprusside and glycine discriminate the level of ketonuria with definite color differences over the range from 5 to 10 mg./dl. (trace to slight), 20 to 30 mg./dl. (moderate), and 60 mg./dl. or above (severe). Symptomatic ketosis occurs at levels of 50 mg./dl. or above, while levels of 20 to 30 mg./dl. signal moderately serious metabolic imbalance. These gradations, therefore, correlate well with clinical usefulness.

Protein

The classic tests for urine protein involve precipitating the proteins, either chemically or by heating. The precipitate includes all types of protein, at a minimum sensitivity of 1 to 10 mg./dl., the quantity of precipitate being roughly proportional to the amount of protein present.

REAGENT STRIP METHODS

Reagent-impregnated strips detect proteinuria with a buffered color indicator (tetrabromphenol blue) which, at pH 3, is yellow when protein is absent and green when protein is present. The advantage of this procedure, besides rapidity, is that turbidity of the specimen or the presence of radiocontrast media or other macromolecules do not affect the results. On the other hand, it detects primarily albumin and does not indicate the presence of globulins, Bence-Jones protein, other globulin fragments, or myoglobin.

PROTEIN QUANTITATION

Reagent strips permit modest quantitation of protein present in random specimens, but other techniques are used for total urinary protein excretion. The turbidity produced with sulfosalicylic acid precipitation can be quantitated fairly accurately, giving a specific figure for protein in all or part of a collected specimen. Either a total 24-hour collection or smaller timed aliquot can be used. Normal excretion is no more than 150 mg. in 24 hours.

The standard curve used for quantitation goes up to concentrations of 100 mg. protein in 100 ml. urine. If the patient's urine has more protein than this, it can be diluted to fall within the range, and appropriate calculations made for actual concentration. Sulfosalicylic acid precipitates polypeptides, Bence-Jones protein, and proteoses (heat soluble glycoproteins) as well as albumin and normal globulins; thus a variety of abnormal constituents may be included in the total figure.

SIGNIFICANCE. Protein excretion above 150 mg. per day is nearly always significant. Most often the protein is albumin. Albuminuria frequently indicates abnormal glomerular permeability, due either to intrinsic glomerular disease or to changes in blood pressure, as in hypertension, pre-eclampsia, or abnormalities of the renal veins. The list of all conditions causing proteinuria of any degree would simply be a list of all possible urinary tract diseases. Massive proteinuria, greater than 4 gm. per day, is the hallmark of the nephrotic syndrome, which can be "idiopathic" or due to lupus erythematosus, amyloid disease, or other conditions. The proteinuria in glomerulonephritis is inconstantly related to the severity or the phase of the process. When glomerular function is severely reduced, as in acute proliferative glomerulonephritis or chronic glomerulonephritis approaching "end-stage" disease, proteinuria may be minimal.

INFLAMMATORY SIGNS. Large numbers of white cells accompanying proteinuria usually signal infection at some level in the urinary tract, the protein originating from the white cells, the bacteria, or the increased capillary permeability that inflammation induces. Noninfectious inflammatory diseases of the glomeruli tend to contribute both red and white blood cells accompanying proteinuria, notably in glomerulonephritis and the nephritis of lupus erythematosus. Proteinuria does not inevitably accompany renal disease. Pyelonephritis, obstructions, nephrolithiasis, tumors, and metabolic nephropathies may cause severe illness without telltale protein leakage.

ORTHOSTATIC PROTEINURIA. Somewhat perplexing is the significance of postural (orthostatic) proteinuria, found in up to 5 percent of healthy adolescents and young adults, usually male. There is evidence[25] that consistent protein leakage, occurring only in the upright position and without other urinary abnormalities, is unlikely to develop into more severe disease later. Persistent proteinuria unrelated to posture and intermittent proteinuria occurring with no predictable physiologic concomitant carry greater likelihood of unfavorable prognosis and existing renal biopsy changes.

Proteins Other Than Albumin

Of increasing significance are the proteinurias not due to albumin. These include the classic example, Bence-Jones protein of multiple myeloma, as well as the proteins or protein components in heavy chain disease, macroglobulinemia and various tubular defects. These will be detected by heat precipitation or sulfosalicylic acid, whereupon specific immunologic, electrophoretic, or chromatographic identification should be undertaken. Reagent-strip testing does not screen adequately for these conditions. The urine found to be negative with strip testing and positive with sulfosalicylic acid signals a need for more detailed investigation.

BENCE-JONES PROTEIN

Bence-Jones protein is the most commonly sought nonalbumin protein in urine. These low molecular weight polypeptides (molecular weight 22,000 to 44,000) are immunoglobulin light chains which circulate and enter the urine as monomers, dimers, and trimers or tetramers. Approximately 60 percent of patients with multiple myeloma have this distinctive form of proteinuria. The Bence-Jones protein precipitates reversibly at temperatures between 45 and 60°C., re-entering suspension at higher or lower temperatures.

HEAT TESTING. The classic test consists of placing the slightly acidified urine sample in a water bath and raising the temperature gradually to the boiling point. If turbidity develops at the mid-range, disappears as the boiling point approaches, reappears as the urine cools, and then disappears on return to room temperature, the demonstration is virtually conclusive. Turbidity may fail to clear when the urine cools if other proteins have been precipitated by the heat or if the urine has been excessively acidified. Filtering the turbid specimen at high temperatures may remove precipitated protein and permit demonstration of the appropriately reacting Bence-Jones material, but some Bence-Jones proteins do not disperse completely at high temperature.

ELECTROPHORESIS. Heat testing may miss as many as one-third of Bence-Jones proteinurias. In patients with suspected myeloma or other dysproteinemias, it is preferable to perform electrophoresis of the urine proteins. Usually, it is necessary to concentrate the urine sample, since electrophoresis is unsatisfactory at protein concentrations below 0.5 to 1 gm./dl. Bence-Jones protein appears as a peak at the α_2-globulin location. Serum electrophoresis usually does not reveal circulating Bence-Jones protein, since the small molecules pass rapidly through the glomerular filter and are, in addition, rapidly destroyed by bodily metabolism.[26] Most myeloma patients also produce whole immunoglobulin in a diagnostically significant monoclonal pattern, although in perhaps 20 percent of patients, the isolated light chains may be the only detectable abnormal secretory product.[26] Bence-Jones proteinuria occasionally may accompany macroglobulinemia and, rarely, some leukemias.[32]

ELECTROPHORETIC PATTERNS

Electrophoresis of urine proteins may demonstrate that abnormal serum constituents, potentially damaging to the kidney, have entered the urine for excretion. Albumin is the predominant urinary protein when glomerular permeability is increased, but with normal glomerular permeability and various prerenal abnormalities, circulating globulins may appear in the urine. Bence-Jones protein is especially important because it does not appear on serum electrophoretograms. Hemoglobins, following intravascular hemolysis, and myoglobin, following extensive muscle damage, appear on urine electrophoretograms at the α_1-globulin band. In conditions of catabolic stress and "inflammatory syndrome," there may be α_1-globulin elevations without increased albumin. If the stress or systemic damage alters glomerular permeability in addition, a high albumin peak accompanies the α_1 peak.

Microscopic Examination of Sediment

The urine sediment, containing cells and other formed elements, constitutes a direct sampling of urinary tract morphology. For best results, urine should be examined within 1 or 2 hours of voiding, and a concentrated urine will contain proportionally more formed elements than a dilute specimen. The first or second voided morning specimen usually gives best results, and the number of organized elements can be roughly quantitated from their number in a centrifuged aliquot. More accurate quantitation sometimes is obtained by the Addis count on a 12-hour timed collection, but more often qualitative judgments provide sufficient information. Significant elements to be sought in all specimens are red blood cells, white blood cells, epithelial cells, casts, trichomonads, bacteria, and yeasts.

COLLECTION TECHNIQUE

Sediment of normal urine may contain occasional white blood cells and squamous epithelial cells but should be virtually free of red blood cells. Cleansing and collection procedures are critical, for urine voided through an inadequately cleansed meatus may contain leukocytes, epithelial cells, bacteria, and red blood cells, especially from menstruating women. Overenthusiastic cleansing, combined with poor collection technique, may introduce red cells, extraneous fibers, epithelial cells, and starch or powder granules. If technique has been satisfactory and the voided urine is examined within 2 or 3 hours, the sediment can be considered representative of the bladder contents. Urine specimens refrigerated for 12 to 24 hours still can provide valid bacteriologic information, but in the absence of preservative, casts and cells begin to deteriorate after about 3 hours.

INFLAMMATION

The usual cause of urinary leukocytosis is acute infection somewhere in the urinary tract. If the infection is in the kidney, the white cells tend to be associated with cellular and granular casts, bacteria, renal epithelial cells, and relatively few red cells. The degree of pyuria need not reflect the severity of the inflammatory process, but rather the proximity of the infection to functioning nephrons, collecting ducts, and the pelvis.

Bladder infections will not produce casts, since the process occurs below the level of renal tubules, the only site where casts are formed. Cystitis frequently produces red cells in the sediment, as well as leukocytes and, often, large epithelial cells of bladder origin. Cystitis may be bacterial or nonbacterial with little distinction in the sediment, although the cultures will provide necessary differentiation. In acute glomerulonephritis there may be significant urinary leukocytosis, although red cells usually predominate. Various noninfectious inflammatory diseases of the kidney, ureters, and bladder may contribute moderate numbers of white cells to the sediment.

RED BLOOD CELLS

Red cells greatly in excess of leukocytes indicate bleeding into the urinary tract. Among other causes, this may be due to trauma, which usually can be elicited by history; tumor, in which case cytologic examination of the urinary sediment may permit positive diagnosis;

or systemic bleeding disorders, such as thrombocytopenia, acquired hemorrhagic diatheses, congenital deficiencies, aspirin ingestion, or anticoagulant therapy. In acute glomerulonephritis, red cells enter the urine because of glomerular capillary damage, and in necrotizing arteriolar nephrosclerosis, there may be intermittent mild hematuria because of small vessel hemorrhage.

CASTS

Casts composed largely or exclusively of cells indicate exudative, hemorrhagic, or desquamative conditions of the nephron. Red cell casts suggest destructive lesions of the glomerulus and are fairly common in acute glomerulonephritis; they are less conspicuous in severe lupus nephritis, arteritis of any cause, or necrotizing arteriolosclerosis. White cell casts may be difficult to distinguish from epithelial cell casts, and both kinds of cells may be intermixed. In acute tubular necrosis, brownish pigment casts and casts of tubular epithelial cells are numerous, along with isolated, often degenerating, epithelial cells.[9] In inflammatory states, leukocytes and epithelial cells tend to be present together. So-called granular casts probably represent degenerated cellular elements embedded in the protein matrix. The nature of *waxy casts*, which are homogeneous, sharply defined, and highly refractile, is uncertain.

CAST FORMATION. Most casts derive from the distal convoluted tubules, where hydrogen ion and electrolyte concentrations are high, and have the narrow caliber of this segment. Occasionally, wide-bore casts are seen which originate from the collecting tubules. Because urine flow in these ducts normally is too swift for casts to form, the development of broad casts indicates severe slowing of the urinary stream and pronounced renal malfunction. Since the ducts where this occurs tend to be those whose contributing nephrons have been damaged or destroyed, these wide casts reflect severe kidney damage and sometimes are called *renal failure casts.*

Crystals

Most crystals or amorphous material have little clinical significance but may obscure other elements in the sediment. Crystalluria becomes important in some disorders of amino acid metabolism, notably cystine, leucine, or tyrosine, or in patients taking poorly soluble sulfa drugs or other medications. The clinician should alert the laboratory that these elements may be present so that special examination and identification can be made. Far more common findings in urinary sediment are crystalline or amorphous urates, calcium oxalate, and crystalline or amorphous phosphates. Bilirubin and cholesterol occasionally may be present as urinary crystals.

Other Findings

Motile trichomonads sometimes are present in urine specimens from women with vaginitis, if collecting technique has been poor. In men, trichomonads can produce urethritis, and occasionally the organisms may be seen in the urine. When fungi or bacteria are present in urine sediment, the cause may be significant infection or multiplication of a few organisms in a specimen that has been standing for too long. Globules of cholesterol and other lipids sometimes are seen in urine from patients with intense proteinuria. Since lipid vacuoles occur in tubular epithelial cells when proteinuria is severe, these globules may derive from coalesced epithelial vacuoles or degenerated cells, or they may result in some way from the high serum lipid levels usually present in these patients.

SPECIAL TESTS

Bilirubin and Urobilinogen

Tests are available for many other substances which may appear in urine under various clinical conditions. The abnormal constituent most often sought, and found, is bilirubin. Since bilirubin is water-soluble only when conjugated, it is posthepatic, direct-reacting bilirubin that appears in urine. This form, normally excreted in the bile, enters urine when blood levels are high; thus jaundice of some degree always accompanies bilirubinuria. With severe jaundice, the renal excretory pathway achieves metabolic significance, and serum bilirubin levels may increase if renal function deteriorates.

The classic cause for bilirubinuria is extrahepatic biliary tract obstruction, but conjugated bilirubin may enter the urine when there is portal inflammation or hepatocellular damage. In viral or toxic hepatitis, bilirubinuria may be conspicuous. Urine color may range from yellow-orange through brown, depending on the concentration, and shaking the specimen produces a yellow foam. Urine pigmented from urobilin and urobilinogen does not have yellow foam when shaken; this permits differentiation of a sort, but there are better tests available for both substances than the "foam test."

UROBILINOGEN

Urobilinogen is formed in the intestine from normally excreted conjugated bilirubin. Bacterial activity produces a series of colorless substances known collectively as urobilinogen (also called stercobilinogen), which, upon oxidation, form orange-brown urobilin (stercobilin), which gives normal feces their color. Some urobilinogen is absorbed from the colon into the blood stream, whence it returns to the liver for re-excretion in bile. This enterohepatic circulation appears to serve no useful function, but the water-soluble urobilinogen enters the urinary filtrate as blood goes through the kidney.

INCREASED URINE LEVELS. Normally, urine contains small quantities of urobilinogen, but pathologic amounts appear if abnormally large amounts are present in the intestine or if the liver cannot re-excrete the absorbed urobilinogen. With increased hemoglobin breakdown, intestinal urobilinogen increases and urinary urobilinogen rises. Urine urobilinogen levels can be a sensitive indicator of hepatic damage, since hepatic urobilinogen excretion is more vulnerable to mild parenchymal damage than is bilirubin excretion. Early hepatitis or mild toxic injury may cause elevated circulating urobilinogen because of decreased biliary-tract excretion, despite unchanged serum bilirubin levels. In such cases, elevated urine urobilinogen points to incipient liver disease. Obviously, if no bilirubin enters the bile, no urobilinogen will be produced. With severe liver damage or obstruction, both urinary and fecal urobilinogen will decline. The classic association of pale stools and dark urine in obstructive jaundice results from diminished intestinal bilirubin being converted to the chromogen, while increased plasma bilirubin enters the urine.

CHEMICAL TESTS

BILIRUBIN. Tests for urinary bilirubin employ either a diazo reaction or the oxidation of bilirubin to biliverdin. Fouchet's test employs the oxidation principle, with trichloroacetic acid and ferric chloride added to the bilirubin remaining when filtered urine is adsorbed onto barium chloride. A positive result is the appearnace of a green spot. Even if exposure to air has oxidized some bilirubin, this test may be positive. Since the diazo test, available in tablet form, reacts only with the somewhat labile nonoxidized form, the age of the specimen may affect the results of tablet testing. Positive tests result in purple or bluish-purple coloration.

Since urine contains only conjugated bilirubin, there is no need to worry about "direct" and "indirect" reactions. Urobilin, the oxidation product of urobilinogen, may produce a red spot with this test, or a muddy purple color on Fouchet's test, but both constitute negative results for bilirubin. Salicylates also may give false positives, and large amounts of ascorbic acid can interfere with both tests.

UROBILINOGEN. Urobilinogen testing uses Ehrlich's aldehyde reagent. Since urobilin will not react, the specimen must be protected from oxidation. Besides urobilinogen, porphobilinogen, sulfonamides, and 5-hydroxyindoleacetic acid (5-HIAA) all react with Ehrlich's aldehyde reagent, but urobilinogen can be separated by chloroform extraction for identification if necessary. Because small amounts of urobilinogen are normal, the results must be quantitated.

The Watson-Schwartz method measures the amount of urobilinogen excreted in a carefully timed 2-hour collection period between the hours of 1 and 3 p.m., and the results are given in Ehrlich units. The classic technique uses spectrophotometric reading for accurate quantitation. A reagent strip method permits semiquantitation by comparing developed color against reference blocks. The normal concentration range is 0.1 to 1 Ehrlich unit per 100 ml. urine, or less than 1 Ehrlich unit in a 2-hour collection. Patients with biliary obstruction or diminished bacterial flora will excrete little or no urobilinogen, but there is no reliable way of documenting abnormally low urinary urobilinogen. Strongly acid urine may give a falsely low test result. Porphobilinogen (see below) also gives positive results with Ehrlich's aldehyde reagent.

Hemoglobin Precursors

Porphobilinogen is a hemoglobin precursor rather than a breakdown product. It is a single-ringed structure which develops from the straight-chain molecule delta-aminolevulinic acid. Heme synthesis progresses from delta-aminolevulinic acid (ALA), through porphobilinogen to the four-ringed precursors uroporphyrinogen, coproporphyrinogen, protoporphyrinogen, and protoporphyrin which finally combines with iron to become heme. The porphyrinogen forms are hematologically active and remain in the marrow. The inactive end products uroporphyrin and coproporphyrin are excreted in urine and feces.

SECONDARY PORPHYRIAS

A group of heritable metabolic diseases, the porphyrias, produce abnormal porphyrin values in both urine and feces. Impaired hematopoiesis or decreased liver function also may cause porphyrin excretion to rise. Rare cases of liver disease and severe lead poisoning may elevate urinary levels of uroporphyrin, but the more frequent urinary metabolite in secondary porphyria is coproporphyrin. Mild coproporphyrinuria may accompany heavy metal poisoning; carbon tetrachloride or benzene toxicity; Hodgkin's disease; some cases of hemolytic, aplastic, or megaloblastic anemia; and, in an unpredictable fashion, liver disease of various kinds. Substantial porphyrinuria, however, usually signifies a primary metabolic disorder.

PRIMARY PORPHYRIAS

ERYTHROPOIETIC PORPHYRIA. The porphyrias are divided into two different groups, classified as erythropoietic and hepatic. In the erythropoietic forms, the major accumulation of porphyrins is in the erythrocytes. Up to 50 mg. of urinary uroporphyrin per day may be excreted in the least rare of these conditions; in the other forms, fecal and urinary uroporphyrin, coproporphyrin, and protoporphyrin levels are not significant. Urinary levels of ALA and porphobilinogen are normal in all the erythropoietic conditions, and definitive diagnosis rests on red cell studies.

HEPATIC PORPHYRIAS. In the hepatic porphyrias, red cell levels of heme precursors are normal, and diagnosis rests on urinary and fecal determinations. The three major forms of hepatic porphyria are *acute intermittent porphyria,* characterized by markedly increased urinary ALA and porphobilinogen, moderate urinary uroporphyrin, and mildly elevated urinary coproporphyrin; *porphyria cutanea tarda*, in which ALA and porphobilinogen are normal, but urinary uroporphyrin and coproporphyrin are both markedly elevated; and *variegate porphyria*, a disease chiefly associated with South Africa, in which porphobilinogen and ALA appear in urine during acute attacks, along with both coproporphyrin and uroporphyrin. Fecal levels of protoporphyrin are markedly elevated in variegate porphyria, a finding distinctive for this condition.

PORPHOBILINOGEN DETERMINATION. Normal porphobilinogen excretion is 1 to 1.5 mg. per day. During active episodes of acute intermittent porphyria, porphobilinogen excretion increases enormously. When the disease is latent, the substance may or may not be present in diagnostic amounts. Porphobilinogen converts to dark red porphobilin and colorless porphyrins on standing. Since these do not react with the aldehyde reagent, fresh specimens should be used for testing. On the other hand, the observation that a specimen turns wine-colored on standing may indicate that porphyria should be considered in a patient's differential diagnosis.

If the Ehrlich's aldehyde test is positive on whole urine, chloroform extraction can be used to remove most extraneous Ehrlich-reactive materials. The aqueous phase remains Ehrlich-reactive if porphobilinogen is present. Subsequent butanol extraction gives even better identification, since butanol removes all the Ehrlich-reactive material except porphobilinogen, which steadfastly remains in the aqueous phase. In porphyria cutanea tarda, another hepatic porphyria, porphobilinogen occasionally may be increased.

SCREENING WITH ULTRAVIOLET LIGHT. The simplest screening test for urinary porphyrins is to view the specimen with ultraviolet light. The porphyrins exhibit orange fluorescence in highly acid urine and orange-red to red fluorescence as the pH rises. Coproporphyrin is extracted from the aqueous urine with ethyl acetate or ether at lower pH, in the range of 3 to 3.5,[5] or by adsorption onto alumina or column chromatography. Quantitation is possible by spectrophotometric or fluorometric measurement, but the degree and shade of fluorescence may permit sufficient estimation for diagnostic purposes.

DELTA-AMINOLEVULINIC ACID. In acute intermittent porphyria, delta-aminolevulinic acid (ALA) is markedly increased, as well as porphobilinogen. At least a part of the metabolic defect in this disease is an increase in the hepatic enzyme. ALA-synthetase, which causes buildup of both substances.[30] Screening batteries to diagnose porphyria usually do not include testing for urinary ALA, because porphobilinogen testing is more productive. Urinary ALA levels, however, are used in screening for lead poisoning, since lead toxicity very early impairs hemoglobin synthesis at the stage at which ALA is converted to porphobilinogen.[13] Thus ALA builds up to be excreted in the urine, where it can be detected and quantified. Normal urine ALA should be below 0.5 mg./dl.; values above that, in populations at risk, suggest toxic damage.

Industrial exposure, either acute or chronic, is a hazard in adults. Childhood plumbism tends to be insidious and associated with pica and with deteriorated housing conditions. Since urinary ALA levels occasionally may be within normal limits despite significant levels of blood lead, the screening test is not ideal. Because measuring blood lead is difficult and expensive, the search continues for a better screening test for early plumbism. One very promising approach is measurement of blood ALA-dehydratase, the enzyme whose reduced activity leads to ALA accumulation,[13] but urinary ALA determination remains, at present, an important tool for evaluating possible lead toxicity.

Calcium

Urinary calcium excretion is largely determined by serum calcium levels and the equilibrium between calcium and phosphates. A normal individual excretes as much as 200 to 400 mg. of calcium daily on diets containing between 500 mg. and 1 gm. of calcium. Marked changes in dietary intake produce only slight variation in urinary calcium excretion. The serum calcium level is far more important than calcium intake in determining excretion. Normally, up to 99 percent of filtered calcium is reabsorbed. When serum calcium levels fall to 7.5 mg./dl. or below, virtually all the filtered calcium is salvaged, leaving practically none in the excreted urine. Calcium excretion rises with high sodium and magnesium intakes, while increasing dietary phosphate reduces calcium excretion. Metabolic acidosis and glucocorticoid excess also increase calciuria.

HYPERCALCIURIA

Increased calcium excretion almost always accompanies elevated serum calcium levels. Hyperparathyroidism produces the most striking hypercalciuria, but increased excretion occurs whenever calcium is mobilized from bone, as in metastatic malignancies, Paget's disease of bone, and prolonged skeletal immobilization. Hypercalciuria also may accompany multiple myeloma, sarcoid, vitamin D intoxication, and some cases of thyrotoxicosis. Since calcium excretion fluctuates throughout the day, being heaviest just after meals and lowest at night, accurate evaluation of total calcium excretion requires a 24-hour determination. The specimen should be collected with 10 ml. of concentrated hydrochloric acid so that calcium salts will not precipitate. Calcium excretion greater than intake is always excessive, and excretion above 400 to 500 mg. in 24 hours is reliably abnormal.

THE SULKOWITCH TEST

The quantitative methods used for serum calcium also can be used for urine determinations. The Sulkowitch test is a simple, time-honored means for qualitative evaluation. Although the results cover a wide range of quantitative equivalents, the test remains useful. In the Sulkowitch test, a calcium oxalate precipitate forms in the presence of acetic acid and oxalates, the amount of precipitate roughly proportional to the amount of calcium present.

RANGE OF RESULTS. The traditional interpretation is that normal urine produces a fine white cloud, neither a clear solution which indicates no calcium at all, nor a heavy precipitate reflecting excessive excretion. If normal excretion is taken as 150 mg. in 24 hours and normal urine volume as 1500 ml., then an average normal specimen should contain roughly 10 mg. per 100 ml. A 2+ Sulkowitch reading corresponds to a mean value of 9 mg./dl., but the range is very wide.[22] Negative results clearly indicate decreased calcium excretion, covering a range from 1 to 3.45 mg./dl., and 4+ is clearly increased (30 to 43 mg./dl.), but between these extremes, the range of scatter is wide.

The Sulkowitch test is used primarily on random specimens to identify the reduced calcium excretion that accompanies decreased serum levels or to document excessive excretion if other signs and symptoms point to hyperparathyroidism. Specimens should be selected with diurnal variation in mind. To rule out hypercalciuria, an early morning specimen should be examined, since excretion is lowest then. If hypocalcemia is suspected, the sample should be taken after a meal, when excretion is maximal. The test is sufficiently simple that repeated determinations are feasible, at home by the patient himself, if necessary.

Amino Acid Abnormalities

Amino acids appear in urine either when metabolic dysfunction presents abnormal amino acid loads to a normal kidney, or when an abnormal kidney is unable to process the normally constituted glomerular filtrate. Most of the abnormal filtered loads result from inborn errors of metabolism, although occasional acquired conditions, such as severe liver disease or intravenous alimentation with protein hydrolysates, may produce generalized aminoaciduria. Inborn renal tubular disorders usually involve specific transport mechanisms, the malfunction of which results in excretion of predictable amino acids. With acquired renal damage, the degree of aminoaciduria reflects the severity of the damage. Chromatography of urine and plasma is essential for accurate diagnosis, although screening procedures are available for several particularly significant conditions.

PHENYLKETONURIA

More urine amino acid tests are done for phenylketonuria, the clinical syndrome arising from phenylalanine hydroxylase deficiency, than for any other amino acid disorder. This is partly because it is less rare than most (an autosomally recessive condition estimated to occur once in every 20,000 live births[17]), and also because prompt recognition and treatment can avert the disastrous consequences of the metabolic abnormality. The enzyme deficiency prevents conversion of phenylpyruvic acid to tyrosine. The accumulating phenylalanine is converted to phenylpyruvic acid and thence to phenyllactic and phenylacetic acids, all of which appear in the urine.

Urinary screening uses ferric chloride, which produces a bluishgray appearance in the presence of phenylpyruvic acid. Blood phenylalanine level is a more distinctive indicator of phenylketonuria than urinary screening. This is most often evaluated by Guthrie's technique[7] of measuring the growth-enhancing effect that phenylalanine has on cultures of B. subtilis. In the test procedure, an inhibiting agent is introduced into the growth medium. Phenylalanine, at levels above 4 mg./dl., overcomes the inhibition; the higher the phenylalanine concentration, the greater the bacterial growth.

FERRIC CHLORIDE TESTING. Ferric chloride-impregnated strips are available for simple, rapid screening. Ferric chloride also signals urinary abnormalities in patients with tyrosinosis, alcaptonuria, "maple-syrup urine disease" (branched chain ketoaciduria), histidinemia, and "oasthouse urine disease" (excretion of β-hydroxybutyric acid, tyrosine, and methionine as well as phenylalanine); thus the screening strips are useful for many of these rare conditions. In most amino acid disorders, abnormal metabolites reliably appear in urine only when postnatal diet and metabolism are stabilized. For best results, screening should be done at several weeks of age, rather than in the immediate newborn period. More detailed study is required of infants with positive or suggestive results.

ALKAPTONURIA

Alkaptonuria, the syndrome accompanying homogentisic acid oxidase deficiency, can be detected by observing that the urine turns black on standing or if alkalinized. The urinary metabolite is homogentisic acid, a fairly late-stage product of phenylalanine metabolism. In affected individuals, this substance is present in urine, but not in serum, shortly after birth and throughout life. The symptoms of connective tissue and joint degeneration do not appear until late in adult life. Homogentisic acid reduces Benedict's reagent, gives a purple-black color with ferric chloride, and blackens a saturated solution of silver nitrate.

CYSTINURIA

In cystinuria, the dibasic amino acids cystine, lysine, arginine, and ornithine are excreted excessively, with cystine predominating. Cystine is poorly soluble, and its lifelong presence at high concentration often leads to urinary tract calculi and renal damage. The screening test is not difficult. Sodium nitroprusside added to alkalinized urine treated with sodium cyanide produces a magenta color proportional to the amount of amino acid present. The flat, hexagonal, cystine crystals also can be recognized on microscopic examination of concentrated urine specimens.

The disease is transmitted as an autosomal recessive, with an incidence of at least 1 in 20,000. Heterozygotes also excrete excessive quantities of cystine, and mass screening has revealed an incidence of presumed heterozygotes of 1 in 200.[4] Therapy is directed toward maintaining a high volume of dilute urine so that crystallization does not occur. Except for the renal damage induced by cystine stones, even the homozygous condition is relatively innocuous. Positive cyanide-nitroprusside tests also occur in cystinosis (a far more damaging but less common condition) and homocystinuria. Urine and plasma chromatography readily distinguish these conditions over and above the differences in clinical presentation.

Products of Melanogenic Neoplasms

Some patients with melanin-producing malignant tumors excrete in urine a colorless precursor, melanogen, which is readily identifiable and specific for the disease. Colorless initially, melanogen darkens spontaneously if left at room temperature for 24 hours. Ferric chloride, with added HCl, turns the urine brownish-black, and sodium nitroprusside (Thormählen test) produces a dark bluish-black or greenish-black reaction. Homogentisic acid behaves somewhat like melanogen in that it darkens spontaneously on standing and blackens ferric chloride and ammoniacal silver nitrate. Melanogen, however, does not darken more rapidly when alkalinized, as does homogentisic acid. Moreover, it reacts more slowly with silver nitrate than homogentisic acid, which starts turning black even before ammonia is added.

Carcinoid Tumors

Another urinary constituent identified with neoplasm is 5-hydroxyindoleacetic acid (5-HIAA), a denaturation product of serotonin. Serotonin is a vasoconstricting and neuroactive indoleamine produced by argentaffin cells of the gastrointestinal tract and present in the blood bound to platelets. Argentaffin tumors, also called carcinoid tumors, elaborate great quantities of serotonin, resulting in large quantities of the metabolic end product 5-HIAA. Determination of urinary 5-HIAA, a fairly simple test, is the diagnostic procedure for hormonally active argentaffin tumors. Normal persons excrete 2 to 10 mg. of 5-HIAA daily, while patients with active carcinoid may excrete 50 to 500 mg. or more. Carcinoid syndrome is the only condition causing pronounced 5-HIAA excretion, although minor elevations may occur in nontropical sprue.

Urinary testing depends upon the reaction of 5-HIAA with nitrosonaphthol to produce a purple color. Phenothiazine drugs interfere with the reaction, and false positives may result from ingestion, within 72 hours, of reserpine, acetanilid-containing preparations, or serotonin-containing foods such as bananas or pineapple. Both the screening and the quantitative procedures employ the same reaction, but in the quantitative technique, potentially interfering ketoacids are removed, and 5-HIAA is twice extracted to enhance specificity and intensity of the reaction.

Drug Metabolites

Urine tests for drug metabolites may be used as guides to the blood level and possible toxicity of the drug in question, or to monitor whether or not a patient has taken certain drugs. Chromatography, either thin-layer or gas-liquid, affords the most accurate and complete information about drug metabolites. Large-scale screening programs for drugs of abuse use thin-layer chromatography, and comprehensive toxicology laboratories use these techniques along with radioimmuno-assay. The older, presumptive tests for toxicology screening continue to be useful, but with limitations. Salicylates, barbiturates, pheno-thiazines, and the morphine derivatives are the substances most often of emergency importance. Chronic ingestion of heavy metals also may be at issue.

BARBITURATES

Urine is not the best specimen for barbiturate testing. Short-acting barbiturates may be lethal before significant quantities are excreted, and with the longer-acting preparations, the urinary level correlates poorly with blood levels. Stomach contents can be tested in the same fashion as urine, often with more useful results for immediate toxicologic diagnosis. Blood levels are essential for monitoring therapy. The screening procedure involves formation of chloroform-soluble mercuric complexes, which turn purple when reacted with diphenylcarbazone. Hydantoins, certain analgesics, and glutethimide (Doriden) also react in this way. If the first chloroform extract is subjected to controlled hydrolysis, barbiturates remain measurable, but the other drugs lose reactivity.

SALICYLATES

Salicylates and phenothiazines both produce a purple reactant with ferric chloride. Ferric chloride-impregnated reagent strips turn purple in the presence of either group, but concentrated sulfuric acid in-tensifies the color produced by phenothiazines, and may diminish the purple produced by salicylates. This procedure is really too sensitive to be useful, since ingestion of as little as 300 mg. (one adult tablet) of aspirin can produce a positive result. If salicylate toxicity is suspected, evaluation of acid-base status and determination of blood salicylate levels are essential, since the quantity of urinary salicylates may not reflect clinical severity.

PHENOTHIAZINES

An effective screening test for documenting phenothiazine derivatives in urine uses a mixture of perchloric acid, nitric acid, and ferric chloride to produce a pink through violet color range which depends on the drug and its dose. Chromatography and ultraviolet spectral absorption are needed for identification of specific drugs.

DRUGS OF ABUSE

Satisfactory identification of morphine, amphetamines, and other organic bases requires chromatographic analysis. Thin-layer techniques which are both rapid and reliable are available for this purpose.

Heavy Metals

To screen for heavy metals, the Reinsch test is simple and valuable. A shiny copper wire is heated in the acidified specimen, which may be urine, blood, or gastric fluid. If arsenic, mercury, bismuth, or antimony is present, a deposit coats the surface in rough proportion to the concentration of the metal. Mercury produces a shiny or silvery deposit, while the others are gray to black. More specific quantitative tests are available if the screening test is positive.

URINARY CALCULI

It is often helpful to analyze stones that occur in the urinary tract, since their composition may highlight a treatable metabolic condition, but in about half the cases of nephrolithiasis, no etiology can be found.[23] The incidence of urinary calculi appears to be increasing,[19] a tendency some have attributed to increasingly sedentary life styles and improper diet or hydration or both.

Calcium

Calcium is the most common constituent of renal stones, and hypercalcemia is often associated with stone formation. Excess calcium absorbed from dietary sources must be excreted through the kidneys. Specific conditions that predispose to calcium stone formation include hypervitaminosis D, milk-alkali syndrome, multiple myeloma, sarcoidosis, and many bone diseases. Most calcium stones occur, however, without complicating illness, the result of a syndrome called idiopathic urolithiasis. Although there is some evidence of overenthusiastic vitamin D metabolism in these patients,[29] modest restriction of calcium intake and a conscientious regimen of overhydration (urine volume of 2500 ml. or more per day) usually are sufficient to reduce or prevent stone formation.

Cystine

Cystine stones comprise less than 1 percent of identified stones,[14] but when found, this observation should prompt a workup for the heritable amino acid abnormality cystinuria. Cystine stones tend to be soft, lustrous, and white or yellowish-white. Several fairly simple chemical tests using sodium cyanide and nitroprusside or naphtho-quinone reagent can identify cystine calculi, and subsequent investigation should include urine chromatography for amino acid analysis. Therapeutically, the prevention of further cystine stones is fairly straightforward. Since prevention requires lifelong awareness and cooperation from the patient, the diagnosis should be made as early and as reliably as possible.

Urates

Uric acid or urate-containing stones accounted for approximately 10 percent of Herring's series of 10,000 analyses.[14] Patients with high serum uric acid are likely to form stones, whether the hyperuricemia results from a gouty diathesis or from cell destruction. When urine is highly concentrated or very acid, urate precipitation is more likely. Alkalinizing the urine from a pH of 5 to 6.5 produces a tenfold increase in solubility of uric acid. This procedure, combined with high fluid intake to maintain large volumes of dilute urine, is the most effective way to prevent formation of urate stones. Moreover, it is far easier, more palatable, and more reliable than attempting to modify the diet to reduce uric acid production.[29] Urate calculi are identified by the murexide test or by development of blue color when a sodium carbonate suspension of the stone is reacted with phosphotungstic acid.

Phosphates

Although phosphate is a common anion in renal stones, it occurred as the principal constituent in only 16 percent of Herring's series. Stones that are predominantly phosphates tend to be friable, pale, and variable in size. "Staghorn" calculi often consist largely of phosphates, as do stones in any location associated with infection, stasis, and alkaline pH. Phosphates produce a yellow precipitate when ammonium molybdate is added to the pulverized stone, and calcium phosphate produces a dense white precipitate when sodium hydroxide reacts with an acid extract of the stone. Other cations that accompany phosphates are ammonium and magnesium, which occur together as part of so-called triple phosphate stones.

Oxalates

Calcium oxalates, in various chemical combinations, are the most common findings when stones are analyzed. These produce a fine white precipitate when sodium hydroxide is mixed with the acid extract. The oxalate constituents produce a slow bluish-green reaction with resorcinol reagent and release gas bubbles when magnesium dioxide is added to an acid extract of pulverized stone.

Very rare stone constituents include xanthine, glycine, silica, and sulfonamide crystals.

REFERENCES

1. Alleyne, G. A. O., and Roobol, A.: *Renal metabolic processes and acid-base changes.* Med. Clin. North Am. 59:781, 1975.
2. Bricker, N. S., and Klahr, S.: *The physiologic basis of sodium excretion and diuresis.* Adv. Intern. Med. 16:17, 1970.
3. Cannon, P. J.: *The kidney in heart failure.* N. Engl. J. Med. 296:26, 1977.
4. Crawhill, J. C., Scowen, E. F., Thompson, C. J., and Watts, R. W. E.: *The renal clearance of amino acids in cystinuria.* J. Clin. Invest. 46:1162, 1967.
5. Fernandez, A. A., and Jacobs, S. L.: *Porphyrins, porphobilinogen and aminolevulinic acid in urine.* Stand. Meth. Clin. Chem. 6:57, 1970.
6. Flocks, R. H.: *Urinary tract infection.* Med. Clin. North Am. 54:397, 1970.
7. Guthrie, R., and Susi, A.: *A simple phenylalanine method for detecting phenylketonuria in large populations of newborn infants.* Pediatrics 32:338, 1963.
8. Hall, P. M., Schuman, M., and Vidt, D. G.: *Laboratory tests of renal function.* Clin. Lab. Sci. 7:33, 1976.
9. Harrington, J. T., and Cohen, J. J.: *Acute oliguria.* N. Engl. J. Med. 292:89, 1975.
10. Hays, R. M.: *Antidiuretic hormone.* N. Engl. J. Med. 295:659, 1976.
11. Hendler, E. D., Kashgarian, M., and Hayslett, J. P.: *Clinicopathologic correlations of primary haematuria.* Lancet 1:458, 1972.
12. Henry, R. J., Cannon, D. C., and Winkelman, J. W. (eds.): *Clinical Chemistry: Principles and Technics.* ed. 2. Harper & Row, Hagerstown, Md., 1974.
13. Hernberg, S., Nikkanen, J., Mellin, G., et al.: *δ-amino levulinic acid dehydrase as a measure of lead exposure.* Arch. Environ. Health 21:140, 1970.
14. Herring, L. C.: *Observations on the analysis of ten thousand urinary calculi.* J. Urol. 88:545, 1962.
15. Jain, N. C.: *Quality control and mass screening of drugs of abuse,* in

Sunderman, F. W. (ed.): *Seminar on the Laboratory Diagnosis and Monitoring of Disorders Caused by Drugs and Toxic Agents.* Association of Clinical Scientists, Philadelphia, 1975.

16. Jamison, R. L., and Maffly, R. H.: *The urinary concentrating mechanism.* N. Engl. J. Med. 295:1059, 1976.

17. Knox, W. E.: *Phenylketonuria,* in Stanbury, J. B., Wyngaarden, J. B., and Frederickson, D. S. (eds.): *The Metabolic Basis of Inherited Disease.* ed. 3. McGraw-Hill, New York, 1972.

18. Levinsky, N. G.: *Pathophysiology of acute renal failure.* N. Engl. J. Med. 296:1453, 1977.

19. Lonsdale, K.: *Human stones.* Science 159:1199, 1968.

20. Miller, A. L., Worsley, L. R., and Chu, P. K.: *Brown urine as a clue to phenacetin intoxication.* Lancet 2:1102, 1970.

21. Nobel, S.: *Toxicology in a general hospital.* Stand. Meth. Clin. Chem. 6:73, 1970.

22. Pitts, R. F.: *Physiology of the Kidney and Body Fluids.* ed. 3. Year Book Medical Publishers, Chicago, 1974.

23. Reiner, M., Cheung, H. L., and Thomas, J. L.: *Calculi.* Stand. Meth. Clin. Chem. 6:193, 1970.

24. Relman, A. S., and Levinsky, N. G.: *Clinical examination of renal function,* in Strauss, M. B., and Welt, L. G. (eds.): *Disease of the Kidney.* ed. 2. Little, Brown, Boston, 1971.

25. Rennie, I. D. B.: *Proteinuria.* Med. Clin. North Am. 55:213, 1971.

26. Roitt, I.: *Essential Immunology.* ed. 2. Blackwell Scientific Publications, Oxford, 1974.

27. Rosenberg, L. E., and Scriver, C. R.: *Disorders of amino acid metabolism,* in Bondy, P. K., and Rosenberg, L. E. (eds.): *Duncan's Diseases of Metabolism.* ed. 7. W. B. Saunders, Philadelphia, 1974.

28. Rutecki, G. J., Goldsmith, C., and Schreiner, G. E.: *Characterization of proteins in urinary casts.* N. Engl. J. Med. 284:1049, 1971.

29. Smith, L. H., Van Den Berg, C. J., and Wilson, D. M.: *Current concepts in nutrition. Nutrition and urolithiasis.* N. Engl. J. Med. 298:87, 1978.

30. Tschudy, D. P.: *Porphyrin metabolism and the porphyrias,* in Bondy, P. K., and Rosenberg, L. E. (eds.): *Duncan's Diseases of Metabolism.* ed. 7. W. B. Saunders, Philadelphia, 1974.

31. Tschudy, D. P., Perlroth, M. G., Marver, H. S., et al.: *Acute intermittent porphyria: the first "overproduction disease" localized to a specific enzyme.* Proc. Natl. Acad. Sci. U.S.A. 53:841, 1965.

32. Wintrobe, M. M., Lee, G. R., Boggs, D. R., et al.: *Clinical Hematology.* ed. 7. Lea & Febiger, Philadelphia, 1974.

CHAPTER 18

FECES

Examination of the feces often receives short shrift in laboratories and clinics. Unlike urine, blood, or spinal fluid, it often cannot be collected on demand, and patients usually dislike collecting and delivering it for examination. Nursing and laboratory personnel tend to share the patient's aversion, and the doctor often excuses himself from contact with excreta. Yet disease of the gastrointestinal tract is widespread, and examination of feces helps elucidate many common clinical dilemmas.

Various means of collecting feces are available. The physician performing a rectal examination should sample whatever fecal material is within finger range. This constitutes a random, rather small sample, chiefly important for documenting unsuspected occult bleeding or striking abnormalities of color or consistency. The specimen collected at the time of defecation, constituting a single evacuation, permits a number of tests and inferences. Conditions suggested from single specimen findings sometimes require documentation by quantitative tests on timed collections.

THE NORMAL SPECIMEN

The average, normal adult excretes 100 to 300 gm. of fecal material per day. Of this, as much as 70 percent may be water, and of the remaining material, up to half may be bacteria and their debris. Vegetable residues, small amounts of fat, desquamated epithelial cells, and other miscellany constitute the rest. The feces are what remains of approximately 10 L. of fluid material entering the intestinal tract each day.[2] Ingested food and fluid, saliva, gastric secretions, pancreatic juice, and bile all contribute to input; the output depends on a complex series of absorptive, secretory, and fermentative processes.

The small intestine is approximately 23 feet long, while the large intestine is between 4 and 5 feet.[4] The small intestine degrades ingested fats, proteins and carbohydrates to absorbable units, and then absorbs them. Pancreatic, biliary, and gastric secretions operate on the luminal contents to prepare them for active mucosal transport. Other vitally important substances absorbed in the small intestine include fat-soluble vitamins, iron, and calcium. Vitamin B_{12}, after complexing with intrinsic factor, is absorbed in the ileum. The small intestine also absorbs, for return to the blood, as much as 9.5 L. of water and associated electrolytes. The large intestine is shorter and performs less complex functions than the small intestine. The right or proximal colon absorbs much of the remaining water. Bacteria within the colonic lumen degrade many of the end products of metabolism, and the distal portion of the colon stores the feces until a convenient time for evacuation.

Normally evacuated feces reflect the shape and caliber of the colonic lumen. The normal consistency is somewhat plastic—neither fluid, mushy, nor hard. The usual brown color results from bacterial degradation of bile pigments into stercobilin, while the odor derives from indole and skatole, degradation products of proteins. In persons with normal gastrointestinal motility, consuming a mixed dietary intake, colonic transit time is 24 to 48 hours. Small intestinal contents (chyme) begin to enter the cecum as soon as 2 to 3 hours after a meal, but the process is not complete until 6 to 9 hours after eating.[8]

LABORATORY EXAMINATION

Gross Appearance

Stool examination should evaluate size, shape, consistency, color, odor, and the presence or absence of blood, mucus, pus, tissue fragments, food residues, or parasites. This examination should be done before the patient is exposed to barium or purges.

Alterations in size or shape indicate altered motility or abnormalities in the colonic wall. Thus very large caliber indicates dilatation of the viscus, while excessively small, ribbon-like extrusions suggest decreased elasticity or partial obstruction. Small, round, hard masses accompany habitual, moderate constipation, but severe fecal retention can produce huge impacted masses with small volumes of pasty material excreted as overflow.

COLOR

Alterations in color may have diagnostic significance but may reflect only dietary peculiarity. Diets high in milk and low in meat produce light-colored stool with little odor. Excessive fat intake may produce a clay-like appearance, and large quantities of green vegetables may color stool green. Black or very dark brown feces may result from iron or bismuth ingestion or from an unusually large proportion of meat in the diet. A good history helps distinguish these adventitious changes from significant abnormalities.

The usual cause of clay-colored stools is that reduced quantities of bile pigments enter the intestine because of intrinsic hepatobiliary disease or obstruction. The presence of excessive fat in a light-colored stool suggests malabsorption, a condition in which accurate dietary history is most important. Black feces suggest bleeding fairly high in the gastrointestinal tract, but this must be confirmed chemically. Unchanged bile pigments in feces indicate intestinal transit too rapid to allow bacterial degradation.

DIARRHEA

Acute, self-limited attacks of mild diarrhea cause little but inconvenience to otherwise healthy adults or older children. In infants, the elderly, or anyone in a precarious fluid or nutritional state, diarrhea alone can be dangerous or fatal, and the conditions that provoke the diarrhea can range from trivial to life-threatening. Although present-day clinicians possess a broader range of diagnostic tools than has ever before been possible, many diarrheal illnesses remain mysterious.

Stool can be cultured for enteropathogens[3] and examined microscopically for protozoal parasites. Immune electron microscopy has made possible direct demonstration of viral agents, notably hepatitis viruses[6] and parvo- and reo-like viruses.[10] Lactose intolerance, achieving prominence as a common cause of both upper and lower gastrointestinal tract symptoms, is evaluated by the lactose tolerance test (see p. 601). Pseudomembranous colitis tends to occur in patients with poor intestinal perfusion and in those whose intestinal flora has been disturbed by antimicrobial medications. When Staphylococcus, Proteus, or Pseudomonas grow as the predominant organisms in a patient with suitable clinical history, pseudomembranous colitis should be strongly considered. Endoscopic, radiographic, and biopsy procedures, which are beyond the scope of this chapter, play an increasingly important role in diagnosing intestinal diseases.

OTHER ELEMENTS

Grossly visible blood is never normal. Blood streaked on the outer surface usually suggests hemorrhoids or anal abnormalities but can also arise from abnormalities higher in the colon. If transit time is sufficiently rapid, blood from the stomach or duodenum may appear as bright or dark red in the feces.

Mucus also is abnormal if grossly visible. Because colonic mucosa secretes mucus in response to parasympathetic stimulation, fecal mucus appears in conditions of parasympathetic excitability. The classic example is *mucous colitis* in which increased motility and mucus secretion occur without bleeding or inflammation. Mucus may signal other diffuse or localized abnormalities of the distal colon, especially the well-differentiated, mucus-producing tumors. If there is sufficient destruction of colonic mucosa, as in severe ulcerative colitis, mucus production ceases in the involved segments. Mucus incorporated within the fecal mass, rather than streaked on the surface, suggests an abnormality more proximal in the colon, and the mucus particles usually are smaller.

Recognizable pus is seldom seen in or on feces unless a draining rectal infection is present. Pus intermixed with tissue fragments and necrotic debris can, however, result from some ulcerating or fungating process. More often, acute inflammation produces excessive numbers of leukocytes which are intermixed with the feces and seen only on microscopic examination.

Microscopic Examination

PARASITES

Microscopic examination of fecal material may augment the observations from gross inspection. Parasites and their ova usually require microscopic examination for diagnosis, although adult nematodes or tapeworm segments occasionally may be only too obvious in the gross material. For significant parasitologic evaluation, the stool specimen must be fresh, and the examiner must be experienced. To diagnose and identify amoebae and other motile parasites, the examiner should observe freshly passed material while it is still warm. Bloody or mucus-containing fragments give the best results, and both a saline emulsion and an iodine emulsion should be examined. Concentrating the stool sample helps in finding helminth ova; their presence in a simple emulsion indicates that large numbers are present. Zinc sulfate flotation of washed, concentrated fecal material is widely used, although various methods of concentration, fixation, or staining find favor in various laboratories.

UNDIGESTED MATERIAL

Besides demonstrating parasites, microscopic examination of feces permits rapid screening of digestive efficiency. If visibly striated meat fibers can be seen, proteolysis is inadequate. The significance of fats in a random specimen is less clear. A certain amount of fecal fat is normal, corresponding to 5 to 7 percent of dietary intake. By no means all, or even most, of this fat comes directly from dietary input,[15] but the approximate proportion is fairly predictable. Recent dietary intake influences the fat content of random or single specimens. A patient with malabsorption problems may restrict his fat intake because of anorexia, resulting in normal excretion at the time of examination. Conversely, a metabolically normal patient with abnormally high intake may excrete more fat than the expected normal. If there is reason to suspect abnormal fat metabolism, evaluation of a random specimen should include available information about recent intake.

CELLULAR ELEMENTS

A certain number of epithelial cells may be present in feces, but large numbers of epithelial cells or of mucus indicate an irritated mucosa. Because white cells are not normal constituents, their presence indicates inflammation at some point in the lower alimentary tract or excretory organs. While large numbers of white cells suggest a fairly serious or extensive inflammatory process, the absence of leukocytes does not mean that inflammation is absent. An inflammatory process deep in the wall or a surface condition which does not attract neutrophils will contribute few leukocytes to the fecal content. Unaltered red blood cells, when present, usually come from the anus or rectum. Intraluminal blood from higher in the gastrointestinal tract undergoes damage to the cells even if the hemoglobin remains undegraded.

Chemical Examinations

Chemical tests performed on feces usually seek blood, abnormal quantities of fats, or rarely, increased protein. Accurate testing for blood in the stool is one of the most significant laboratory tools available, since both positive and negative results have important implications.

BLOOD

Most tests for blood in biologic specimens utilize the catalytic effects of heme compounds on the oxidation of such organic substances as benzidine or guaiac. Of the hemoglobin breakdown products, only hematin retains this peroxidase activity, which also is present in myoglobin and certain plant enzymes. Since small amounts of fecal peroxidase activity may derive from dietary meat or, rarely, vegetable substances, and since small quantities of blood may not have clinical significance, tests for fecal blood must have appropriate sensitivity. Too many false positives wreak havoc with patients. False negatives may prevent early diagnosis of extremely important diseases.

Perfectly normal individuals lose between 1 and 3 ml. of blood daily in the feces,[13,14] presumably from minimal abrasions of naso-pharyngeal and oral surfaces as well as from the gastrointestinal tract. Quantities of blood larger than 50 ml. arising high in the gastro-intestinal tract darken the feces to the black appearance known as *melena*. To detect quantities between these two levels and to confirm that black stools really do contain blood, the peroxidase tests are essential.

POSSIBLE FALSE INFERENCES. The location of bleeding cannot always be inferred from the stool color. Black stools are said to be due to conversion of hemoglobin to hematin by gastric acid, but melena can occur when blood enters the intestine below the pylorus.[9] Similarly, bright or dark blood may be seen in feces with bleeding points above the pylorus, if motility is sufficiently rapid. The general rule that black stools mean gastric bleeding and bright blood means low colonic bleeding is suggestive but hardly absolute. Similarly, superficial blood streaking on formed stool often means hemorrhoidal bleeding but does not preclude colonic lesions, nor does it exclude simultaneous existence of a more proximal, more significant bleeding point. The existence of melena does not necessarily imply active bleeding. Up to 5 days after a single instillation of blood into the stomach, tarry stools still can be noted,[9] and tests for occult blood remain positive for several weeks.

TESTS EMPLOYED. Of the reagents commonly used for demonstrating blood in the feces, orthotoluidine is the most sensitive. Benzidine produces somewhat fewer false positives, but it is a potential carcinogen and is not in routine laboratory use. Gum guaiac solution is much less sensitive than either of these others. It is probably best for routine screening use, since there is less problem of false positives, and a meat-free diet is unnecessary. Properly made up and stored, the guaiac reagents can detect 0.5 to 1 percent of hemoglobin in an aqueous solution, compared with 0.01 to 0.1 percent concentrations detected with orthotoluidine.[1] These figures cannot be used to estimate fecal blood loss, since fecal findings depend not only on the amount of blood, but also on the net balance of heme degradation, competitive activity of fecal reducing substances, and the presence of interfering pigments. In addition, the test reagents must be of proper concentration. Even when stored so that deterioration is slowed, they should be made up fresh at monthly intervals.

SIGNIFICANCE. With a test suitably standardized to avoid false positives, the finding of occult blood is nearly always diagnostically significant. Of upper gastrointestinal bleeding sites, peptic ulcers, bleeding varices, gastritis, and gastric carcinoma are the usual causes, in approximately that order,[7,9] while colitis, colon carcinoma, and diverticulitis are the commonest causes of lower intestinal bleeding. Patients can lose surprising amounts of blood without noticing—as much as 150 ml. of blood per week in one study.[13] Prolonged loss of relatively small, daily quantities can produce anemia and persistently positive tests for occult fecal blood without localizing symptoms.

One precipitating factor in chronic, or sometimes acute, blood loss is aspirin ingestion. This medication, so common that patients often do not consider it a drug and fail to mention it when asked about medications, is increasingly implicated as a gastric irritant. As many as 70 percent of patients regularly taking large doses of aspirin may have blood in their stools, averaging 5 ml. per day.[11] Occasional patients, especially those with pre-existing atrophic gastritis, develop massive acute hemorrhagic gastritis after aspirin ingestion.[16]

MALABSORPTION PROBLEMS

A variety of disorders may cause excessive fecal fat excretion. Staining a fecal smear to find increased fat globules is a useful screening device but is nonquantitative. Often the patient's history of bulky, light-colored, floating stools provides the presumptive diagnosis, although in one series of children with celiac disease, 38 out of 40 had excessive fat on a stained smear, while only 21 reported bulky or foul stools.[5]

Fat Excretion

To quantitate fat excretion, there must be known dietary intake and timed stool collection. The usual technique involves a diet containing 100 gm. of fat daily, with a 3-day stool collection to measure total fat excretion. Excretion of more than 5 gm. per day is abnormal, and values may range upwards to 50 gm. or more. In feces, most lipids are present as fatty acids, both saturated and unsaturated, since neutral fats are hydrolyzed by lipases high in the small intestine. Lipase deficiency, usually due to pancreatic disease, increases the proportion of neutral fat. In these cases, the stool usually contains excessive quantities of undigested protein, because pancreatic proteases also are deficient. Disease of liver and biliary tract severe enough to produce steatorrhea usually causes jaundice and abnormalities of blood chemistry before the steatorrhea becomes a diagnostic problem.

Fatty acids of normal fecal lipids are not precisely those of the diet. Apparently bacterial activity, epithelial desquamation, and mucosal transport mechanisms modify the excreted elements. With altered intestinal bacterial flora, increased motility, abnormal mucosal metabolism, decreased enzyme or bile salt content, or simple loss of absorbing surfaces (as from resections or fistulas), fecal fat content increases markedly and may approach more nearly the lipid composition of the diet.[15] Fecal calcium also increases, due partly to soap formation with the fatty acids and partly to decreased transport resulting from faulty absorption of vitamin D, which is fat-soluble.

Carbohydrate Utilization

When celiac disease, nontropical sprue (adult celiac disease), tropical sprue, and infiltrative diseases intrinsic to the small intestine cause steatorrhea, other malabsorption problems also may be present. Carbohydrate absorption often is decreased, exacerbating the patient's nutritional problems. The complete investigation of steatorrhea usually includes one or more studies of carbohydrate metabolism.

Comparing oral glucose tolerance results with intravenous glucose tolerance testing may demonstrate that intestinal malfunction is at fault rather than pancreatic deficiency. Patients with intestinal malabsorption raise their blood sugar little more than 35 mg. per 100 ml. after orally ingesting 100 gm. of glucose, but they have a normal curve after parenteral glucose infusion. Since diabetes sometimes can cause diarrhea and malabsorption, the glucose tolerance tests may be valuable in differential diagnosis. Other metabolic abnormalities, especially excessively rapid peripheral glucose utilization, can give a potentially confusing flat GTT curve, but the intravenous GTT then has the same shape as the oral test results.

LACTOSE INTOLERANCE

Most dietary carbohydrate, besides starch which is a polysaccharide, is in the form of disaccharide, two simple sugars joined together. For absorption, enzymic cleavage is necessary. The intestinal mucosa possesses a variety of disaccharidases, several of which can manifest congenital or acquired deficiency. The commonest deficiency involves *lactase*, the enzyme that cleaves lactose into its constituent sugars, glucose and galactose. Since intestinal lactase activity declines with age, milk intolerance is far commoner in adults than in children. There is also racial difference in lactase activities, many blacks having lower levels at all ages than other populations.

Defective lactase activity is associated with diarrhea, abdominal cramping, "gas," and general gastrointestinal uneasiness after ingesting milk or milk products. Lactose tolerance can be tested by administering either pure lactose (50 gm., the usual dose, is the amount present in a quart of milk) or by having the patient drink a large quantity of milk. If adequate lactase is present, blood glucose levels in the next 60 minutes rise at least 20 mg./dl. over basal levels, as the constituent glucose is absorbed. The lactase-deficient patient who fails to achieve increased blood glucose usually will have pronounced diarrhea and cramping as additional confirmation of the diagnosis.

Protein Loss

There is no satisfactory technique for quantitating fecal proteins, and for very few patients is this a problem. The protein loss with generalized malabsorption does not require separate documentation. In occasional patients, however, severe fecal protein loss may occur, a condition to which the descriptive term *protein-losing enteropathy* has been applied.

Proteins within the intestinal lumen are reduced enzymatically to their component amino acids, which are then reabsorbed. If mucosal abnormalities prevent reabsorption, or if protein leakage exceeds reabsorptive capacity, hypoproteinemia may result. Severe ulcerative colitis, Whipple's disease, disturbances of lymphatic circulation, and intestinal lymphomas may produce this syndrome, which is suggested by hypoalbuminemia in the absence of hepatic disease or urinary protein loss. The fecal protein excretion can be documented by administering isotopically labeled albumin or polyvinylpyrrolidone (PVP), rather than by chemical analysis of feces.

Patients with severe malabsorption may have low serum albumin levels, due partly to general malnutrition and partly to excessive fecal loss. Inadequate absorption of the fat-soluble vitamins can produce low vitamin A levels, coagulation abnormalities due to vitamin K deficiency, and osteoporosis with elevated alkaline phosphatase levels due to reduced vitamin D activity.

Fecal analysis is not applied to suspected pancreatic enzyme deficiencies, except in very young children. Below age 2, stool normally manifests tryptic activity; although trypsin and chymotrypsin activity is sometimes noted in adult feces, the presence or absence of enzyme activity cannot be correlated reliably with pancreatic disease. Some of the fecal enzymes may be of bacterial origin. Analysis of duodenal aspirates is more informative for pancreatic disease.

Definitive diagnosis of intestinal mucosal abnormality now can be made by histologic examination of biopsies obtained by peroral techniques. Biopsies, when available, are especially useful for following response to therapy, since histologic changes in most of the more common problems are reversible.

REFERENCES

1. Beeler, M. F., and Kao, Y. S.: *The examination of feces,* in Davidsohn, I., and Henry, J. B. (eds.): *Todd-Sanford Clinical Diagnosis by Laboratory Methods.* ed. 15. W. B. Saunders, Philadelphia, 1974.
2. Carey, W. D.: *Colon physiology. A review.* Cleve. Clin. Q. 44:73, 1977.
3. Ewing, W. H., and Martin, W. J.: *Enterobacteriaceae,* in Lennette, E. H., Spaulding, E. H., and Truant, J. P. (eds.): *Manual of Clinical Microbiology.* ed. 2. American Society for Clinical Microbiology, Washington, D.C., 1974.
4. Goss, C. M. (ed.): *Gray's Anatomy of the Human Body.* ed. 27. Lea & Febiger, Philadelphia, 1959.
5. Hamilton, J. R., Lynch, M. J., and Reilly, B. J.: *Active celiac disease in*

childhood. *Clinical and laboratory findings in forty-two cases.* Q. J. Med. 38:135, 1969.

6. Melnick, J. L., Dreesman, G. R., and Hollinger, F. B.: *Viral hepatitis.* Sci. Am. 237:44, 1977.

7. Palmer, E. D.: *The vigorous diagnostic approach to upper gastrointestinal tract hemorrhage.* J.A.M.A. 207:1477, 1969.

8. Peterson, M. L.: *Constipation and diarrhea,* in MacBryde, C. M., and Blacklow, R. S., (eds.): *Signs and Symptoms: Applied Pathologic Physiology and Clinical Interpretation.* ed. 5. J. B. Lippincott, Philadelphia, 1970.

9. Schiff, L.: *Hematemesis and melena,* in MacBryde, C. M., and Blacklow, R. S. (eds.): *Signs and Symptoms: Applied Pathologic Physiology and Clinical Interpretation.* ed. 5. J. B. Lippincott, Philadelphia, 1970.

10. Schreiber, D. S., Trier, J. S., and Blacklow, N. R.: *Recent advances in viral gastroenteritis.* Gastroenterology 73:174, 1977.

11. Scott, J. T., Porter, I. H., Lewis, S. M., and Dixon, A. St. J.: *Studies of gastrointestinal bleeding caused by corticosteroids, salicylates, and other analgesics.* Q. J. Med. 30:167, 1961.

12. Spiro, H. M.: *Clinical Gastroenterology.* ed. 2. Macmillan, New York, 1977.

13. Stack, B. H. R., Smith, T., Hywel Jones, J., and Fletcher, J.: *Measurement of blood and iron loss in colitis with a whole-body counter.* Gut 10:769, 1969.

14. Stephens, F. O., Milverton, E. J., Hambly, C. K., and Van Der Ven, E. K.: *The effects of food on aspirin-induced gastrointestinal blood loss.* Digestion 1:267, 1968.

15. Wiggins, H. S., Howell, K. E., Kellock, T. D., and Stalder, J.: *The origin of fecal fat.* Gut 10:400, 1969.

16. Winawer, S. J., Bejar, J., McCray, R. S., and Zamchek, N.: *Hemorrhagic gastritis. Importance of associated chronic gastritis.* Arch. Intern. Med. 127:129, 1971.

CHAPTER 19

SPUTUM

Sputum is the material secreted in the tracheobronchial tree and brought up by coughing. Although the submucosal glands and secretory cells in the lining mucosa normally elaborate up to 100 ml. of viscoelastic fluid daily, the healthy individual does not produce sputum.

NORMAL PHYSIOLOGY

Mucus secretion is part of normal bronchopulmonary cleansing. The secretions form a layer perhaps 5 μm. thick,[11] immediately overlying the ciliated epithelium. By ciliary action, this semisticky mantle of fluid moves upward toward the oropharynx, carrying with it inhaled particles which have found their way down to the respiratory bronchioles. From the oropharynx, the secretions are swallowed, so that the normal person is not aware of their presence. Coughing or expectorating tracheobronchial secretions is abnormal, the quantity of material roughly paralleling the severity of the abnormality.

Besides its mechanical cleansing action, mucus attacks inhaled bacteria directly. The antibacterial effect of normal tracheobronchial mucus results largely from antibody activity, although lysozymes and slightly acid pH conditions also help maintain sterility. The antibodies are predominantly IgA, entering the mucus by direct glandular secretion rather than by transudation from plasma.[13] Despite daily inhalation of innumerable organisms, the contents of the lower respiratory tract are sterile in normal individuals.

Response to Injury

Respiratory tract disease alters the tracheobronchial secretions, and these altered secretions in turn influence the pathophysiologic process. In bacterial infections, the volume of sputum increases, the pH becomes more acid, and the chemical composition changes. Acidic pH, below 6.5, inhibits ciliary action, thereby reducing one important defense mechanism. Sputum viscosity increases, further reducing normal flow, and the number of leukocytes also rises. As in all inflammatory conditions, membrane permeability increases, so that antibiotics and other normally intravascular elements may enter the sputum. Bacterial infections result in increased DNA content, to some extent replacing normal mucopolysaccharides.[6] Besides increasing sputum viscosity, DNA also inhibits proteolytic activity. This reduces the effectiveness of drugs intended to liquefy sputum.

Sputum in quantities sufficient to be coughed up is abnormal. Some patients expectorate a mixture of nasopharyngeal secretions and saliva, but this is not sputum. Patients with chronic postnasal drip may complain of cough and expectoration, but the quality of the cough and watery nature of the material distinguish this condition from true productive coughing. In addition, microscopic examination reveals squamous epithelial cells and such characteristically oral flora as *Fusobacterium fusiforme,* oral spirochetes, and nonpathogenic acid-fast organisms.

SPUTUM EXAMINATION

Collecting the Specimen

True sputum originates from below the larynx. Some patients need instruction in deep breathing and coughing before they produce an adequate specimen. An aerosol of mucolytic agents may be helpful, as may the simple mechanical maneuver of reclining the patient with his head lower than his lungs for a few minutes. Good oral hygiene improves the quality of the sputum specimen, and the patient should rinse his mouth thoroughly before coughing. Brushing the teeth is desirable when feasible.

Sputum usually is collected for microbiologic culture or for cytologic examination or both. In certain conditions, gross examination of the sputum and microscopic examination of stained smears are helpful. If the patient reports a change in the quantity or appearance of his sputum, this may be significant. In chronic bronchitis, which has been defined as the presence of a productive cough for at least 3 consecutive months a year for 2 consecutive years,[8] patients tend to observe the sputum closely. Since changing cough may signal carcinoma in these high-risk patients,[9] their complaints should be accorded appropriate diagnostic attention.

QUANTITY AND COLLECTION

Quantitating sputum rarely is necessary. A good sputum specimen can, and in most cases should, be collected from a single episode of deep coughing. This usually results in 0.5 to 5 ml. of material. An early morning specimen is best, since it represents overnight accumulation and is unlikely to contain food particles. Persons who handle the specimen should avoid contaminating themselves and introducing organisms into material destined for microbiologic examination. The collecting vessels should be clean, wide-mouthed, and capable of secure closure. If day-long or 24-hour collections are made, usually when *Mycobacterium tuberculosis* is sought, the container should be kept closed when not immediately in use, and the patient should be especially careful not to soil the exterior. Sputum examination is indicated for suspected lower respiratory tract infections or tumors, although infarcts and noninfectious infiltrates sometimes can be spotted from sputum findings.

Gross Appearance

Descriptive terms applied to sputum include mucoid, mucopurulent, frankly purulent, blood-tinged, frankly bloody, or dust-flecked, and these characteristics correlate moderately well with the cause of cough. Purulent sputum usually accompanies acute bacterial pneumonias. In a patient with chronic bronchitis, change from mucoid to purulent or mucopurulent indicates bacterial infection overlying the chronic inflammatory process. Gradual progression from scant, sticky sputum to more abundant, loose, purulent material may signal the development of bronchiectasis. Rupture of a pulmonic abscess causes sudden expectoration of abundant purulent, often foul-smelling, pus.

MICROBIOLOGIC FINDINGS

The classical stages of pneumococcal pneumonia may be followed as the sputum changes from pink to mucoid, through reddish-brown to purulent, often with gross streaks of blood. Treated pneumococcal pneumonia does not always follow this pattern, but despite changing clinical features and nonspecific sputum appearance, pneumococcus (now formally called *Streptococcus pneumoniae*[4]) remains one of the commonest pathogens in lower respiratory tract infections.[3] Other common bacterial pathogens, both in adults and children, are *H. influenzae*,[3,12] the gram-negative bacilli, especially in debilitated patients with other primary diseases;[2] staphylococci,[5] and sometimes nonpneumococcal streptococci, although these derive more often from the pharynx than from the lung as a primary source.

Sputum cannot be cultured effectively for anaerobic organisms because it is in contact with air. Anaerobic infection should be suspected, however, when sputum is copious, foul-smelling, and contains much necrotic material.[1] A mixed aerobic flora often is present in addition to anaerobes, which can be identified if the empyema or abscess is approached surgically.

Mycoplasma pneumoniae and the respiratory viruses are very frequent pathogens, especially when lower respiratory tract disease occurs acutely in previously healthy individuals.[3] These are difficult to isolate in the routine laboratory. The sputum in nonbacterial pneumonias tends to be less abundant and nearly always contains fewer polymorphonuclear leukocytes than in bacterial pneumonia. Serologic study of acute and convalescent serum samples may facilitate viral and mycoplasmal diagnosis, albeit in retrospect. Skin testing, as well as serologic evaluation, can be helpful in diagnosing fungal infections, especially if cultures are unrevealing. If cultures are negative, the presence of eosinophils in the sputum sometimes distinguishes an asthmatic etiology from viral or mycoplasmal involvement.

Problems With Cultures

Interpreting sputum cultures requires judgment, since some organisms, saprophytic and nonpathogenic in the oropharynx, acquire distinct significance when found in the lung. Candida, Actinomyces, and *Klebsiella pneumoniae* are particular offenders, since the pulmonary infections tend to be severe and often difficult to treat. Despite obvious pulmonary infection, sputum cultures may be negative, owing to irregular distribution of organisms in the sputum. Selecting purulent or particulate material for inoculation helps to circumvent this sampling error, especially when similar particles are examined on Gram-stained and acid-fast stained smears. Conversely, Candida often is present in sputum cultures from patients whose infection is merely superficial and who have pulmonary disease on some other, non-monilial basis.[7]

Homogenizing and liquefying the specimen improves sampling, especially with very viscid material. Sometimes the laboratory can treat the specimen, but intratracheal aerosol of N-acetylcysteine can result in a more voluminous, less viscid sample at the time the patient coughs. When the patient, especially a child, cannot produce an adequate specimen at all, a cough swab may be helpful. The swab is held above the larynx, while the tongue and epiglottis are depressed, and the patient coughs directly onto the swab. Bacteriologically active material can be obtained in this way, even if sputum production is minimal.

HEMOPTYSIS

Massive hemoptysis indicates blood vessel erosion by a neoplastic or inflammatory process, usually a granuloma. Streaks of blood in an otherwise purulent or mucoid sputum usually accompany more diffuse pneumonic processes—bacterial, mycoplasmal, viral, or sometimes fungal. Occasional patients with inactive tuberculosis cough up blood-streaked sputum, but in general this suggests active disease. Distinct from blood-streaking or massive hemoptysis is uniform discoloration of the sputum. "Rusty" sputum accompanies chronic passive congestion, while abundant pink, frothy sputum is an immediate danger sign of acute pulmonary edema. Following non-fatal infarcts, the sputum may progress from blood-streaked, through bloody, to a uniform brown tinge reflecting hemoglobin breakdown. Sputum findings, however, are not consistently helpful when infarction is part of the differential diagnosis.

MICROSCOPIC EXAMINATION

Formed elements in sputum are best studied by cytologic techniques, using the Papanicolaou stain or an appropriate modification. If detailed cellular examination is not needed, routine staining techniques are valuable. Leukocytes can be classified tentatively on Gram-stained smears, and morphology alone often permits distinction between polymorphs, found in infection, and eosinophils, characteristic of asthmatic attacks. Wright's stain or other Romanowsky-type stains provide conclusive distinction. PAS and silver stains sometimes are applied to sputum in suspected pulmonary alveolar proteinosis. The characteristic compacted protein may be inside

mononuclear cells or free in round or laminated clumps or in aggregates with cleft-like spaces. When round and laminated, these resemble the cysts of *Pneumocystis carinii*. Although both are PAS-
positive, only Pneumocystis takes a silver stain.

Curschmann's spirals can be identified readily on Gram-stained
smears. These coiled, mucus filaments, once considered pathognomonic of asthma, are casts of small bronchi and may occur whenever increased mucus production accompanies bronchial obstruction.
Since bronchospasm and excessive secretions characterize asthmatic
attacks, Curschmann's spirals are particularly to be expected, but
they also can occur in other types of acute bronchitis or in bronchopneumonia and may be found in sputum arising from small bronchi
adjacent to lung carcinomas.

The cytologic evaluation of sputum specimens is beyond the scope
of this chapter.

REFERENCES

1. Briggs, D. D., Jr.: *Pulmonary infections*. Med. Clin. North Am. 61:1163, 1977.
2. Eickhoff, T. C.: *Nosocomial infections,* in Hoeprich, P. C. (ed.): *Infectious Diseases.* ed. 2. Harper & Row, Hagerstown, Md., 1977.
3. Hers, J. F. P., Masurel, N., and Gans, J. C.: *Acute respiratory disease associated with pulmonary involvement in military servicemen in The Netherlands.* Am. Rev. Respir. Dis. 100:499, 1969.
4. International Committee on Nomenclature of Bacteria (Subcommittee on Streptococci and Pneumococci): Minutes of the Moscow meeting, July 21, 1966. Int. J. System. Bacteriol. 17:281, 1967.
5. Kuperman, A. S., and Fernandez, R. B: *Subacute staphylococcal pneumonia.* Am. Rev. Respir. Dis. 101:95, 1970.
6. Lieberman, J.: *The appropriate use of mucolytic agents.* Am. J. Med. 49:1, 1970.
7. Masur, H., Rosen, P. R., and Armstrong, D.: *Pulmonary disease caused by Candida species.* Am. J. Med. 63:914, 1977.
8. Mitchell, R. S., and Pierce, J. A.: *Cough,* in MacBryde, C. M., and Blacklow, R. S. (eds.): *Signs and Symptoms: Applied Pathologic Physiology and Clinical Interpretation.* ed. 5. J. B. Lippincott, Philadelphia, 1970.
9. Rimington, J.: *Smoking, sputum, and lung cancer.* Br. Med. J. 1:732, 1968.
10. Stinghe, R. V., and Mangiulea, V. G.: *Hemoptysis of bronchial origin occurring in patients with arrested tuberculosis.* Am. Rev. Respir. Dis. 101:84, 1970.
11. Teager, H., Jr.: *Tracheobronchial secretions.* Am. J. Med. 50:493, 1971.
12. Tillotson, J. R., and Lerner, A. M.: *Hemophilus influenzae bronchopneumonia in adults.* Arch. Intern. Med. 121:428, 1968.
13. Tomasi, T. B.: *The gamma A globulins: first line of defense,* in Good, R. A., and Fisher, D. W. (eds.): *Immunobiology.* Sinauer Associates, Stamford, Conn., 1971.

CHAPTER 20

GASTRIC AND DUODENAL CONTENTS

The stomach's purely mechanical functions of storing, mixing, and gradually emitting ingested food and fluid usually are evaluated roentgenographically and are not subject to direct laboratory investigation. The gastric mucosa has several secretory products which can be subjected to study but rarely are, namely rennin, lipase, mucus, and small amounts of nondigestive enzymes. The proteolytic enzymes, principally pepsin, undoubtedly have considerable physiologic significance, but no well-defined or generally accepted pathophysiologic tests are currently in use. Hydrochloric acid, which the gastric mucosa is capable of elaborating at concentrations as high as 160 mEq./L,[2] is the one element of gastric origin regularly evaluated in the laboratory.

MEASURING GASTRIC ACIDITY

The complete role of gastric HCl in normal and pathologic physiology is a topic too complex for this chapter. Hydrochloric acid along with gastric proteolytic enzymes, is important in initiating protein digestion. In the clinical syndrome called peptic ulcer disease, gastric or duodenal mucosa or both are attacked by these proteolytic activities, and gastric acidity measurements often can be correlated with clinical findings and prognosis. Measurement of gastric acid secretion is essential in diagnosing the special subgroup of peptic ulcer disease known as Zollinger-Ellison syndrome and is often contributory in those hematologic and sometimes neurologic maladies characterized by impaired absorption of vitamin B_{12}, folic acid, or iron. Gastric hydrochloric acid is not, itself, implicated in these transport mechanisms, but deficiencies in absorptive cofactors often are mirrored in deficiencies of gastric acid secretion, a function more directly measurable.

Gastric secretions are collected by aspiration through a tube passed through the mouth or the nasopharynx. Fluoroscopic monitoring helps insure good intragastric placement. The tip should be at the most dependent portion of the stomach, without curling or twisting. Most gastric aspiration is performed in the morning, after an overnight fast. At this time the stomach should contain no more than 50 ml. of clear or opalescent fluid, free of food particles, blood, or bile. The usual bacterial flora have little clinical significance, but tuberculous patients whose sputum contains no organisms sometimes have *M. tuberculosis* in cultures of overnight gastric contents. Cytologic examination of native gastric juice usually is unsatisfactory, since desquamated cells are poorly preserved. After the gastric contents have been aspirated, gastric washings can be extremely useful in documenting the presence, and sometimes the nature, of gastric neoplasms.

Normal Physiology

Under resting, unstimulated conditions, the stomach secretes a small amount of acid. Increased acidity results, physiologically, from neural and humoral stimulation; actual food intake is not required. Psychic phenomena, including emotional stimuli and the sight and smell of food, induce gastric secretion by stimulating the vagus nerve. Vagal impulses affect parietal cells directly and also induce cells in the antrum to produce gastrin, an intense hormonal stimulus to parietal cell activity.[3] Antral gastrin secretion is further enhanced by distention of the stomach wall or by contact with protein breakdown products. A third, but weaker, stimulus to gastric acidity occurs when the duodenal mucosa, in contact with intraluminal digestive products, releases humoral activators. Feedback inhibition also exists, since pH levels of 1.5 or below inhibit gastrin production.[2]

UNITS OF MEASUREMENT

In the older literature, gastric acidity was expressed as "degrees," one degree standing for each milliliter of 0.1 N NaOH needed to titrate 100 ml. of gastric juice to the desired end point. Two end points were in common use: pH 3.5, the end point of Topfer's reagent, and the pH 7.0 to 9.4 range obtained with phenolphthalein and neutral red. At pH levels below 3.5, all the HCl was thought to exist as dissociated or "free" acid, while above that point, the hydrogen ion was thought to be buffered by organic acids and peptides.

TITRATABLE ACIDITY. The concept of free and combined acid has been shown[15,18] to have neither physiologic nor physicochemical validity, and gastric acidity is now increasingly reported simply as titratable acidity. The single end point of titration is neutrality (pH 7.0) or physiologic neutrality (pH 7.4), and the result is expressed as milliequivalents of acid. Since 1 ml. of 0.1 N NaOH (the usual titrant) neutralizes 0.1 mEq. of HCl, calculations are very simple. The volume of 0.1 N NaOH needed to neutralize an aliquot of gastric juice, divided by 10, gives the milliequivalents of acid in the aliquot. The milliequivalents in the total specimen are calculated easily from the milliequivalents in the measured sample. The acid concentration, in milliequivalents per liter, also can be calculated from the measured number of milliequivalents in the aspirated material. The pH of gastric juice can be measured with a pH meter or, at the bedside, with pH paper. Electrometric measurement is easier and more reliable,[18] and the results can be converted to milliequivalents per liter by use of conversion tables.

TEST MEALS. In older investigations, the volume and acidity of the fasting overnight collection were compared against volume and acidity of gastric juice aspirated after ingestion or intragastric instillation of a *test meal*. Besides the variability of the overnight collection period and the wide range of individual response to test meal stimulation, the crackers, meat, alcohol, or whatever was used to stimulate acid secretion introduced uncontrollable error through unpredictable buffering effect. More reproducible and intrinsically more accurate is basal collection of gastric juice during a timed period when no secretory stimuli are active. This is followed by administration of some pharmacologic stimulus known to evoke maximal or near-maximal secretion in virtually all patients.

BASAL AND STIMULATED SAMPLING

Basal collection begins after removal of the fasting contents. The volume, color, and gross composition of the overnight collection should be observed, but the acid content is not measured. Once the tube is positioned and the patient is comfortable, timed collection begins. Better volume recovery occurs when suction is applied continuously, either with a pump or manually with a syringe, rather than relying on interval removal of accumulated secretions. Ordinarily, the 1 hour of basal observation is divided into four separate 15-minute collections, with the acid content of each combined for the report of milliequivalents per hour.

PHARMACOLOGIC STIMULI. Two stimulants are widely used to evoke maximal acid production. Histamine, usually given as histamine acid phosphate (0.04 mg./kg. body weight), is the usual stimulant in the United States, while synthetic gastrin (Pentagastrin) is widely used in Great Britain and Europe. Gastrin evokes a somewhat greater acid response than histamine[19] and tends to produce fewer side effects.[14] Antihistamine given 30 minutes before histamine injection reduces the uncomfortable side effects of that drug. After stimulation, 15-minute collections continue, usually for a total of 60 minutes. The acidity of each specimen is measured separately, and two different values may be reported. The maximal acid output (MAO) is the total amount of acid produced in the hour after pharmacologic stimulation. This is reported as milliequivalents per hour or as the percentage of increase over basal output. The peak acid output (PAO) is the sum of the two highest consecutive 15-minute values and is reported as milliequivalents per 30 minutes.

DIAGNOSTIC FINDINGS. This test of acid output after maximal stimulation provides certain types of information but not others. The principal diagnostic usefulness is demonstration of anacidity. Anacidity is best defined as failure of gastric pH to fall below 6.0 at any time, even after maximal stimulation. A modest number of individuals lose their basal acidity with advancing age, but failure to secrete acid after maximal stimulation indicates loss of parietal cell mass and strongly suggests atrophic gastritis.[12] Anacidity nearly always accompanies pernicious anemia, but it can occur without the hematologic diseases. Since gastric anacidity never accompanies active peptic ulcer,[18] epigastric pain associated with anacidity must have an etiology other than peptic ulcer disease, often, but not always, gastric carcinoma.

ZOLLINGER-ELLISON SYNDROME. The histamine test also is useful in evaluating suspected Zollinger-Ellison syndrome. In this condition, gastrin-secreting pancreatic tumors bombard the parietal cells with continuous, high-level stimulation. The expected findings, then, are large volume and high acid concentration in the basal collection, with relatively little rise following exogenous histamine or gastrin. While basal acid output above 15 mEq./hr. is suggestive of Zollinger-Ellison syndrome, as many as 10 percent of patients with simple peptic ulcer disease may have outputs this high.[11] In normally responsive individuals, maximal stimulation leads to appreciably increased acidity even when basal output is high. If basal acidity is 60 percent or more of the level attained after maximal stimulation, it suggests that abnormal endogenous gastrin production is eliciting a continuous state of near-maximal secretion.

PEPTIC ULCER DISEASE. The histamine test cannot, by itself, distinguish gastric from duodenal peptic ulcer, nor can it reliably separate benign from malignant gastric ulceration. While patients with gastric carcinoma tend, as a group, to have lower basal and maximal acid production than patients with benign ulcers, test results cannot have absolute significance in any individual patient. Compared with normal individuals, patients with peptic ulcer disease have moderately high basal secretion and excessively active maximal histamine response. The normal mean basal acid output is approximately 4 or 5 mEq./hr., while several series of patients with duodenal ulcer give means of 7.1 or between 6 and 7 mEq./hr.[11] The range and standard deviation in all series are extremely large, however, so comparison of basal figures offers only minimally suggestive information. The extent of maximal secretory rise tends to be higher in patients with duodenal ulcer (35 to 40 mEq./hr.) than in controls (22 to 26 mEq./hr.), but again the ranges overlap markedly and up to half of patients with proven ulcer have values well below 40 mEq./hr.[18] Patients with hiatal hernia do not differ significantly from controls, nor does the postoperative prognosis of peptic ulcer patients correlate reliably with the preoperative histamine test results.

The Insulin Test

Postvagotomy gastric analysis has an intent and technique different from histamine testing to diagnose ulcer. The vagus nerve is highly important in acid secretion, mediating both direct parietal cell stimulation and gastrin production. Most operations for peptic ulcer disease include sectioning the vagus nerves in the expectation that neural stimulation to acid production will be diminished. Because of anatomic variations and the peculiarities of operative conditions, complete vagotomy often is difficult to accomplish or evaluate. The

Hollander insulin test[10] attempts to document vagus inactivation by demonstrating failure to evoke gastric acid response under conditions which normally produce vagal stimulation.

PHYSIOLOGIC EFFECTS

One known, powerful stimulus to vagal activation is hypoglycemia. In the intact individual, a significant drop in the blood sugar produces increased gastric acidity by vagus-mediated stimulation. If the vagi have been completely sectioned, hypoglycemia produces little change in acid secretion. The vagotomy does not produce basal anacidity; it simply abolishes the neural stimulus to increased acid production.

Before measuring the acid response to hypoglycemia, one should determine that the patient is capable of acid production. Failure to increase posthypoglycemic acidity over a low basal level could be due to parietal cell loss or nonreactivity, rather than to absent vagal stimulation. Many workers believe that if the basal acid output is zero, histamine stimulation should be performed to document parietal cell reactivity. Once this capacity has been documented, insulin provocation can be interpreted meaningfully.

PROCEDURE

The insulin test is performed after an overnight fast, and the fasting blood glucose level is determined as well as the basal acidity. In this test, comparisons usually are made on the basis of acid concentration, expressed in milliequivalents per liter in each of eight 15-minute collections, rather than on volume or total output. Blood sugar must be tested at intervals, since blood glucose levels remaining above 45 mg./dl. (some workers say 50 mg./dl.) prove that hypoglycemia has not been adequate. Patients with low fasting blood glucose levels should manifest a drop to one-half the fasting value. The usual dose is either 0.2 unit per kilogram body weight or 20 units, administered intravenously.

Hollander originally proposed that if any of the 15-minute aliquots had an increment of 20 or more mEq./L. over basal acid concentration, then vagus function persisted. If the initial sample was anacid, then a rise to 10 mEq./L. in any postinsulin sample was considered a positive result. Most later workers have used these criteria, although the time at which the test is performed and the size and sex of the patient may affect the results. It has become common to separate positive responses according to whether they occur in one of the first four collection periods (i.e., during the first hour) or in the latter four collections. Since hypoglycemia-induced secretion depends on vagal innervation, provocation of significant acidity in either period indicates integrity of at least some vagal fibers.

INTERPRETATION

The timing of postoperative testing is important, for it appears that false-negative results are fairly common in tests done 1 week to 3 months after vagotomy.[13] Whether this is due to regeneration of marginally traumatized nerve fibers or to temporary aberrations of motility and secretion is difficult to say.

Another problem is evaluating the patient with high postoperative acid secretion. The results of insulin testing are given in concentration of acidity per liter. The total amount of acid is not recorded. Mason and Giles[13] have found that if total acid output is high (above 20 mEq. per hour), the comparison of concentration before and after hypoglycemia has much less predictive value. As a rule, vagotomy and pyloroplasty reduce, but do not abolish, basal and stimulated acidity. Persistence of high total acid output carries a poor prognosis for recurrence.

Among ulcer patients with normal or reduced basal acidity after vagotomy, the value of the insulin test in predicting recurrence is somewhat questionable. A negative test done at a suitably late time after the operation carries a good but not absolute prognosis for no recurrence, but positive results are more difficult to interpret.[5, 13, 20] As complex as are the etiologic factors in peptic ulcer disease, it is hardly surprising that a single test of a single variable provides no absolute answer. A variety of selective vagotomy procedures have been used in attempts to reduce acid output to acceptable levels without impairing motility or producing abnormal patterns of gastric emptying.[4]

DUODENAL FLUID

Collecting duodenal secretions is more difficult and time-consuming than gastric aspiration, since the tube must pass the pylorus and locate itself close to the ampulla of Vater. Fluoroscopic monitoring is virtually essential. A double lumen tube is customary, with one portion remaining in the stomach to aspirate acidic gastric juice which, if it passed the pylorus, would contaminate the alkaline duodenal secretions.

Physiology

The duodenum normally secretes 1200 to 1500 ml. per day of enzyme-rich clear fluid with a pH of 8 to 8.5 and containing up to 145 mEq./L. of bicarbonate ion.[6] Pancreatic enzymes split fats, carbohydrates, and proteins, the major constituents being lipase, amylase, trypsin, and chymotrypsin. Secretions of bicarbonate ion and of enzymes have different physiologic provocation, although both are mediated hormonally.

When acidic gastric contents enter the duodenum, the fall in pH stimulates mucosal cells to produce secretin. Secretin calls forth watery pancreatic secretion with high bicarbonate content. Enzyme production is provoked by pancreozymin, also elaborated by small intestinal mucosa, but the stimulus to pancreozymin secretion is the presence of digestive products in the lumen. Distention by volume alone inspires a small amount of pancreozymin secretion, but sustained pancreozymin production is best evoked by polypeptides or micellar fatty acids or both in the small intestinal contents.[7]

Secretin Testing

Both secretin and pancreozymin are available in pharmacologic forms. Secretin usually is cheaper and gives as good results as pancreozymin, which finds more use in Europe.[18] Prior to intravenous injection, intradermal tests should be done to ensure that there is no sensitivity to these foreign proteins. The usual dose of secretin is one clinical unit per kilogram body weight, but the dose of pancreozymin, when this is used, is more subject to individual preference.

The secretin test is performed after a 20-minute basal collection of duodenal secretions, the initial fasting contents having been aspirated and examined. The presence of bile, blood, undigested food particles, and cholesterol crystals in the duodenal fluid is abnormal. The postinjection samples are collected in 20-minute aliquots, with the volume and bicarbonate concentration measured separately for each sample. Dreiling and Janowitz originally collected for 80 minutes, but many workers now use a 60-minute collection. Since the volume and, to some extent, the bicarbonate output vary with the size of the patient, results usually are expressed per kilogram body weight.

VOLUME

Dreiling and Janowitz[6] consider a cumulative volume of 2 ml. output per kilogram body weight over the total collecting period to be the lower limit of normal. Another group,[9] using a larger secretin dose by constant infusion, reached approximately the same lower limit. Patients with chronic pancreatitis tend to secrete reduced volumes, but the range of variation is wide.[17] Thus secretion of less than 2 ml./kg. points to fairly severe pancreatic destruction, either inflammatory or neoplastic, but values above that do not invalidate these diagnoses.

BICARBONATE

The concentration of bicarbonate in secretin-stimulated pancreatic secretion usually reaches a peak value of 90 to 100 mEq./L. during at least one of the collection periods.[6, 9, 17] This value is significantly and reliably lower in patients with chronic pancreatitis, often in the range of 40 mEq./L. Since the reserve capacity of the pancreas is considerable, a lower figure once again has affirmative value, while a normal or low-normal result must be interpreted along with clinical findings. The total output of bicarbonate can, of course, be calculated from the concentration and the volume. Diagnostically this offers no advantage over determining the peak concentration[9] but may provide more reproducible results if serial testing is done on the same individual.[17]

ENZYME CONTENT

Secretin does not stimulate enzyme release. If enzyme activity is to be measured, pancreozymin must be administered, usually after the secretin-stimulated secretions have been collected. The results ordinarily parallel the findings in secretin testing (i.e., reduced enzyme activity in patients with pancreatic damage due to inflammation or widespread neoplastic destruction). The combination of pancreozymin with secretin may afford slightly increased diagnostic sensitivity.[8] Amylase is the easiest of the pancreatic enzymes to assay accurately, although trypsin and lipase also can be measured.

In evaluating pancreatic insufficiency, fecal enzyme determinations tend to be difficult and variably reliable; thus when the clinical condition suggests enzyme abnormalities, pancreozymin provocation may be valuable. A simpler and reasonably effective way to estimate enzyme production is to ɪook for abnormal quantities of fat and inadequately digested meat in feces.[1] The usefulness of this procedure depends upon the experience of the examiner in evaluating normal and abnormal observations, but in skilled hands, simple microscopic examination gives good correlation with more detailed tests of pancreatic function.[16]

REFERENCES

1. Brooks, F. P.: *Testing pancreatic function.* New Engl. J. Med. 285:300, 1972.
2. Cannon, D. C.: *Gastric analysis,* in Henry, R. J., Cannon, D. C., and Winkelman, J. W. (eds.): *Clinical Chemistry: Principles and Technics.* ed. 2. Harper & Row, Hagerstown, Md., 1974.
3. Cooperman, A. M.: *Gastric physiology.* Cleve. Clin. Q. 44:65, 1977.
4. Cooperman, A. M.: *Selective and highly selective vagotomy with and without gastric drainage.* Cleve. Clin. Q. 43:51, 1976.
5. Dignan, A. P.: *A laboratory appraisal of the effects of truncal and selective vagotomy.* Br. J. Surg. 57:249, 1970.
6. Dreiling, D. A., and Janowitz, H. D.: *The laboratory diagnosis of pancreatic disease: secretin test.* Am. J. Gastroenterol. 28:268, 1957.
7. Go, V. L. W., Hofmann, A. F., and Summerskill, W. H. J.: *Stimulation of pancreozymin secretion by digestive products in man.* J. Clin. Invest. 49:1558, 1970.
8. Hanscom, D. H.: *Diagnostic tests in pancreatic disease.* Med. Clin. North Am. 52:1483, 1968.
9. Hartley, R. C., Gambill, E. E., Engstrom, G. M., and Summerskill, W. H. J.: *Pancreatic exocrine function.* Am. J. Dig. Dis. 11:27, 1966.
10. Hollander, F.: *Laboratory procedures in the study of vagotomy (with particular reference to the insulin test).* Gastroenterology 11:419, 1948.
11. Kaye, M. D., Rhodes, J., and Beck, P.: *Gastric secretion in duodenal ulcer, with particular reference to the diagnosis of Zollinger-Ellison syndrome.* Gastroenterology 58:476, 1970.
12. Kirkpatrick, J. R., Davis, G. T., Jacobs, A., and Williams, S. W.: *The recognition of atrophic gastritis.* Br. J. Surg. 56:742, 1969.
13. Mason, M. C., and Giles, G. R.: *The postoperative insulin test: failure to detect incomplete vagotomy in patients with high acid levels.* Br. J. Surg. 55:865, 1968.
14. Mason, M. C., and Giles, G. R.: *Evaluation and simple modification of the gastrin test.* Gut 10:375, 1969.
15. Moore, E. W., and Scarlata, R. W.: *The determination of gastric acidity by the glass electrode.* Gastroenterology 49:178, 1965.
16. Moore, J. G., Englert, E., Jr., Bigler, A. H., et al.: *Simple fecal tests of absorption: a prospective study and technique.* Am. J. Dig. Dis. 16:97, 1971.
17. Petersen, H.: *The duodenal aspirate following secretin stimulation. A variance study in man.* Scand. J. Gastroenterol. 4:407, 1969.

18. Spiro, H. M.: *Clinical Gastroenterology.* ed. 2. Macmillan, New York, 1977.
19. Thompson, J. C.: *Gastrin and gastric secretion.* Annu. Rev. Med. 20:291, 1969.
20. Weinstein, V. A., Hollander, F., Lauber, F. U., and Colp, R.: *Correlation of insulin tests studies and clinical results in a series of peptic ulcer cases treated by vagotomy.* Gastroenterology 14:214, 1950.

CHAPTER 21

THE CEREBROSPINAL FLUID

Lumbar puncture and examination of the aspirated fluid ordinarily are diagnostic tools, though at times the entire procedure itself may have therapeutic implications. Lumbar puncture, a procedure which inspires more respect in physicians and trepidation in patients than many other manipulations, constitutes a vitally important technique in many conditions.

ANATOMY AND PHYSIOLOGY

Origin of the Fluid and Its Contents

The cerebrospinal fluid (CSF), originating from the choroid plexus of the ventricles, occupies the ventricles and the subarachnoid space over the surfaces of the brain and around the spinal cord. Whether the CSF is a dialysate of plasma or a secretion of the choroid plexus is a debate which need not concern us unduly.

The concentration of many but not all of the CSF electrolytes varies with changes in plasma levels, but some appear to be independent. Most constituents of the CSF are present in equal or lower concentrations than in plasma, but the chloride concentration normally is higher. Under pathologic conditions, elements ordinarily restrained by the so-called blood-brain barrier may enter the spinal fluid.

Red cells and white cells can enter the CSF either from rupture of vessels or from meningeal reaction to irritation. Bilirubin, normally absent from CSF, may be found in the spinal fluid of nonjaundiced

patients after intracranial hemorrhage. The bilirubin is the unconjugated prehepatic form, suggesting that hemoglobin can be cata-
bolized locally within the central nervous system.

Pressure Relations

The brain, spinal cord, and cerebrospinal fluid are enclosed in a
rigid container composed of skull and vertebral column. Normal
pressure is maintained by absorption of CSF in amounts equal to
production, the absorption occurring primarily through the arachnoid
villi and pacchionian corpuscles. Many factors regulate the level of
CSF pressure, but the venous pressure is the most important, for
ultimately the resorbed fluid drains into the venous system.

Anatomic Relations

Despite continuous production and resorption of the fluid and exchange of substances between CSF and blood, considerable stagna-
tion occurs in the lumbar sac. For this reason, the protein concentration and cell count of lumbar fluid exceed the values found in
ventricular or cisternal fluid. The lumbar sac, however, is the usual
site for routine puncture, since in this caudal area only the filum
terminale occupies the spinal canal, and damage to the nervous
system is unlikely to occur. In children, the spinal cord persists more
caudally than in the adult, and therefore a low lumbar puncture
should be made.

INDICATIONS FOR LUMBAR PUNCTURE

Before undertaking lumbar puncture, the physician should define
his diagnostic objectives. This will avoid unnecessary manipulation
and permit rational selection of laboratory tests. In many conditions,
the primary goal is examination of the spinal fluid itself. This goal
is paramount in cases of suspected meningitis, in subarachnoid or
other intracranial hemorrhage, in certain cases of suspected tumor
or brain abscesses, and in cases of undiagnosed neurologic disease
when these conditions must be ruled out.

In other patients, the level of CSF pressure is sought, and the
goal may be to document impairment of CSF flow or to lower pressure by removing a volume of fluid. Still another reason for entering
the subarachnoid space is to introduce anesthetics or other medication or radiographic contrast media.

Danger from Increased Pressure

Lumbar puncture should be done with extreme caution, if at all, when intracranial pressure is elevated, especially when papilledema is present. The reason for caution is that rapid removal of fluid from the lumbar sac alters the pressure relationships within the subarachnoid space, and the brain stem can be dislocated from a region of high pressure (within the skull) to a region of lower pressure (through the foramen magnum into the spinal canal), a potentially fatal phenomenon known as herniation or "coning." In some cases of increased intracranial pressure, the need to establish a diagnosis outweighs the danger of the procedure, so that each case must be decided individually. An example of this dilemma is the comatose patient in whom intracranial bleeding or meningitis is suspected. If removal of just a few milliliters of fluid causes pressure to drop 25 to 50 percent, the procedure should be stopped immediately.[8] Many clinicians would follow this with prompt intravenous infusion of a solute diuretic, such as urea or mannitol, as a means to reduce intracranial pressure.

Other Problems

Serious spinal deformities or extreme age may make lumbar puncture difficult, and infection or severe dermatologic disease in the lumbar area also should contraindicate the procedure. Cisternal puncture can be used in such cases or in cases of spinal block, but this procedure requires a sure and experienced hand. A relative, though certainly not absolute, contraindication to lumbar puncture is the existence of severe personality problems in the patient. Many patients point to a previous lumbar puncture as the origin of "the miseries" for years afterward.

EXAMINATION OF CEREBROSPINAL FLUID

Certain observations should be made every time lumbar puncture is performed. The pressure should be measured, and in a few cases it may be desirable to document the dynamic relationships with the Queckenstedt procedure (see p. 625). The CSF should be examined for general appearance, consistency, and tendency to clot. A cell count should be performed, along with an attempt to distinguish the types of cells present. In many cases, protein and sugar concentrations are desirable. Other tests done when the patient's condition dictates include examination of Gram-stained or acid-fast stained smears of the CSF sediment; culture for pyogenic bacteria, tubercle bacilli, or fungi; differential tests employing colloidal suspensions or protein partition; serologic tests for syphilis; and miscellaneous chemical determinations such as bilirubin, urea, chlorides, bromides, or various enzymes.

Table 21 shows some of the normal values for CSF examination in which a difference may exist between adults and children.

General Appearance

Normal spinal fluid has the clarity and consistency of water. Slight color change may be difficult to note, and it is helpful to compare a sample of the CSF with a tube of water. Ordinarily, the consistency need not be specially examined, because conditions which increase the viscosity nearly always cause fairly conspicuous color change. Turbidity signifies the presence of leukocytes, usually neutrophils, in considerable numbers; lymphocytes alone rarely produce a grossly visible change. Yellowish discoloration, called xanthochromia, usually signifies previous bleeding. The pH tends to be slightly lower than that of blood, a pH of 7.31 being normal in CSF when the arterial pH is 7.41.[1]

BLOOD IN CSF

It may be difficult to evaluate the significance of fresh blood in the specimen, since damage to an intraspinal vessel may cause a "bloody tap," even though the spinal fluid is intrinsically clear. If the blood is due to local trauma, the admixture diminishes as CSF is removed, and the fluid in the third tube tends to be appreciably lighter than

Table 21. Normal CSF Values for Children and Adults

	Adults	Infants and Young Children
Quantity (Total)	100–150 ml.	Varies with size
Appearance	Clear	Clear
Pressure	75–200 mm. H_2O	50–100 mm. H_2O
Cells	0–5	0–20
	All lymphocytes	All lymphocytes

in the first. If the proportion of blood remains constant, it is probable that the bleeding preceded the puncture.

Subsequent examination of the specimen may clarify the problem of bloody tap versus genuinely bloody fluid. After centrifugation, the supernatant fluid is colorless if the blood came from traumatic lumbar puncture and is pale to deep yellow if the blood was in the fluid initially. Xanthochromia begins within 4 or 5 hours after subarachnoid hemorrhage and usually clears approximately 3 weeks after the event.

CLOTTING

In conditions of spinal subarachnoid block, the fluid may be dark yellow with a tendency toward rapid and spontaneous clotting, but spontaneous clotting can occur whenever the protein content is high. It is conversion of fibrinogen to fibrin that produces the clot. Fibrinogen is absent from the normal CSF, but when protein increases significantly, fibrinogen as well as globulins and increased quantities of albumin cross the blood-brain barrier.

CSF Pressure

In recumbent adults, the CSF pressure in the lumbar sac varies from 75 to 200 mm. of water, with a mean normal value of 120 mm. If lumbar puncture is done with the patient seated, the fluid in the manometer normally approaches the level of the foramen magnum. Slight elevation of spinal fluid pressure may occur if an anxious patient involuntarily holds his breath or tenses his muscles. If the knees are flexed too firmly against the abdomen, venous compression may cause spurious elevation, especially in obese patients.

Pathologic decrease of CSF pressure is rare but may occur in conditions of dehydration or following previous aspiration of CSF.

More significant is elevation of CSF pressure, which may be a conspicuous finding in patients with intracranial tumors or with purulent or tuberculous meningitis. Less marked elevation to approximately 250 to 500 mm. of water may accompany low-grade inflammatory processes, encephalitis, or neurosyphilis.

THE QUECKENSTEDT PROCEDURE

Since the ventricular spaces, intracranial subarachnoid space, and vertebral subarachnoid space are part of the same closed system, pressure change in one area should be reflected in other areas as well. If local change is not transmitted, existence of a block can be inferred. In the Queckenstedt test, the jugular veins are compressed while lumbar CSF pressure is monitored. Temporary occlusion of both jugular veins impedes the absorption of intracranial fluid and produces an acute rise in intracranial CSF pressure. If CSF flow is unobstructed, the pressure elevation is transmitted to the lumbar fluid, which rises in the manometer and then returns to previous levels when venous occlusion is released. Total or partial spinal block is diagnosed if the lumbar pressure fails to rise when both jugular veins are compressed or if the pressure requires more than 20 seconds to fall after compression is released. This procedure is risky in patients with increased intracranial pressure or with highly reactive carotid body receptors. Radiologic examination with contrast material (myelogram) is safer and gives far more information.

OPENING AND CLOSING PRESSURES

Removal of cerebrospinal fluid produces a drop in CSF pressure. Although no absolute figure can apply, an expected range of decline is 5 to 10 mm. for every milliliter of fluid removed from the lumbar sac. If, for example, 10 ml. are removed for examination, the closing pressure would be 50 to 100 mm. of water less than the opening pressure. A conspicuously small drop in pressure suggests that the total quantity of spinal fluid is increased, as in hydrocephalus; a disproportionately large pressure drop indicates a small CSF pool, as might occur with tumors or spinal block.

Cell Count

The normal spinal fluid is virtually free of cells, although as many as five small lymphocytes per mm.^{3} are considered normal. In children, the upper limit of normal may be as high as 20 lymphocytes per mm.^{3} The presence of granulocytes or large mononuclear cells is never normal, nor should red cells be present. If red cells are present in the CSF, they may be due to a hemorrhagic process or to trauma during the puncture. In distinguishing these events, the red cells should be examined closely. Crenation of the cells indicates that they have been in the CSF for some little time. A decrease in the RBC count between the first and last fluid to be aspirated indicates a traumatic puncture.

Sometimes it is necessary to evaluate the leukocyte or protein content of spinal fluid known to be contaminated by traumatic bleeding. A rough rule for discounting adventitious blood is that simple contamination adds one or two white cells for every 1000 red cells, so that a bloody spinal fluid that contained, for example, 20,000 red cells per mm.³ should be expected to contain no more than 30 to 40 white cells. Unless the blood has an unusually high white cell count, demonstration of more than 45 cells in such a fluid would indicate pre-existing pleocytosis.

DIFFERENTIAL WHITE COUNT

When cells are counted, they also should be identified as to type. Spinal fluid for cell counts usually is diluted with some compound that accentuates the nucleus and permits rapid differentiation between mononuclear cells and granulocytes. For more detailed morphologic study, the centrifuged sediment can be smeared and examined, and techniques are available for concentrating cells on a fine-gauge filter or in an induced fibrin clot.

SIGNIFICANCE OF ELEVATION

White cell counts below 300 to 500 per mm.³ usually consist largely of mononuclear cells and may indicate viral infection (including poliomyelitis and "aseptic meningitis"), syphilitic involvement of the central nervous system, tuberculous meningitis, multiple sclerosis, or some localized irritative process such as a tumor or abscess. Above 500 per mm.³, the white cells tend to be predominantly granulocytes arising from a purulent infection, although cell counts to 1000 per mm.³, including many neutrophils, can occur in neuromyelitis optica, a rapidly progressive form of demyelinization.[1]

NEUTROPHILS PLUS MONOCYTES. A puzzling finding may be a mildly or moderately elevated count with significant numbers of both lymphocytes and neutrophils. This may reflect developing tuberculous meningitis or can be found in the CSF when there is a brain abscess. Localized tumors contribute relatively few cells to the CSF, but massive leukemic infiltration of the central nervous system may cause significant pleocytosis.

CRYPTOCOCCUS. In occasional cases, an erroneous diagnosis of "moderate numbers of lymphocytes" may be made if cryptococcal organisms are in the CSF. These fungi are small and round and may be numerous without provoking a significant cellular response. Cryptococci are easily demonstrated by adding India ink to the spinal fluid, for the cryptococcal capsule stands out as a transparent disk surrounded by black carbon particles.

CHEMICAL TESTS

Spinal Fluid Proteins

The spinal fluid normally contains very little protein, inasmuch as serum proteins are large molecules which do not cross the blood-brain barrier. The normal concentration—15 to 45 mg./dl.—is well below 1 percent of the normal serum levels of 5 to 8 gm./dl. (see Table 22). The proportion of albumin to globulin is even higher in spinal fluid than in plasma, since the albumin molecule is significantly smaller and can pass more easily through endothelial barriers. This situation is comparable to the passage of serum proteins across the glomerular filter, and urinary protein tends to be largely albumin in all but the most florid renal disorders.

SOURCE OF ABNORMAL PROTEINS

Protein concentration may rise for a number of reasons. One source is increased permeability of the blood-brain barrier due to inflammation. In severe meningitis, all types of serum protein may enter the CSF, including fibrinogen which is a very large molecule indeed. In purulent meningitis, the CSF protein is further increased because bacteria and cells, both intact and disintegrated, contribute protein to the medium. In most diseases, cell count and protein concentra-

Table 22. Normal Values for Some Commonly Measured Substances in Cerebrospinal Fluid.

	CSF Level	Compared with Plasma Level
pH	7.32–7.35	Very slightly lower
Glucose	45–85 mg./dl.	50–80 percent
Protein	15–45 mg./dl.	0.2–0.5 percent
A/G Ratio	8:1	3–4 times higher
Chloride	110–125 mEq./L.	115–125 percent
Urea nitrogen	10–15 mg./dl.	Same

tion tend to change in parallel, although in multiple sclerosis there may be an increase in the amount and the percentage of immunoglobulin G as a protein constituent, with very little increase in cells.[7]

EFFECT OF ADDED BLOOD. When there is blood in the spinal fluid, the CSF protein level is necessarily elevated, but pre-existing protein levels sometimes must be evaluated in a spinal fluid contaminated by a bloody tap. The rough calculation of 1 mg. protein for every 1000 red cells can be subtracted from the measured protein concentration. A chronic subdural hematoma may contribute a small amount of protein to the CSF without introducing red cells.

PROTEIN WITHOUT CELLS

When protein concentration rises and relatively few cells are present, degenerative disease of the central nervous system should be suspected. The Guillain-Barré syndrome, or ascending polyneuritis, characteristically affects the spinal fluid proteins, and multiple sclerosis and neurosyphilis may increase the globulin content, adding only a few mononuclear cells. Conditions of subarachnoid block, especially when caused by a spinal tumor, permit protein accumulation in the fluid distal to the block, and the fluid may clot upon aspiration. Superficially located tumors, notably acoustic neuroma and meningioma, may cause a moderate increase in CSF protein.

TECHNIQUES

Since the protein concentration in CSF is so much lower than in blood, different means must be used for measurement. The most popular quick qualitative test for increased protein is the Pandy test, in which dilute phenol solution added to the specimen produces turbidity proportional to the protein concentration. Greater accuracy can be achieved by using sulfosalicylic acid and quantitating the turbidity with a colorimeter.

ELECTROPHORESIS. More detailed information about proteins can be achieved by electrophoresis. The CSF proteins derive largely from serum proteins, and, as might be expected from molecular sizes, albumin is the predominant protein in normal CSF. The gamma globulin fraction is normally very low, but when serum globulin levels are high, the CSF gamma peak may increase. Occasionally, elevated CSF immunoglobulin without parallel serum levels suggests a central nervous system plasmacytoma, and multiple sclerosis may cause an increase specifically in CSF IgG without altered serum composition.[7] Increased CSF levels of all plasma proteins characterize the *capillary permeability pattern,* a finding associated with, but hardly specific for, inflammation, neoplasms, diabetes, Guillain-Barré syndrome, and some cerebrovascular disease. A so-called degenerative pattern has been described in which the β_2-globulins are disproportionately increased. This has been reported in some cases of cerebral atrophy, syringomyelia, and amyotrophic lateral sclerosis but cannot be considered a reliable diagnostic finding.

Glucose

Cerebrospinal fluid glucose concentration normally is 50 to 80 percent of the blood glucose level, and changes in the blood sugar are reflected in the CSF after a 30- to 60-minute lag.[1] The normal CSF glucose level is between 40 and 80 mg. per 100 ml., but critical evaluation of CSF glucose determination requires comparison against a blood sample drawn, if possible, 30 to 60 minutes before lumbar puncture is done.

The most dramatic drop in CSF sugar occurs with purulent meningitis, when the combination of bacterial and leukocytic activity may reduce the CSF glucose to zero. Glucose metabolism is an active process which continues after the sample has been aspirated, so that sugar should be determined promptly in samples that are suspected to contain granulocytes or microorganisms. Because all types of organisms consume glucose, a decreased sugar content may indicate the presence of fungi, protozoa, or tubercle bacilli, as well as pyogenic bacteria. Less change in CSF sugar accompanies lymphocytic meningitis, brain abscesses, degenerative diseases, and most tumors. Occasional superficial tumors may lower the sugar content, and the glucose level in neurosyphilis may vary slightly from normal in either direction.[11]

Chlorides

Unlike most other CSF constituents, chlorides are present in higher concentration than in plasma. The ratio is approximately 1.2 to 1, so that normal CSF chloride values are 110 to 125 mEq./L. The plasma chloride level is quite labile, and changing plasma values are reflected promptly in the CSF; thus any condition that alters the plasma chloride also will affect the CSF level. Spinal fluid chloride determination receives less attention now than in the past. Its chief diagnostic value is in tuberculous meningitis, in which there may be nonspecific neurologic findings and mild elevation of proteins and mononuclear cells in the CSF. The CSF levels of sugar and chlorides in these cases are significantly depressed. Other types of meningitis may cause a decrease in the CSF chloride, while syphilis, tumors, encephalitis, and brain abscesses do not affect this ion. If the patient is receiving an intravenous infusion of electrolyte solutions, the chloride values in the CSF are invalidated.

Urea

The urea levels in blood and spinal fluid are approximately equal, and CSF urea increases in uremia. Urea is sometimes injected intravenously in patients with acutely elevated intracranial pressure. In such cases, the induced uremia results in markedly increased CSF osmolality, which may relieve cerebral edema by shifting fluid from brain to hyperosmolar spinal fluid. Following infusion of 0.5 to 1.0 gm. of urea per kilogram of body weight, the urea levels of blood and spinal fluid require 24 to 48 hours to return to physiologic levels.

Calcium

The spinal fluid contains only half as much calcium as the blood contains. This is entirely predictable, since approximately one-half of the serum calcium is bound to protein, and protein does not diffuse freely into the spinal fluid. When CSF protein is increased, the calcium level increases as well.

Enzymes

Such serum enzymes as lactic dehydrogenase (LDH), glutamic oxalacetic transaminase (GOT), and glutamic pyruvic transaminase (GPT) have been measured in the spinal fluid and are present in slightly lower concentrations in the CSF than in serum. Although many workers have found that mild to moderate enzyme changes accompany various neurologic disorders, CSF enzyme levels, at present, are not measured under routine conditions. The enzyme most often affected is glutamic oxalacetic transaminase, which rises in inflammatory, hemorrhagic, or degenerative diseases of the central nervous system.[11]

MICROORGANISMS

Significant numbers of bacteria, fungi, or protozoa in the CSF can be identified by examining the stained sediment after centrifugation. Whenever there is a question of meningitis or central nervous system infection, smears of the CSF sediment should be stained with a Gram stain and with an acid-fast stain. The pyogenic bacteria and many fungi can be demonstrated by examination of a good smear, but failure to isolate organisms on smear should not be interpreted to mean that organisms are absent. Unless the cause of the central nervous system disorder is self-evident, steps should be taken to rule out the presence of tubercle bacilli, because tuberculous meningitis can develop insidiously and presents few clear-cut diagnostic signs.

Culturing CSF

The spinal fluid should be cultured on several media since it is always advisable to rule out bacterial, fungal, and tuberculous infections, and more than one organism may be present. The meningococcus (*Neisseria meningitidis*) prefers a high carbon dioxide atmosphere and special media, so that separate plates should be inoculated to isolate this organism. Sometimes an aliquot of the original sample can be incubated at 37°C. for 24 hours, permitting the organisms to multiply in the spinal fluid before incubation of a second set of cultures.

IMMUNOLOGIC TESTS

Immunologic techniques are now being applied to CSF microbiology in some laboratories. The cryptococcal antigen test[5] uses a strong, specific anticryptococcal antibody to identify antigenic elements which may be in CSF even when organisms are undetectible. Several bacterial antigens have been demonstrated by counterimmunoelectrophoresis,[2] a technique which can give extremely specific documentation of bacterial invasion in little more than an hour. This technique is still experimental but has tremendous potential application.

LIMULUS ASSAY

The presence, in the central nervous system, of gram-negative infection can be demonstrated rapidly with the Limulus assay. The lipids that constitute gram-negative endotoxin have the property of co-agulating the blood-like fluid of the horseshoe crab of the genus Limulus. Very small amounts of endotoxin exert this effect, and the test has been proposed as a quick means of diagnosing gram-negative endotoxemia. Results of clinical tests on blood have been rather mixed,[9,10] but in the relatively uncomplicated setting of spinal fluid, the procedure has been fairly successful.[12] Gram-negative rods are, however, an uncommon agent for meningitis.

SEROLOGIC TESTS FOR SYPHILIS

Blood tests used in diagnosing syphilis are of two types: the non-specific types which demonstrate syphilitic reagin and the specific types which demonstrate antitreponemal antibodies. The nonspecific tests, which are cheaper, more readily available, and do not require a specialized laboratory, are most widely used for spinal fluid test-ing. Biologic false positives are fairly rare on CSF specimens. The pronounced alterations in protein proportions that accompany encephalitis, hemorrhage, acute meningitis, or even a bloody tap, sometimes may give reactive results in flocculation tests, such as the Venereal Disease Research Laboratory (VDRL) test.[6] The older tech-niques of colloidal gold or gum mastic testing relied upon these syphilis-induced protein alterations to produce diagnostic changes in suspension stability. These tests largely have been abandoned, since syphilis can be diagnosed immunologically with a greater degree of accuracy, and other protein aberrations are documented more effi-ciently by electrophoresis.

Although nonspecific tests usually are applied to CSF, they are considerably less sensitive than the fluorescent treponemal antibody (FTA) test for detecting neurosyphilis.[4] Because of the low antibody levels involved, absorption with nonsyphilitic treponemal antigen (FTA-ABS) may remove CSF reactivity. If neurosyphilis is a serious diagnostic consideration, the FTA constitutes a more reliable screen-ing test than the VDRL.

REFERENCES

1. Adams, R. D., and Victor, M.: *Principles of Neurology.* McGraw-Hill, New York, 1977.
2. Coonrod, J. D., and Rytel, M. W.: *Determination of aetiology of bacterial meningitis by counterimmunoelectrophoresis.* Lancet 1:1154, 1972.
3. Edwards, E. A., Muehl, P. M., and Peckinpaugh, R. O.: *Diagnosis of bacte-*

rial meningitis by counter immunoelectrophoresis. J. Lab. Clin. Med. 80:449, 1972.

4. Escobar, M. R., Dalton, H. P., and Allison, M. J.: *Fluorescent antibody tests for syphilis using cerebrospinal fluid: clinical correlations in 150 cases.* Am. J. Clin. Pathol. 53:886, 1970.

5. Goodman, J. S., Kaufman, L., and Koenig, M. G.: *Diagnosis of crypto-coccal antigen.* New Engl. J. Med. 285:434, 1971.

6. Holmes, K. K.: *Syphilis,* in Thorn, G. W., Adams, R. D., Braunwald, E., et al. (eds.): *Harrison's Principles of Internal Medicine.* ed. 8. McGraw-Hill, New York, 1977.

7. Johnson, K. P., and Nelson, B. J.: *Multiple sclerosis: diagnostic usefulness of cerebrospinal fluid.* Ann. Neurol. 2:425, 1977.

8. Krieg, A. F.: *Cerebrospinal fluid and other body fluids,* in Davidsohn, I., and Henry, J. B. (eds.): *Todd-Sanford Clinical Diagnosis by Laboratory Methods.* ed. 15. W. B. Saunders, Philadelphia, 1974.

9. Levin, J., Poore, T. E., Young, N. S., et al.: *Gram-negative sepsis: detection of endotoxemia with the Limulus test.* Ann. Intern. Med. 76:1, 1972.

10. Martinez, G. L. A., Quintiliani, R., and Tilton, R. C.: *Clinical experience on the detection of endotoxemia with the Limulus test.* Infect. Dis. 127:102, 1973.

11. Spiegel-Adolf, M.: *Cerebrospinal fluid.* Prog. Neurol. Psychiatry 20:455, 1965.

12. Tuazon, C. U., Perez, A. A., Elin, R. J., and Sheagren, J. N.: *Detection of endotoxin in cerebrospinal and joint fluids by Limulus assay.* Arch. Intern. Med. 137:55, 1977.

INDEX